VASCULAR AND ENDOVASCULAR SURGICAL TECHNIQUES

An Atlas

VASCULAR AND ENDOVASCULAR SURGICAL TECHNIQUES

An Atlas

Third Edition

Edited by

ROGER M. GREENHALGH MA, MD, MChir, FRCS

Professor of Surgery, Charing Cross and Westminster Medical School, London, UK

W. B. Saunders Company

London · Phildelphia · Toronto · Sydney · Tokyo

W. B. Saunders Company Ltd 24–28 Oval Road
London NW1 7DX, England

The Curtis Center
Independence Square West
Philadelphia, PA 19106–3399, USA

Harcourt Brace & Company
55 Horner Avenue
Toronto, Ontario M8Z 4X6, Canada

Harcourt Brace Jovanovich & Company Australia
30–52 Smidmore St
Marrickville, NSW 2204, Australia

Harcourt Brace & Company Japan Inc.
Ichibancho Central Building, 22–1 Ichibancho
Chiyoda-ku, Tokyo, 102, Japan

This book is printed on acid-free paper

A catalogue record for this book is available from the British Library.

ISBN 0 720 1901 1

Editorial and Production Services by Fisher Duncan
10 Barley Mow Passage, London W4 4PH

Typeset by Paston Press Ltd, Loddon, Norfolk
Printed and bound in Great Britain by The Bath Press, Avon

CONTENTS

Treatment of varicos veins

Deep venous surgery

CONTRIBUTORS

G. Andros, MD
Vascular Laboratory,
Saint Joseph Medical Center,
2601 West Almeda Avenue, Suite 302,
Burbank, California CA 91505,
USA

E. Ascer, MD
Associate Professor of Surgery,
Albert Einstein College of Medicine,
111 East 210th Street, Bronx,
New York NY 10467-2490,
USA;
Vascular Surgeon in Charge,
North Central Bronx Hospital, New York,
USA

R. N. Baird, ChM, FRCS
Consultant Surgeon,
Bristol Royal Infirmary,
Bristol BS2 8HW,
UK

G. Biasi, MD, FACS
Professor of Vascular Surgery,
Department of Vascular Surgery, Bassini Hospital,
Via Massimo Gorki 50,
I-20092 Cinisello Balsamo, Milan,
Italy

N. K. Barrett, MRCP FRCR
Consultant Radiologist,
Charing Cross Hospital,
Fulham Palace Road,
London W6 8RF,
UK

A. A. B. Barros D'Sa, MD, FRCS, FRCSEd
Consultant Vascular Surgeon,
Vascular Surgical Unit,
Royal Victoria Hospital,
Grosvenor Road,
Belfast,
Northern Ireland
UK

Y. Bensaid
Service de Chirurgie Vasculaire,
Groupe Hospitalier,
Pitie-Salpetriere,
47–83 Boulevard de L'Hospital,
Paris,
France

J. J. Bergan, MD
Clinical Professor of Surgery,
North Coast Surgeons Medical Group Inc.,
La Jolla, California,
USA

S.-E. Bergentz, MD
Department of Surgery,
Lund University,
Malmo General Hospital,
S 21401 Malmo,
Sweden

M. Birnstingl, MS, FRCS
Consulting Surgeon,
St Bartholomew's Hospital,
London,
UK

B. J. Brener, MD
Director of Vascular Surgery,
Newark Beth Israel Medical Center,
201 Lyons Avenue,
Newark, New Jersey NJ 07112,
USA

N. Browse, MD PRCS
President,
Royal College of Surgeons,
London,
UK

K. G. Burnand, MS, FRCS
Professor of Vascular Surgery,
Department of Surgery,
St Thomas' Hospital,
Lambeth Palace Road,
London SE1 7EH,
UK

B. B. Chang, MD
Assistant Professor of Surgery,
Department of Surgery,
Albany Medical College,
47 New Scotland Avenue,
Albany, New York NY 12208,
USA

T. Chuter
Department of Surgery,
College of Physicians and Surgeons of Columbia University,
630 West 168th Street,
New York NY 10032,
USA

F. B. Cockett, MS, FRCS
Consulting Surgeon,
St Thomas's Hospital,
Lambeth Palace Rd,
London SE1 7EH,
UK

M. Colonna, MD
Department of Vascular Surgery,
University Hospital of Rome,
Cattedra de Chirurgia Vascolare, Dell'Universita di Roma, "La Sapienza",
Policlinico Umberto 1,
00161 Rome,
Italy

R. Courbier
Emeritus Professor Agrégé à la Faculté de Medicine,
Hôpital St Joseph,
Marseille,
France

F. J. Criado, MD
Maryland Vascular Institute,
The Union Memorial Hospital,
201 East University Parkway, Suite 650,
Baltimore, Maryland MD 21218-2895,
USA

H. Dardik, MD, FACS
Chief, General and Vascular Surgery,
Englewood Hospital and Medical Center,
350 Engle Street,
Englewood, New Jersey NJ 07631,
USA;
Clinical Professor of Surgery,
Mt Sinai Medical Center,
New York City,
USA

R. C. Darling, III, MD
Assistant Professor of Surgery,
Department of Surgery,
Albany Medical College,
47 New Scotland Avenue,
Albany, New York NY 12208,
USA

M. E. DeBakey, MD
Olga Keith Wiess Professor of Surgery and Chairman,
Cora and Webb Mading Department of Surgery and Chancellor,
Baylor College of Medicine,
Houston, Texas,
USA

R. G. DePalma, MD
Department of Surgery,
George Washington University Medical Center,
HB Burns Memorial Building,
2150 Pennsylvania Avenue,
Washington DC 20037,
USA

A. C. De Vries, MD
St Antonius Hospital,
Nieuwegein,
The Netherlands

Do-Dai-Do
Medical Department of the University of Berne,
CH3010 Berne,
Switzerland

L. B. Dulawa, MD
Vascular Surgeon,
Vascular Laboratory,
Saint Joseph Medical Center,
Burbank, California CA 91505,
USA

W. K. Ehrenfeld, MD
Professor of Surgery,
University of California at San Francisco,
505 Parnassus Avenue,
San Francisco, California CA 94143,
USA

B. C. Eikelboom, MD, PhD
Department of Surgery,
Section of Vascular Surgery,
Utrecht University Hospital,
PO Box 85500,
3508 GA Utrecht,
The Netherlands

H. Ellis, CBE, DM, MCh, FRCS
Professor of Surgery,
Division of Anatomy and Cell Biology,
UMDS Guy's Hospital Campus,
London Bridge, London SE1 9RT,
UK

G. F. Fadda, MD
Department of Vascular Surgery,
University Hospital of Rome,
Cattedra de Chirurgia Vascolare Dell'Universita di Roma, "La Sapienza",
Policlinico Umberto 1, 00161 Rome,
Italy

V. Faraglia, MD
Department of Vascular Surgery,
University Hospital of Rome,
Cattedra de Chirurgia Vascolare Dell'Universita di Roma, "La Sapienza",
Policlinico Umberto 1, 00161 Rome,
Italy

P. Fiorani, MD
Professor of Vascular Surgery,
University Hospital of Rome,
Cattedra de Chirurgia Vascolare Dell'Universita di Roma, "La Sapienza",
Policlinico Umberto 1, 00161 Rome,
Italy

L. J. Greenfield, MD
Department of Surgery,
University of Michigan,
2101 Taubman,
Box 0346,
1500 East Medical Center Drive,
Ann Arbor, Michigan MI 48109,
USA

R. M. Greenhalgh, MA, MD, MChir, FRCS
Professor of Surgery and Chairman,
Department of Surgery,
Charing Cross and Westminster Medical School,
Fulham Palace Road,
London W6 8RF,
UK

S. J. Gupta, MD
Associate Professor of Surgery and Associate Chief of Vascular Surgery,
Albert Einstein College of Medicine and Montefiore Medical Center,
111 East 210th Street, Bronx,
New York NY 10467-2490,
USA

E. J. Gussenhoven, MD
University Hospital Dijkzigt,
Erasmus University Rotterdam,
40 Molewaterplein,
3015 GD Rotterdam,
The Netherlands;
The Dutch Heart Foundation and the Interuniversity Cardiology Institute

P. L. Harris, MD, FRCS
Consultant in Vascular Surgery,
Broadgreen Hospital,
Liverpool,
UK;
Lecturer in Clinical Surgery,
University of Liverpool,
Liverpool,
UK

R. W. Harris, MD
Vascular Surgeon,
Vascular Laboratory,
St Joseph Medical Center,
2601 West Almeda Avenue,
Suite 302,
Burbank, California CA 91505,
USA

W. P. Hederman, MCh, FRCSI
Consultant Surgeon,
Mater Misericordiae Hospital,
92 Upper Leeson Street,
Dublin 4,
Ireland

F. H. W. M. van der Heijden, MD
Department of Surgery,
Section of Vascular Surgery,
Utrecht University Hospital,
PO Box 85500, 3508 GA Utrecht,
The Netherlands

L. H. Hollier, MD, FACS, FACC
Chairman,
Department of Surgery and Executive Director of Clinical Affairs,
Health Care International,
Beardmore Street,
Clydebank, Glasgow G81 4DY,
Scotland

C. Jamieson, MS, FRCS
Consultant Surgeon,
St Thomas' Hospital,
Lambeth Palace Road,
London SE1 7EH;
Honorary Consultant Surgeon,
Hammersmith Hospital and Royal Postgraduate Medical School,
London,
UK

J. M. Jausseran
Chef due Service de Chirurgie,
Cardio-Vasculaire,
Hopital St Joseph,
Marseille,
France

D. L. Jicha, MD
Vascular Fellow,
Department of Surgery,
University of California at San Francisco,
505 Parnassus Avenue,
San Francisco, California CA 94143,
USA

E. Kieffer
Service de Chirurgie Vasculaire,
Groupe Hospitalier,
Pitie-Salpetriere,
47–83 Boulevard de L'Hopital,
Paris,
France

G. Kretschmer, MD
University Clinics of Surgery,
University of Vienna,
Währinger Gürtel 18–20,
A-1090 Vienna,
Austria

R. J. Lane, MS, FRCS, FRCSE, DDU, FRACS
Visiting Vascular Surgeon,
The Royal North Shore Hospital,
St Leonards,
New South Wales,
Australia;
Visiting Vascular Surgeon,
North Harbour Private Hospital,
Harbord,
New South Wales,
Australia

R. P. Leather, MD
Professor of Surgery,
Albany Medical College,
47 New Scotland Avenue,
Albany, New York NY 12208,
USA

A. van der Lugt, MD
University Hospital Dijkzigt,
Erasmus University Rotterdam,
40 Molewaterplein,
3015 GD Rotterdam,
The Netherlands;
The Dutch Heart Foundation and the Interuniversity Cardiology Institute

F. Mahler
Medical Department of the University of Berne,
CH3010 Berne,
Switzerland

J. A. Mannick, MD
Moseley Professor of Surgery,
Harvard Medical School;
Surgeon,
Brigham and Women's Hospital,
75 Francis Street,
Boston, Massachusetts, MA 02115,
USA

A. O. Mansfield, ChM, FRCS
Professor of Surgery,
St Mary's Hospital,
Praed Street,
London W12 1NY;
Honorary Senior Lecturer in Vascular Surgery,
Royal Postgraduate Medical School,
London,
UK

M. L. Marin, MD
Assistant Professor of Surgery,
Division of Vascular Surgery,
Albert Einstein College of Medicine and Montefiore Medical Center,
111 East 20th Street, New York NY 10467,
USA

C. N. McCollum, MD, FRCS
Professor of Surgery,
University of South Manchester,
Research and Teaching Bldg,
Nell Lane, West Didbury,
Manchester M20 8LR,
UK

J. McIvore, FRCR, FFR, FDSRCS
Clinical Director of Diagnostic Imaging,
Charing Cross Hospital,
Fulham Palace Road,
London W6 8RF,
UK

J. H. Miller, MB BS, FRCS, FACS
19 High Street,
Unley Park,
South Australia 5061,
Australia

P. Mingazzini
Assistant Professor,
Department of Vascular Surgery,
Bassini Hospital,
Via Massimo Gorki 50,
I-20092 Cinisello Balsamo, Milan,
Italy

W. S. Moore, MD
Department of Surgery,
UCLA Medical Center,
10833 LeConte Avenue,
Los Angeles, California CA 90024,
USA

H. O. Myhre, MD, PhD
Professor and Chairman,
Department of Surgery,
Trondheim University Clinic,
Trondheim 7006,
Norway

B. Nachbur
Department of Thoracic and Cardiovascular Surgery,
University of Berne,
CH3010 Berne,
Switzerland

J. Natali
Service de Chirurgie Vasculaire,
Groupe Hospitalier,
Pitie-Salpetriere,
47–83 Boulevard de L'Hôpital,
Paris,
France

B. Niederle, MD
University Clinics of Surgery,
University of Vienna,
Währinger Gürtel 18–20,
A-1190 Vienna,
Austria

R. W. Oblath, MD
Vascular Surgeon,
Vascular Laboratory,
St Joseph Medical Center,
2601 West Almeda Avenue,
Burbank, California CA 91505,
USA

M. J. Olding, MD
Department of Surgery,
George Washington University Medical Center,
HB Burns Memorial Building,
2150 Pennsylvania Avenue,
Washington DC 20037,
USA

J. C. Palmaz, MD
Professor and Chief of Cardiovascular and Special Interventions,
The University of Texas Health Science Center at San Antonio, Texas TX 78282,
USA

J. C. Parodi, MD
Instituto Cardiovascular de Buenos Aires,
Blanco Encalada 1543/47,
1428 Capital Federal, Buenos Aires,
Argentina

P. Patten, RN
Maryland Vascular Institute,
The Union Memorial Hospital,
201 East University Parkway, Suite 650,
Baltimore, Maryland MD 21218-2895,
USA

M. O. Perry, MD
Department of Surgery,
Division of Vascular Surgery,
Texas Tech University,
Health Sciences Center,
School of Medicine,
3601 4th Street, Lubbock, Texas TX 79430,
USA

C. Petitjean
Service de Chirurgie Vasculaire,
Groupe Hospitalier,
Pitie-Salpetriere,
47–83 Boulevard de L'Hôpital,
Paris,
France

H. Pieterman, MD
University Hospital Dijkzigt,
Erasmus University, Rotterdam,
40 Molewaterplein,
3015 GD Rotterdam,
The Netherlands

M. C. Proctor, MS
Department of Surgery,
University of Michigan,
2101 Taubman,
Box 0346,
1500 East Medical Center Drive,
Ann Arbor, Michigan MI 48109,
USA

L. A. Queral, MD
Maryland Vascular Institute,
The Union Memorial Hospital,
201 East University Parkway, Suite 650,
Baltimore, Maryland MD 21218-2895,
USA

T. K. Ramos, MD
Vascular Division,
Department of Surgery,
University of California at San Francisco,
505 Parnassus Avenue,
San Francisco, California CA 94143,
USA

M. K. Reilly, PhD, MD
Department of Surgery,
Division of Vascular Surgery,
Texas Tech University,
Health Sciences Center,
School of Medicine,
3601 4th Street, Lubbock, Texas TX 79430,
USA

N. M. Rich, MD, FACS
Professor and Chairman, Department of Surgery, USUHS and Chief Division of Vascular Surgery,
F. Edward Herbert School of Medicine,
Uniformed Services University of the Health Sciences,
4301 Jones Bridge Road,
Bethesda, Maryland MD 20814-4799,
USA

L. Rizzo, MD
Department of Vascular Surgery,
University Hospital of Rome,
Cattedra de Chirurgia Vascolare Dell'Universita di Roma, "La Sapienza",
Policlinico Umberto 1, 00161 Rome,
Italy

J. V. Robbs, ChM (CT), FRCSEd
Chief, Vascular Surgery and Head, Division of Surgery,
University of Natal Medical School,
Box 17039 Congella 4013,
Durban,
South Africa

K. Robinson, MS, FRCS
Consultant Surgeon,
Chelsea and Westminster Hospital,
London,
UK

S. S. Rose, FRCS
Consulting Surgeon,
University Hospital of South Manchester,
Withington Hospital,
Manchester,
UK

J. P. Royle, MB BS, BS, FRCS(Ed), FRCS, FRACS, FACS
Director of Vascular Surgery Unit,
Austin Hospital,
Heidelberg, Victoria,
Australia;
Senior Associate, University of Melbourne,
Victoria,
Australia;
Consultant Vascular Surgeon,
Fairfield Hospital,
Victoria,
Melbourne,
Australia

U. Ruberti, MD
Professor and Chief,
Institute of General and Cardiovascular Surgery,
University of Milan,
Milan,
Italy

O. D. Saether, MD
Consultant Vascular Surgeon,
Department of Surgery,
Trondheim University Clinic,
Trondheim 7006,
Norway

W. Sandmann, MD
Professor of Surgery,
Chirurgische Universitatsklinik Dusseldorf,
Heinrich-Heine-Univ, Moorenstrasse 5, Dusseldorf,
Germany

E. Schneider
Division of Angiology,
Medical Department of the University of Zurich,
Zurich,
Switzerland

P. A. Schneider, MD
Vascular Surgeon,
Vascular Laboratory,
Saint Joseph Medical Center,
2601 West Almeda Avenue, Suite 302,
Burbank, California CA 91505,
USA

D. M. Shah, MD
Professor of Surgery,
Department of Surgery,
Albany Medical College,
47 New Scotland Avenue,
Albany, New York NY12208,
USA

F. Speziale, MD
Department of Vascular Surgery,
University Hospital of Rome,
Cattedra de Chirurgia Vascolare Dell'Universita di Roma, "La Sapienza",
Policlinico Umberto 1, 00161 Rome,
Italy

R. J. Stoney, MD
Professor of Surgery,
University of California at San Francisco,
505 Parnassus Avenue,
San Francisco, California CA 94143,
USA

M. Taurino, MD
Department of Vascular Surgery,
University Hospital of Rome,
Cattedra de Chirurgia Vascolare Dell'Universita di Roma, "La Sapienza,
Policlinico Umberto 1, 00161 Rome,
Italy

P. R. Taylor, MA, FRCS
Consultant Vascular Surgeon,
Guy's Hospital Medical School,
London Bridge, London SE1 9RT,
UK

Th. Theodorides, MD
Department of Surgery,
Section of Vascular Surgery,
Utrecht University Hospital,
PO Box 85500, 3508 GA Utrecht,
The Netherlands

N. A. Theodorou, MS, FRCS
Consultant Surgeon,
Gastrointestinal Unit,
Charing Cross Hospital,
Fulham Palace Road,
London W6 8RF,
UK

J. E. Thompson, MD, FACS
Attending Surgeon,
Baylor University Medical Center,
Dallas, Texas, USA;
Clinical Professor of Surgery,
University of Texas Southwestern Medical School,
Dallas, Texas,
USA

R. W. H. van Reedt Dortland, MD
Department of Surgery,
Section of Vascular Surgery,
Utrecht University Hospital,
PO Box 85500, 3508 GA Utrecht,
The Netherlands

H. Van Urk, MD
Professor and Chief, Vascular Surgery,
University Hospital Dijkzigt,
Erasmus University Rotterdam,
40 Molewaterplein,
3015 GD Rotterdam,
The Netherlands

F. J. Veith, MD
Professor of Surgery,
Division of Vascular Surgery,
Albert Einstein College of Medicine and Montefiore Medical Center,
111 East 210th Street, Bronx,
New York, NY 10467-2490,
USA

O. Wagner, MD
Professor of Surgery,
Krankenhaus der Barmherzigen Bruder,
Chirurgische Abeteilung, Grosse Mohrengasse 9,
A1020 Vienna,
Austria

K. R. Wengerter, MD
Assistant Professor of Surgery and Assistant Attending Vascular Surgeon
Albert Einstein College of Medicine and Montefiore Medical Center,
111 East 20th Street, Bronx,
New York, NY 10467-2490,
USA

D. Westaby, MA, FRCP
Consultant Physician,
Gastrointestinal Unit,
Charing Cross Hospital,
Fulham Palace Road,
London W6 8RF,
UK

A. D. Whittemore, MD
Associate Professor of Surgery,
Harvard Medical School;
Surgeon,
Brigham and Women's Hospital,
75 Francis Street,
Boston, Massachusetts MA 02115,
USA

S. G. J. Williams, MA, MRCP
Research Registrar,
Gastrointestinal Unit,
Charing Cross Hospital,
Fulham Palace Road,
London W6 8RF,
UK

J. H. N. Wolfe, MS, FRCS
Consultant Vascular Surgeon and Honorary Senior Lecturer,
St Mary's Hospital Medical School, Praed Street,
London W2 1NY;
Consultant Vascular Surgeon and Honorary Senior Lecturer,
Royal Postgraduate Medical School,
Hammersmith Hospital, London,
UK

M. Wunderlich, MD
Department of Surgery,
General Hospital,
A-2020 Hollabrunn,
Austria

J. S. T. Yao, MD, PhD
Professor of Surgery and Director,
Blood Flow Laboratory,
Northwestern University Medical School,
251 East Chicago Avenue, Suite 628,
Chicago, Illinois IL 60611,
USA

PREFACE

There is a long-standing perception that the techniques in vascular surgery are well established. In the last five years, however, it is evident that many apparently standard procedures have required review. Advances in endovascular techniques have been so dramatic as to call into question the future practice of traditional procedures. The single most significant report was that of Juan Parodi and Julio Palmaz who employed an expandable metal stent for holding a prosthetic tube on the inside of an artery to repair an aneurysm. This appeared in the literature in 1991, a year in which most of us first heard about this possibility. The third edition of this Atlas necessarily incorporates these new endovascular surgical techniques as they are being practised at the time of going to press. We have managed to assemble the world's best in this section. Parodi and Palmaz give chapters and techniques of their own and Bruce Brener who describes his own stent also describes his techniques of ultrasound guided angioplasty. Frank Criado now at Baltimore, also shows his techniques of stenting in vascular surgery. Wesley Moore and Tim Chuter describe their method with Dacron fixation and a metal device. The endovascular section is given pride of place to indicate the importance of these advances.

Standard procedures still have their place and every trainee vascular surgeon must know exactly how the masters perform these procedures. The extracranial arterial section has been updated in all cases but there have been more changes to the section on surgery of the aorta, visceral and renal arteries. We welcome Ron Stoney, current President of the Society for Vascular Surgery in the United States, as an author of the first chapter of this section. The other chapters have been thoroughly overhauled. In the upper limb section, thoracic endoscopic sympathectomy has now become an essential skill in many hospitals as the transaxillary and cervical approach require longer hospitalization. The lower limb section has been totally reconsidered and amended where appropriate. It is perhaps gratifying that there have been few changes in the techniques of amputations, although it would appear that despite a rising population in the over 60s, fewer amputations are being performed in this country and one would hope that this is becauseof the interventions of expert vascular surgeons.

The remaining sections on vascular trauma, portal hypertension and venous surgery have been assessed most carefully and thoroughly edited. At the time of going to press, Frank Cockett has been involved with a serious motor accident, but is recovering rapidly. I have edited his chapter on perforating veins in a way that I was not able to discuss with him completely. The long incision for ligation of perforating veins is seldom performed these days since duplex scanning can pinpoint such veins accurately and the incisions reduced appropriately. It is hoped that he will recover extremely fast and also that he will find it in his heart to forgive me for the changes in this important chapter. To those who have found the second edition very helpful and are just getting used to it, I apologise for the enormous changes which have been necessary in this edition which only reflect the rather unexpected leap forward that has occurred recently in the techniques available to the vascular surgeon.

R. M. Greenhalgh *February 1994*

Planning the intervention

ROGER M. GREENHALGH MA, MD, MChir, FRCS

Professor and Chairman, Department of Surgery, Charing Cross & Westminster Medical School, London, UK

Introduction

Before a procedure is chosen, the vascular surgeon must always consider if the patient really requires an operative procedure at all. It is absolutely essential to be certain that the odds are very good that any operative procedure is likely to produce the desired effect. It takes much less time to learn a technique than to learn the indications for the application of the technique and when it is better not to intervene at all.

At first consultation, the patient and the referring doctor expect to learn the intentions of the vascular specialist. In order to give a sensible opinion, it is necessary to achieve accurate diagnosis at the first consultation which is achievable these days by improved non-invasive vascular imaging. Secondly, if an operation or operative technique is contemplated, it is important to know if the patient is fit for the procedure.

First consultation assessment

There is no substitute for a very careful history. It is absolutely essential to understand the patient's complaints and how these effect the quality of life relative to age and occupation. Patients with arterial disease are usually smokers over many years and may have concomitant arterial disease elsewhere. In the history it is important to establish if concomitant arterial disease is symptomatic and if the patient suffers from diabetes or hypertension.

The cardiac status is particularly important if a patient requires a general anaesthetic and operative procedure. More than half of patients with peripheral arterial disease have resting electrocardiographic changes indicating ischaemic heart disease and a greater number have abnormalities on the ECG after a period of exercise. At least 10% of patients with peripheral arterial disease are diabetic and more than 30% are likely to be hypertensive. It is important that hypertension is controlled from the point of view of reducing risk of stroke. In addition, the use of β-blocker drugs can exacerbate intermittent claudication and there are usually better alternative ways of controlling hypertension.

Complete physical examination is essential, recognizing the generality of arterial disease and the importance of the heart and chest in terms of mortality risk at operative procedures. Careful examination of a patient with an abdominal aortic aneurysm is vital and it should be noted if any pulsating and expansile swelling is tender. Peripheral pulses are graded normal 2, reduced 1 and absent 0. Patients with venous disease and venous ulceration must always be examined in the standing position in a good light. There it can be noted if there are obviously clinically incompetent long or short saphenous veins or obvious perforating veins on the medial or lateral aspects of the leg relating to any ankle ulcers.

1

Vascular imaging is now possible at first consultation. Ideally, colour coded duplex scanning is available close to the consultation area for patient convenience. Where necessary the arterial tree can be scanned from the diaphragm downwards including the iliac, femoral popliteal and proximal tibial vessels. From the history and physical examination, the clinician can indicate to the vascular technologist the expected diagnosis and appropriate imaging can be performed. The images are transferred ideally to a simple chart as shown. For suspected renal or visceral artery stenoses, images of these vessels can also be performed with the appropriate duplex probe.

Illustration 1 which shows a colour duplex scan of aorta, visceral, renal and peripheral arteries is an example of disease demonstrated at first consultation in a patient presenting with symptoms of peripheral arterial disease. The patient complained of bilateral buttock claudication and right calf claudication and the image shows a 75% stenosis of the right common iliac and a 50% stenosis of the left common iliac artery with disease in more peripheral vessels, including a long occlusion of the left superficial femoral artery with already well developed collateral circulation. There is also evidence of early aortic dilatations, a small abdominal aortic aneurysm, which must be taken into account.

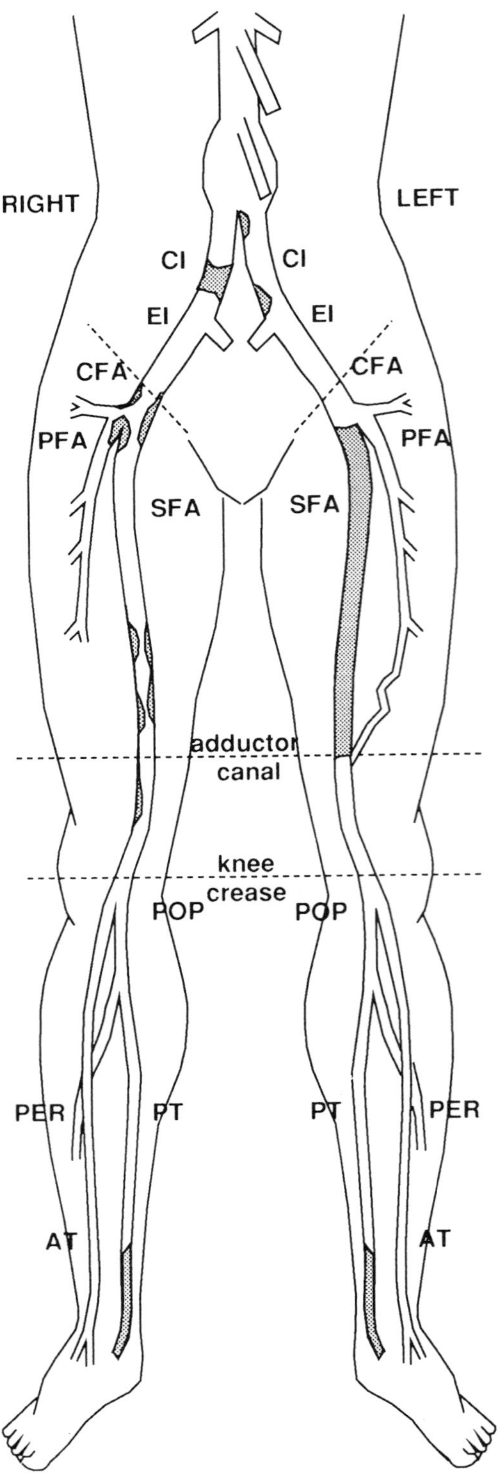

1

2

Illustration 2 shows palpable pulses, Doppler segmental pressures and velocity profiles of aorta, visceral, renal and peripheral arteries. Alongside the peripheral arterial image (*Illustration 1*), it is useful to have segmental pressure readings and an opportunity to recall the pulse findings. The normal pulse is shown as 2, reduced pulse as 1 and absent pulse as 0. Pulses are felt at the femoral, popliteal posterior tibial and dorsalis pedis positions. On the chart are also indicated segmental pressure findings in the thighs, calves and ankles and waveforms of the velocity profiles are indicated. This provides additional numerical data relating to the severity of the disease whereas the Doppler imaging merely shows distribution of disease. It is still useful to express ankle pressures as a proportion of the right brachial pressure (pressure index, PI) and these are indicated on the chart also. For patients with a pressure index of >0.9, it is appropriate and more sensitive to use the 1 minute exercise test (Laing and Greenhalgh, 1980). After walking on a treadmill for 1 minute at 4 kilometres per hour on a 10 degrees slope, a fall of Doppler pressure of >30 mm of mercury indicates abnormality. This implies that somewhere between the ankle and infrarenal aorta, there is significant disease contributing to this fall of pressure with exercise. For patients with suspicious symptoms, normal pressures at rest and normal exercise tests, it is highly unlikely that they have significant arterial disease and the clinician should consider very carefully any possible alternative diagnosis, such as sciatica. Today such definitive assessments are at first consultation alongside the clinician. In

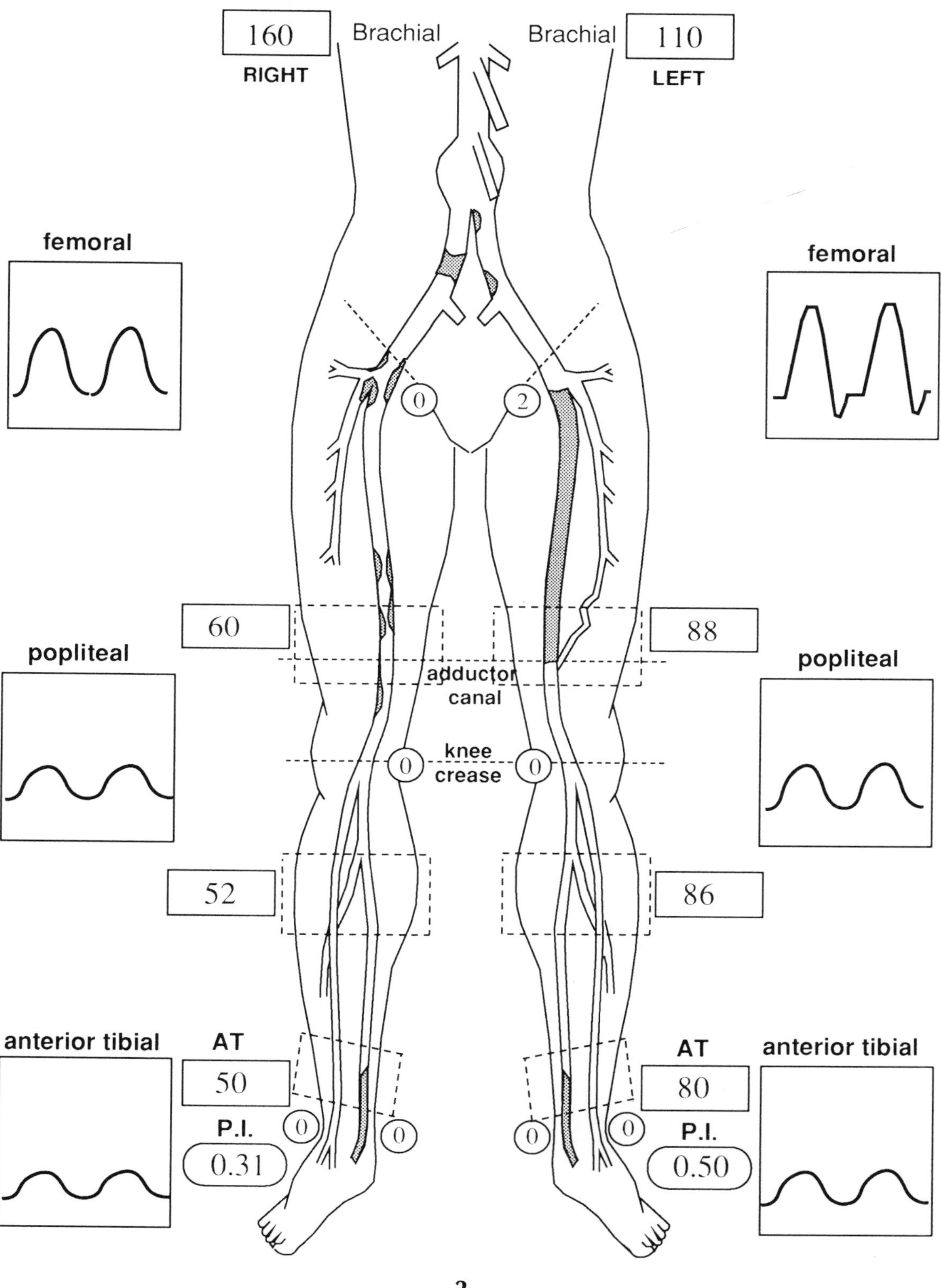

2

the illustration the right femoral pulse velocity waveform is monophasic or 'damped' which relates to the common iliac occlusion above and absent femoral pulse. The pressure readings in the right leg, 60, 52 and 50 mmHg respectively, are consistent with the scan finding or relatively little disease below the right groin. On the left, the femoral pulse velocity waveform is triphasic and normal and coincides with a normal feeling pulse.

3

For patients with asymptomatic carotid arterial disease, transient ischaemic attack, transient stroke, established stroke, progressing stroke or crescendo transient ischaemic attacks, it is appropriate to perform duplex scanning of the carotid and vertebral arteries at once. Also for patients with peripheral arterial disease, the carotid arteries are scanned for presence of asymptomatic arterial disease. It is now well within the compass of vascular technologists to scan accurately the carotid bification, assess disease in the proximal common carotids and even using the appropriate probes, proximal subclavian and innominate vessels. The direction of blood flow in vertebral arteries is well within the compass of the investigation these days and retrograde flow in a vertebral in association with an occluded first part of the subclavian is picked up reliably at once. Transcranial Doppler can give further information about the middle cerebral artery, the whole of the circle of Willis, basilar artery and distal vertebral vessels but this is seldom required at first consultation.

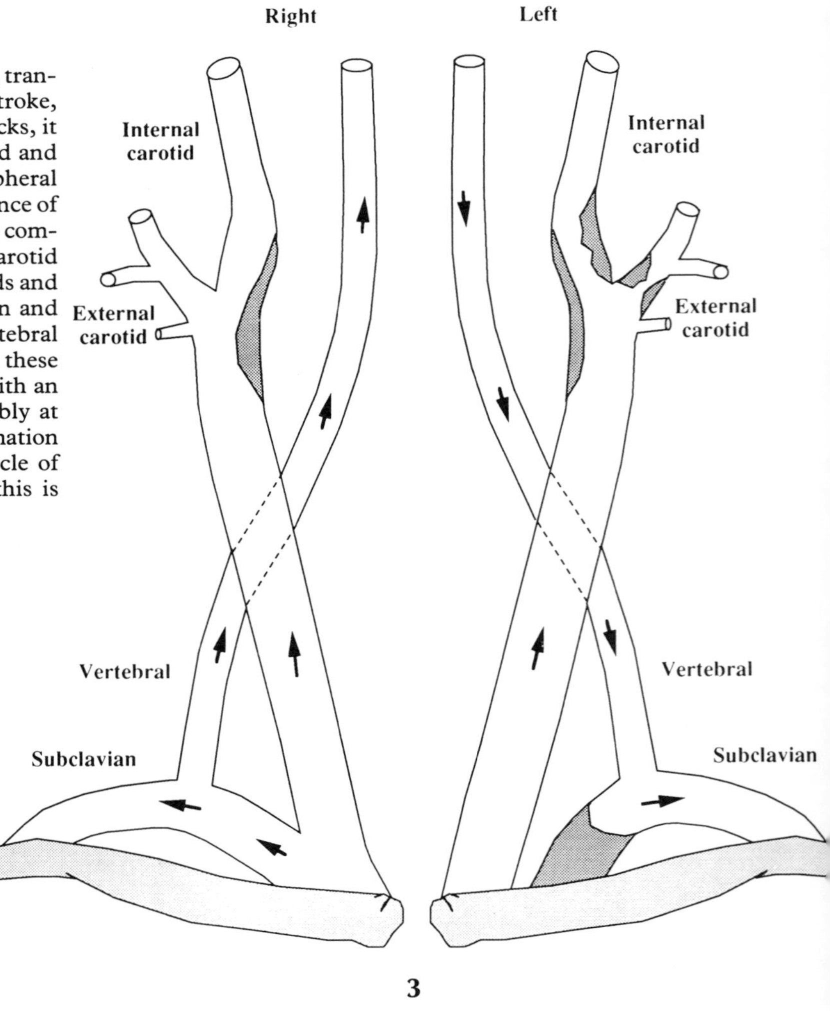

3

4

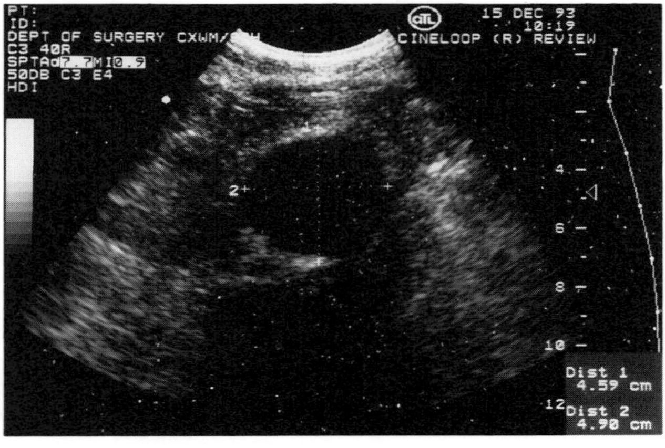

4

Approximately 10% of patients with intermittent claudication or symptomatic carotid artery disease have an abdominal aortic aneurysm by ultrasound (external diameter of >3 cm), (MacSweeney *et al.*, 1993). The abdominal aorta is scanned with simple B mode ultrasound at first consultation. The colour duplex scan can be used for this but a simpler B mode ultrasound scan is perfectly satisfactory. In this illustration an abdominal aortic aneurysm has been discovered at first consultation.

5

For patients with arterial disease, the Harp-Nasor classification of category and severity at first consultation is a useful summary. This can then be upgraded on future occasions. This classification stresses that for any patient with arterial disease there is likely to be concomitant disease elsewhere. The categories of disease are Heart, Aneurysm, caRotid and Peripheral (HARP). Within a category of disease are various severities Normal Asymptomatic Symptomatic Operation Recurrence. In the associated chart, it can be seen how the classification is used and encourages the clinician to think about arterial disease elsewhere and to note from time to time if there is progression of arterial disease in a particular category or whether another part of the body has become affected.

The HARP NASOR system for category and severity of arterial disease

← Arterial disease categories →

	Heart	Aneurysm	CaRotid	Peripheral
Normal	↓	↓	↓	↓
Asymptomatic		↓	↓	↓
Symptomatic		↓		↓
Operation				↓
Recurrence				

5

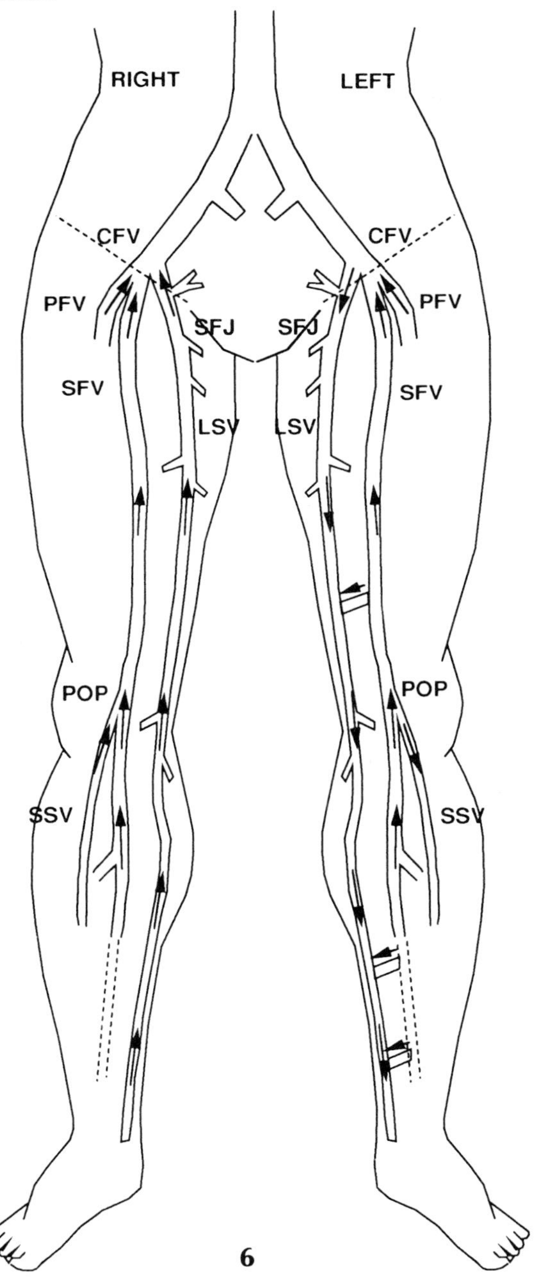

6

6

Venous scanning has become as sophisticated as arterial scanning and this chart shows the type of information which can now be available at first consultation. Colour duplex scan can follow the direction of flow and whether the deep veins are competent, incompetent or obstructed. It is possible to see with the colour code system, exactly where the blood passes through the deep fascia into the superficial system. Perforating veins can be marked accurately and sites of incompetence into the long and short venous system can be pin-pointed. This is particularly helpful for patients with venous ulceration or complex venous problems, such as complex recurrent varicose veins. The venous scans are most revealing and on many occasions, for patients who have had years and years of venous ulceration and previous surgery, it has been possible to remedy problems such as an incompetent vein coming from a medial or lateral aspect of a common femoral vein. The high pressure blood can be traced on many occasions to immediately above where ankle ulceration of long standing exists. With this careful pin-pointing of the underlying problem, it is possible to reduce the size of operation incisions to an absolute minimum and patients can be admitted on the same day as operations, sometimes discharged as a day case or at most kept over night for 24 hours. Healing of most venous ulceration is the four layer bandage technique used at the Riverside Venous Ulcer project (Moffatt *et al.*, 1992) and is achieved without hospital admission.

Contrast imaging of veins and arteries

Venography is required less and less these days and for patients with suspected venous thrombosis, colour duplex scan is ideal. The calf vein and pelvic veins can be scanned in rapid time. This is also a vital investigation for patients with suspected thromboembolism. In planning deep venous surgery, ascending and descending venography is still advocated by many and will be discussed in the appropriate chapter later in this Atlas. Arteriography and CT scanning can be performed as an outpatient procedure these days. Indications for arteriography vary somewhat in different parts of the world and some are moving towards avoiding arteriography for symptomatic carotid disease and relying entirely upon duplex scanning. Personally I am still persuaded that an arch flush angiogram with 5 French gauge catheter releasing a small amount of contrast from the arch of the aorta and using digital subtraction angiography produces excellent confirmatory visualization of the major vessels and intracranial views. It may be that we are close to abandoning some of these techniques for regular use but for the present, a majority of surgeons use contrast studies before planning surgery. There is no indication for translumber aortography these days. Gone are the days when a patient needed to be admitted to hospital for a general anaesthetic and a needle was driven through the back for this outmoded procedure. Often the patient was not fit for the investigation but would have been fit to have limb and life saving procedures. It is remarkable that this procedure is still being practised.

Arteriography for aortic aneurysm is somewhat controversial, particularly as CT scans show such fine detail and can show exactly the upper and lower extremities and sometimes details of renal and visceral vessels. The intravenous digital subtraction angiogram is helpful, particularly for looking at the vessels off the aorta, enabling operation planning. Magnetic resonance imaging for all at affordable costs is awaited.

Decision of procedure for the patient and referring doctor

At first consultation it has been seen that a very precise diagnosis is possible. It should be communicated at once to the patient and the referring doctor. All of the benefit of this superb first consultation diagnosis is that the various options for management can be discussed. Endovascular procedures should always be preferred and applied where possible. These enable the patient to be admitted to hospital for the shortest possible period of time. They are cost-effective and are considered for lesser degrees of arterial disease for which a formal bypass would not be appropriate. If the only option is a full bypass, this should be considered against the patient's symptoms and the hospital stay expected and the age and condition of the patient. For an elective procedure, the patient should be asked to stop smoking before the elective procedure is undertaken. If the patient is at risk of stroke or bursting of aneurysm or has severe ischaemic rest pain, then of course the operation should go ahead nevertheless and the patient advised not to smoke. If the patient has mild intermittent claudication for example and an endovascular procedure or say femoropopliteal bypass is contemplated, then it is known that recurrence is more likely if the patient smokes (Wiseman *et al.*, 1990). Consequently, it is reasonable to expect the patient to stop smoking before the procedure is offered.

It is one of the great advances of vascular surgery in the last 5 years that instant diagnosis and imaging at the first consultation has become possible with the opportunity to discuss all options with a patient from the start.

Acknowledgement

Illustrations by Rachel Cuming.

References

Laing, S. P. and Greenhalgh, R. M. (1980). Standard exercise test to assess peripheral arterial disease. *British Medical Journal* **280**, 13.

MacSweeney, S. T. R., O'Meara, M., Alexander, C., Powell, J. T. and Greenhalgh, R. M. (1993). High prevalence of unsuspected abdominal aortic aneurysm in patients with confirmed symptomatic peripheral or cerebral arterial disease. *British Journal of Surgery* **80**, 582.

Moffatt, C. J., Franks, P. J., Oldroyd, M., Bosanquet, N., Brown, P., Greenhalgh, R. M. and McCollum, C. N. (1992). Community clinics for leg ulcers and impact on healing. *British Medical Journal* **305**, 1389.

Wiseman, S., Kenchington, G., Dain, R., *et al.* (1989). Influence of smoking and plasma factors on patency of femoropopliteal vein grafts. *British Medical Journal* **299**, 643.

Wiseman, S., Powell, J. T., Greenhalgh, R. M., *et al.* (1990). The influence of smoking and plasma factors on prosthetic graft patency. *European Journal of Vascular Surgery* **4**, 57.

Techniques of anastomosis

ROGER M. GREENHALGH MA, MD, MChir, FRCS

Professor and Chairman, Department of Surgery, Charing Cross & Westminster Medical School, London, UK

Introduction

The various techniques of anastomosis, or joining of blood vessels, fall into two main types: end-to-end anastomosis and end-to-side anastomosis. Various graft materials are preferred for bypass in different parts of the body and these are described in detail in subsequent chapters. For replacement of large vessels such as the aorta, Dacron has become the material of choice. Essentially, Dacron prostheses are of two main types, woven and knitted. The woven variety has the advantages that it does not require any preclotting of the Dacron and it does not leak blood. Its disadvantage is that it is rather stiff and when cut it frays. It is advisable to cut woven Dacron with an electric diathermy needle so that the ends are sealed, but this can be quite a tricky procedure compared with the precise cutting of a knitted Dacron graft which can be performed with scissors. The great advantage of knitted Dacron is that it can be shaped exactly as required but must be preclotted. Preclotting can be achieved by taking approximately 100 ml of blood from a nearby vein such as the vena cava and syringing it down through the graft so that the blood pours through the holes. The blood is then caught in a dish and syringed through the graft again and again with some pressure until the interstices become blocked by the clotting blood. The blood is then squeezed out of the Dacron which should be leak-proof and it is ready for anastomosis. To dispense with or minimize preclotting, collagen impregnation and albumen coating of Dacron has been introduced. An externally supported Dacron graft has gained much favour and may prove ideal in sites where it is important that the graft should not be squashed, such as for axillofemoral bypass.

Dacron is perhaps the material of choice for the replacement or bypass of arteries ranging in size from the aorta to the common femoral artery. Expanded polytetrafluoroethylene (PTFE) is mainly used in long straight tubes for the replacement of smaller arteries than is ideal for Dacron. However, a bifurcated graft of PTFE is now available to replace or bypass the aortic bifurcation; it does not require preclotting and is easy to work. Patients who are expected to have a PTFE graft should begin aspirin and dipyridamole 48 h before surgery to minimize postoperative graft thrombosis. It is an excellent graft material for femorofemoral cross-over, axillobifemoral bypass and bypass of the femoral artery in the thigh.

Human umbilical vein does not require preclotting and remains an alternative to autologous vein for bypass from the groin to below the knee. It is also advisable to give aspirin and dipyridamole 48 h before the insertion of this graft as this is thought to reduce the risk of graft thrombosis.

Antibiotics and suture materials

When a prosthetic graft material is to be used it is advisable to commence prophylactic antibiotics either the day before surgery or at the time of the premedication 1 h before the operation. Some surgeons prefer to begin a day early, but virtually all would agree that it is essential to have satisfactory antibiotic levels in the blood at the time the graft material is implanted. The most threatening organism is *Staphylococcus aureus* and flucloxacillin is effective against this, but if this is used on its own there is a small risk of infection of the graft from Gram-negative organisms and it is, therefore, wise to combine ampicillin with flucloxacillin. Some prefer to use a cephalosporin prophylactic antibiotic which has antistaphylococcal ability as well as providing cover for the Gram-negative organisms.

Fashions have changed for the choice of suture for vascular anastomosis. Only recently silk was in common usage but it is now used very rarely. It fragments after some time, but those who use it maintain that the strength of the anastomosis is in the healing of the graft to the vessel. Mersilene handles like silk; it is a braided material made of Dacron and so, in many respects, is ideal for anastomosing a Dacron graft to a large vessel. It has the advantages that is does not slip and it is easy to use. Polypropylene is a slippery monofilament suture which is without doubt the most commonly used suture material for vascular anastomoses. Using a double-ended atraumatic needle of polypropylene, great flexibility of anastomotic technique is achieved. A disadvantage of this material, however, is that when it is tied it slips and it is wise to place up to six knots to guarantee a secure anastomosis. The slippery quality of polypropylene can however be used to advantage; sutures can be left long and the graft slid down along their length before tying.

Lighting and magnification

It is essential to perform any anastomosis in good light. Not every operating room has an excellent lighting system and the best can be adjusted by the surgeon himself. The types which have sterile handles are the easiest to use, and at least two and preferably four lights, which can all be adjusted by the surgeon, are ideal. Few vascular surgeons have this facility. The absolute minimum is two good lights, but, all too frequently, it is not possible for the surgeon to adjust them himself. In such instances an alternative is for the surgeon to wear a fibre optic headlight. The best variety have a sterile adjuster so that once again the surgeon can direct the light exactly where it is required.

It takes time to adjust to any form of magnification but × 2.5 magnification with a simple loupe is easy to use. The focal length is usually about 50 cm but this can be varied according to the particular circumstances. For anastomoses to vessels of 2 or 3 mm diameter such as tibial vessels, this degree of magnification is essential. For smaller vessels of 1–2 mm diameter an operating microscope is required and a triploscope is ideal. This has a split beam, enabling the surgeon and assistant and a television camera to view to the same work through one prism. Microvascular anastomoses require special training in a laboratory and should not be attempted in theatre by the novice surgeon.

All vascular anastomoses are either end-to-end or end-to-side. The different techniques described here are variations of end-to-end and end-to-side techniques. *It is a vital principle of all anastomoses, whether end-to-end or end-to-side, that the edges should always be everted. In this way the intima of the artery and lining of the graft material are brought into apposition.*

Techniques

End-to-end anastomosis of a graft to a large vessel

1

For an end-to-end anastomosis of large vessels (such as the aorta) it is convenient to use a polypropylene suture and place the first four or five sutures before pulling down the graft. This facilitates careful placement of the sutures in the back row. It is much easier to do this rather than to place anchoring stitches which make the subsequent adjacent suturing more difficult. It is important to take a deep bite of the posterior wall in the artery and pull it up into a ridge. It is not necessary to cut the vessel right across. Rather it can be cut approximately half-way to two-thirds across and opened like the leaves of a book. The posterior sutures are then placed long as shown.

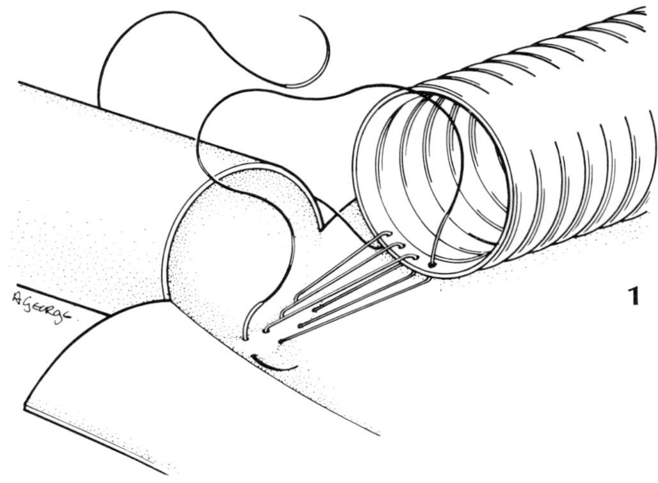

1

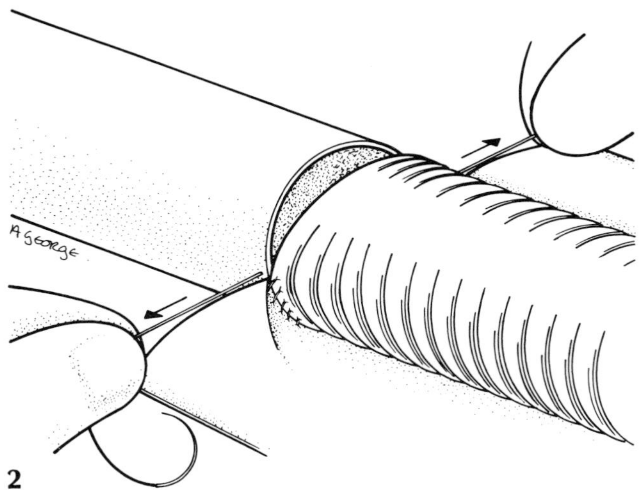

2

2

After the graft is pulled down the suturing is continued to the mid-point, the polypropylene sutures being pulled tight in opposite directions as suturing proceeds to avoid slippage. Slippage will lead to leakage around the back of the anastomosis which is difficult to correct subsequently.

3 & 4

The suturing is continued over and over until the sutures meet. Frequently, it does not matter if the needle passes from the Dacron to the artery or from the artery to the Dacron. Whichever is the more comfortable should be performed. However, if it is anticipated that passing the needle from aorta to Dacron will dissect atheroma it is then essential to pass the needle in the conventional method from Dacron to aorta at all times.

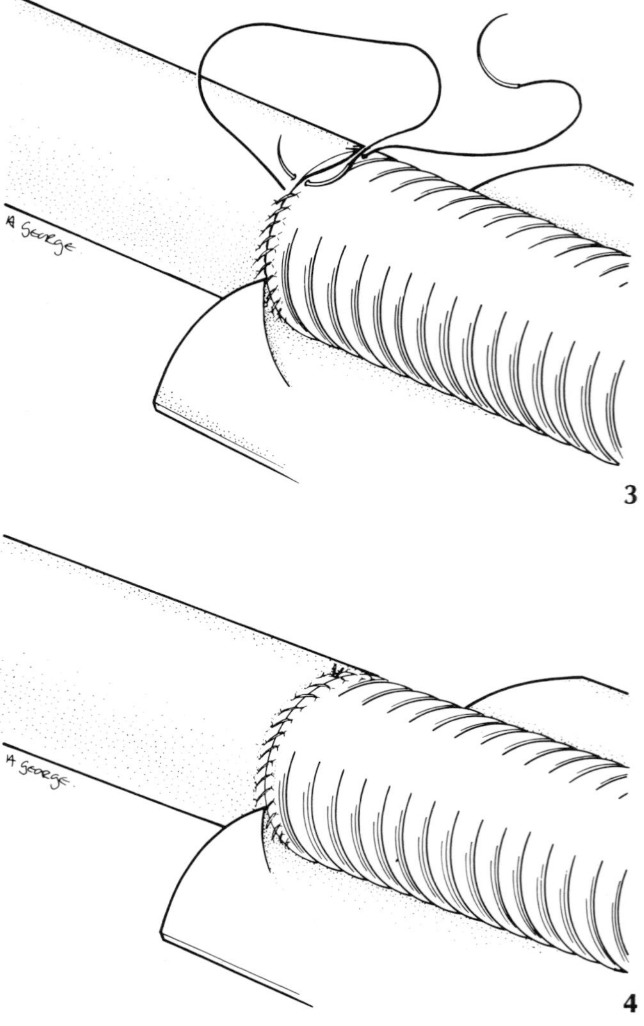

3

4

End-to-end anastomoses of smaller vessels

5

Wherever smaller vessels are to be anastomosed end-to-end, the vessel should be cut obliquely as shown. This will increase the length of the suture line thus reducing tension and will minimize the risk of stenosis.

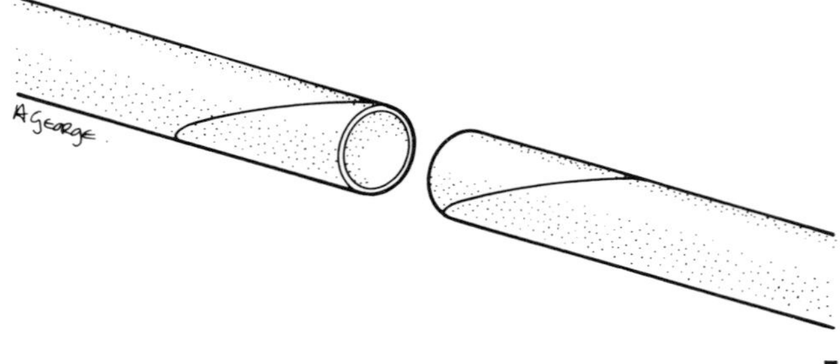

5

6

Two double-ended polypropylene sutures are passed through the opposing cut ends of the vessels.

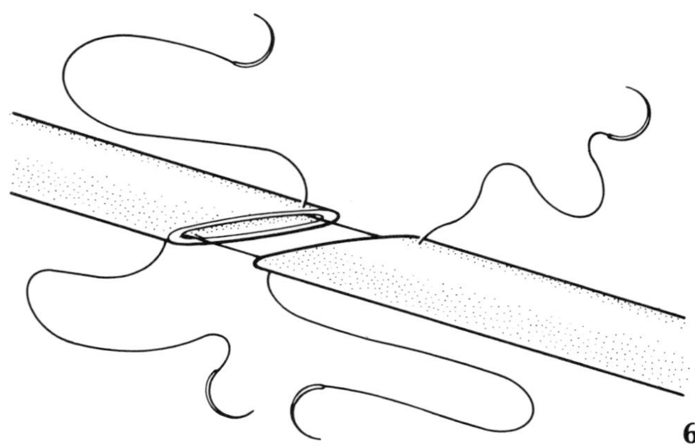
6

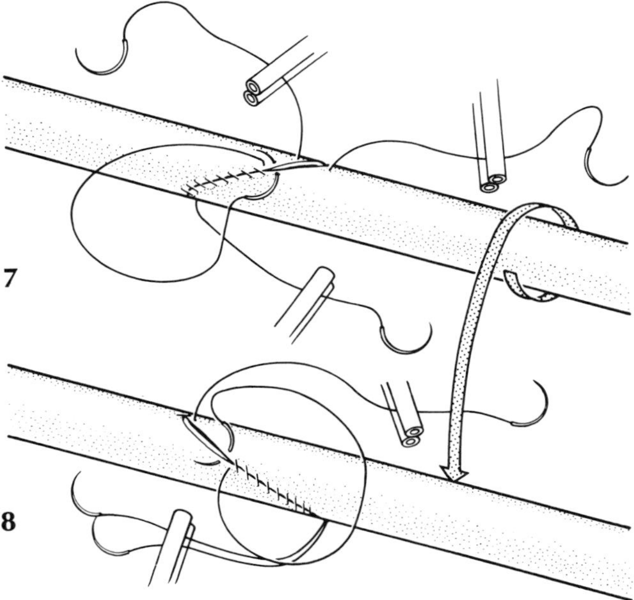
7

8

7 & 8

One end is tied and the other is held with rubber-shod mosquito forceps. One end of the tied suture is used to sew over and over towards the other corner, while the other is held as a stay suture with rubber-shod mosquito forceps. On completion of one side, the vessel is rotated as shown.

The other side is sewn over and over between the held suture ends. At the end of the procedure the polypropylene sutures are cut long to avoid slippage.

End-to-side anastomosis

9

This illustration shows a conventional method of anastomosis of a Dacron limb to the side of the common femoral artery. The arteriotomy is cut to match the length of the obliquely cut Dacron tube and sutures are passed through each apex and tied and held with rubber mosquito forceps.

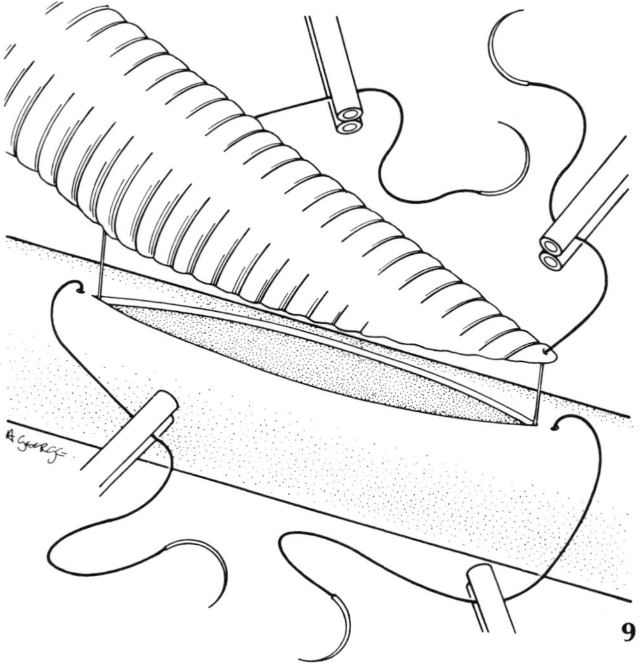
9

10

Suturing progresses forwards from the heel and backwards from the toe. Again, most surgeons sew from Dacron to artery to avoid freeing atheroma from the artery wall, but in some instances this is not essential. The disadvantage of this technique is that the toe end can pull away from the apex and once the sutures are pulled down it is difficult to place the adjacent sutures, particularly at the heel end. This technique is perfectly satisfactory when performed on the common femoral artery but when the Dacron is angled into the origin of the profunda artery this recipient vessel can be very thin and the Dacron frequently pulls away from the apex causing tearing of the vessel.

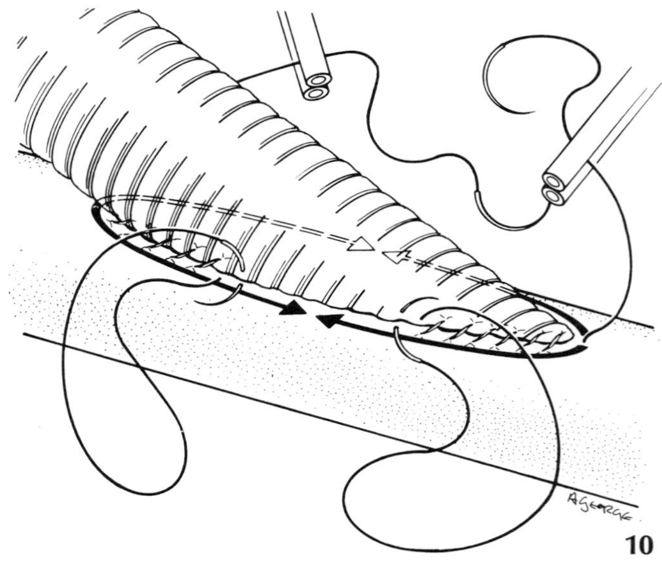

10

11

Alternative end-to-side method with eccentric stitch

11

The illustration shows autologous reverse vein with carefully placed dots along its length so that twisting is avoided when it is tunnelled. In this illustration the first double-ended suture is placed at the heel of the anastomosis as before but the second is placed eccentrically rather than at the apex. The suturing progresses as before, forwards from the heel suture and backwards from the eccentric stitch. The other eccentric stitch is continued forwards around the toe of the graft to meet the other suture. This minimizes the risk of the graft tearing from the apex.

Alternative end-to-side anastomoses using a loose stitch at the heel end

12 & 13

This method is commonly used for anatomosing the end of expanded PTFE to the side of the popliteal artery. It is very convenient, especially for the more experienced vascular surgeon, to place the sutures at the heel end of the graft and leave them long as shown. When the first suture is pulled down and tied as described above, it can be quite difficult to place sutures on either side. This method shown here makes the rest of the anastomosis very easy. It is essential that the sutures be placed without any crossing and it is also vital to use polypropylene because of its slippery quality.

The rest of the anastomosis is either with one double-ended polypropylene suture carried around the toe of the anastomosis to meet the other suture or else a second double-ended suture can be adopted and tied in the eccentric position as shown. With practice a single double-ended polypropylene suture is the fastest way of anastomosis and is technically satisfactory.

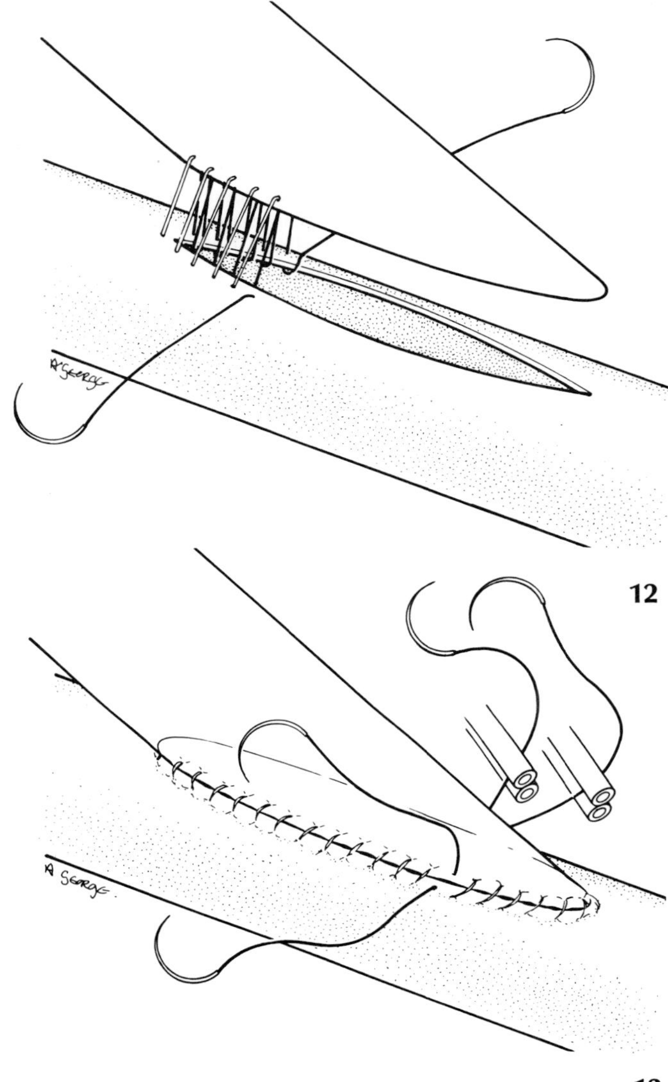

12

13

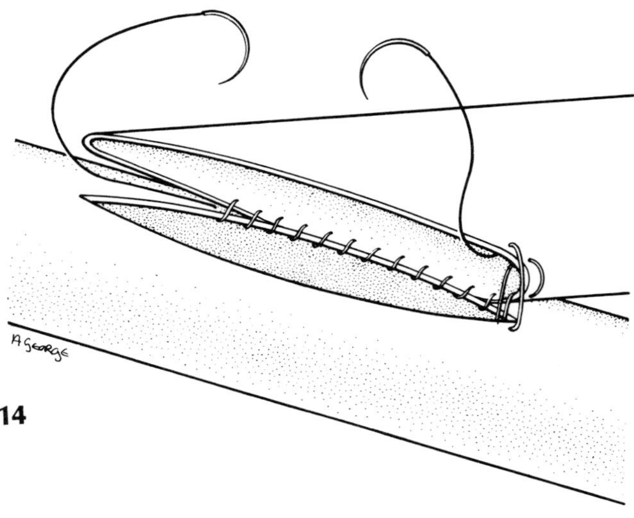

14

14

In *Illustration 12* a long suture is sewn over and over so that on one side the sewing is from graft to artery and from the other side it is from artery to graft. Some surgeons prefer to avoid this and instead insert the first suture as a mattress stitch so that it then becomes possible to complete the anastomosis by sewing with both needles from graft to artery. This is more like the conventional approach and will pin the atheroma to the artery wall. However, the disadvantage is that it leads to many 'backhand' sutures and this prolongs the anastomosis. If the surgeon is prepared to turn so that he always sews 'forehand' and does not mind whether he sews from graft to artery or artery to graft the whole procedure can be completed much more easily, but this is not possible if there is any risk of dissecting the diseased artery wall.

End-to-side anastomoses in a small vessel using interrupted sutures

15

The example shown is the umbilical vein with its Dacron sheath being anastomosed to a small vessel. The heel of the graft is sewn in the usual way. It is essential to pick up the whole thickness of the graft material including the intima and the Dacron mesh with each stitch. For the toe end of the graft it may be preferable to use interrupted stitches so that they can be placed accurately before being tied. It is a very useful technique and provides an alternative method of ensuring accurate placement of the sutures in this vital part of the anastomosis.

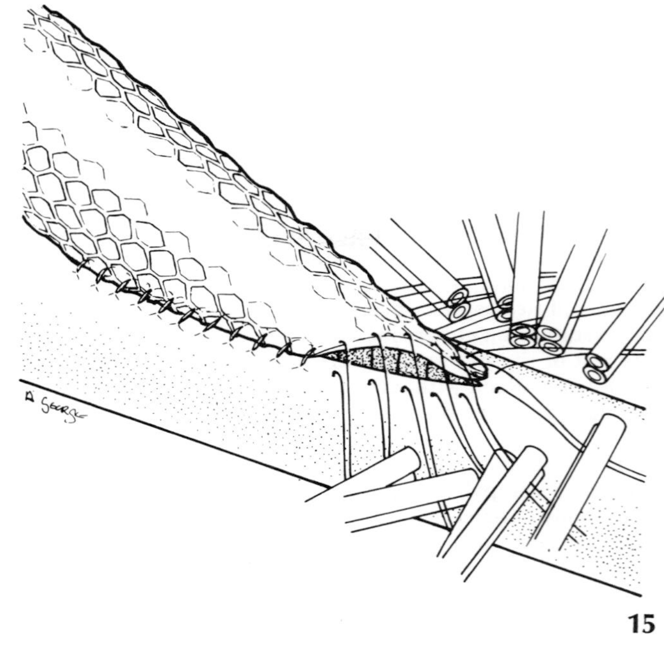

15

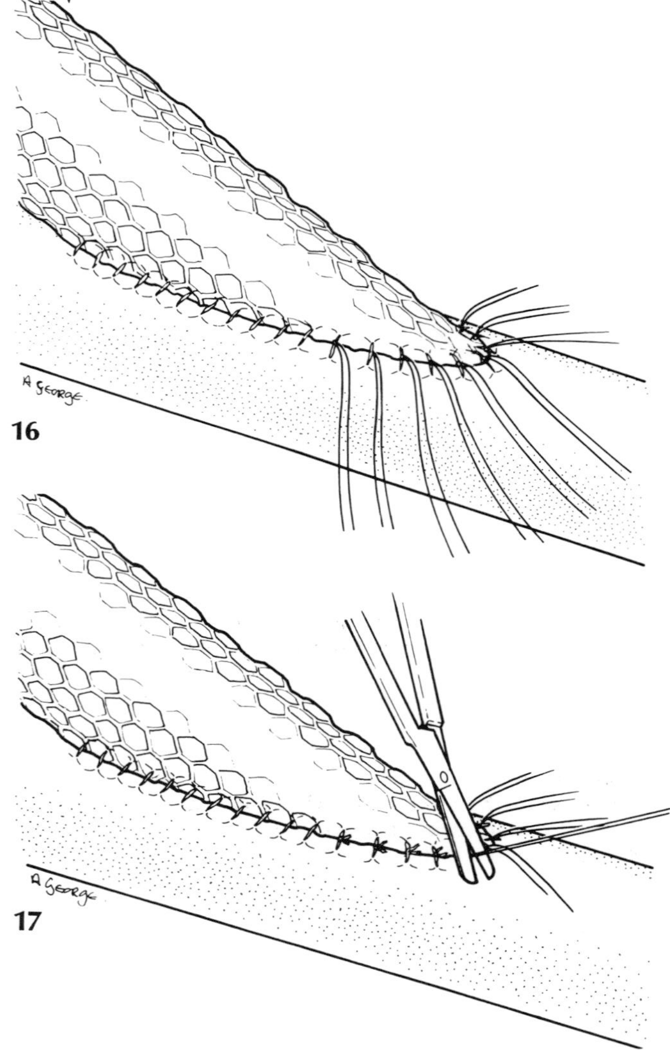

16

17

16 & 17

On completion of the anastomosis the interrupted sutures are tied, held long and then cut one by one.

Confirming patency

Patency must be assessed before the wound is closed. Each surgeon has his own method of doing this and the subject cannot be dealt with in any detail here. The most conventional test, however, is to perform an on-table operative arteriogram. This will demonstrate the anatomy of the anastomoses and if nothing else it is a very useful teaching manoeuvre. Many anastomoses which were thought to be satisfactory are discovered by this method to be unsatisfactory. Such quality control leads to improved surgery.

The electromagnetic flow probe provides physiological data and is very much quicker than the operative arteriogram. The flow probe is placed around the graft and the volume flow per minute is measured. Additionally, a waveform of the flow is printed out for a permanent record.

Another method of checking an anastomosis is by direct pressure readings above the inflow and below the outflow. The needle can be connected to a thin polythene catheter which the anaesthetist attaches to a three-way tap to which the radial line is attached for monitoring. This technique is in its infancy and is probably best used in conjunction with flow readings.

Duplex scanning is now used in the operating room. A sterile Doppler probe may be used to image the vessel and assess the velocity of the blood flow in it.

Digital subraction angiography is also of tremendous value. It enables operative arteriography to be performed much more easily and can play back the result in order to minimize the problem of the timing of taking the film.

Wound closure

Clearly, meticulous aseptic technique is vital whenever prosthetic material is introduced into the body because if any infection is present the graft will be rejected. Wound infection can be minimized by closing the wound very carefully in several layers and it can be helpful to mop the wound edges with an aqueous solution of chlorhexidine. Before the final placement of the skin sutures a spray of povidone-iodine is given. Groin wounds are the most difficult and a subcuticular polypropylene suture fixed in place with beads is an ideal method of closure. This suture is removed after 7 days and leaves a good cosmetic result.

Intraoperative proof of patency

BERT C. EIKELBOOM MD, PhD
Department of Surgery, University Hospital, Utrecht, The Netherlands

ALEXANDER C. DE VRIES MD
St Antonius Hospital, Nieuwegein, The Netherlands

Introduction

Technical errors during vascular reconstructive surgery should be detected intraoperatively because they are partly responsible for the failure of these procedures. Graft failure of up to 18% within 1 month of femorocrural bypass surgery, and complications like stroke and restenosis after carotid endarterectomy, are to some degree caused by technical inaccuracies such as intimal flaps, anastomotic and endarterectomy suture line strictures, and intraluminal thrombi.

Intraoperative detection of these imperfections will enhance quality and patency in vascular surgery. The two most common and readily available techniques — angiography and Doppler flow assessment — will be described in detail. Other techniques, such as vascular endoscopy, outflow resistance measurement, as well as the more sophisticated forms of ultrasound assessment (e.g. spectral analysis and duplex scanning), will be discussed briefly.

Angiography

Intraoperative angiography is considered to be the best form of intraoperative assessment, especially in lower limb bypass surgery. In general, we prefer to use Doppler ultrasound, as described in the next section, because we find it a less time-consuming screening technique before angiography. We perform prebypass intraoperative angiography if more information is required regarding the outflow tract.

Modern X-ray facilities in the operating room include fluoroscopy, a reference monitor, immediate replay, subtraction and roadmapping. A free-standing radiolucent operating table facilitates the investigation.

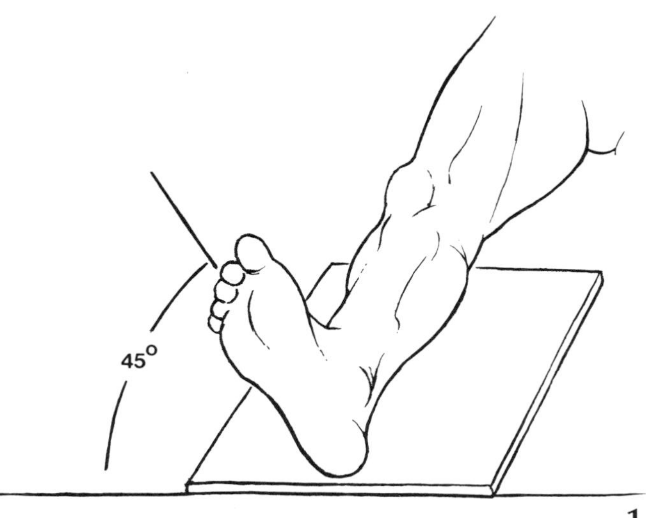

1

1, 2 & 3

The foot lies at an angle of 45° and the plate is placed flat on the table so that the angiogram is effectively shot obliquely through the leg. Depending on the type of bypass surgery, slightly different access routes are utilized. For the most common – angiography of autologous reversed saphenous vein bypass – we prefer to perform the proximal anastomosis first, allowing arterial blood pressure to straighten the graft and thus avoid kinking and rotation. In this way graft inflow can also be checked. After completion of the distal anastomosis, angiography is performed as shown, via a proximal side branch of the vein in the functioning graft.

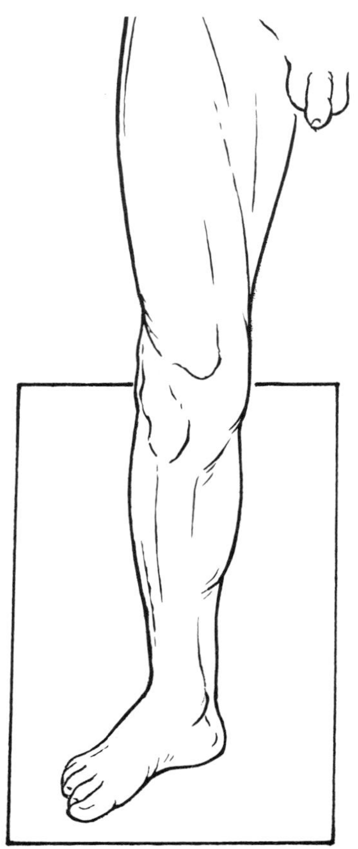

2

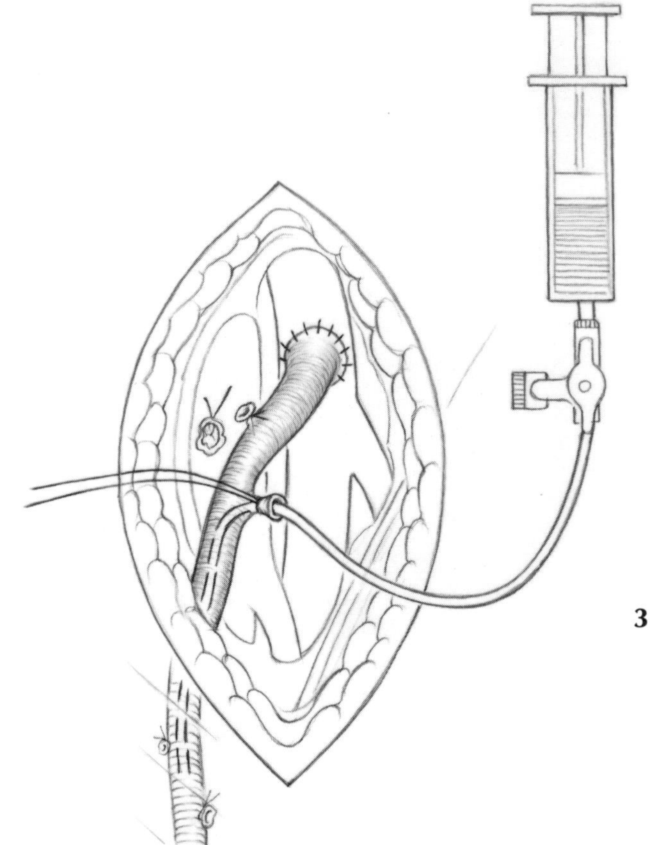

3

4

Alternatively, a vein bypass can be punctured using a standard infusion needle system (venflon 1.4 mm o.d.) as advocated for synthetic graft assessment. *In situ* bypass can be assessed in exactly the same way as reverse vein, but Doppler techniques are our preferred procedures.

Even in experienced hands, erroneous anastomosis to the venous system is possible on occasions and a distal bypass outflow angiogram will alert the surgeon to this mistake. Sometimes, the distal anastomosis is performed first to allow better exposure. The angiogram is then performed before the upper anastomosis is completed.

Following distal outflow angiography, flushing with heparinized saline is advised. If necessary, additional X-rays are performed of the foot region or the graft itself.

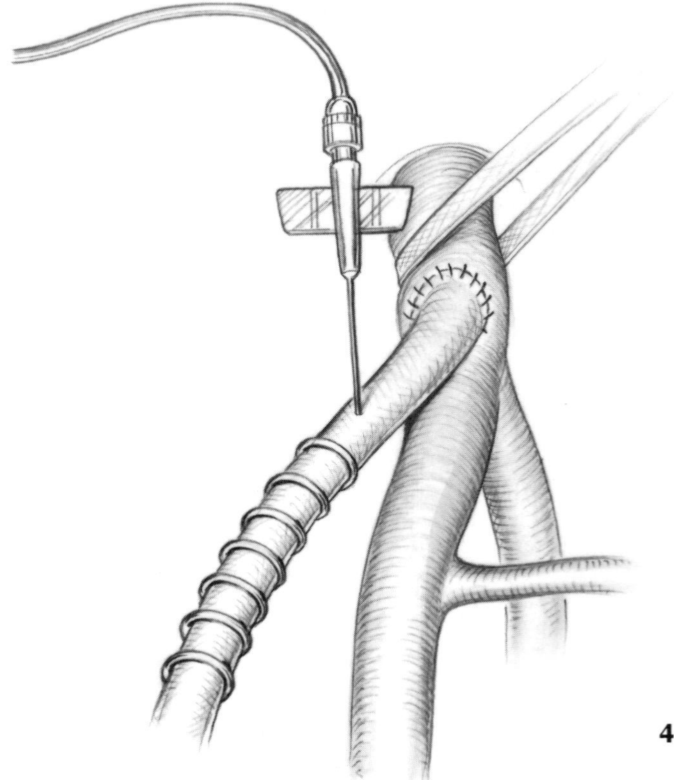

4

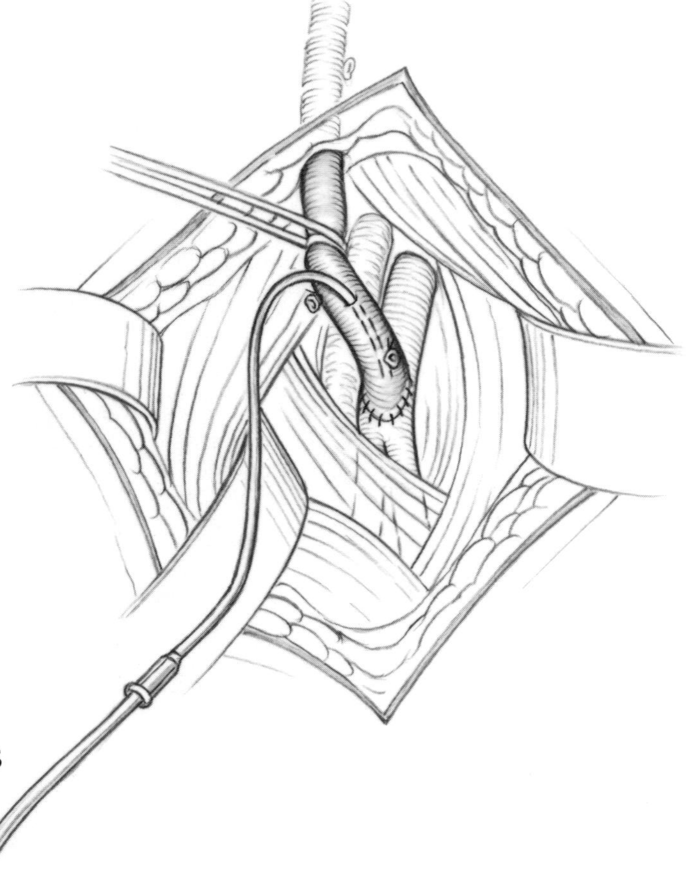

5

5

In the previous illustration an externally supported PTFE bypass is cannulated with a simple butterfly needle. Alternatively, as is shown here, at the end of both anastomoses a bypass (vein or prosthesis) can be occluded and a distal silastic catheter can be passed towards the lower anastomosis to allow good contrast delineation of the critical run-off area.

Doppler flow assessment

6

The Doppler system is a valuable tool for screening technical difficulties during vascular reconstructive surgery. We use this system in the most simple form, which comprises sterilizable probes connected to the basic apparatus which remains outside the operative field. Only audible processing is used. The apparatus remains on standby during all vascular surgery. It is less time-consuming and there are no disadvantages. It is used before or in some instances instead of angiography.

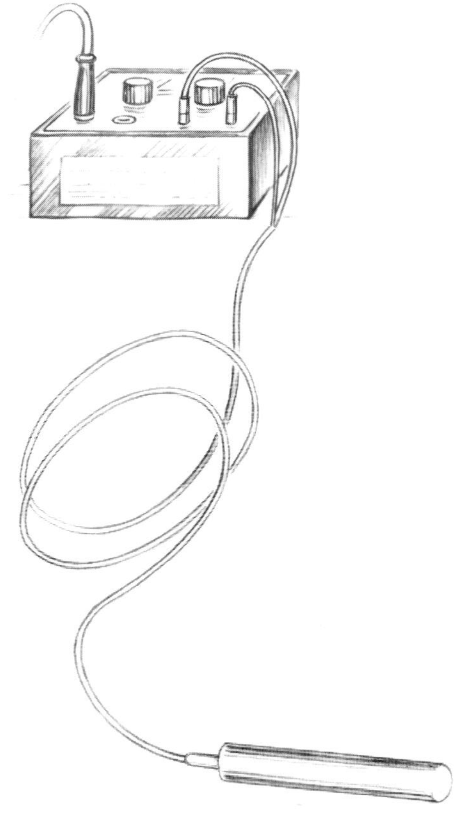

6

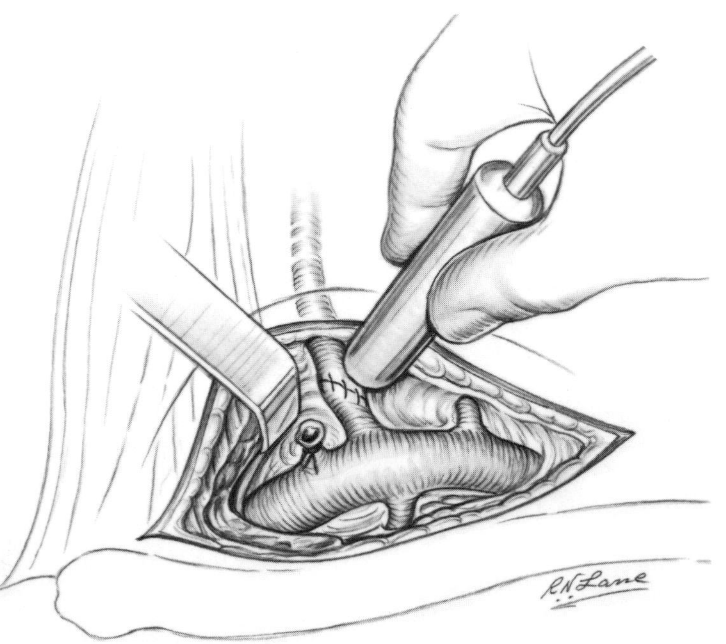

7

7

During surgery the functioning graft or reconstructed area is checked. The probe is placed near to the vessel to be assessed, preferably at an angle of 60°. Conduction of ultrasound is easily achieved by placing both the probe and the vessel under heparin saline solution in a vertebral-truncus thyrocervical transposition, as shown. In this way audible signals are processed. These sounds are easily recognized, even by untrained ears. A 'good' signal is characterized by an uninterrupted flow with three components, i.e. a triphasic pattern. A 'poor' signal consists of so-called 'damped' signals of short systolic peaks of low frequency with intermissions without any recognizable flow. The haemodynamic equivalent of this is a stepwise, slow flow through the assessed vessel. The traces are shown from a directional Doppler trace but the ear can tell the difference. Stenoses are recognized by frequency shifts, while at the site of anastomoses some turbulence must be accepted. For *in situ* bypass surgery, it can be used to locate side branches as previously described (Greenhalgh *et al.*, 1985).

Miscellaneous techniques

Spectrum analysis of directional Doppler ultrasound

Doppler-derived signals can be interpreted more accurately by means of computer processing, i.e. spectral analysis. The spectrum is then visualized and can be further analysed by means of indexes. These analyses require meticulously obtained samples and are therefore not always ideal for intraoperative use. Moreover, the indexes obtained are not easily interpreted.

Duplex scanning

Duplex scanning combines Doppler with B-mode ultrasound. This image allows visualization of reconstructed areas (Flanigan, 1985). The apparatus is expensive and requires its operators to be highly trained. The scan heads used are large in comparison to the operative site to be analysed. They are not sterilized but covered by plastic bags. The instrument itself needs constant operation and adjustment, which means that a technician and a skilled surgeon skilled in the use of ultrasound are required in the operating theatre. On the other hand, it offers all ultrasound possibilities, which makes this system the most versatile for the trained operator. When this system is operational, it offers the best information possible, especially for carotid surgery.

Angioscopy

Angioscopy has become increasingly accepted as an adjunct to *in situ* bypass grafting. It helps to identify valves, which can be destroyed under direct vision, and it helps to occlude side branches either externally through small incisions or from within the lumen using coils. The value of these techniques has not yet fully been established. Other applications include technical control after bypass, endarterectomy or thrombectomy.

Outflow resistance measurement

This technique offers outflow resistance measurements (Ascer and Veith, 1985). The value of this parameter is limited and the system is not yet commercially available.

Flow measurement

Electromagnetic flow measurement has been largely abandoned owing to technical problems (difficult probe fit) and because results have been of limited value. In the future, it will probably be replaced by Doppler-derived volume flow measurement which offers greater technical simplicity.

Summary

Doppler ultrasound, where simple audible processing is satisfactory for intraoperative use, offers a valuable tool in vascular reconstructive surgery. It is less time-consuming and requires little experience. It is advocated for screening and technical inaccuracies. We prefer its use before angiography, especially in peripheral bypass surgery. Of the other techniques mentioned, duplex scanning is the most promising. It offers all ultrasound-derived possibilities, including true visualization. However, its complexity makes its use in intraoperative application limited as yet.

References

Ascer, E. and Veith, F. J. (1985). Outflow resistance measurements in infrainguinal bypass operations by injecting saline and measuring the integral of pressure. In *Diagnostic Techniques and Assessment Procedures in Vascular Surgery*. Greenhalgh, R. M., ed. London and Orlando: Grune and Stratton.

Flanigan, D. P. (1985). Peroperative Doppler testing and imaging in patients with lower limb ischaemia. In *Diagnostic Techniques and Assessment Procedures in Vascular Surgery*. Greenhalgh, R. M., ed. London and Orlando: Grune and Stratton.

Greenhalgh, R. M., Heather, B. P., Green, I. L. and McCollum, C. N. (1985). Intra-operative detection of arteriovenous fistulae after *in situ* vein bypass. In *Diagnostic Techniques and Assessment Procedures in Vascular Surgery*. Greenhalgh, R. M., ed. London and Orlando: Grune and Stratton.

Loeprecht, H., Weber, H. and Monnig, J. (1985). Vascular endoscopy. In *Diagnostic Techniques and Assessment Procedures in Vascular Surgery*. Greenhalgh, R. M., ed. London and Orlando: Grune and Stratton.

Conventional percutaneous transluminal angioplasty

NIGEL K. BARRETT MRCP, FRCR, *Consultant Radiologist*
JAMES McIVOR FRCR, FFR, FDSRCS, *Clinical Director*
Charing Cross Hospital, London, UK

Introduction

Despite the introduction into the market place of devices such as thermal high frequency ablators (Gould, 1990), numerous different types of laser tips including bare tips, different types of metal probes, and sapphire tipped probes (Yang *et al.*, 1991), high speed rotating catheters (Kensey *et al.*, 1987) and even different designs of atherectomy catheters, percutaneous transluminal balloon angioplasty still remains the proven method of choice for dilating stenotic and occluded arterial segments.

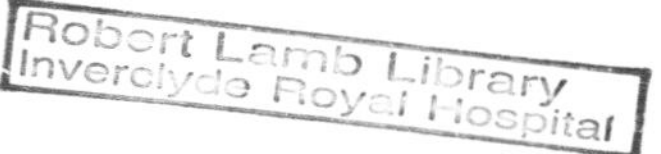

1

In 1974 Gruntzig and Hopff described a technique whereby a double lumen catheter, with an inflatable cylindrical polyvinyl balloon near its tip, was passed through a stenotic segment and the balloon was inflated on several occasions before being withdrawn. Ten years earlier Dotter and Judkins (1964) had described a technique for dilating stenotic arteries using a series of catheters of increasing diameter. Although there were some successes the incidence of complications at the puncture site, which required an arteriotomy, and at the site of the lesion, was high and the technique was not widely accepted. There were two technical advantages to the Gruntzig balloon. The first was that the deflated balloon could be applied tightly to the shaft of a normal sized arterial catheter and introduced percutaneously over a guidewire without resorting to an arteriotomy, and secondly that the inflated balloon applied a dilating force to the artery but no shearing force to the stenotic lesion.

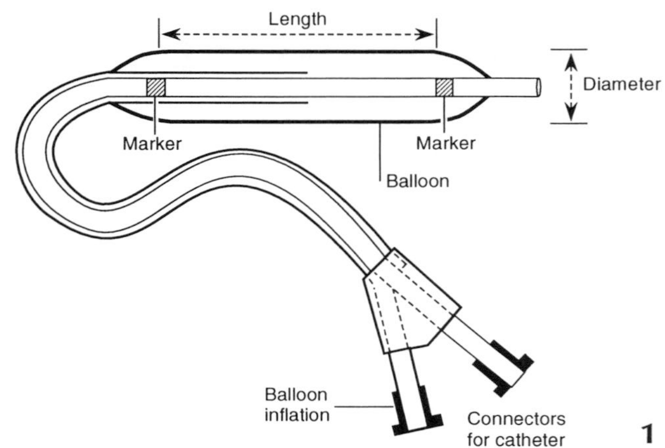

1

2

The original theory about the mechanism of angioplasty consisted of compression and remodelling of atheromatous plaques. These original theories have had to be modified by more recent investigations which have shown that transluminal angioplasty is effected by controlled damage of the arterial wall layers with subsequent healing and by stretching. Over 60% of atherosclerotic lesions are eccentric and this asymmetrical location results in dilation of the normal portion of the vessel wall with preservation of the media behind the plaque (*Illustration 2*).

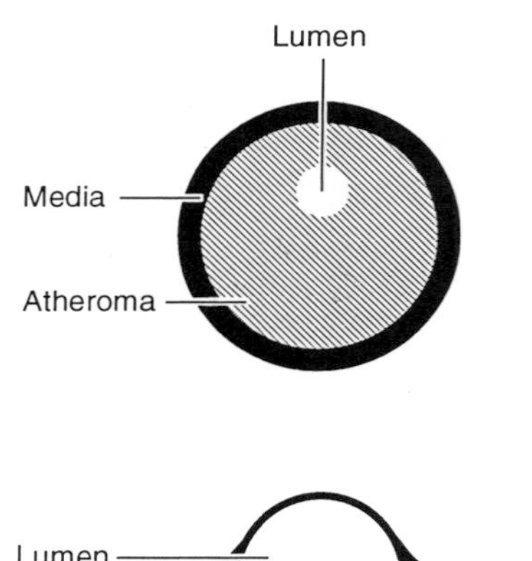

2a

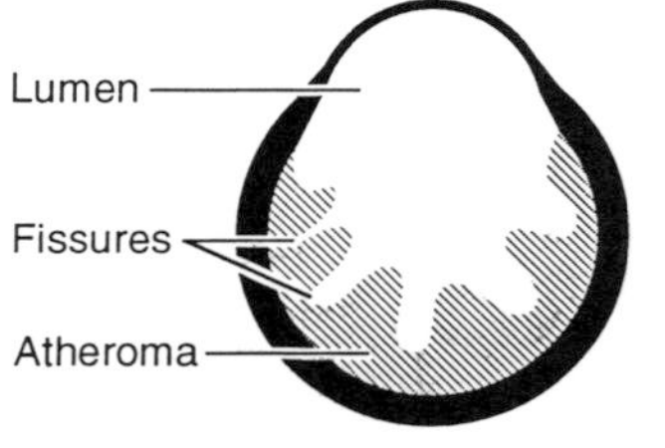

2b

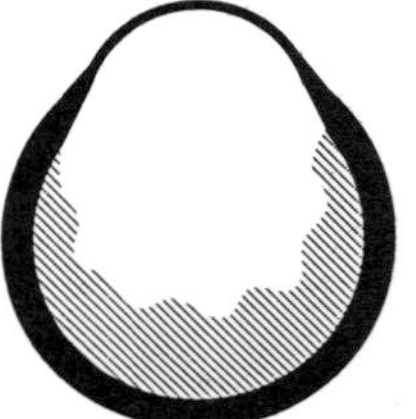

2c

Pathophysiology

Following the trauma of dilatation, platelets aggregate on the denuded luminal surface followed by proliferation and invasion of smooth muscle cells, resulting in a hypertrophied neointima which is covered by a neoendothelium. Destruction of the muscle layers also results in scarring and intimal hyperplasia and multinucleated macrophages and fibroblasts eventually reconstitute the entire vessel wall. The internal elastic lamina is not reconstituted and with marked overdilatation of the artery adventitial tears may be demonstrated which may lead to vessel rupture. Repair of the dilated arterial walls occurs with organization of the thrombus, intimal hyperplasia and fibrosis (Zollikofer *et al.*, 1984). It is thought that thrombus organization and intimal hyperplasia have a compensatory function in cases of extensive wall damage with advantitial stretching, so that healing without aneurysm formation may occur. Because of the vulnerability of atherosclerotic vessels, overdistension has to be avoided because vessel rupture may occur (Salomonowitz *et al.*, 1991).

Balloon design

There has been extensive research into angioplasty balloon catheters since Gruntzig's first double lumen balloon catheter was designed, when both the catheter shaft and the balloon were constructed from polyvinyl chloride. The importance of the balloon research is that the dilating force applied to a stenotic lesion is dependent on several factors including balloon diameter, balloon inflation pressure, compliance of the balloon, balloon length, and length and degree of stenotic segment (Zollikofer *et al.*, 1988). According to the law of Laplace, the tension exerted on the wall of an inflated balloon is directly proportional to the pressure within the balloon and the radius of the balloon. the dilating force generated by a balloon therefore, is directly proportional to the balloon diameter and the inflation pressure, so that larger balloons will require less pressure than smaller balloons to generate substantial dilating forces and similarly larger vessels, such as the abdominal aorta or the common iliac arteries, require less pressure to dilate and rupture.

The compliance of the balloon is a measure of how much it will stretch beyond a predetermined diameter when a force is applied to it. Totally non-compliant balloons will not stretch beyond a predetermined diameter despite increases in inflation pressures, whilst maintaining its profile and shape with repeated inflations. Balloons made from compliant materials, however, will continue to increase their diameter as the inflation pressure increases, particularly in the areas of least resistance. This can result in the adjacent normal vessel lumen being overdilated and the area of stenosis being non-dilated and a greater chance of rupture of the artery at this site (Matsumoto *et al.*, 1993).

Balloon manufacturers are therefore now making balloons from derivatives of one of five basic classes of plastic polymers, namely, polyvinyl chloride, polyethylene, polyethylene teraphthalate, nylon, or reinforced polyurethane.

Catheter technology

Hand in hand with the balloon technology goes the catheter technology. The balloon has to be firmly attached to the catheter and there are various different mechanisms for supplying channels for both the guidewire and the inflating liquid used during the procedure. The different catheter designs all have variable advantages which must be taken into consideration when performing the angioplasty. Of equal importance is the fact that manufacturers are now able to apply their balloons to smaller and smaller shafts so that the 7 and 9 French shafts have now been replaced by balloons being mounted on 4 and 5 French shafts (1.3–1.6 mm). This enables the angioplasty balloon catheter to be introduced over a guidewire without the need of an introducer sheath, thus keeping the hole made in the artery at the puncture site to a minimum. Another advantage of these high tech balloons is that they will follow guidewires round acute angles and reach vessels that were hitherto unreachable with the older systems. They also have a much higher working inflation pressure of up to 12 atmospheres, a pressure that will dilate up the majority of tight stenoses.

Indications for angioplasty

As angioplasty balloon catheter design has improved over the years, so have the indications and potential sites for angioplasty increased. The technique is of proven value in the treatment of atheromatous narrowing and occlusion of the iliac, femoral and popliteal arteries (Zeitlar *et al.*, 1983; Cumberland, 1983) and in atheromatous narrowing of the coronary arteries (Gruntzig, 1981; Cumberland, 1983). The initial patency rates for iliac artery stenosis are reported as 95% or more and 5-year patency rates of up to 57% (Jeans *et al.*, 1990).

Transluminal angioplasty of renal artery stenosis is a successful alternative to surgery in the treatment of reno-vascular hypertension (Tegtmeyer *et al.*, 1984; Martin *et al.*, 1986), and in lesions produced by fibromuscular dysplasia or short isolated atherosclerotic stenoses renal angioplasty should be considered the treatment of choice. Successful dilatation of atheromatous lesions in other sites, including the aorta (Kumpe, 1981) and other branches such as the axillary (Cumberland, 1983), subclavian (Erbstein *et al.*, 1988), coeliac (Saddekni *et al.*, 1980) and mesenteric (Novelline, 1980) arteries has been reported. Angioplasty has also been used to treat arterial narrowing due to therapeutic radiation, takayasus arteritis and surgery (Saddekni *et al.*, 1980).

Balloon angioplasty can also be used in the venous system and is routinely used to treat venous stenoses distal to haemodialysis fistulae (Gmelin *et al.*, 1989) and there are reports of successful dilatation of venous narrowing following venous anastomosis, such as splenorenal and mesocaval shunts (Cope, 1980; Novelline, 1980) and even portal vein stenoses following liver transplantation (Olliff *et al.*, 1991).

The success rate of second angioplasty procedures after complete or partial failure on the first attempt is roughly similar to the success rate of first attempts, but it is usual to leave an interval of 6 weeks between procedures to allow for epithelial regeneration.

Drug therapy

Intra-arterial heparin is usually administered prior to inflation of the balloon with the aim of reducing the chances of thromboembolism. A dose of 5000 i.u. is given, which has a low risk with high potential benefits. It is not common to continue on long-term heparin unless there is evidence of distal embolization at the time of angioplasty, or unless the flow rates are so slow as to provoke thrombosis when the patient may be placed on oral anticoagulation.

Acetylsalicylic acid (aspirin) 300 mg per day inhibits platelet aggregation, but the benefits of this drug following balloon angioplasty are still not proven.

Access to vascular tree

3

The Seldinger technique may be used to obtain access to the femoral artery, brachial artery or axillary artery. The brachial artery at the elbow can be entered using a cut-down technique and a catheter introduced directly.

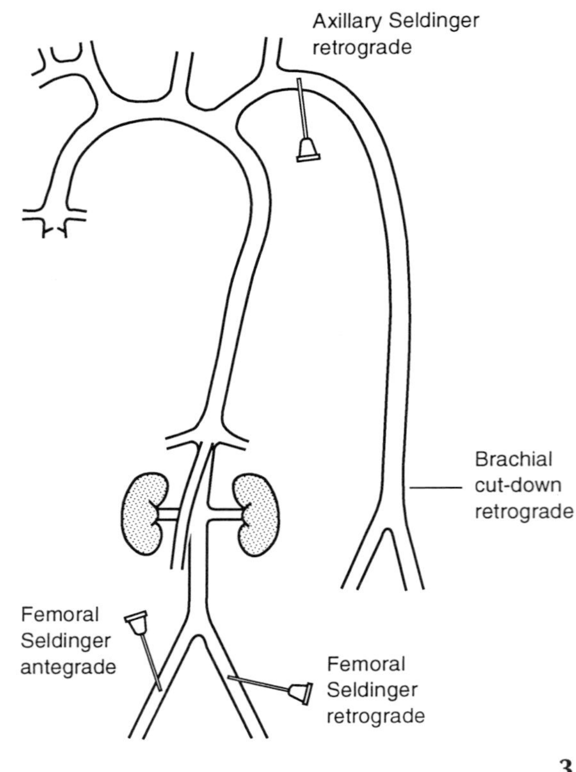

3

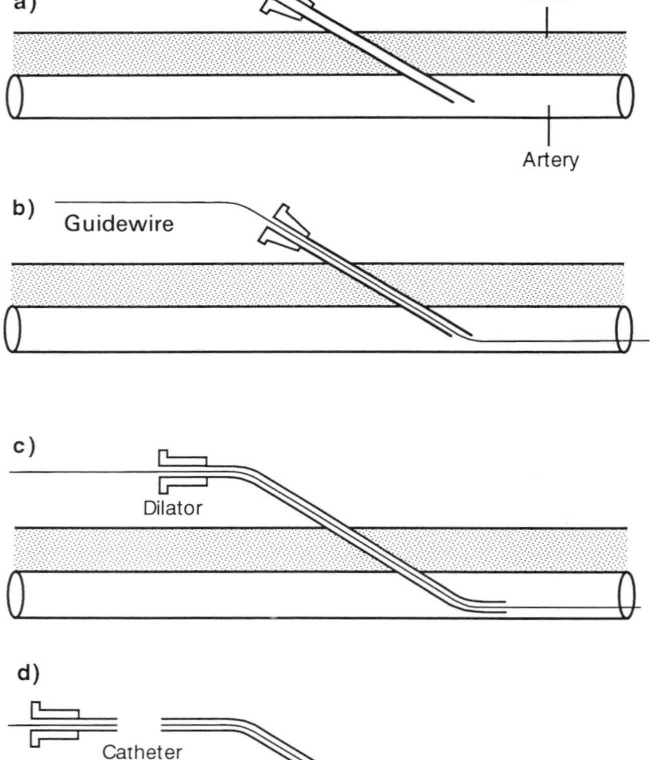

4

4a, b, c & d

After puncturing the artery with either a one-part or two-part needle (*a*), a standard guidewire with a soft flexible tip is inserted and advanced in the correct direction (*b*). The tract is dilated through soft tissues and arterial wall if required (*c*) and the angioplasty catheter is then passed over the guidewire (*d*).

Selective catheterization using the wire exchange technique

5

Most angioplasty catheters are straight and therefore cannot be passed directly into branches of the aorta. The stenotic artery is therefore catheterized initially using an arterial catheter with a pre-formed curve and a long (200 cm) exchange guidewire is passed through this catheter and beyond the stenosis. The arterial catheter is removed leaving the guidewire across the stenosis and the angioplasty catheter is then passed over the wire, into the artery, and through the stenosis. The guidewire must always be kept through the angioplasty catheter and beyond the stenosis so that the balloon can be returned to the site easily should a complication occur, or the dilatation be unsatisfactory.

In the event of a rare, but life-threatening, rupture of the angioplastied arterial wall, limitation of haemorrhage can be performed by passing a balloon catheter over the wire and placing it in the vessel proximal to the site of rupture. If the balloon is the same size or slightly larger than the artery that has ruptured, inflation at this site will cause complete occlusion of the lumen and reduce further haemorrhage, allowing time for surgical intervention to take place.

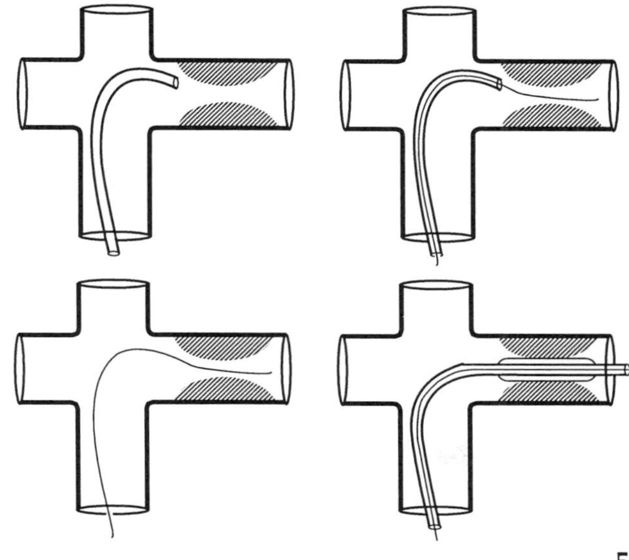

5

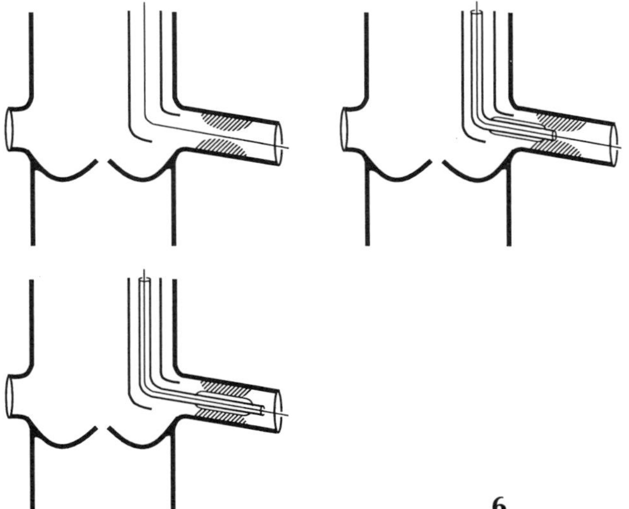

6

Selective catheterization using a coaxial system

6

A catheter with a preformed end near its tip is passed into the orifice of the artery which is to be dilated and a guidewire passed through the stenosis. The angioplasty catheter is then passed over the wire, through the guiding catheter, until it lies across the stenosed segment. As catheter design improved, so the size of the balloon catheters decreased and 5 French angioplasty catheters are able to pass through 6 or 7 French guiding catheters. This technique is in general use for coronary artery angioplasty (as shown here) and is often used for renal artery angioplasty.

Long or multiple stenoses

7

Angioplasty, like surgery, is most effective when used to treat a single short stenotic segment. However, stenotic lesions that exceed the length of the angioplasty catheter can be treated by dilating one segment at a time, beginning with the end furthest from the puncture site and gradually withdrawing the balloon catheter whilst inflating it at different sites. As the length of lesions that are being angioplastied has increased, so the manufacturers have developed balloon catheters to cope with these and it is now possible to obtain catheters with 15 cm length balloons on them. These longer balloons decrease the time taken to angioplasty long segments.

Multiple stenoses can be managed in a similar fashion by either dilating the individual stenoses one at a time, beginning with the lesion furthest from the puncture site, or using a long balloon to angioplasty all the lesions simultaneously. The tip of the guidewire should never be advanced through a recently dilated stenotic segment owing to the risk of dissection and it is therefore important that the wire is always maintained distal to the stenosis, so that the stenosis does not have to be retraversed.

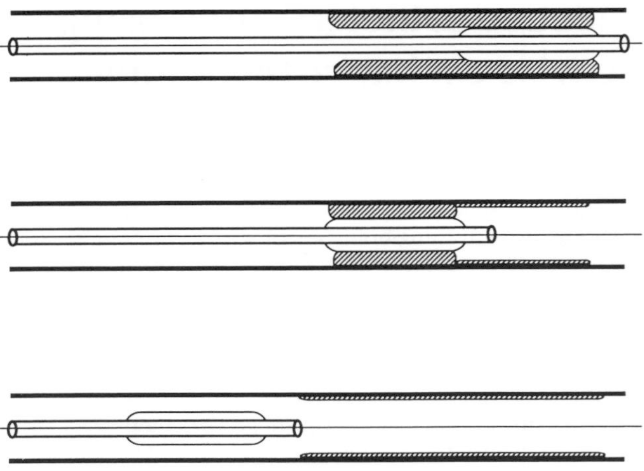

7

8

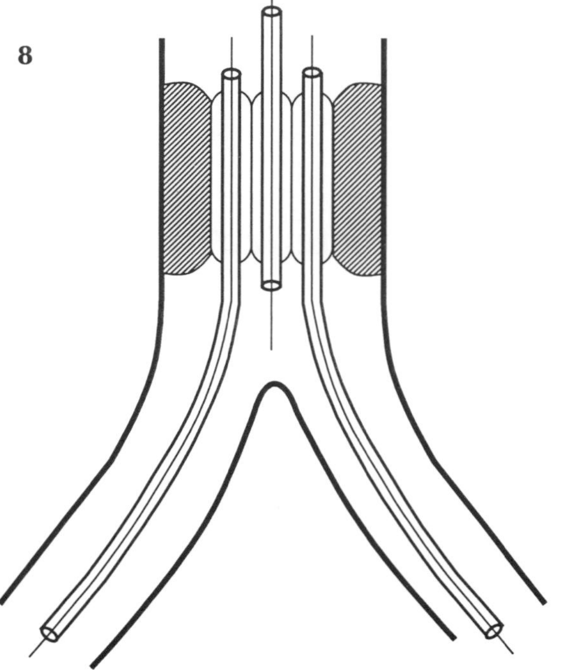

Stenosis of the infrarenal abdominal aorta

8

In cases where the arterial lumen is wider than the diameter of a single balloon, then two or more catheters can be passed through the stenosis and inflated simultaneously. If two catheters have been passed up either femoral artery and a third catheter is required, this can be passed down from the axillary artery.

Occluded arteries

9

Complete occlusions of the iliac, femoral and popliteal arteries can often be re-canalized by advancing a guidewire through the occluded arterial lumen, followed by a thin straight catheter and finally by the angioplasty catheter. The occluded segment is then dilated, beginning at the end furthest from the puncture site. An initial success rate of 78% and 5-year patency rate of 63% has been recently reported for iliac occlusions and the length of the occlusion did not affect the initial and long-term results (Gupta *et al.*, 1993). It has been suggested that re-canalization of femoro-popliteal occlusions should be limited to occlusions of less than 10 cm in length.

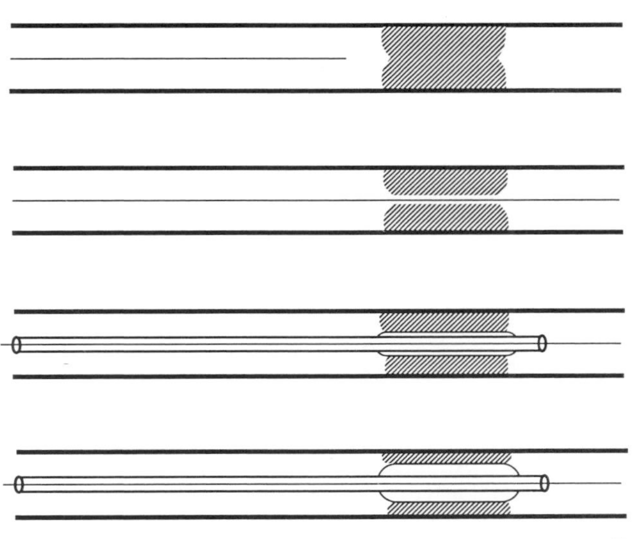

9

Balloon inflation

10

The balloon should be inflated with dilute ionic contrast medium containing 10–15% iodine concentration. The use of viscous contrast material should be avoided as it cannot be completely aspirated from the angioplasty balloon at the end of the procedure, especially with the smaller bore catheters that have narrower channels within them. The manufacturers' guidelines for the pressures that the balloons can withstand should be closely adhered to. Most modern catheters can now take pressures of 10–12 atm (1010–1212 kPa) without rupturing. It is important to use non-compliant balloons that will not overstretch and will continue to apply the dilating force to the stenotic area and not to the adjacent normal vessel. There are several commercially available pressure gauges that can be used to monitor the pressure in the inflated balloon, so that over-inflation and risk of balloon rupture does not occur (*Illustration 10*). Most authors would recommend inflation periods of 10–30 seconds which can be repeated until the fluoroscopically visible waisting of the balloon has vanished.

Following successful balloon dilatation a postdilatation arteriogram should be performed to obtain a permanent record, and this can usually be carried out through the angioplasty catheter. However, if there is any possibility of further dilatation being attempted at the same session, the guidewire should be kept in position through the stenosis so that the

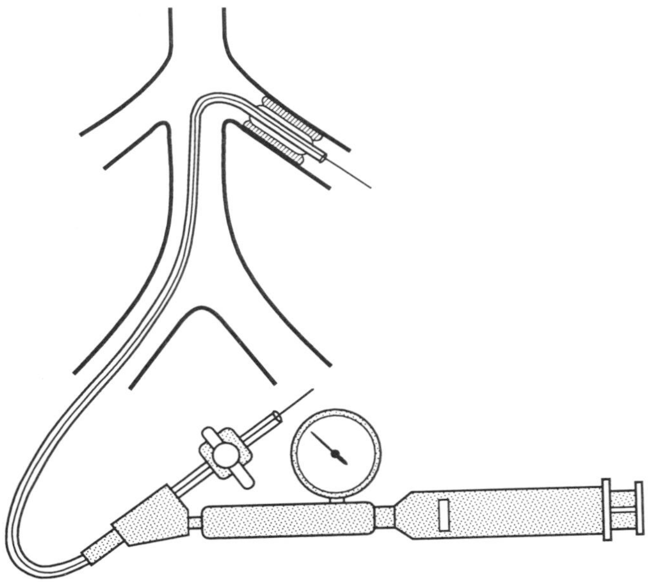

10

balloon catheter may be passed over it again into the stenotic segment. The tip of the guidewire or the tip of the catheter, by itself, should never be passed through a recently dilated artery, owing to the risk of dissection.

A 30% narrowing or less is an acceptable result following angioplasty (except in the coronary arteries) as the lumen of the artery would almost certainly become wider and smoother during the following 6 weeks.

Complications

The most serious complication is sudden occlusion at the site of angioplasty. An incidence of 1–5% has been reported for the ilio-femoral arteries with a higher complication rate following angioplasty of the renal arteries of between 6 and 15% (Billström *et al.*, 1988). The clinical significance of these technical disasters depends on the artery that has been damaged. Sudden occlusion of a coronary artery is a surgical emergency and the possibility of this complication should restrict coronary angioplasty to centres with facilities for immediate cardiac bypass surgery. Even with these facilities, coronary artery angioplasty has a mortality currently estimated at 1%. Occlusion of the renal, mesenteric or coeliac arteries usually requires immediate surgery and occlusion of an upper or lower limb artery may require early surgery. Complications at the angioplasty site can be kept to a minimum by never passing the tip of the guidewire or catheter through a recently dilated artery, as this is likely to cause dissection, and by accepting a less than perfect cosmetic result on the postdilatation arteriogram.

Haematomas are not uncommon at the puncture site, particularly in hypertensive patients. Complications at the puncture site can be kept to a minimum by puncturing the artery as it runs over a bony landmark so that it is easily compressible following catheter removal. The smaller gauge catheters make a smaller hole in the artery enabling more effective haemostasis. Immobilization of the limb for 12 hours following the procedure is to be advocated. Late aneurysm formation at the puncture site is associated with use of larger bore catheters and aneurysm formation at the angioplasty site has been reported.

Conclusion

Balloon angioplasty and the development of newer devices are enabling the radiologist to maintain the patency of vessels with minimal intervention and shorter patient hospitalization. Working jointly with the vascular surgeon, the planning and course of treatment for these patients is being refined and speeded up and as a result of this close co-operation, luminal patency and improvement in the patient's condition is being greatly improved.

References

Billström, A., Ekelund, L. and Hietala, S. O. (1988). Complications of percutaneous transluminal renal angioplasty. *Journal of Interventional Radiology* **3**, 45.

Cope, C. (1980). Balloon dilatation of closed mesocaval shunts. *American Journal of Roentgenology* **135**, 989.

Cumberland, D. C. (1983). Percutaneous transluminal angioplasty: a review. *Clinical Radiology* **34**, 25–38.

Dotter, C. T. and Judkins, M. P. (1964). Transluminal treatment of arteriosclerotic obstruction. Description of a new technique and a preliminary report of its application. *Circulation* **30**, 654.

Erbstein, R. A., Wholey, M. H. and Smoot, S. (1988). Subclavian artery steal syndrome: treatment by percutaneous transluminal angioplasty. *American Journal of Roentgenology* **151**, 291.

Gmelin, E., Winterhoff, R. and Rinast, E. (1989). Insufficient haemodialysis access fistulas: late results of treatment with percutaneous balloon angioplasty. *Radiology* **171**, 657.

Gould, D. A. (1990). Thermal angioplasty using a high frequency ablator. *Journal of Interventional Radiology* **5**, 147.

Grüntzig, A. R. (1981). Percutaneous transluminal coronary angioplasty. *Seminars in Roentgenology* **16**, 152.

Gupta, A. K., Ravimandalam, K., Rao, V. R. K., Joseph, S., Unni, M., Rao, A. S. and Neelkandhan, K. S. (1993). Total occlusion of iliac arteries: results of balloon angioplasty. *Cardiovascular and Interventional Radiology* **16**, 165.

Jeans, W. D., Armstrong, S. A., Cole, S. E. A., Horrocks, M. and Baird, R. N. (1990). Fate of patients undergoing a transluminal angioplasty for lower limb ischaemia. *Radiology* **177**, 559.

Joffre, F., Rousseau, H., Bernadet, P., Nomblot, C., Montoy, J. C., Chemali, R. and Knight, C. (1992). Mid term results of renal artery stenting. *Cardiovascular and Interventional Radiology* **15**, 313.

Kensey, K. R., Nash, J. E., Abrahams, C. and Zarins, C. (1987). Recanalisation of obstructed arteries with a flexible rotating tip catheter. *Radiology* **165**, 387.

Kumpe, D. A. (1981). Percutaneous dilatation of an abdominal aortic stenosis: 3 balloon technique. *Radiology* **141**, 536.

Martin, L. G., Casarella, W. J., Alspaugh, J. P. and Chuang, V. P. (1986). Renal artery angioplasty: increased technical success and decreased complications in the second 100 patients. *Radiology* **159**, 631.

Matsumoto, A. H., Barth, K. H., Selby, J. B. Jr and Tegtmeyer, C. J. (1993). Peripheral angioplasty balloon technology. *Cardiovascular and Interventional Radiology* **16**, 135.

Novelline, R. A. (1980). Percutaneous transluminal angioplasty: newer applications. *American Journal of Roentgenology* **135**, 983.

Olliff, S. P., Pain, J. A., Karani, J. B., Mowat, A. P. and Williams, R. (1991). Percutaneous transhepatic dilatation of late portal vein stenosis following orthotopic liver transplantation. *Journal of Interventional Radiology* **6**, 29.

Saddekni, S., Sniderman, K. W., Hilton, S. and Sos, T. A. (1980). Percutaneous transluminal angioplasty of non atherosclerotic lesions. *American Journal of Roentgenology* **135**, 975.

Salomonowitz, E., Antonucci, F. and Zollikofer, C. L. (1991). Pathophysiology of angioplasty. *Journal of Interventional Radiology* **6**, 57.

Tegtmeyer, C. J., Kellum, C. D. and Ayes, C. (1984). Percutaneous transluminal angioplasty of the renal artery. *Radiology* **153**, 77.

Yang, X. M., Manninen H., Naukkarinen A., Ji, H. X., Karkola K. and Soimakallio S. (1991). Laser ablation ability of the sapphire probe: an experimental comparison with different laser fibretips. *Journal of Interventional Radiology* **6**, 17.

Zeitler, E., Richter, E. I., Roth, F. J. and Schoop, W. (1983). Results of percutaneous transluminal angioplasty. *Radiology* **146, 57.**

Zollikofer, C. L., Salmonowitz, E., Sibley, R., Chain, J., Brühlmann, W. F., Castaneda-Zuniga, W. R. and Amplatz, K. (1984). Transluminal angioplasty evaluated by electron microscopy. *Radiology* **153**, 169.

Zollikofer, C. L., Cragg, A. H., Hunter, D. W., Castaneda-Zuniga, W. R. and Amplatz, K. (1988). Mechanism of transluminal angioplasty. In *Interventional Radiology*. Castaneda-Zuniga, W. R. and Tadavarthy, S. M., eds. Baltimore: Williams and Wilkins, pp. 236–265.

Endovascular ultrasound

HERO VAN URK MD
ELMA J. GUSSENHOVEN* MD
HERMAN PIETERMAN MD
AAD VAN DER LUGT* MD

*University Hospital, Rotterdam, * also The Dutch Heart Foundation and the Interuniversity Cardiology Institute, The Netherlands*

Introduction

Endovascular ultrasound is a rapidly evolving imaging technique most commonly employed in coronary and iliofemoral arteries. The technique has the potential to facilitate the study of the pathomorphology of atherosclerosis and to outline the effect of endovascular intervention in more detail than angiography.

Initially, because of the contrast between angiographic success following intervention and the clinical outcome, endovascular ultrasound was employed to examine the reasons for restenosis. It is now used in association with any endovascular technique.

Technique of endovascular ultrasound

1

The presently used intravascular ultrasound systems fall into two categories: 'electronic' and 'mechanical' systems. The catheter of the 'electronic' device contains multiple (32 or 64) small acoustic elements which are positioned cylindrically around the catheter tip. By introducing electronically switched time delays, subgroups of elements may together form an echo image. Structures close to the catheter are not imaged due to limited resolution and dynamic range of this system. The advantage of the system is that the catheter is very flexible and a central lumen is available for guidewire insertion. No distortion of the image due to inhomogeneous mechanical rotation is present.

Conversely, the single element 'mechanical' devices are either based on the rotating mirror principle or on the principle that the ultrasound element itself is rotated. Realizing a driving mechanism while keeping the catheter fully flexible and steerable as well as its miniaturization are challenging problems. Distortion of the image due to an unequal rotation of the element/mirror at the catheter tip is a limitation of these systems. Advantages of the mechanical probes are imaging of high resolution and absence of near field artifact. Both phased array and mechanical systems operate at either 20 or 30 MHz. The newest development in this area is the positioning of a micro-motor in the tip of the catheter – thus avoiding mechanical problems.

In the departments of Radiology and Vascular Surgery at the Erasmus University Hospital Rotterdam, a mechanical 30 MHz imaging system is used (Du-MED, Rotterdam, The Netherlands). The transducer, mounted on a 4.1 French catheter, rotates up to 16 images per second. The axial resolution of the system is 80 μm at a depth of 1 mm. The resulting images are displayed on a monitor via a video-scanned memory and stored on a VHS system. Sterilization of the ultrasound catheter is accomplished with ethylene oxide.

Illustration 1 shows: (*A*) Electronic multi-element device with central guidewire. 1. integrated electronic circuitry; 2. circumferential array with 64 elements; 3. central guidewire. (*B*) Single element mechanical device rotated by an external motor. 1. flexible drive shaft with coaxial cable in catheter lumen connected to proximal motor unit; 2. ultrasonically transparent dome; 3. ultrasound transducer. (*C*) Single element mechanical device is fixed and the ultrasound beam is deflected by a rotating mirror. 1. flexible drive shaft; 2. ultrasonically transparent dome; 3. ultrasound transducer; 4. mirror body. (Courtesy of N. Bom.)

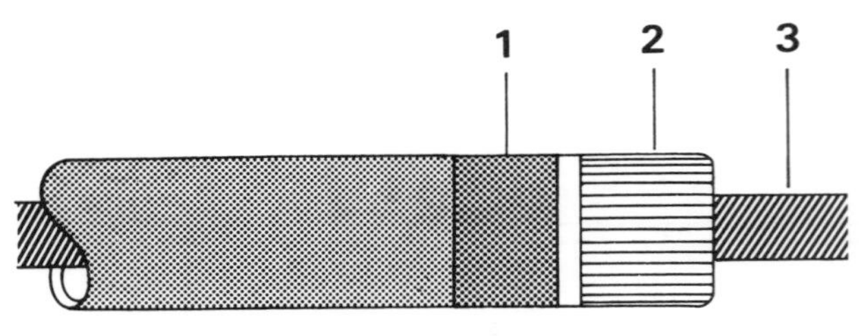

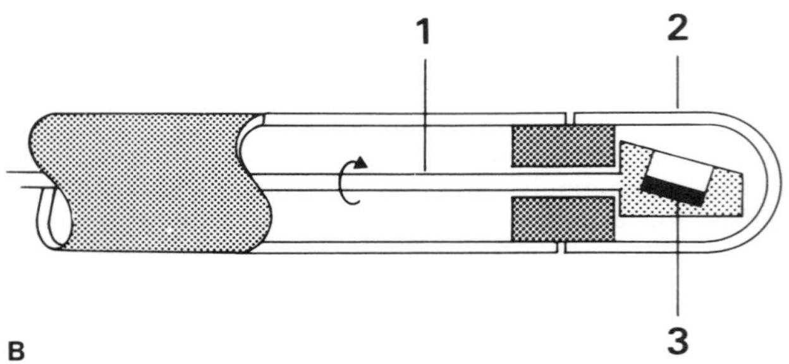

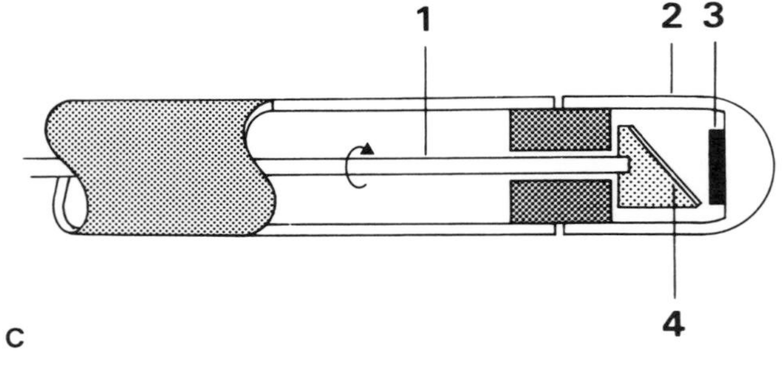

1

2
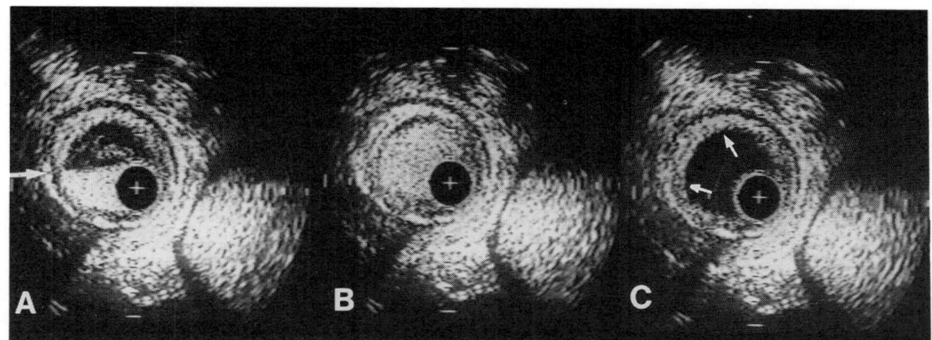

3
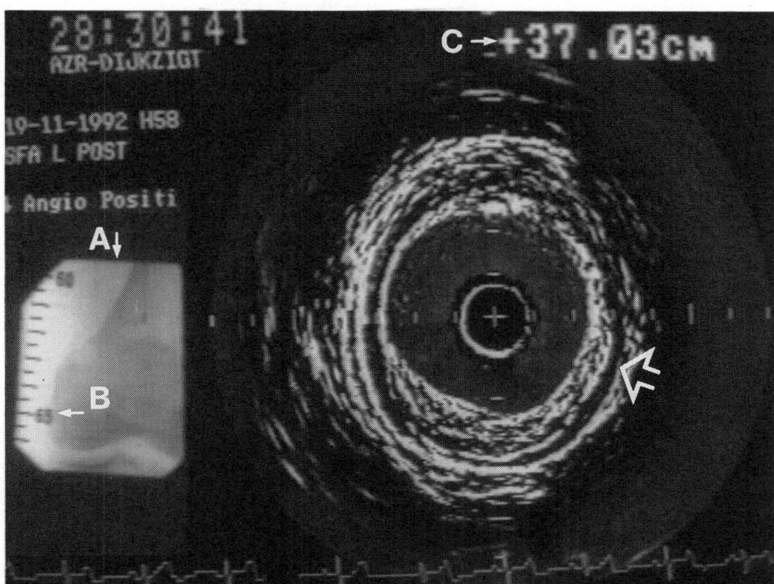

Procedure

2 & 3

The ultrasound catheter is advanced over a guidewire (monorail system) via a 7 French sheath into the common femoral artery to the level of the obstruction and, if possible, beyond the obstructive lesion. Subsequently, a series of cross-sections are recorded during pull-back of the catheter. At each level the catheter is kept in position for a period of time sufficient for recording. In order to eliminate the effects of echogenic blood, saline can be injected via the side-port of the sheath; this procedure facilitates off-line analysis of the still-frames.

The ultrasonic cross-sections in *Illustration 2* show that blood stagnation in the presence of saline enables the determination of the ventral and dorsal sites of the vessel. (*A*) A clear demarcation (arrow) is seen between blood (hyperechoic: dorsal) and saline (black: ventral). (*B*) The same vessel completely filled with blood. (*C*) The echogenic blood is replaced by saline. The arterial muscular media is typically hypoechoic. Note diffuse intimal thickening (arrows) (+ = catheter; calibration = 1 mm).

The position of the ultrasound catheter tip within the artery is documented using a radiopaque ruler (B) as reference. In addition split-screen (A) videotaping real-time cineangiography or fluoroscopy can be combined instantaneously with ultrasound imaging. Finally, a displacement sensing device (C) indicated in cm can be used providing instantaneous online orientation of the exact location where the ultrasound images were derived from within the vascular tree, with known interslice distance. The anatomy displayed by ultrasound reveals the hyperechoic media (open arrow) and a superimposed eccentric soft lesion at 6 o'clock (+ = catheter; calibration = 1 mm). Documentation of the position of the ultrasound catheter tip compared with the radiopaque ruler facilitates comparison of the ultrasound data before and after intervention, and comparison of these results with the angiographic records.

4

In order to understand the potential of intravascular ultrasound the technique was validated extensively *in vitro*. For this purpose vascular specimens obtained at autopsy were used. *Muscular arteries* are recognized by three contiguous layers encircling the lumen: the hypoechoic media seen between the inner echodense layer (intima and internal elastic lamina) and outer echodense layer (external elastic lamina and adventitia). Examples of muscular arteries are coronary, ilio-femoral, popliteal, renal and mesenteric arteries. The arterial wall of *elastic arteries* is recognized by a homogeneous bright echostructure (aorta, carotid artery). Similarly, veins are echographically recognized by a homogeneous vessel wall, while ePTFE (Gore-tex®) prosthesis is seen as a thin but highly reflective echo structure. Prior to the endovascular intervention, intravascular ultrasound distinguishes hypo-echoic with little lipid (top left), soft echo showing thrombus (bottom left), bright echo with excess fibrous tissue (middle top), and bright echo with shadowing representing calcium (bottom middle). The sensitivity and specificity for a lesion are high, whether it is concentric or eccentric, hard or soft, but the sensitivity for lipid is low partly due to calcification of lipid deposits. Following (middle panel) balloon angioplasty dissection, plaque rupture and internal elastic lamina rupture (top right and bottom right) can occur.

Illustration 4 shows that by using a displacement sensing device the positions 4.1 and 5.1 cm could reproducibly be documented. Prior to intervention ultrasound evidenced a lesion that was soft partly hard (4.1 cm) and probably containing lipid deposits (5.1 cm). Following balloon dilatation using a 5 mm balloon the presence of a dissection (arrows) seen on ultrasound was validated with the corresponding histologic cross-sections (+ = catheter; calibration = 1 mm).

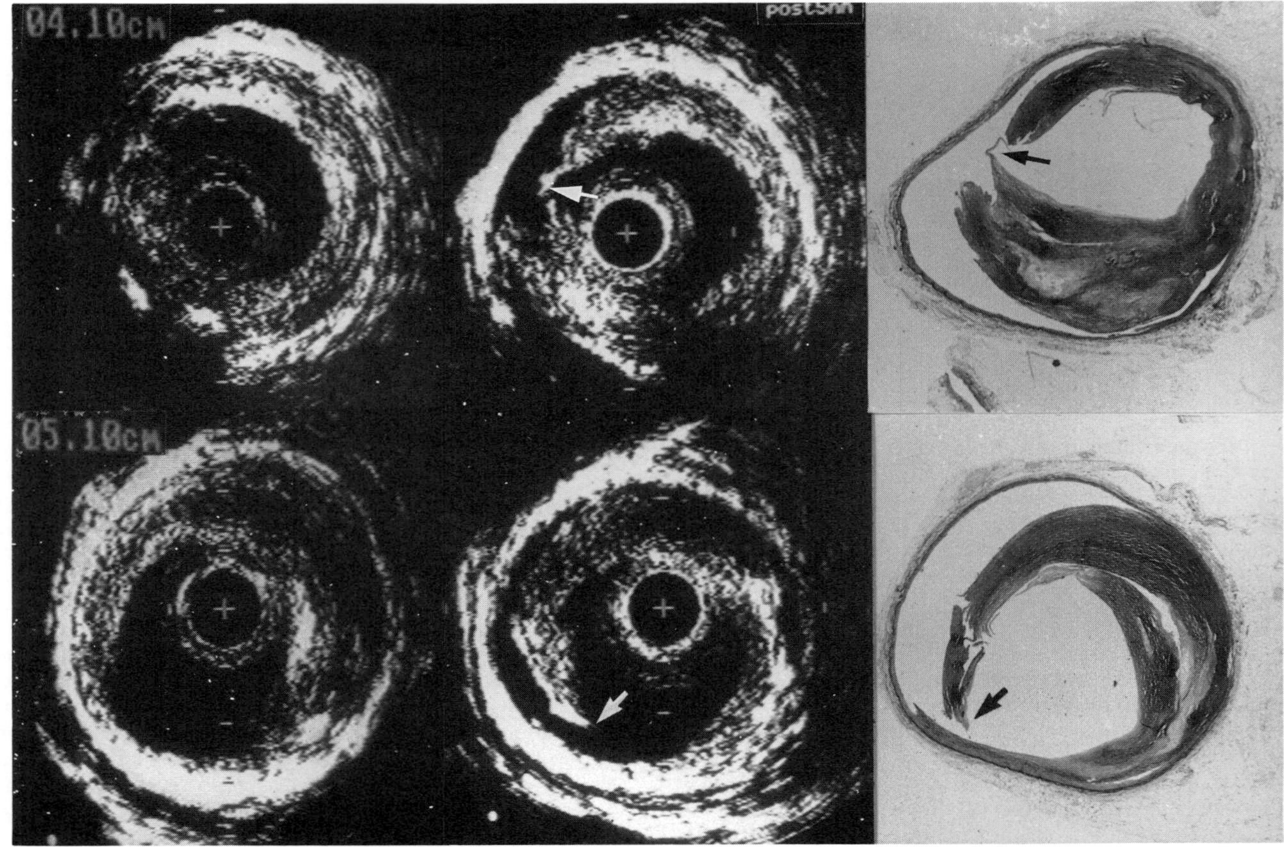

4

Quantitative analysis

5

In order to understand the ultimate effect of an intervention, corresponding ultrasound images prior to and following intervention can be analysed with a digital video analyser. Each image reproduced on the analyser videoscreen can be contour traced. To facilitate the quantitative analysis, real-time images can be replayed on a separate video monitor. The following parameters can be analysed:
Free lumen area (mm^2) defined as the area encompassed by the inner boundary of the intimal surface (characterized also by the presence of blood flow).
Media-bounded area (mm^2) defined as the native vessel area bounded by the hypoechoic medial layer.
Lesion area (mm^2) calculated as the difference between media-bounded area and free lumen area.

Illustration 5 shows intravascular ultrasound cross-sections of the superficial femoral artery obtained before and after intervention traced for free luminal and media-bounded contours. The region enclosed by the two contours represents the eccentric lesion. The hypoechoic media is used as landmark for the media-bounded area. Qualitatively as result of the intervention a plaque rupture and dissection is seen. Quantitatively the free lumen area and media bounded area increased. The lesion area slightly decreased (+ = catheter; calibration = 1 mm).

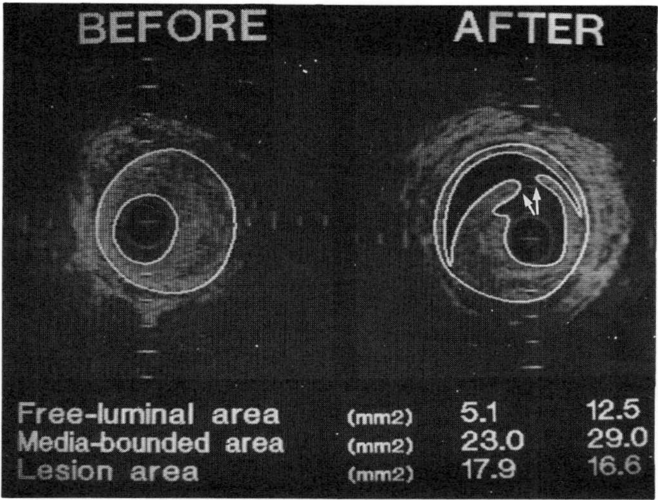

5

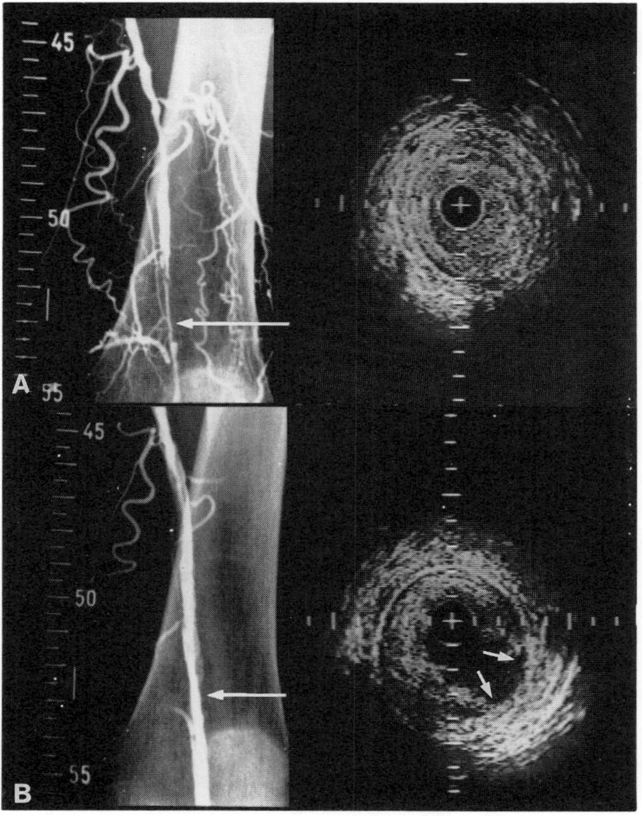

6

Endovascular ultrasound and balloon angioplasty

6

The application of ultrasound *in vivo* reveals new insights into the vessel structure before and after intervention. Intravascular ultrasound shows atherosclerotic lesions in regions in which angiography reveals an apparently normal vascular tree and the percentage obstruction caused by a stenotic lesion measured by intravascular ultrasound is higher than measured by angiography. After intervention more extensive effects are seen with ultrasound than with angiography and by comparing corresponding ultrasound cross-sections before and after balloon angioplasty, it is found that luminal enlargement is achieved primarily by overstretching the arterial wall whilst the lesion volume remains practically unchanged. Overstretching is accompanied almost always by dissection, plaque rupture and rupture of the internal elastic lamina and embolization of the lesion can occur in a small minority probably related to the presence of thrombus.

Illustration 6 shows angiograms and intravascular ultrasound cross-sections obtained before and immediately after balloon angioplasty. (A) Before intervention a more than 90% stenosis was evidenced at level 53. Intravascular ultrasound at this level revealed a soft lesion concentric in nature. The residual lumen is encompassed by the ultrasound catheter. (B) Intervention angiography revealed a less than 50% diameter stenosis whereas quantitative analysis of the intravascular ultrasound cross-section revealed a 64% area stenosis. Plaque rupture and media rupture were seen at 4 o'clock (arrows) (+ = catheter; calibration = 1 mm).

Endovascular ultrasound during bypass surgery

7 & 8

The evaluation of venous bypass anastomoses includes identification of proximal and distal anastomotic site, anatomy of valves inside the vein, presence or absence of intimal hyperplasia and diameter of the vein bypass. Based on these data one may obtain full insight of the anatomy involved and perhaps about the mechanisms of early and late restenosis. *Illustration 7* shows intravascular ultrasound cross-section obtained during a venous bypass procedure showing thickening of the intimal layer (arrows) (+ = catheter; calibration = 1 mm).

Illustration 8 shows angiogram after intervention revealing a patent bypass graft anastomosis. Intravascular ultrasound images (A–C) correspond to positions indicated on the angiogram. (A) The vein is recognized as a homogeneous vessel

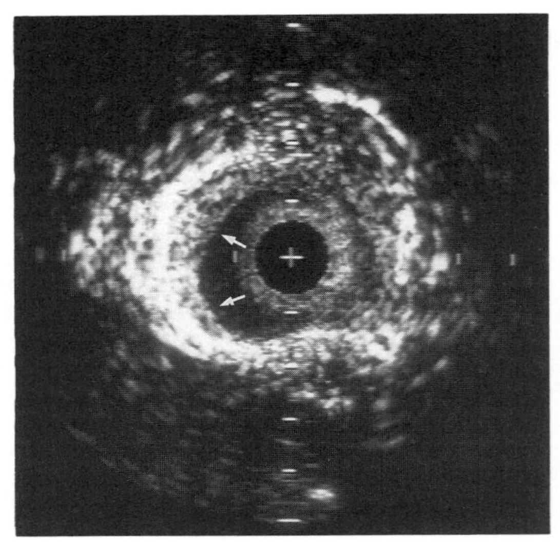

7

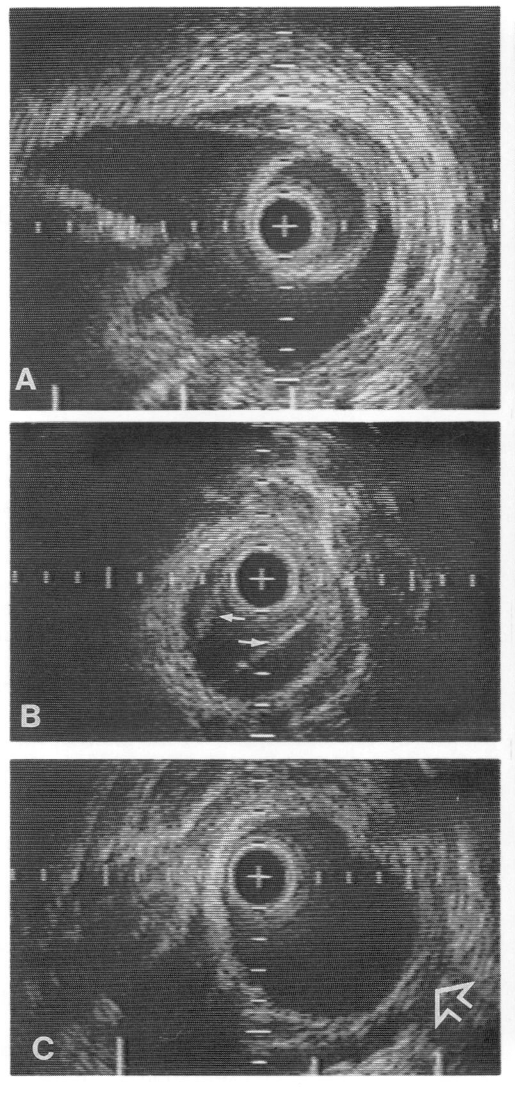

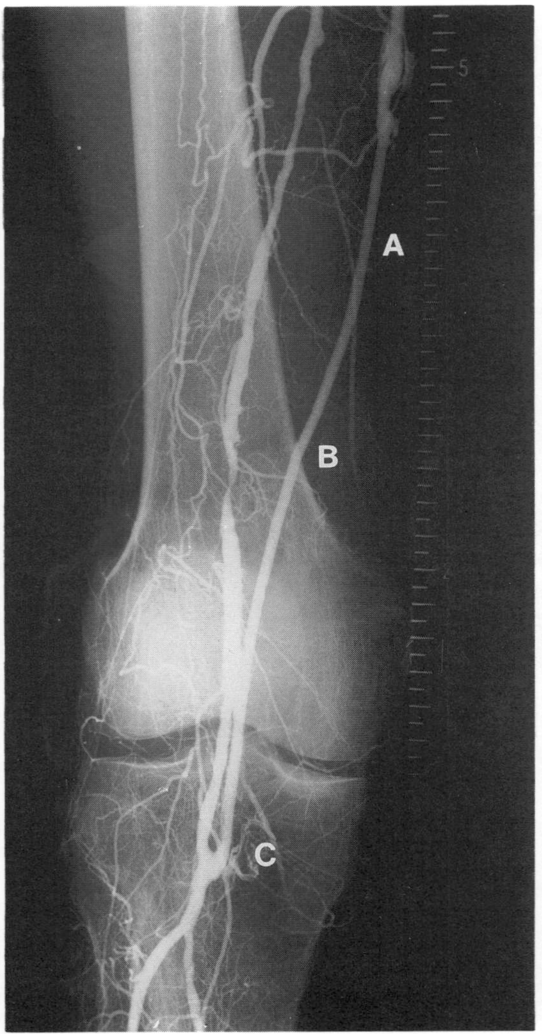

8

wall amidst oedema as result of the intervention. (B) Patent valves of the vein (arrows) are visualized as straight echogenic lines. (C) The anastomosis is seen to be patent. Note that at this junction the muscular nature of the popliteal artery is characterized by a hypoechoic media (open arrow) (+ = catheter; calibration = 1 mm).

9

The *in situ* venous bypass technique can be monitored with endovascular ultrasound: persisting competent valves after valve-cutting procedures can easily be identified. The effect of a repeated passage of the valvulotome can then be confirmed. *Illustration 9* shows intravascular ultrasound cross-sections showing the characteristics of a vein together with valves before (A) and after (B) repeat valve-cutting procedure (arrow) (+ = catheter; calibration = 1 mm).

10

Synthetic grafts (ePTFE) produce a typical echo pattern of a thin single layer of hard echoes, which can be easily discriminated from the three-layered pattern of the proximal and distal arterial parts of the anastomoses after completion of the bypass. *Illustration 10* shows intravascular ultrasound cross-section obtained at the site of anastomosis following synthetic graft (ePTFE) procedure for relief of superficial femoral artery obstruction. The synthetic graft presents as a typical hyperechoic structure (arrow). The femoral artery is recognized by the hypoechoic media (open arrow). Note the echogenicity of blood (+ = catheter; calibration = 1 mm).

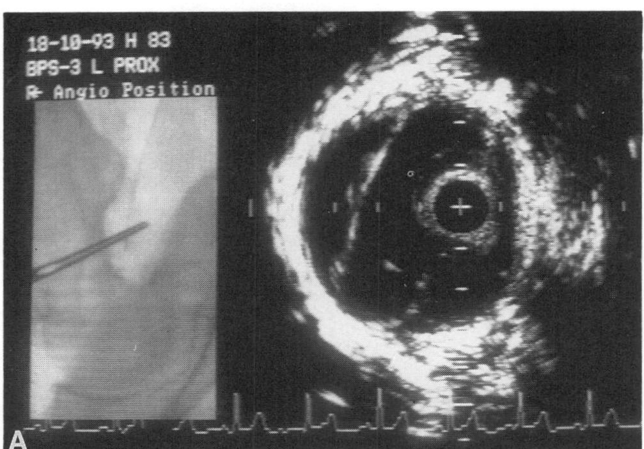

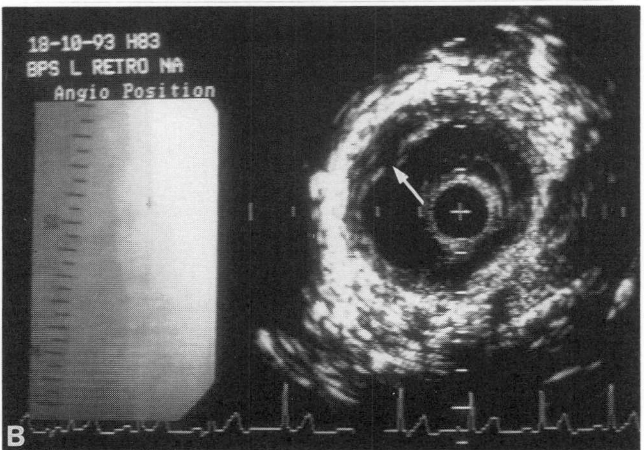

9

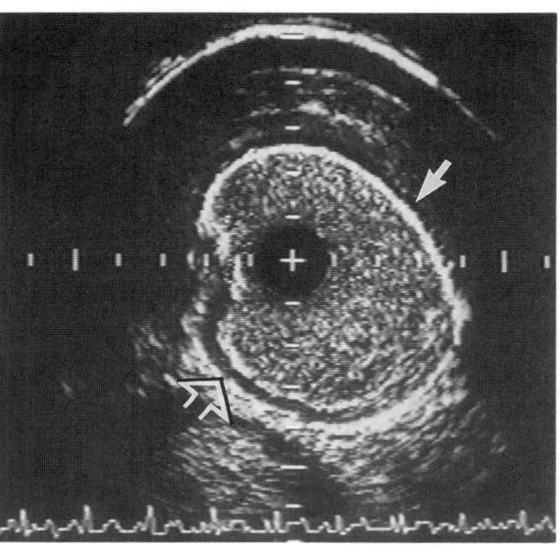

10

References

Gerritsen, G. P., Gussenhoven, E. J., The SHK, Pieterman, H., van de Lugt, A., Li, W., Bom, N., van Dijk, L. C., Du Bois, N. A. J. J. and van Urk, H. (1993). Intravascular ultrasound before and after intervention: *in vivo* comparison with angiography. *Journal of Vascular Surgery* **18**, 31.

Gussenhoven, E. J., Essed, C. E., Frietman, P., Van Egmond, F., Lancée, C. T., van Kappellen, W. H., Roelandt, J., Serruys, P. W., Gerritsen, G. P., van Urk, H. and Bom, N. (1989a). Intravascular ultrasonic imaging: histologic and echographic correlations. *European Journal of Vascular Surgery* **3**, 571.

Gussenhoven, E. J., Essed, C. E., Lancée, C. T., Mastik, F., Frietman, P., Van Egmond, F. C., Reiber, J., Bosch, H., van Urk, H., Roelandt, J. and Bom N. (1989b). Arterial wall characteristics determined by intravascular ultrasound imaging: an in vitro study. *Journal of the American College of Cardiology* **14**, 947.

Gussenhoven, E. J., van der Lugt, A., The SHK, de Feyter, P., Serruys, P. W., van Suylen, R. J., Lancée, C. T., van Urk, H. and Pieterman, H. (1993). Similarities and differences between coronary and iliofemoral arteries related to intravascular ultrasound. In *Intravascular Ultrasound*, Roelandt, J. R. T. C., Gussenhoven, E. J. and Bom, N., eds. London: Kluwer/Academic Press, pp. 45–62.

The SHK, Gussenhoven, E. J., du Bois, N. A. J. J., Pieterman, H., Roelandt, J. R. T. C., Wilson, R. A. and van Urk, H. (1991). Femoro-popliteal bypass grafts studied by intravascular ultrasound. *European Journal of Vascular Surgery* **5**, 523.

The SHK, Gussenhoven, E. J., Zhong, Y., Li, W., van Egmond, F., Pieterman, H., van Urk, H., Gerritsen, G. P., Borst, C., Wilson, R. A. and Bom, N. (1992). The effect of balloon angioplasty on the femoral artery evaluated with intravascular ultrasound imaging. *Circulation* **86**, 483.

van Urk, H., Gussenhoven, W. J., Gerritsen, G. P., Pieterman, H., The SHK, van Egmond, F., Lancée, C. T. and Bom, N. (1991). Assessment of arterial disease and arterial reconstructions by intravascular ultrasound. *International Journal of Cardiac Imaging* **6**, 157.

Uses of balloon expandable stents in combination with PTFE

JULIO C. PALMAZ MD

Professor and Chief of Cardiovascular and Special Interventions, The University of Texas Health Science Center at San Antonio, Texas, USA

Introduction

The effectiveness and safety of stents for recanalization of stenotic or completely occluded blood vessels has been demonstrated in clinical trials in the USA and Europe (Palmaz *et al.*, 1992; Richter *et al.*, 1993). Stents have been particularly useful in focal lesions of the coronary arteries (Serruys *et al.*, 1993). Iliac arteries and aortic bifurcation (Palmaz *et al.*, 1991), superior vena cava syndrome (Carrasco *et al.*, 1992), and for the creation of transjugular intrahepatic portocaval stent shunts (Conn, 1993). Their role in the treatment of localized disease of ostial renal artery stenosis, superficial femoral artery, intrathoracic aortic arch branches and SVC tributaries is still under study.

The use of stents in combination with polytetrafluoroethylene (PTFE) offers the possibility of treating focal vascular lesions other than stenosis or occlusions in patients who cannot otherwise undergo surgical repair for any reason. This is feasible in aneurysms, pseudoaneurysms and arteriovenous fistulas by excluding the abnormal vascular lumen with PTFE coaxially placed over stents as illustrated below.

1

Balloon inflation expands stent and PTFE material simultaneously occluding the lumen of the arteriovenous fistula. It is understood that many of the materials needed to perform these procedures have not been designed for endovascular application and are not yet approved for clinical use as depicted here. However, because of their potential life-saving nature, it may be useful to review these techniques in some detail in case the need arises to use them in a critical situation.

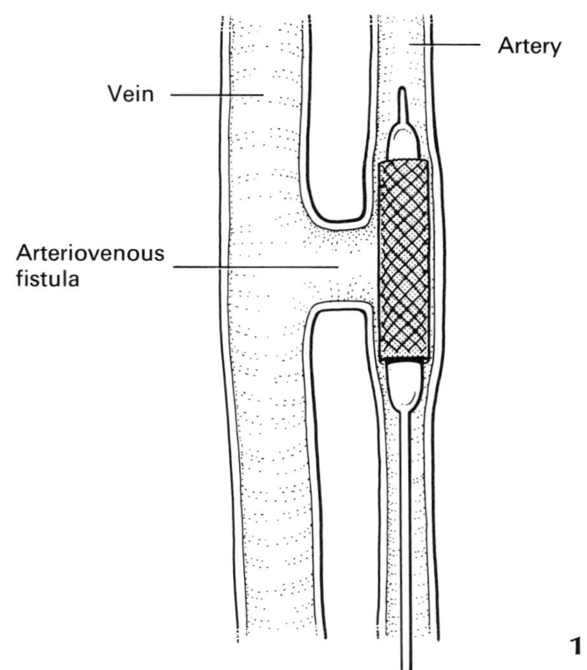

1

Materials and method

Because of its plastic characteristics and the lack of a reinforcing layer Impragraft PTFE is radially expansile if a coaxial balloon is inflated within its lumen. This material may radially elongate with little elastic recoil several times its original diameter before rupture. This typically occurs after stretching 600–700% (McClurken, McHaney and Colone, 1986). The experience provided by bench and animal testing and the limited clinical endovascular use of this material suggests that radial expansion within 350–450% of the original diameter may be adequate for practical use because the physical and mechanical characteristics of the material are not profoundly altered in this range. This ideal expansion ratio must be kept in mind during the selection of the diameter of the bypass material for a given target lesion.

2

We mount Impragraft (TW) on balloon expandable stents (Johnson and Johnson Interventional Systems) by placing the graft material coaxially over the stent and cutting it with a scalpel blade to match the length of the stent. We select the stent type trying to match its expansion range to that of the graft. Grafts of 3 mm expand to 7–8 mm, use a medium 2.5 stent in a 106 g sheath. Grafts of 3.5 and 4 mm use a larger stent and sheath size. The graft is affixed to the stent with 6-0 polypropylene suture with non-cutting needle. The sutures are placed on each quadrant of the stent circumference, 5 mm from the ends as depicted.

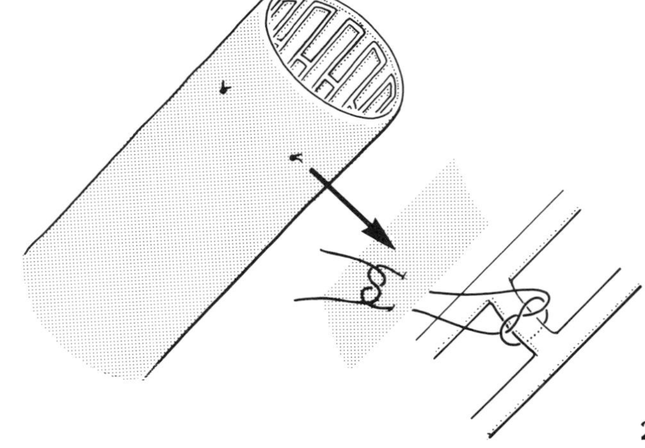

2

3

The choice of the balloon catheter is critical for two reasons: a) the need to maintain the lowest possible profile to allow the smallest introducer sheath diameter; b) the length of the balloon in relationship to the length of the stent-graft assembly. If the balloon is longer than the stent-graft the balloon will adopt a dumb-bell configuration at the beginning of the inflation causing retraction of the graft material and possible tear of the PTFE material at the site of the sutures. These tears may result in longitudinal splitting of the material at higher inflation pressures. If the balloon length is matched with the stent-graft the expansion begins at the centre of the assembly preventing suture disruption. In selecting the appropriate balloon length it is important to remember that the nominal balloon length reflects the length of the cylindrical portion of the balloon and disregards the tapered portions at the ends. This indicates that for a 3 cm stent-graft the ideal balloon length should be 2 cm and have short tapered ends. For a stent-graft assembly composed of two 3 cm stents in tandem with a single piece of coaxially mounted graft the balloon should be 4 cm long. After complete expansion, the stent-graft may have tapered ends, requiring repositioning of the balloon and reexpansion of both ends to attain a cylindrical configuration as illustrated.

Illustration 3a shows an excessively long balloon with dumb-bell expansion causing retraction of the graft over the stent with damage at the suture sites. *Illustration 3b* shows that a shorter balloon expands the stent-graft from the centre out. This produces tapered ends. *Illustration 3c* shows that balloon repositioning and inflation expands the tapered end.

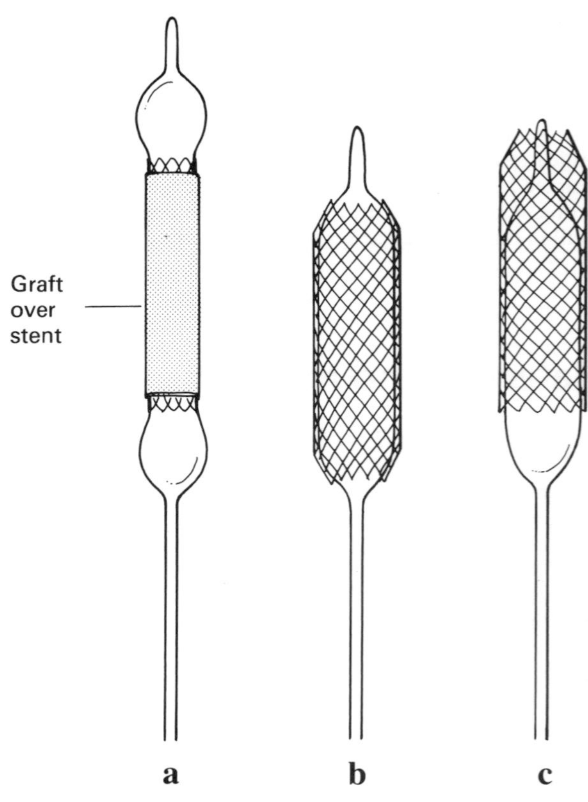

3

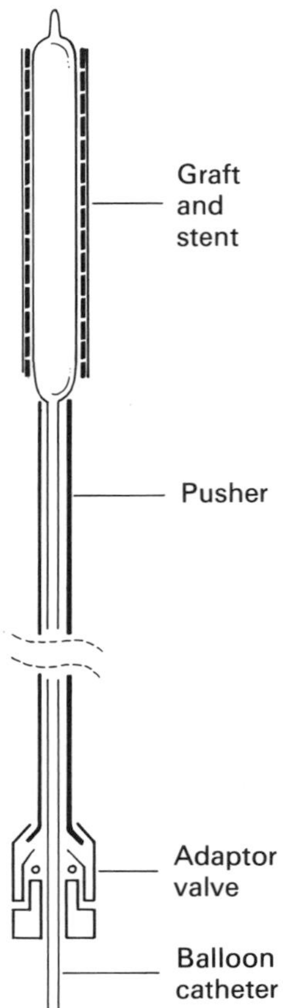

4

4

To stabilize the stent-graft on the balloon during withdrawal of the sheath a 'pusher' catheter can be coaxially mounted over the shaft of the balloon angioplasty catheter. This provides an edge on the back of the balloon that prevents backward displacement. For balloon catheters with 5 French shafts a pusher can be fashioned out of an 8 French Van Andel catheter with the tapered tip cut off. Balloon catheters with a 6 French shaft accept 9 French Van Andel catheters.

5

Stent-graft combinations larger than 15 mm in diameter require pre-expansion of the PTFE because larger balloons generate lower pressures. This determines a smaller margin of safety between the pressure needed to expand the stent-graft and the burst limit of the balloon. The pre-expanded graft must be folded around the stent and balloon catheter like an umbrella and loaded inside a delivery sheath with a haemostatic valve, as illustrated. The assembly may be sterilized with ethylene oxide before use.

A large balloon angioplasty catheter is used to pre-expand PTFE (*left*). The resulting material is sutured to a bridge approximately in the middle of a stent. Therefore, half of the stent is not covered by PTFE (*centre*). The redundant PTFE is folded with two longitudinal folds running along the catheter shaft, inside a sheath with a haemostatic valve (*right*).

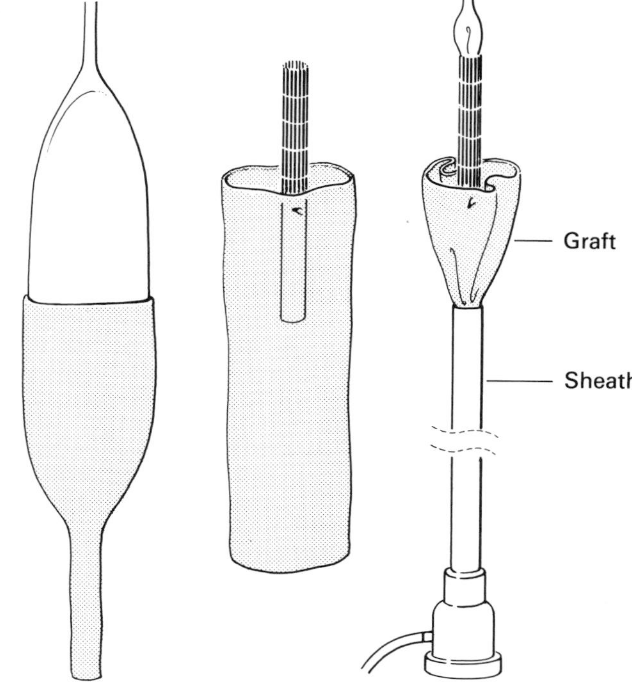

5

6

Unlike stent-graft combinations of 15 mm in diameter or smaller, the large counterparts are delivered to the target site pre-loaded. This means that the sheath is introduced into the vessel with the balloon and the stent-graft inside its lumen. After reaching the desired position, the sheath is withdrawn and the balloon is inflated to deploy the stent. Because using graft material of larger diameter usually involves using greater lengths only part of the graft is supported by stent. The graft ends are applied against the arterial wall by the expanded stent which functions as a friction seal. Only one stent is affixed to the PTFE material prior to placement. A distal stent may be placed immediately after the stent graft is deployed.

A large stent-graft is expanded with partial withdrawal of the delivery sheath (*left*). Complete withdrawal of the sheath allows the PTFE conduit to expand (*centre*). Introduction of a second stent through the sheath is positioned and expanded at the distal end (*right*).

Balloon angioplasty catheters 15–30 mm in diameter are not available for arterial use. In exceptional situations, valvuloplasty and prostatic dilation balloons could be used for these purposes. These balloons should have shafts no larger than 7 French to fit the suggested sheaths and overall lengths of 100 cm.

Intrarterial placement of the large vascular access sheaths, size 12 French and larger, requires direct exposure of the vessel. Occasionally, 12 French sheaths may be introduced percutaneously in patients with large, non-tortuous vessels because these procedures may be done, in general, with small doses of heparin. Introduction of 12 and 14 French sheaths into surgically exposed common femoral arteries should begin with a needle puncture followed by over-the-wire exchange. This technique preserves blood flow around the sheath in contrast with the use of arteriotomy and vessel loops. For sheath sizes 16 French and larger, arteriotomy and vessel loops may be used without disadvantage since these diameter sheaths usually interrupt blood flow.

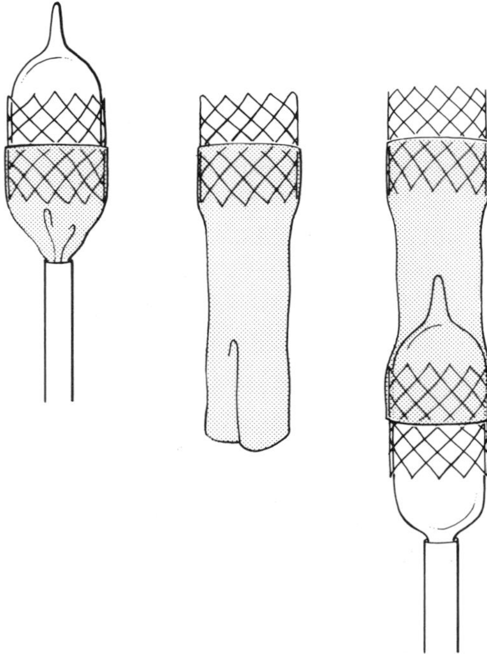

6

Patient examples

7a, b, c & d

A 38-year-old White male was admitted with seminoma metastatic to the retroperitoneum. Following a course of chemotherapy the patient suddenly developed a large, pulsatile, abdominal mass and hypotension. Mid abdominal computed tomographic (CT) scan (*a*) following intravenous bolus of contrast shows rapid enhancement of the mass, suggesting the presence of aortic pseudoaneurysm. Pelvic CT sections demonstrated the presence of haemorrhage at this level. Flush abdominal aortogram (*b*) shows rapid opacification of the mass during the early phase of the injection consistent with a large fistula between the anterolateral aspect of the aorta and the pseudoaneurysm. Because of the emergent situation and the poor operative risk, endovascular treatment was considered for the obliteration of the pseudoaneurysm. Abdominal aortogram following placement of a balloon expandable stent below the renal arteries (*c*). The stent is attached to a 10 cm segment of 6 mm Impragraft which has been previously dilated to 18 mm. The bulge on the lateral aspect of the aorta (arrows) demonstrates the extent of the aortic defect. The distal end of the graft is not affixed by a stent but rather by the windsock effect of the aortic flow. Notice that the significant loss of volume of the pseudoaneurysm following internal bypass is reflected in decreased displacement of the aorta. Follow-up aortogram 6 months later (*d*), shows patency of the bypass. The numbers on the top and bottom of the figure represent mean aortic pressure. The presence of surgical clips around the abdominal aorta correspond to interval exploratory surgery to resect the necrotic tumour. The exploration was negative for remaining neoplastic tissue.

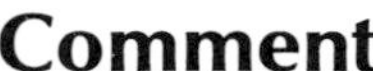

Comment

The rapid onset of the pulsatile abdominal mass was attributed to rapid tumour necrosis following chemotherapy and rupture of the involved abdominal aortic wall. The extravasation was not contained within the pseudoaneurysm as demonstrated by the presence of free blood in the pelvis. This desperate clinical situation was adequately solved by transluminal aortic bypass. The patient recuperated rapidly and was discharged on the fifth postoperative day.

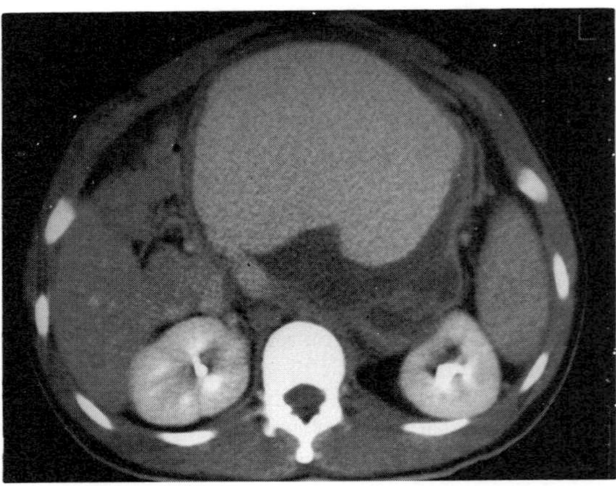

7a

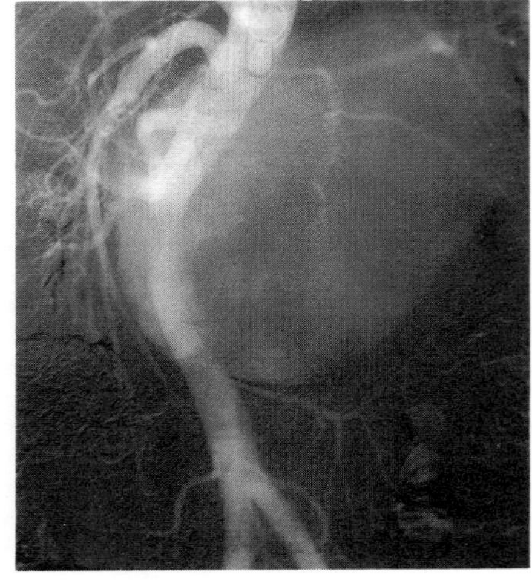

7b

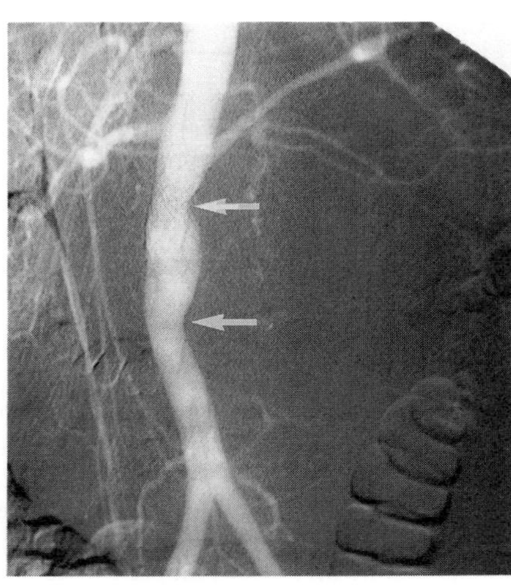

7c

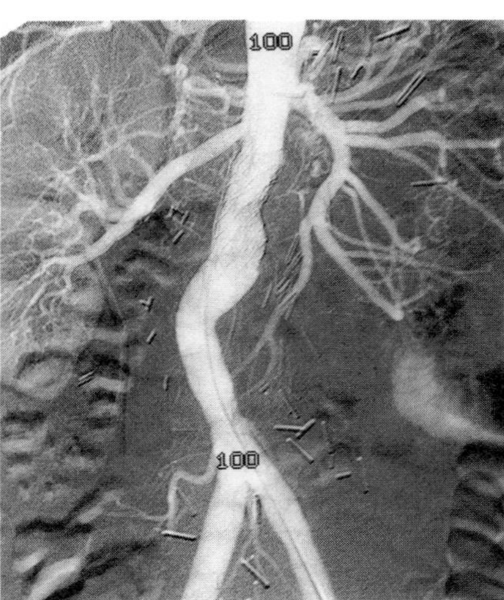

7d

8a, b, c & d

The patient was a 34-year-old White male with previous history of i.v. drug abuse who had suffered a stab wound to the back with resulting right renal artery to inferior vena cava fistula. A previous attempt at surgical repair was unsuccessful. He experienced high output cardiac failure and aortic valvular insufficiency from subacute bacterial endocarditis. Flush abdominal aortogram (*a*) showed an arteriovenous fistula between an enlarged right renal artery and the inferior vena cava through an intervening pseudaneurysm. Selective placement of a 10 French vascular sheath in the right renal artery was performed via percutaneous right femoral approach (*b*). The balloon markers (arrows) indicate the limits of the stent (P-294, Johnson and Johnson Interventional Systems, Warren, NJ). A piece of 3 mm Impragraft TW is sutured to the stent. Following withdrawal of the sheath proximal to the arteriovenous malformation (AVM), contrast injection confirms adequate positioning of the stent-graft assembly (*c*). Following balloon inflation and deployment of the assembly, control arteriogram (*d*) demonstrates patency of the renal artery and exclusion of the AVM.

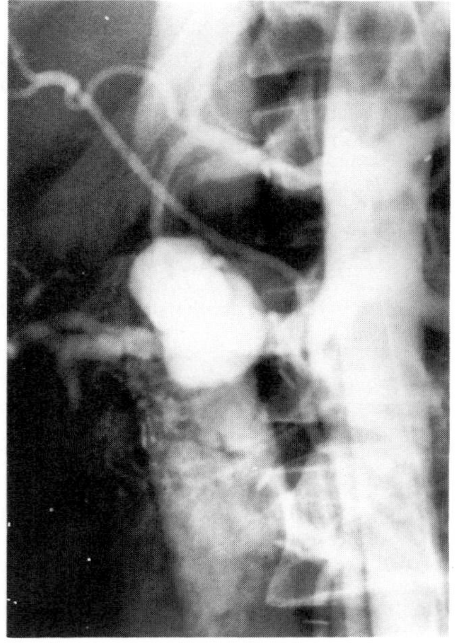

8a

Comment

Given the clinical situation, this form of therapy was deemed as the only alternative for this patient. Unlike embolic techniques, the use of a covered stent maintained patency of the renal artery while excluding the pseudoaneurysm and fistulous communication with the inferior vena cava (IVC). The enlargement of the renal artery due to the high output fistula was fortuitous in regard to the use of intrarenal catheterization with a 10 French sheath which is normally too large for this vessel. Likewise, this patient's lack of peripheral vascular disease facilitated percutaneous placement of this sheath transfemorally. Following transluminal bypass, the patient's symptoms of cardiac failure were greatly improved. The patient was discharged and later lost to follow-up.

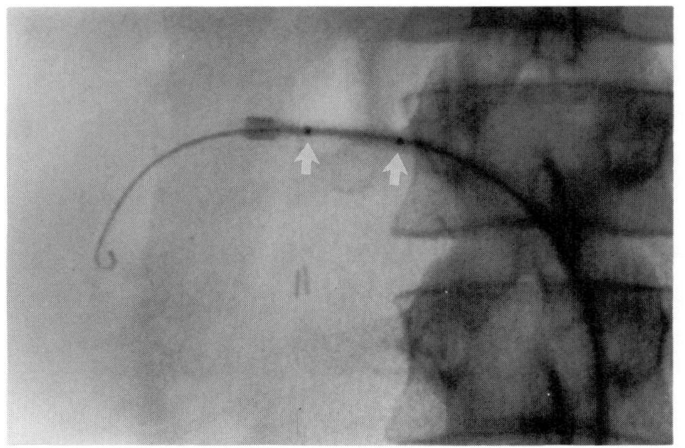

8b

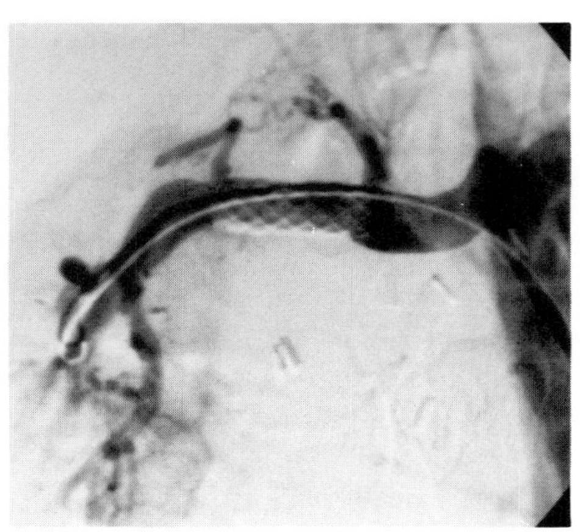

8d

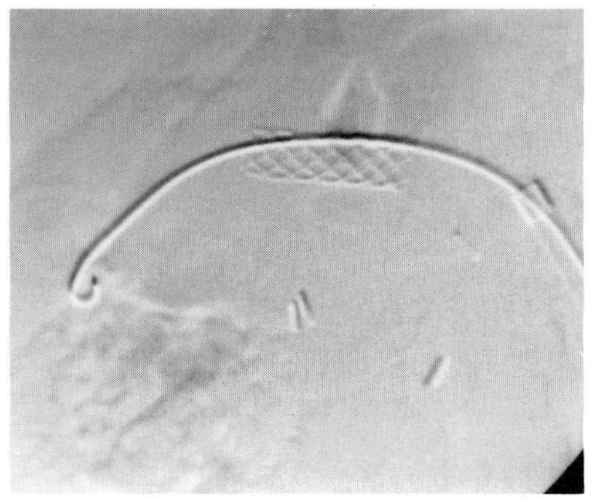

8c

References

Carrasco, C. H., Charsangave, J. C., Wright, K. C., Wallace, S. and Gianturco, C. (1992). Use of the Gianturco self-expanding stent in stenoses of the superior and inferior venae cavae. *Journal of Vascular and International Radiology* **3**, 409.

Conn, H. O. (1993). Transjugular intrahepatic portal-systemic shunts: The state of the art. *Hepatology* **17**, 148.

McClurken, M. E., McHaney, J. M. and Colone, W. M. (1986). Physical properties and test methods for expanded polytetrafluorethylene (PTFE) grafts. ASTM. Special Technical Publication **898**, 82.

Palmaz, J. C., Encarnacion, C. E., Garcia, O. J. *et al.* (1991). Aortic bifurcation stenosis: treatment with intravascular stents. *Journal of Vascular and International Radiology* **2**, 319.

Palmaz, J. C., Laborde, J. C., Rivera, F. J., Encarnacion, C. E., Lutz, J. D. and Moss, J. G. (1992). Stenting of the iliac arteries with the Palmaz stent: Experience from a multicenter trial. *Cardiovascular Interventional Radiology* **15**, 291.

Richter, G. M., Roeren, T., Brado, M. and Noeldge, G. (1993). Further update of the randomized trial: iliac stent placement versus PTA. Morphology clinical success rates and failure analysis. 18th annual meeting of the SCVIR. New Orleans, LA, March 1993.

Serruys, P. W., Macaya, C., de Jaegere P. *et al.* (1993). Interim analysis of the Benestent Trial (abstract). *Circulation* **88**, 1.

Techniques of ultrasound guided angioplasty

BRUCE J. BRENER MD

Director of Vascular Surgery, Newark Beth Israel Medical Center, Newark, New Jersey, USA

Introduction

It is generally agreed that short segmental stenoses of the iliac and superficial femoral arteries are amenable to percutaneous balloon angioplasty. While angioplasty of iliac lesions is associated with excellent long-term patency, this procedure is less successful with superficial femoral artery disease. The procedure is commonly performed in angiographic suites by radiologists using radiographic imaging and contrast agents. Ultrasound guided angioplasty is a technique established in 1990 to reduce the adverse effects of radiation and contrast agents. It allows angioplasty to be performed using a duplex scanner to guide and position the balloon. The scanner provides on-line real-time physiological information verifying the efficacy of the angioplasty procedure before the patient leaves the treatment facility.

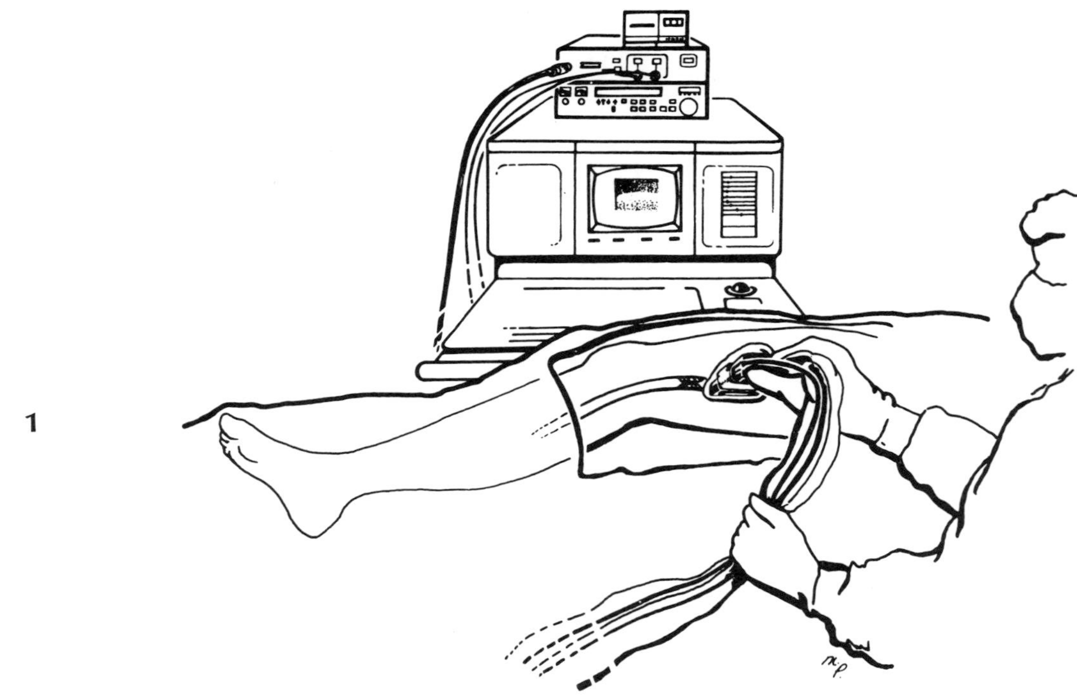
1

1

The patient is evaluated by taking a careful history and performing a thorough examination which includes non-invasive studies. If the patient is considered a candidate for angioplasty, an ultrasound examination with B-mode images and velocity determinations is performed. The location, nature, and length of the stenotic or occluding lesion is identified. If the lesion is found suitable for angioplasty a confirmatory angiogram is obtained – a step that may be eliminated in the future.

The patient is then admitted to an operating room, angiogram suite, or vascular laboratory. The limb is prepared in a sterile manner and draped. The ultrasound probe, covered by a sterile plastic bag, is used to re-identify the location of the lesion.

2

The principles and technique of angioplasty are identical to the usual type of procedure. The main differences are first, the method of guiding the catheter, and second, the real-time monitoring with physiological parameters, rather than morphological imaging.

Iliac lesions are approached through a retrograde puncture of the femoral artery. If the superficial femoral artery is diseased, an antegrade puncture is made in the affected limb below the inguinal ligament but above the bifurcation. The position of the puncture can be guided by ultrasound imaging as well. A guidewire is advanced down the superficial femoral artery.

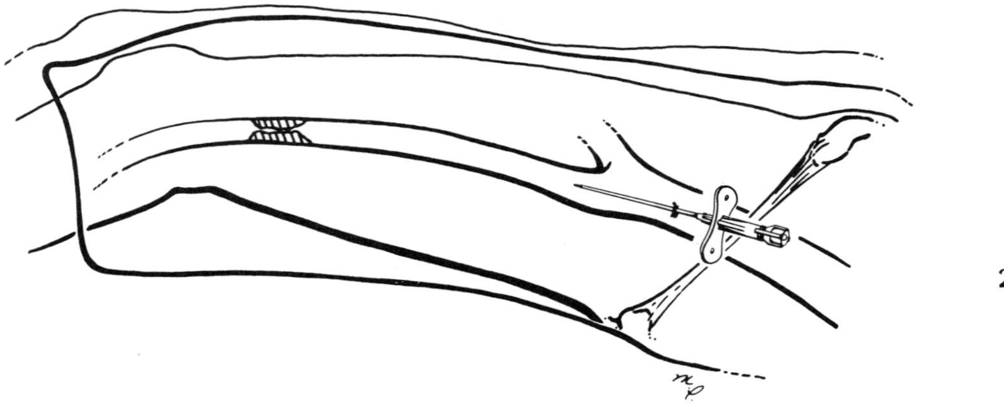
2

3

At times the guidewire will preferentially glide down the deep femoral artery; the sterile ultrasound probe can help localize the direction of the superficial femoral. A guidewire with an isodiametric sensor at its tip has recently been developed which will simplify the directing of that wire.

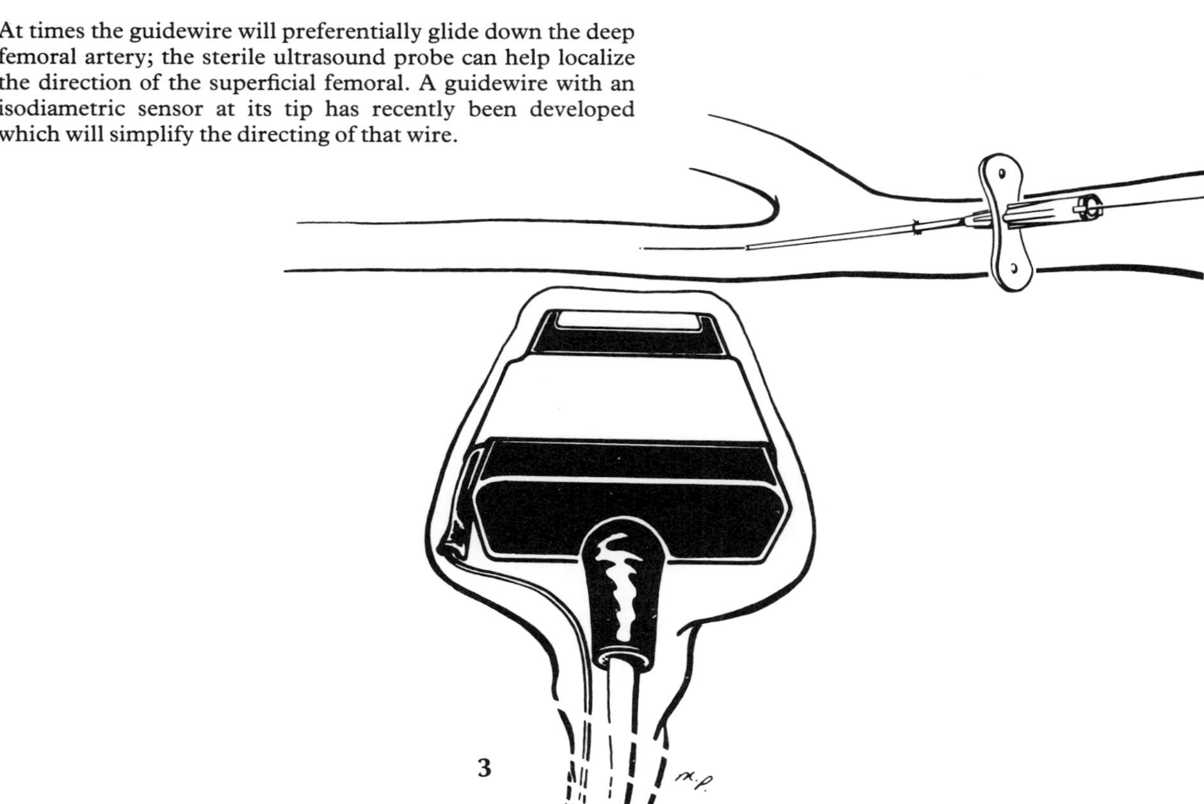

3

4

Once the wire is situated in the superficial femoral artery a haemostatic sheath and introducer are placed in the vessel. The introducer is removed, leaving the sheath in the superficial femoral artery.

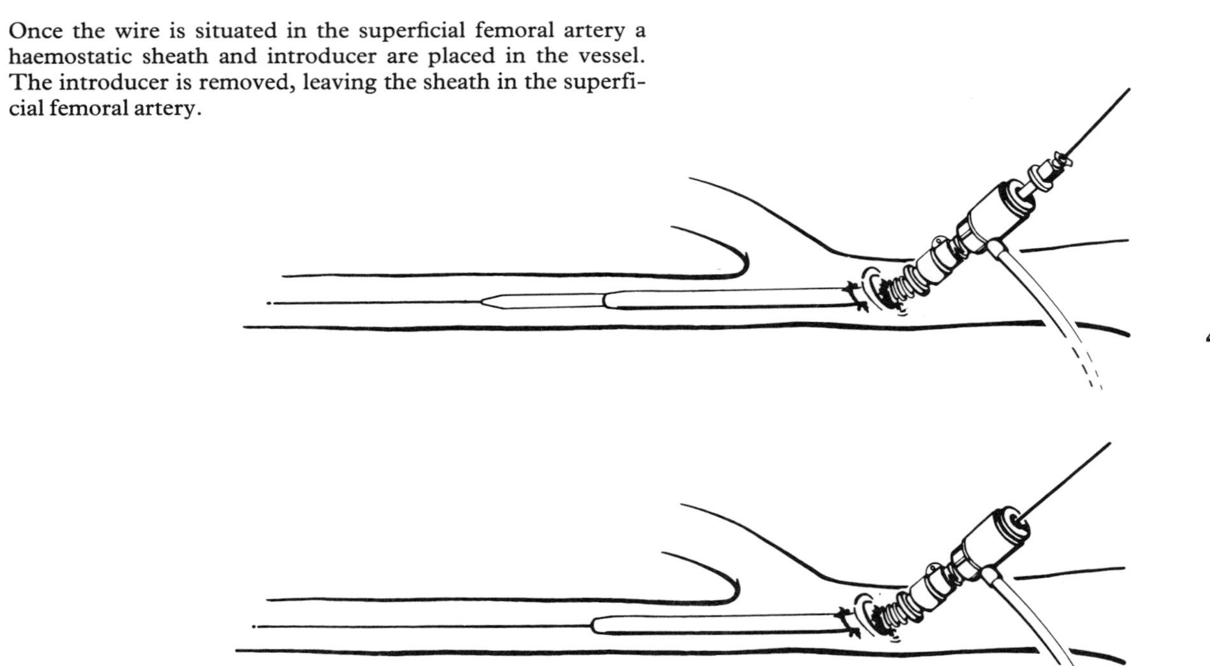

4

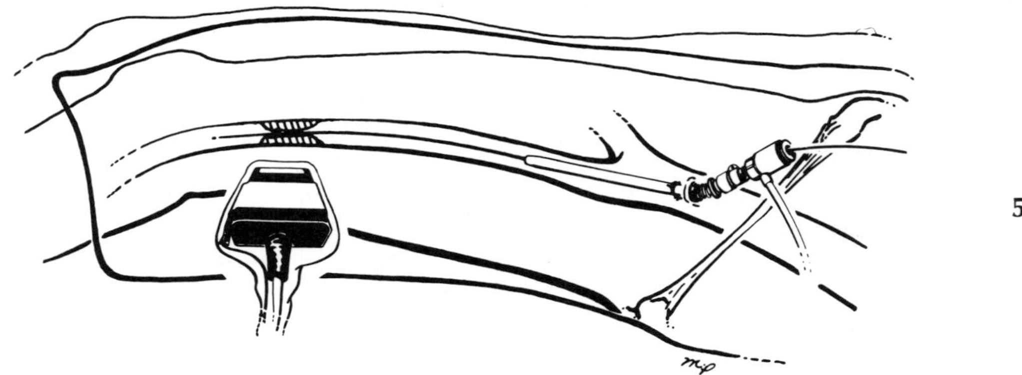

5

5

The guidewire is advanced through the lesion, again using the duplex scanner to track its progress. Until the ultrasound sensor was added to the guidewire, fluoroscopy was used.

6

The balloon catheter is advanced through the sheath and guided in place by the ultrasound probe. A new 6 French balloon catheter has become available, allowing the use of a 7 French sheath. This smaller sized sheath allows greater flow down the vessel, making velocity measurements at the lesion more accurate.

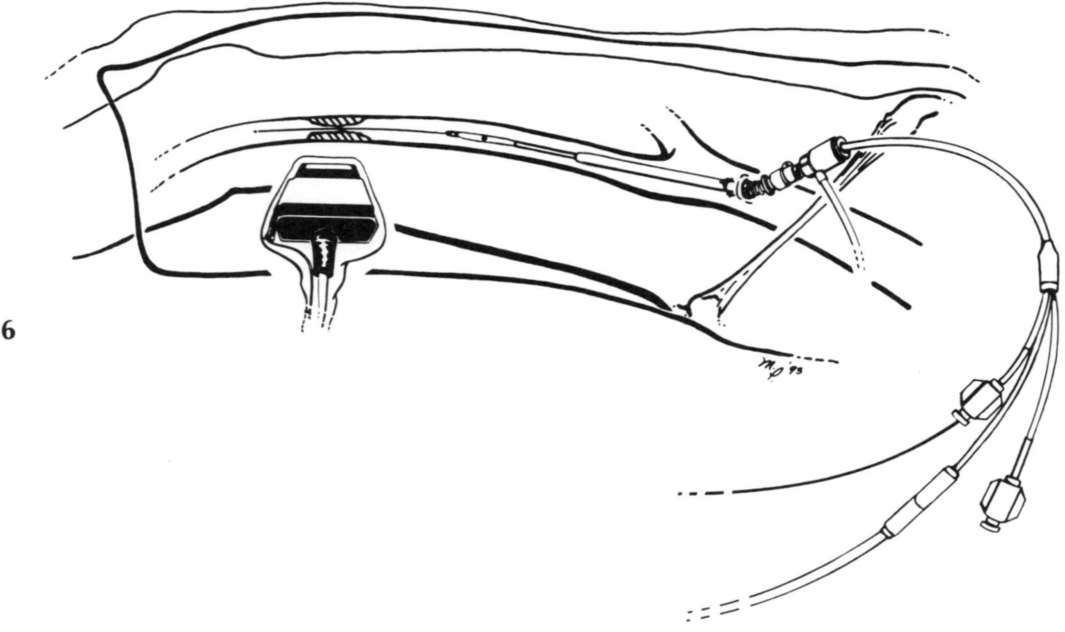

6

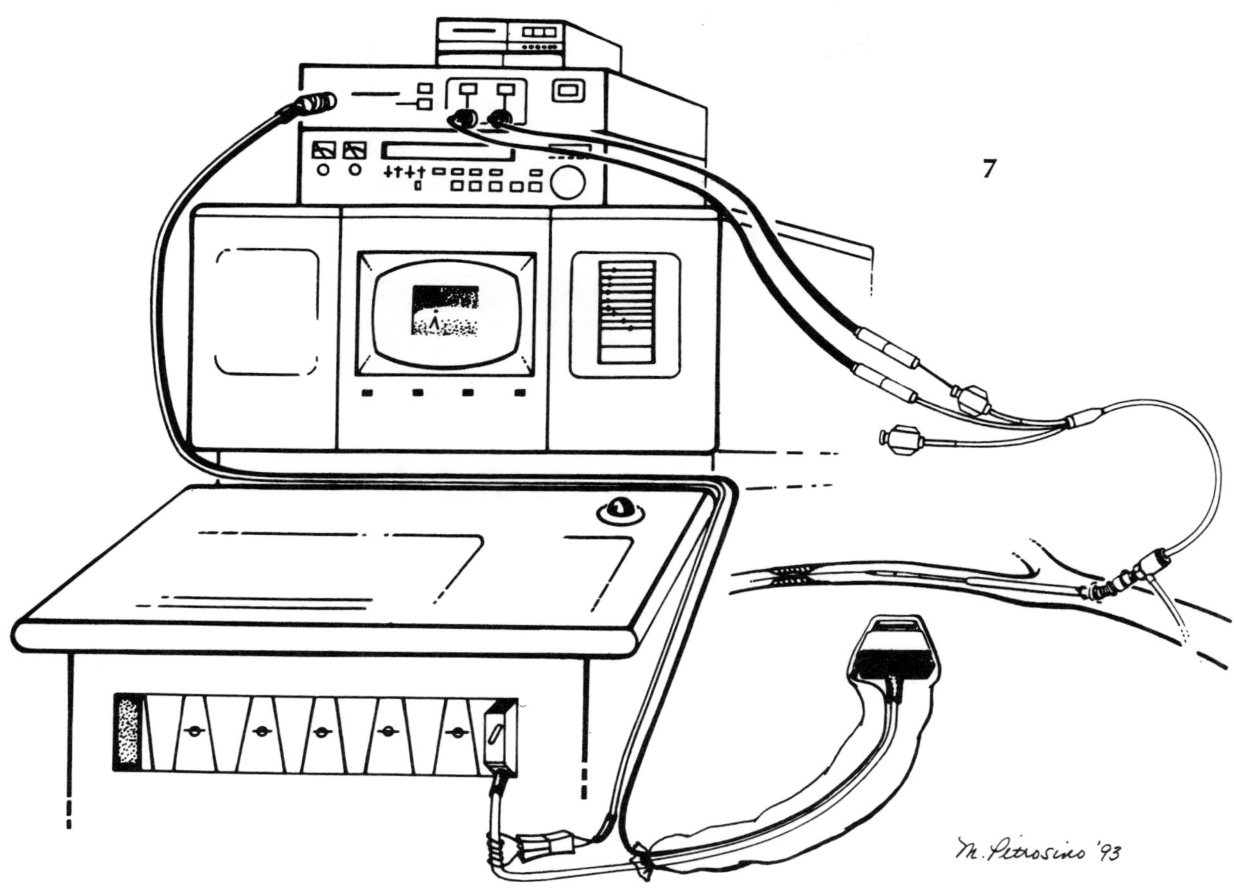

7

The catheter and guidance system was developed by Dr David Vilkomerson and colleagues in 1990. A small brass bead covered with a piezoelectric material is attached to the catheter shaft in the centre of the balloon. Two small wires attached to the piezoelectric membrane lead out of the catheter and are connected to an electronic module called the catheter system interface. In addition two antennae placed around the scan head and its cable are connected to the interface module. The antennae pick up electronic signals that the scan head converts into the ultrasonic beams which form the image on the monitor. When the sound signals strike the piezoelectric material surrounding the brass bead, an electronic current is sent to the module. The module is able to determine which ultrasound beam hits the brass bead; the time of emission and detection determines the depth of the sensor in the tissues. Thus the position of the ultrasound sensor on the catheter can be determined in two planes; it can be electronically represented on the screen by a blinking arrow.

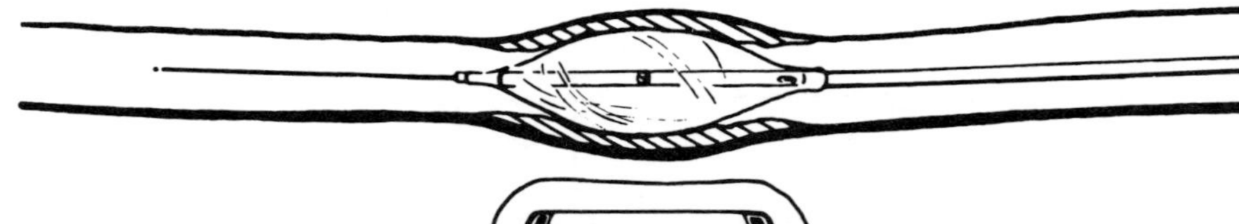

8

The balloon is centred within the lesion in the superficial femoral artery, using the pulsating arrow to identify the middle of the balloon. The balloon is inflated under monitoring of the ultrasound system. The lesion is cracked; the walls of the artery are seen to expand and stretch.

9

The balloon is deflated and withdrawn. The peak velocity is determined and compared with the value before dilatation. The final velocity should be less than twice the velocity recorded at a nearby arterial segment. The guidewire is left in place. If a residual lesion is detected, it should be treated again. Angiography may be used to confirm the result.

The ultrasound system has been successfully employed to accurately guide balloon angioplasty in 37 instances in six medical centres. The distribution of lesions was as follows: iliac 9, superficial femoral 25, popliteal 2, graft 1. Thirty-one lesions were treated satisfactorily with the catheter alone; six lesions required additional treatment with atherectomy or high pressure balloons. Real-time ultrasound appeared to be more sensitive to residual lesions than angiography. The real-time evaluation of the physiological result of angioplasty may complement and perhaps replace the morphological confirmation seen on angiography. Whether this technique eliminates residual stenoses and leads to improved long-term patency remains to be proven.

8

9

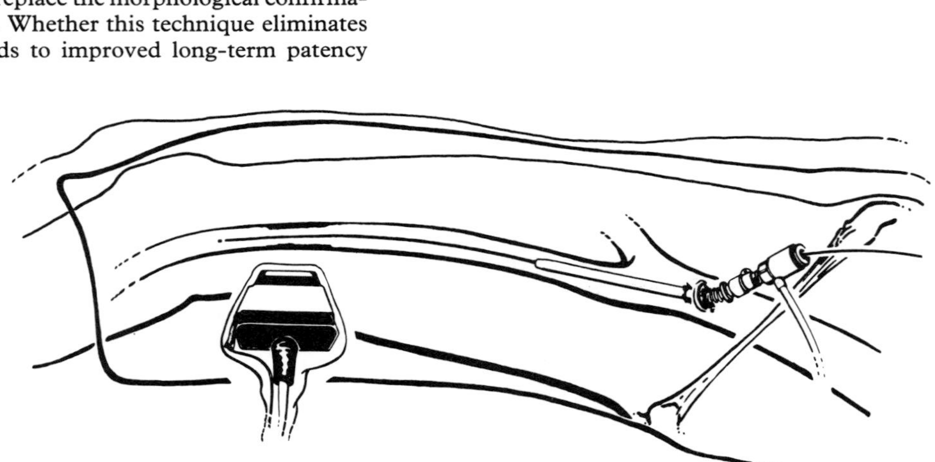

References

Brener, B. J., Cluley, S. R., Hollier, L., Shoenfeld, R., Novick, A., Vilkomerson, D., Parsonnet, V. and Ferrara-Ryan, M. (1993). Ultrasound guided balloon angioplasty: What is its role? In *Current Critical Problems in Vascular Surgery* Vol. 5. Veith, F., ed. St. Louis, MO: Quality Medical Publishers, Chapter 34.

Cluley, S. R., Brener, B. J., Hollier, L. H. *et al.* (1991). Ultrasound-guided balloon angioplasty is a new technique for vascular surgeons. *American Journal of Surgery* **162**, 117.

Cluley, S. R., Brener, B. J., Hollier, L., Shoenfeld, R., Novick, A., Vilkomerson, D. Ferrara-Ryan, M. and Parsonnet, V. (1993). Transcutaneous ultrasonography can be used to guide and monitor balloon angioplasty. *Journal of Vascular Surgery,* **17**, 23.

Hollier, L. H., Brener, B. J., Cluley, S. R., White, C. J. and Ramee, S. R. (1991). Peripheral percutaneous transluminal angioplasty with ultrasound imaging. In *Technologies in Vascular Surgery*. Yao, J. S. T. and Pearce, W. H., eds. Philadelphia: W. B. Saunders, 439.

Vilkomerson, D., Gardineer, B. and Lyons, D. (1992). Theory and practice of beacon-guided interventional ultrasound. *Journal of Ultrasound Medicine* **11**, (suppl) 44.

Transluminal recanalization, angioplasty and stenting in endovascular surgery: techniques and applications

FRANK J. CRIADO MD
LUIS A. QUERAL MD
PEGGY PATTEN RN
Maryland Vascular Institute at The Union Memorial Hospital, Baltimore, Maryland, USA

Introduction

When first introduced 30 years ago, percutaneous transluminal angioplasty was received by most vascular surgeons as a near-inconceivable, dramatic departure from established principles. Instead, albeit unrecognized at the time, the work of Dotter initially and Gruentzig a decade later signalled the dawning of a new era in angiology. The balloon catheter was created, and became the first sophisticated tool of the endovascular interventionist. It has been refined and improved considerably in recent years, and remains the most versatile and cost-efficient device for transluminal intervention. A myriad of 'advanced-generation' catheters and devices have been proposed and developed over the past 10 years. The majority of these have proven no better or worse than the Gruentzig balloon. Several of these techniques are undergoing clinical trials and their application can only be justified in such context.

Endovascular therapy (or surgery) is a relatively new subspecialty which concerns a group of devices and procedures, both diagnostic and therapeutic, sharing in common their catheter-based nature. Access to the vascular lumen is usually attained percutaneously, but there are situations where an open surgical approach is preferable or necessary. Three techniques, namely angioplasty, stenting and thrombolysis are emerging as fundamental in the endovascular interventionist's armamentarium. Clinical indications are becoming clearer as experience accumulates and long-term results become available. Focal stenotic lesions in high-flow, large-calibre arteries carry the best prognosis following endovascular treatment. In selected instances, occlusions can also be recanalized successfully.

What follows is a description of the basic endovascular techniques which have proven most useful in the authors' 6-year experience with over 1000 therapeutic transluminal interventions.

General considerations

1

With few exceptions, local infiltrative anaesthesia (at the puncture site) supplemented with intravenous sedation are utilized for all percutaneous repairs. Low molecular weight Dextran is infused at the rate of 40 ml/h during, and after the intervention for 24 hours. Anticoagulation with intravenous heparin is used in the course of all endovascular transluminal techniques, except when treating iliac stenotic lesions.

In endovascular surgery, aside from one's training and experience, nothing is more important than adequate X-ray fluoroscopy and angiography. The concept of a vascular (or endovascular) suite has thus evolved: that is, a specially designed operating room equipped with a dedicated ceiling-mounted C-arm, and a carbon-fibre radiotranslucent operating table. The system, created by International Surgical Systems (Phoenix, Arizona, USA), is ideal for the performance of all types of endovascular catheter-based interventions, and any form of reconstructive vascular surgery requiring angiography (i.e. distal bypass grafting).

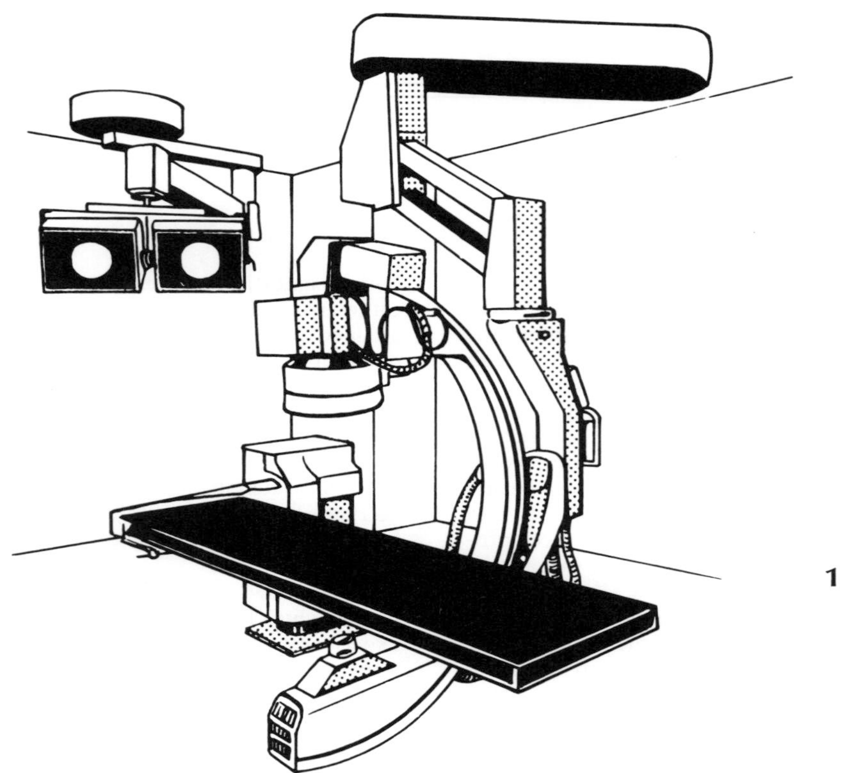

1

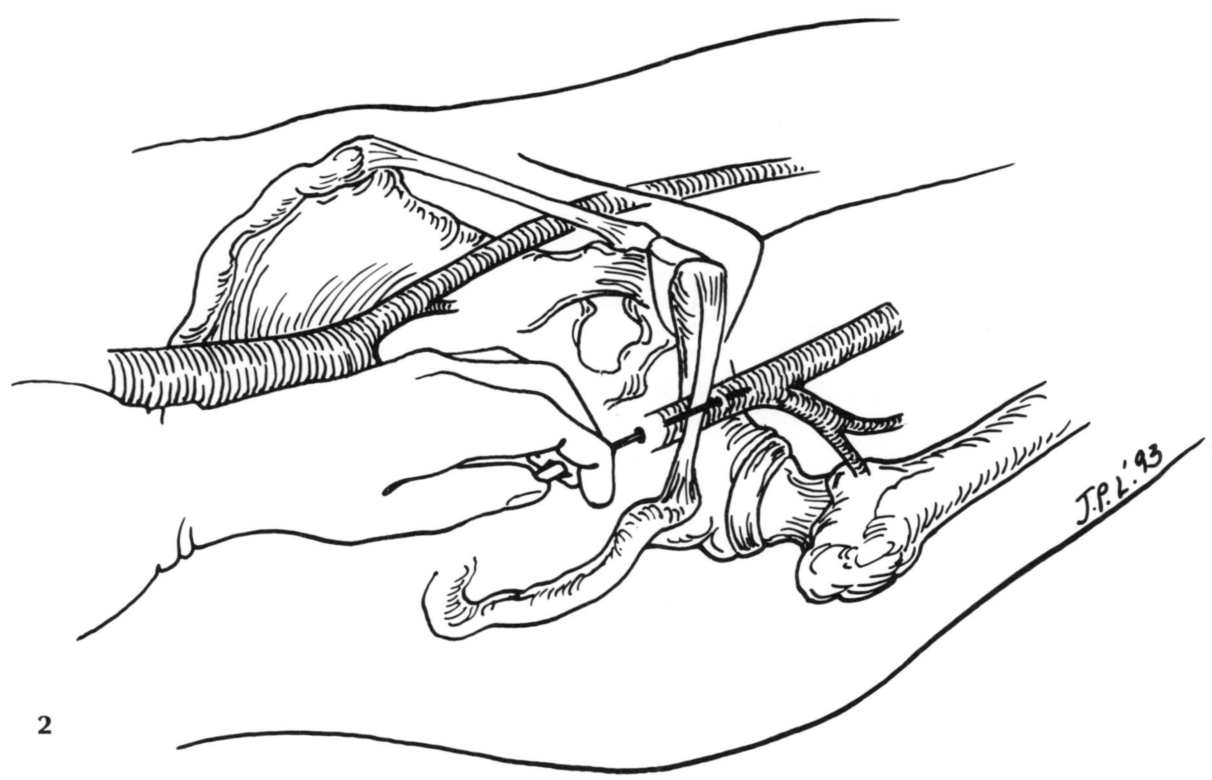

2

Percutaneous access to the vascular lumen

2

Percutaneous arterial puncture is performed with the Potts-Cournand needle. Femoral arterial puncture, whether antegrade or retrograde, should always be below the inguinal ligament. Suprainguinal puncture arterial holes cannot be compressed effectively after removal of the sheath, and troublesome bleeding may result.

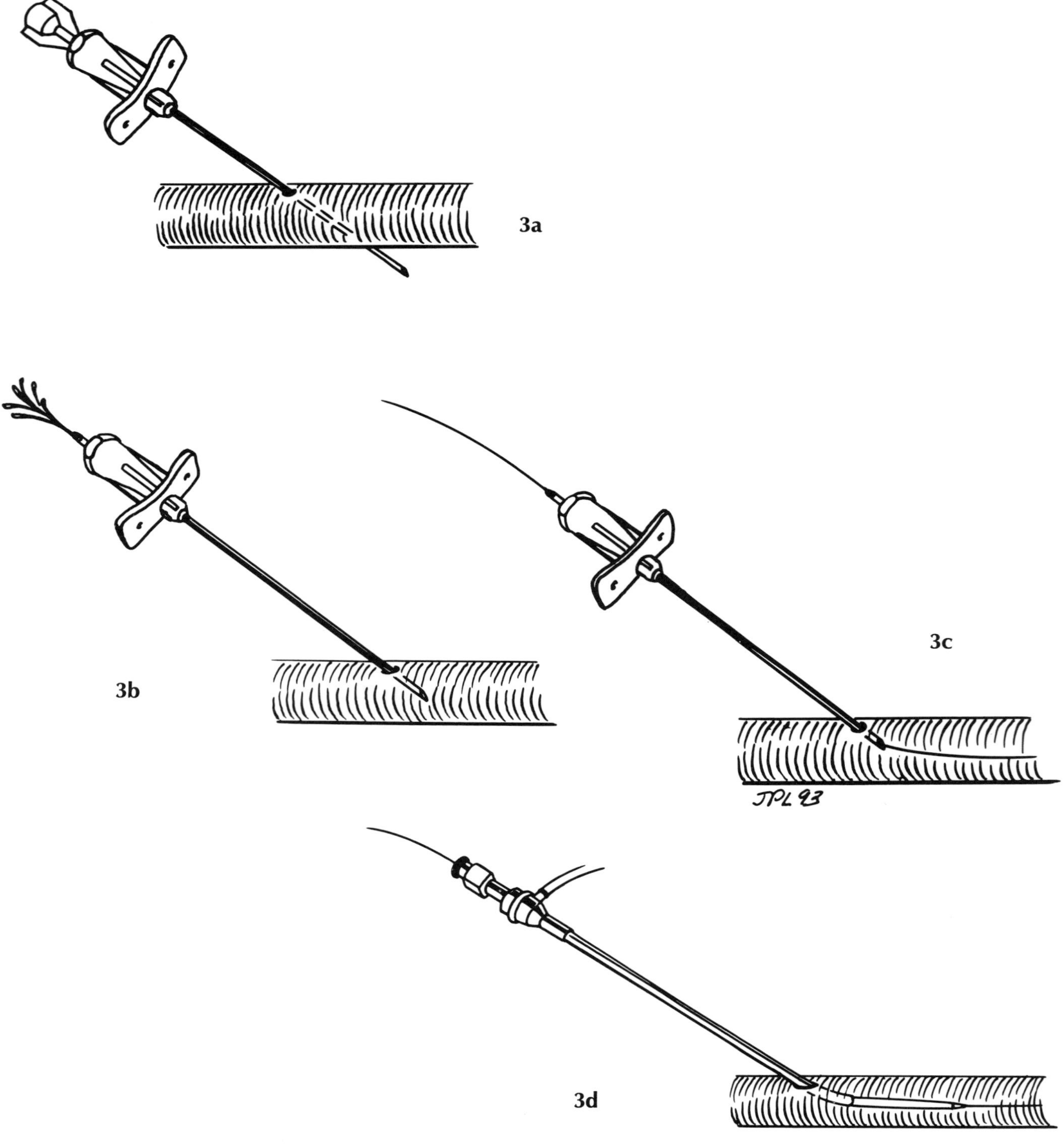

3a, b, c & d

Two-wall needle puncture is routine (*a*); the intraluminal position is secured and determined as the needle is gradually withdrawn (*b*). Single-wall puncture is advisable when anticipating the infusion of thrombolytic agents, and in the course of open surgical access. An angled, steerable guidewire is introduced through the needle and advanced under fluoroscopic control (*c*): a 0.035 inch Terumo glidewire is preferred in most instances. The needle is withdrawn, the skin opening enlarged a bit at the wire entry point with a number 11 blade, and the introducer sheath inserted over the wire into the vascular lumen (*d*). Proper positioning is confirmed angiofluoroscopically.

4a & b

Retrograde puncture of the common femoral artery is a simple technique even when the pulse is barely palpable or absent (*a*). Using the contrast-filled vein as reference may be useful (*b*). Note the infrainguinal course of the needle.

5a & b

Unlike the above-described, antegrade femoral puncture (*a*) is one of the most difficult skills to acquire in endovascular surgery. In a significant number of procedures, direct puncture of the superficial femoral artery is necessary and desirable when the femoral bifurcation lies high in the groin (*b*). 'Roadmapping' fluoroscopic capabilities are extremely helpful in performing this technique. A *test-injection* of radiocontrast material will serve to define the vascular anatomy and ascertain proper positioning of the needle *before* introduction of the wire and sheath (*inset*).

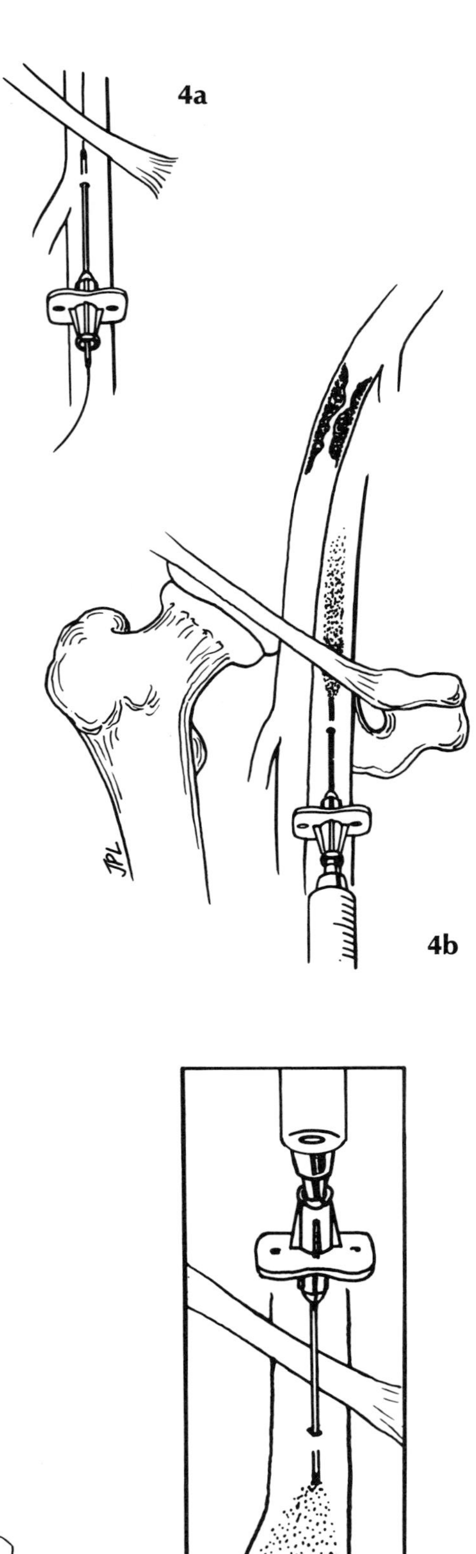

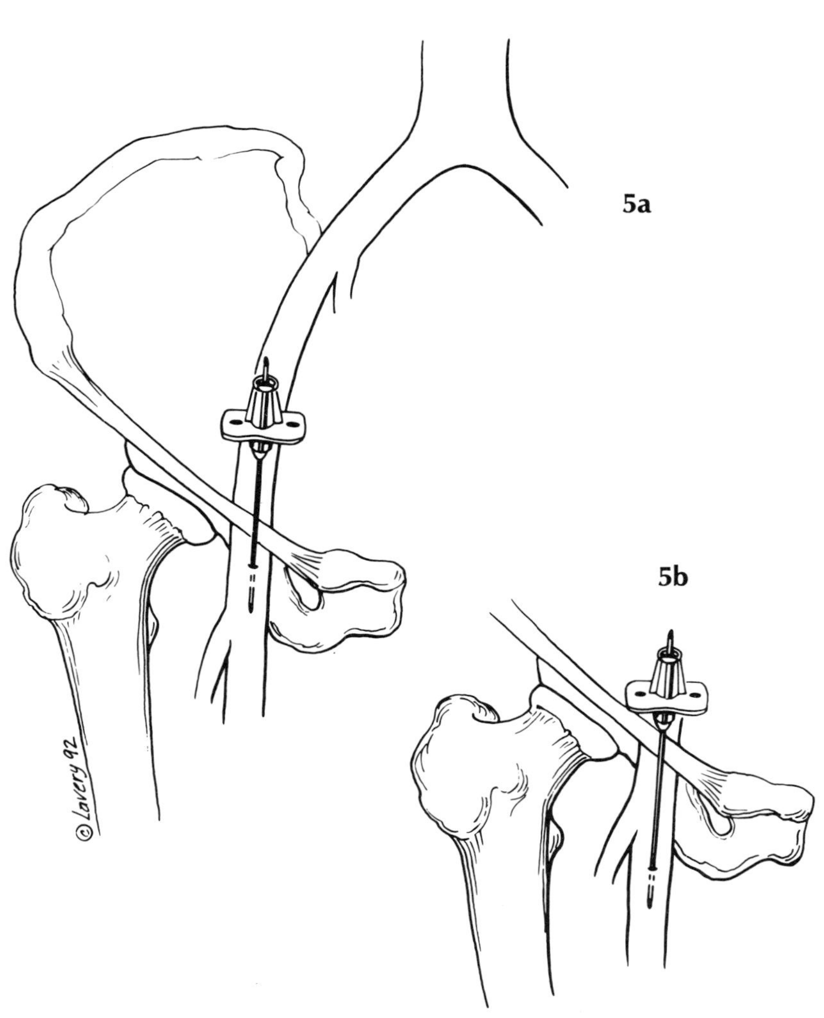

5 (inset)

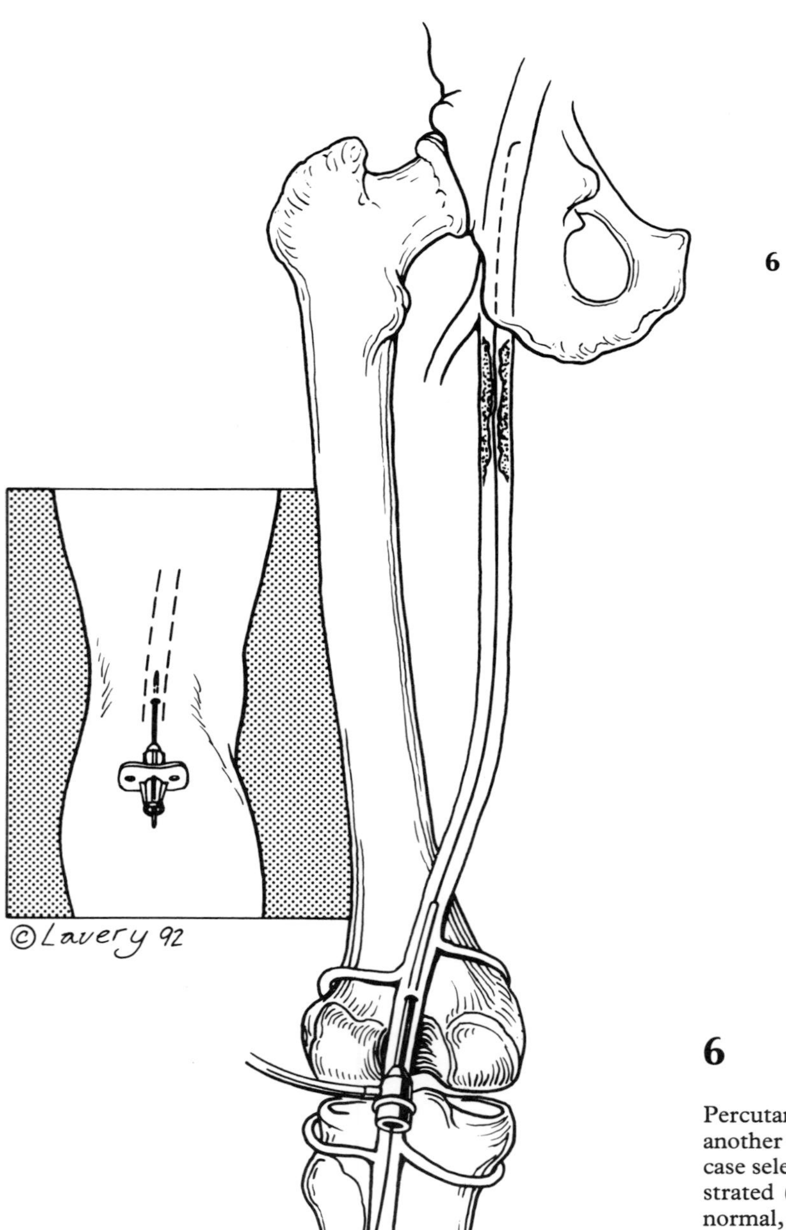

6

6

Percutaneous retrograde puncture of the popliteal artery is another useful technique in selected circumstances. Proper case selection is paramount: only patients who can be demonstrated (on pre-procedure angiography) to have a relatively normal, large-calibre proximal popliteal artery are eligible. Lesions in the proximal segment of the superficial femoral artery, and in the common femoral artery constitute the best applications of this technique. The patient is first positioned supine for the insertion of a small-calibre retrograde femoral sheath. The sheath is secured in place, and the patient turned prone. As radiocontrast material is injected proximally, the 'visualized' popliteal artery is punctured under 'direct vision' as seen on the fluoroscopy monitor. The subsequent steps are exactly the same as described for femoral access. Due to the potentially serious nature of haematomas in this location, *systemic heparin is not utilized* in popliteal-access interventions.

Open surgical access

7a & b

A femoral cutdown is employed infrequently, best indications being significant obesity, and patients with dense, multiple scars in the groin. The exposure need not be wide: complete vessel control is not necessary. Aside from single-wall needle puncture, the technical steps are identical to those already described. Following withdrawal of the sheath, haemostasis is secured with a single figure-of-eight suture while 'pinching' the segment between two DeBakey forceps (*a*). Upstream (iliac) and downstream (fem-pop) procedures, if done concomitantly, require separate punctures as shown (*b*).

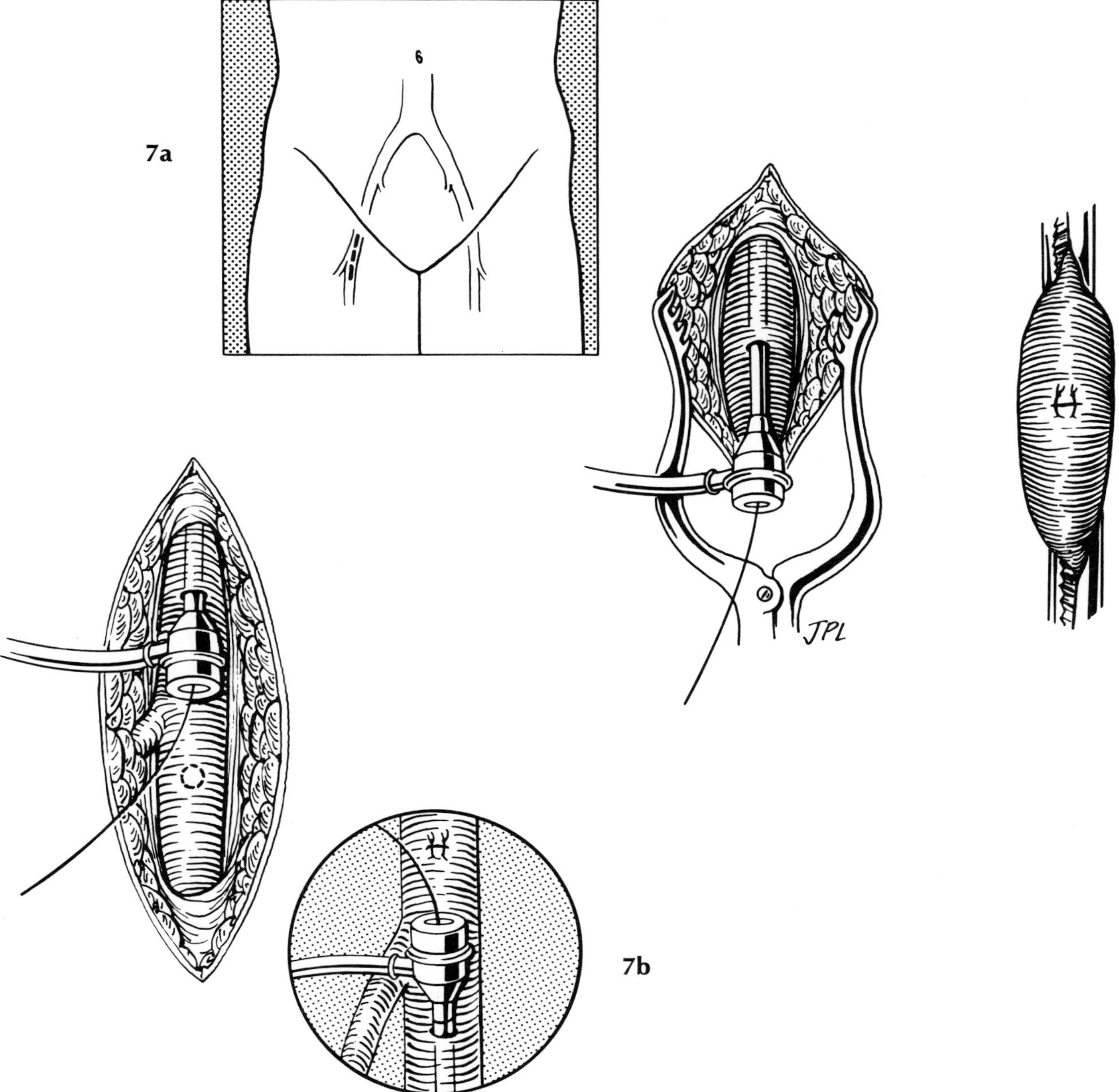

7a

7b

8

More complete exposure is needed when performing a combined surgical reconstruction.

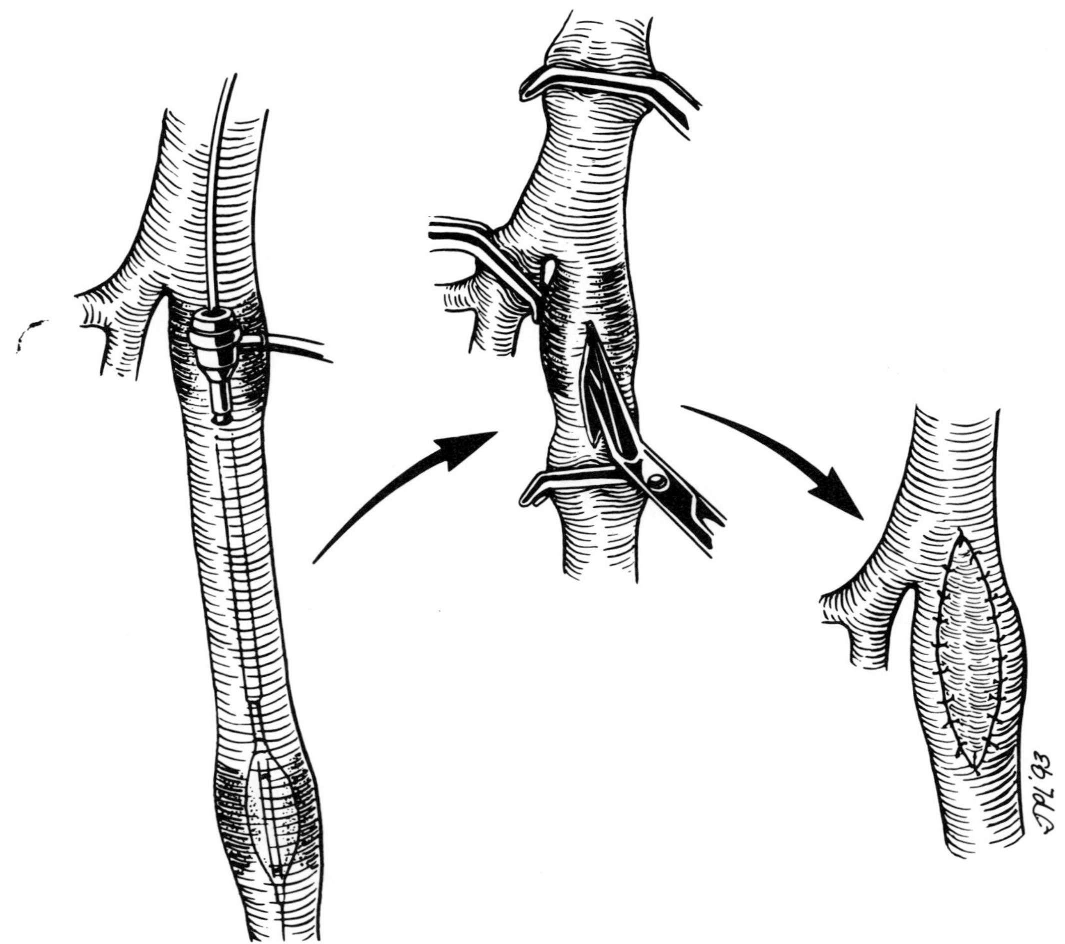

Transluminal navigation and lesion crossing

9a, b, c, d & e

Advancement of the guidewire to the target lesion is an important component of all intraluminal procedures. Fluoroscopic control is required. The Terumo hydrophilic glidewire can cross most tight stenoses and even occlusions. When facing a difficult lesion, *guiding and centring* the wire with a straight angiographic catheter is a very useful manoeuvre to facilitate crossing (*a*) Allowing the wire to form a J is also quite helpful in this regard (*b*, *c*).

Total occlusions are often made up of much clot and an underlying flow-limiting atherosclerotic plaque. It is possible to traverse these occlusions much in the same way as in the case of stenoses (*d*). Clot that is easily penetrated by a wire can often be lysed successfully.

Subintimal recanalization is another possible route (*e-inset*). This is viewed as disadvantageous by most experts, but such opinion is not unanimous. No matter what the specific situation or technique of crossing, *once the guidewire has been placed in its proper position, it must not be removed until the end of the procedure*. This is a fundamental principle applicable to all transluminal interventions.

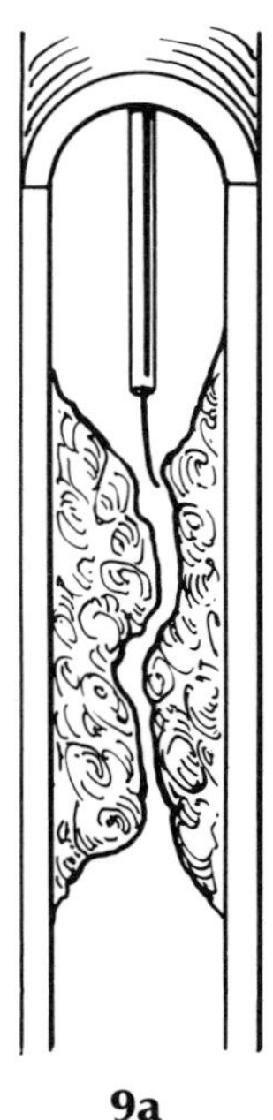

9a

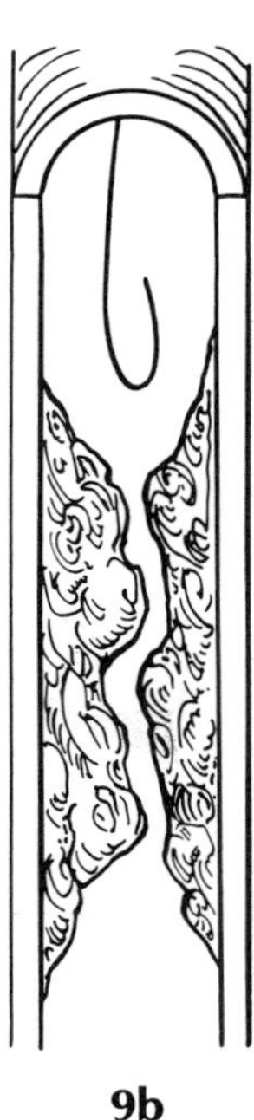

9b

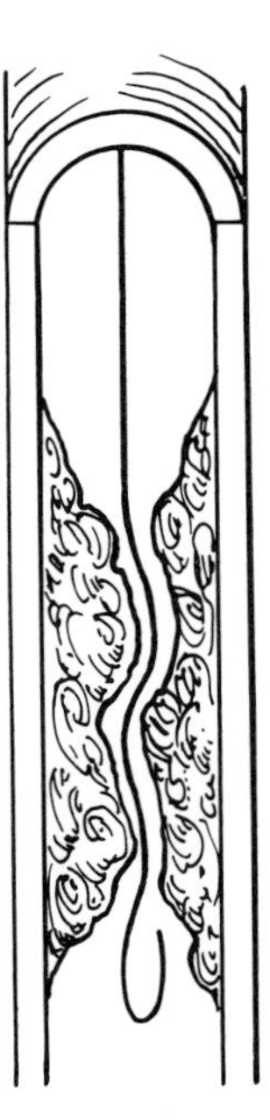

9c

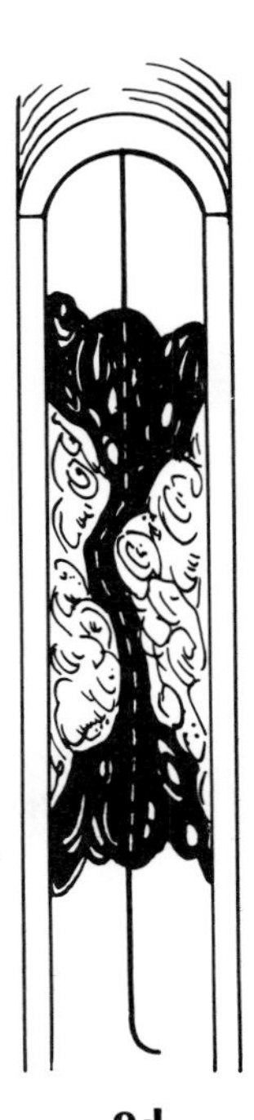

9d

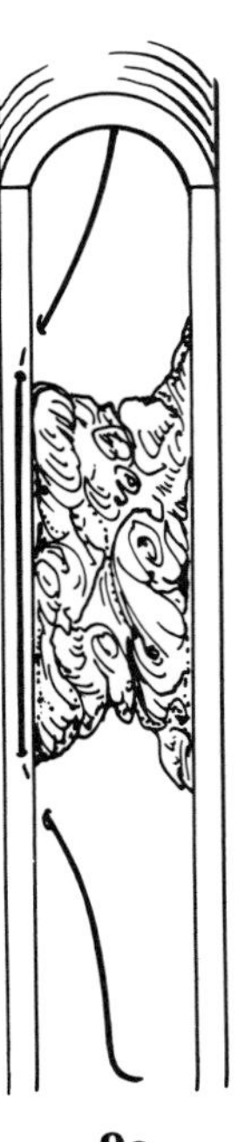

9e

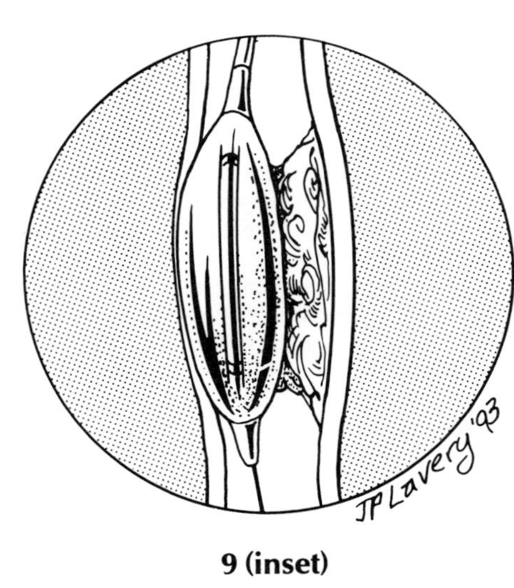

9 (inset)

Haemostasis at puncture site

10

Care of the puncture site is a very important aspect in endovascular surgery. Manual compression for 10–20 minutes is necessary, performed by an experienced team member: this manoeuvre should never be left to the uninitiated. When systemic heparin in full doses has been administered, it is advisable to leave the sheath in place for 45–60 minutes, when it is removed in the recovery room. We have recently found the Femostop device to be extremely helpful and now use it routinely.

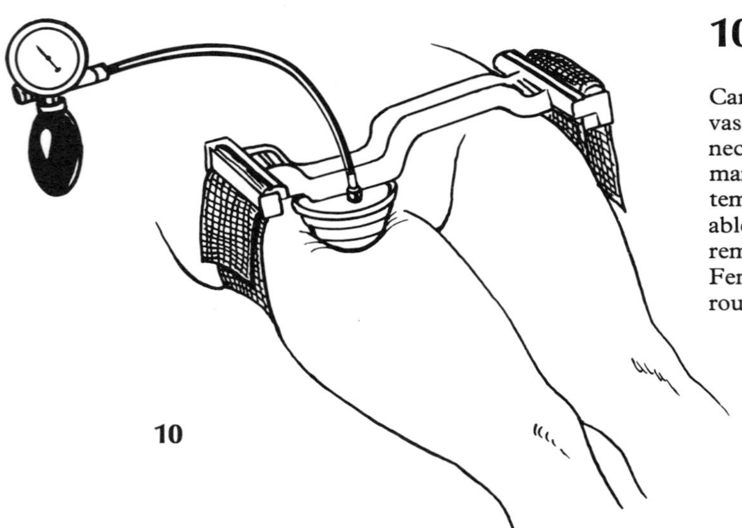

10

Balloon angioplasty

11

The Gruentzig balloon catheter remains the essential tool for endovascular intervention. Recent refinements of significance include improved trackability, lower profile and smaller-size catheters. In nearly every instance, 5 French catheters can now be utilized to dilate lesions in the lower extremities and other territories. Controversy persists regarding the duration of balloon inflation, and whether use of a pressure-gauge inflator is any better than a simple syringe. Balloon sizing is important and, at times, crucial. Overdilation and stretching of the vessel wall beyond its normal diameter is of little practical value, except – perhaps – during implantation of a balloon-expandable stent. Moreover, balloon-induced vessel rupture is a rare but not unknown complication. The subclavian and renal arteries are especially delicate vessels in this regard. When in doubt, it is best to 'undersize' a little and then dilate further if necessary.

Iliac angioplasty is the most successful endovascular procedure. The 'kissing-balloon' technique is a useful modification in cases of aortic bifurcation 'spill-over' lesions involving both iliac artery ostia; stents are frequently added at present (*inset*). While a 'good angiographic result' is a desirable outcome, the complete obliteration of translesional pressure gradients constitutes the most important therapeutic endpoint in all iliac interventions.

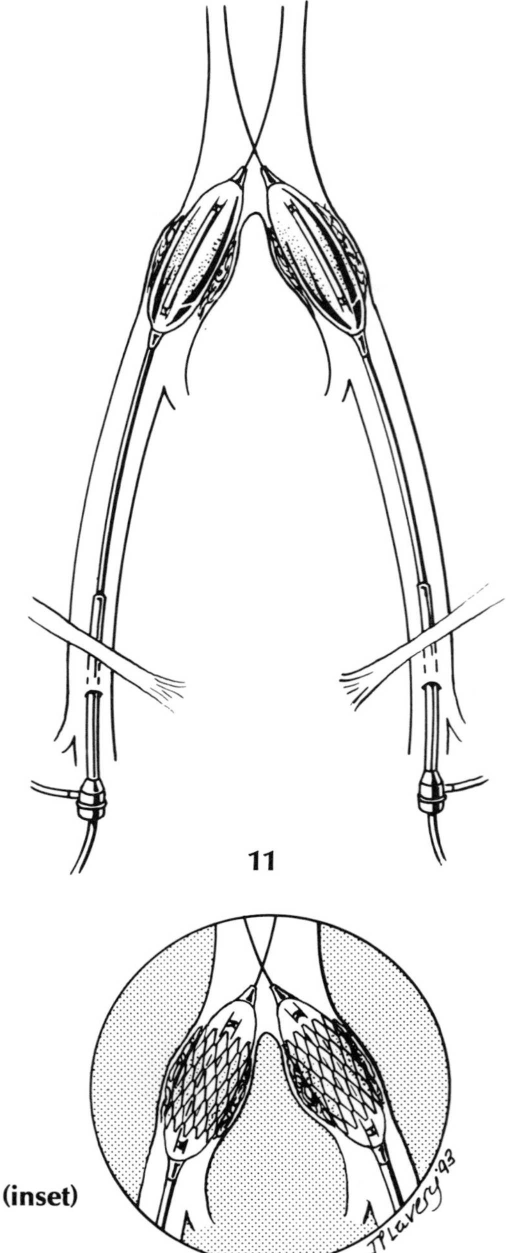

11

11 (inset)

12a, b & c

The cross-over (over-the-hump) approach (*a, b, c*) is a useful alternative in some situations such as mid and distal external iliac artery lesions (too close to where the ipsilateral puncture site would be), common femoral artery stenoses, and other iliac artery lesions resistant to conventional retrograde crossing. This approach is also preferred for preliminary thrombolysis of total occlusions. The technique involves the introduction of a curved catheter into the aorta, passed over an Amplatz superstiff wire. The wire is then withdrawn allowing the curve to re-form, and engage the contralateral iliac ostium as the catheter is pulled down while injecting small amounts of radiocontrast material. A standard wire is then introduced and passed downstream the opposite iliac system.

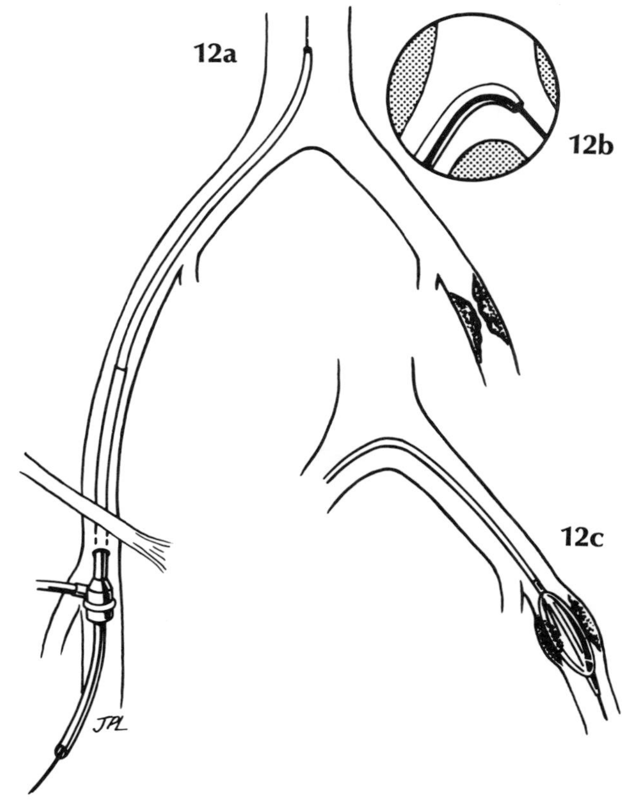

13

Long, 10 cm balloons are often necessary for angioplasty of the superficial femoral artery. Here again, lower profile, ultrathin catheters are preferred.

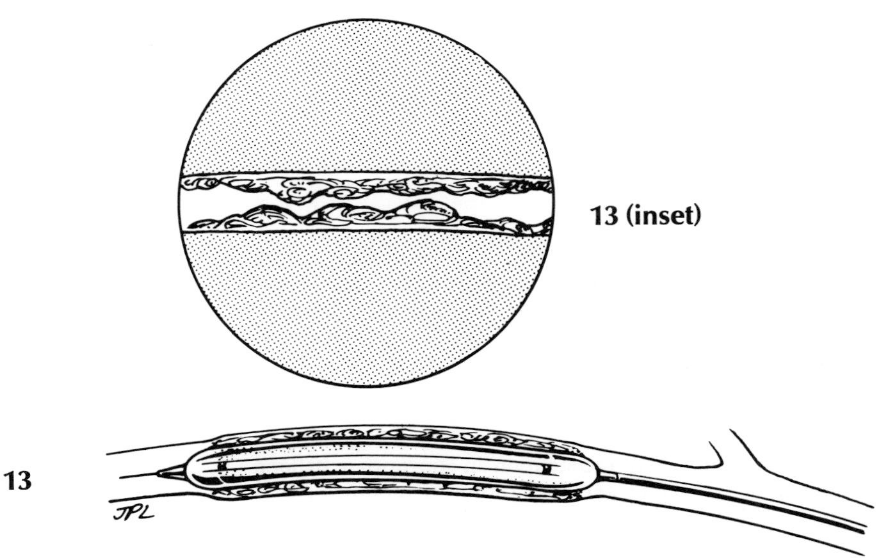

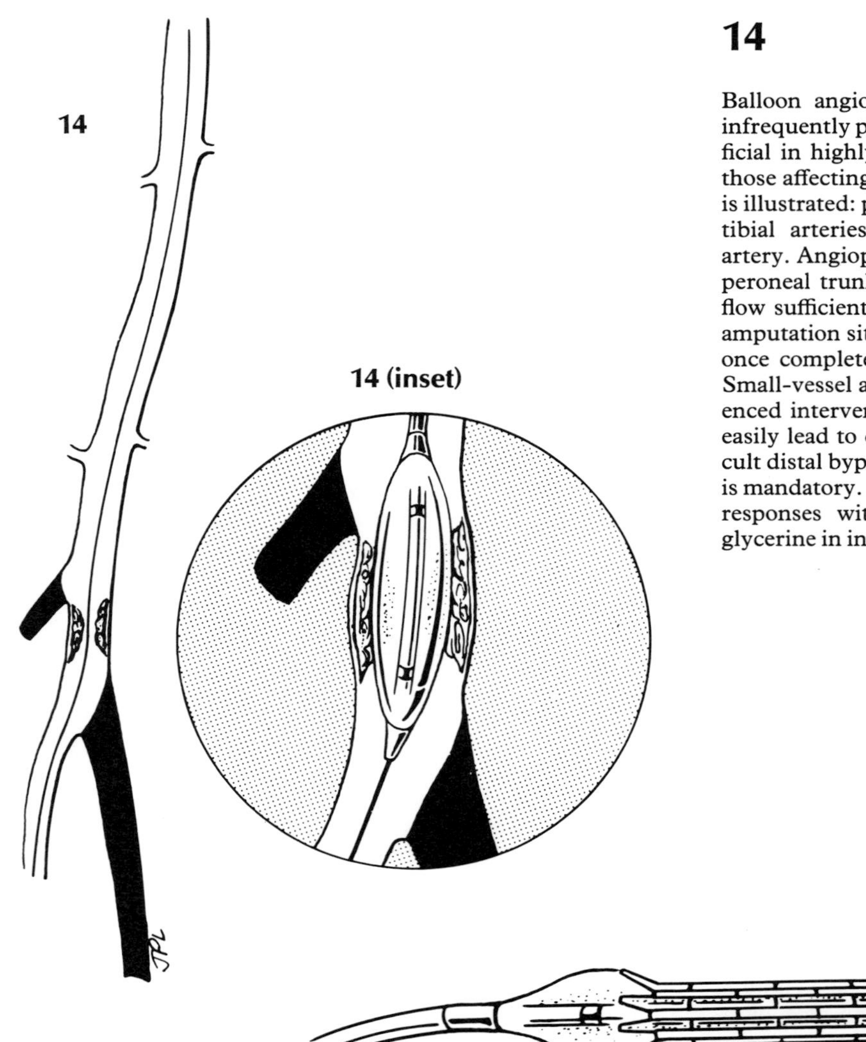

14

Balloon angioplasty of the small tibial-peroneal vessels is infrequently performed. The technique can be clinically beneficial in highly selected instances of focal lesions, especially those affecting the proximal calf vessels. One typical situation is illustrated: patients (usually diabetic) with occlusion of both tibial arteries, and single-vessel run-off via the peroneal artery. Angioplasty of a flow-limiting focal lesion in the tibioperoneal trunk or peroneal artery is likely to improve distal flow sufficiently as to promote healing of an ulcer or minor-amputation site. Long-term patency is relatively unimportant once complete skin coverage has been obtained at the foot. Small-vessel angioplasty should only be attempted by experienced interventionists. Potential technical complications can easily lead to critical limb ischaemia and the need for a difficult distal bypass operation. Full anticoagulation with heparin is mandatory. It is also helpful to prevent frequent vasospastic responses with the administration of intra-arterial nitroglycerine in increments of 100 μg.

Stents

15 & 16

Stenting as an adjunct to angioplasty is a practically useful technique capable of preventing or correcting the mechanical problems associated with conventional balloon dilatation. Dissections, deep fissures into the media, and intimal flaps can all be neatly smoothed out and tacked down with implantation of an intravascular stent.

The Palmaz device (*15*) is a balloon-expandable stent with which we have had a great deal of experience beginning in 1989. Secure mounting of the stent on an appropriate balloon is paramount. A simple personal technical modification is shown (*16*). Nowadays, manufacturer-premounted stents are available.

While indications and notions regarding clinical benefit continue to evolve, a number of well-established principles can be enunciated.

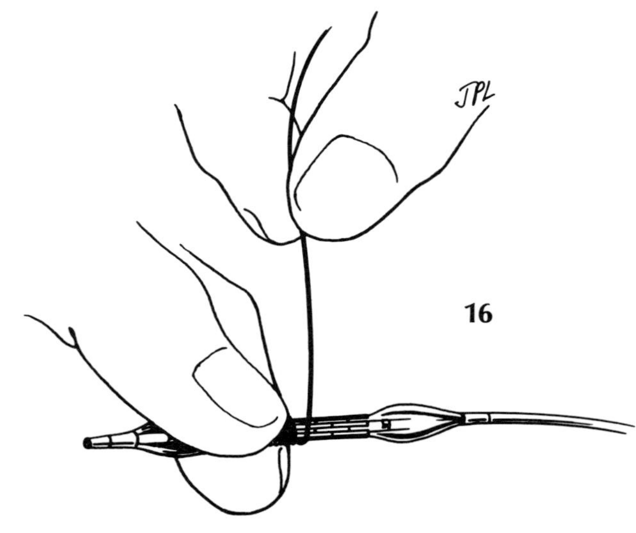

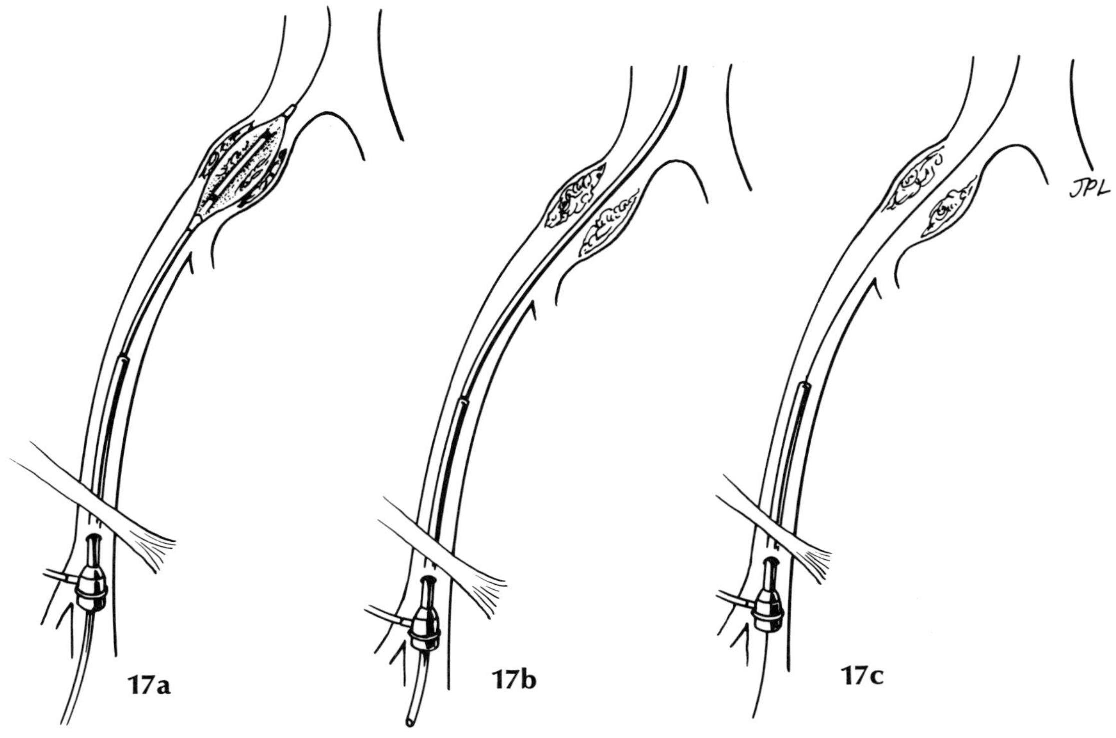

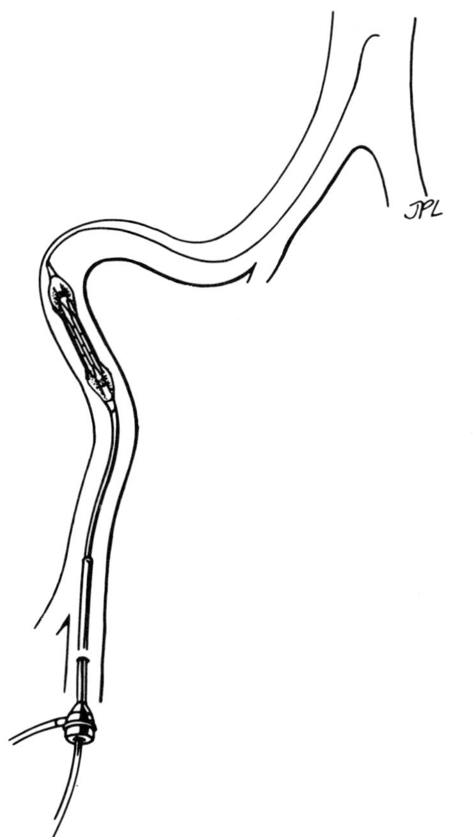

17a, b & c

'Standard' iliac artery stenting involves, first, preliminary conventional balloon angioplasty (predilatation) (*a*). Angiographic control at this juncture must rule out extravasation of contrast, for this constitutes an absolute contraindication to stent implantation. The standard guidewire is then exchanged for an Amplatz superstiff wire with the aid of a small (4–6 French) angiographic ('exchange') catheter (*b*, *c*). This is an important technical step designed to provide a firm track on which to advance the rigid stent. Moreover, with such stiff wire one can 'straighten' moderately tortuous iliac arteries.

18

Severe tortuosity and angulation, however, preclude stenting with this device: it is the second contraindication.

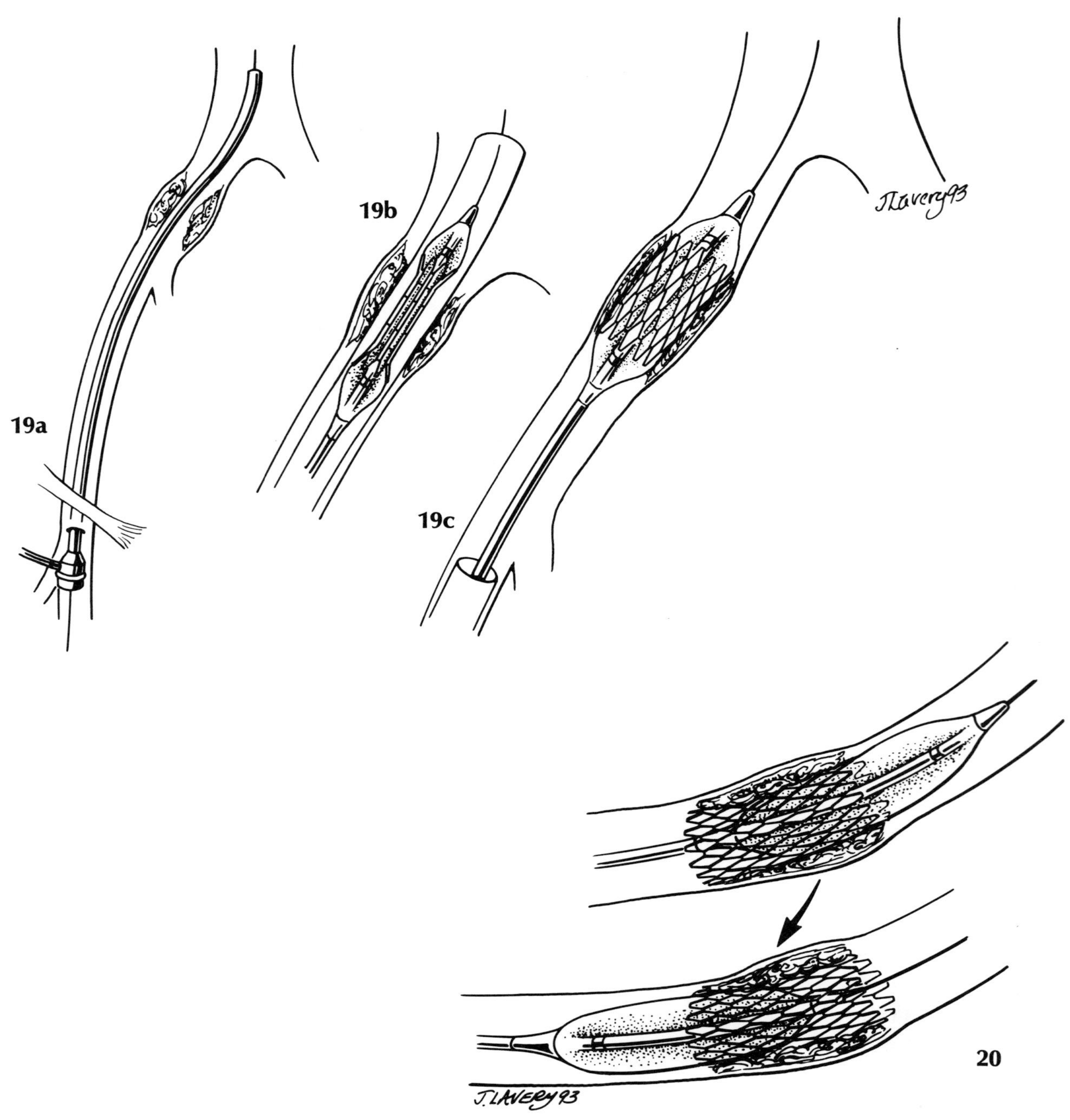

19a, b & c

The next step involves introduction of the special long sheath, whose internal end should be positioned within the aortic lumen (*a*). This sheath (9 French in diameter) serves as a protective conduit for insertion and advancement of the stent mounted on the angioplasty (*b*). Once the stent has been positioned exactly where desired (under fluoroscopy), the sheath is pulled down to allow unimpeded balloon inflation with full expansion of the stent and incrustation into the vessel wall (*c*).

20

On occasion, it is advisable to effect two further balloon inflations at either end of the stent to ensure optimal deployment.

21

If more than one stent is deployed, the devices should be imbricated over 20% of their lengths, beginning with the most distal (from the introducer) and proceeding proximally.

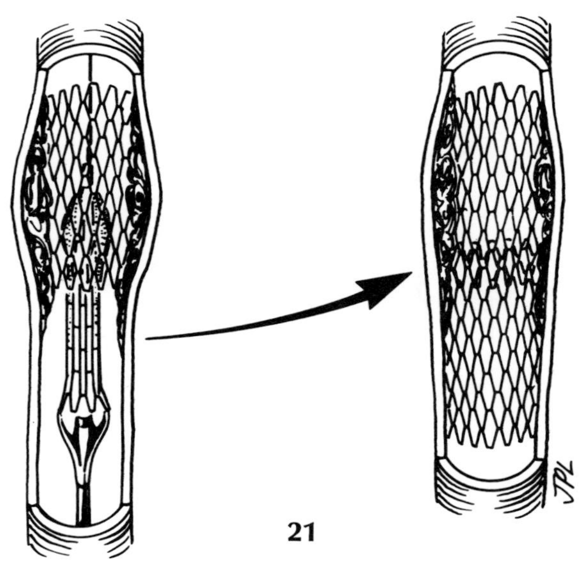

21

A modified simpler technique has evolved more recently. It consists of primary stenting, without pre-dilation, and utilizing a conventional 7 French short introducer sheath. These modifications are not recommended to the inexperienced. However, the availability of low-profile, pre-mounted stents have made these changes logical and quite safe. Omitting the preliminary angioplasty can be troublesome, though. One must learn to distinguish those lesions which are heavily calcified and so hard that they are not amenable to balloon expansion, or likely to perforate the balloon upon inflation (see below). In addition, extremely tight stenoses may not easily be crossed with a balloon/stent catheter: it pays to be cautious and predilate in all such circumstances.

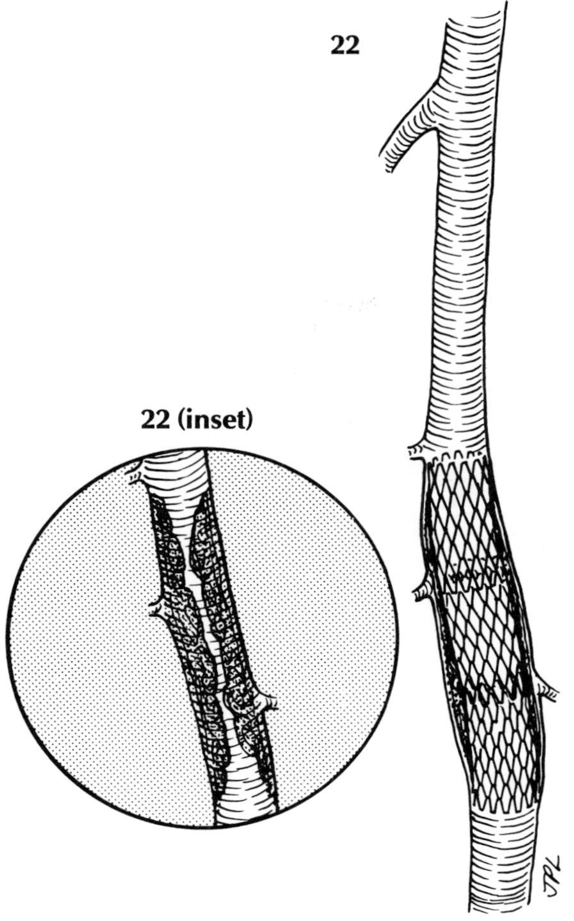

22

22 (inset)

22

Stenting of the superficial femoral and popliteal arteries has yielded results which are much inferior to those obtained in the iliac system. In fact, it may not be any better than conventional balloon angioplasty. It is only in selected lesions and circumstances that stenting can be justified for those segments. The access is the same as with simple angioplasty. Multiple stents are often needed. Prolonged anticoagulation with warfarin may improve mid/long-term results for those patients.

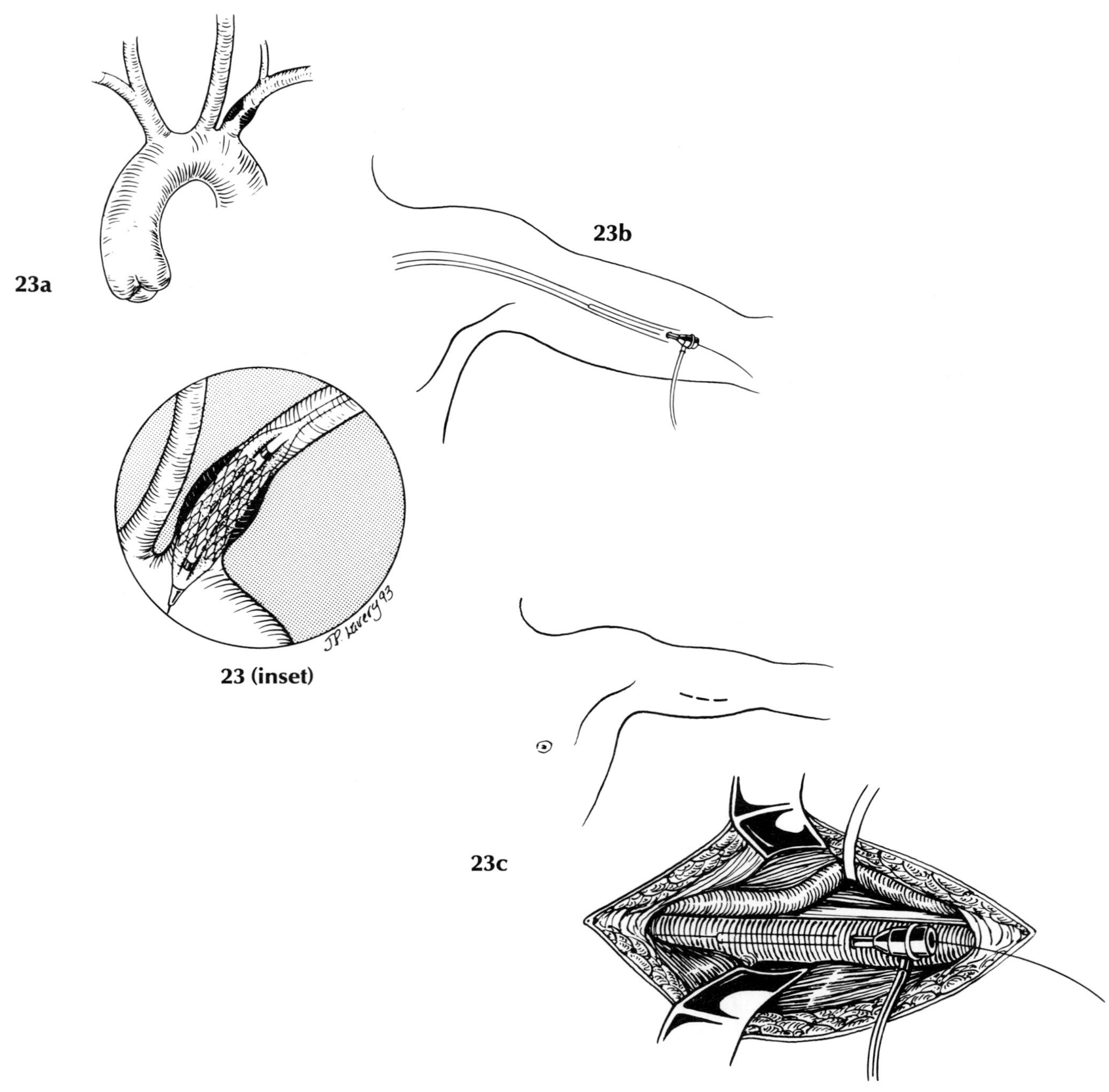

23a, b & c

Focal lesions of the proximal subclavian artery (*a*) lend themselves well to endovascular therapy. Balloon angioplasty, with or without stenting, is rapidly becoming an important therapeutic alternative for these patients. Retrograde access through the brachial artery is preferred. Although percutaneous puncture (*b*) is quite simple, the potential for serious peripheral nerve complications make it less attractive. Open surgical approach requires a small incision and local anaesthesia only (*c*). Direct and indirect (haematoma-induced) nerve injury can be avoided reliably. Markedly curved subclavian arteries can be very difficult for advancement and deployment of the Palmaz device; simple angioplasty, or a more flexible stent (i.e. wallstent) may be a better choice in such instances.

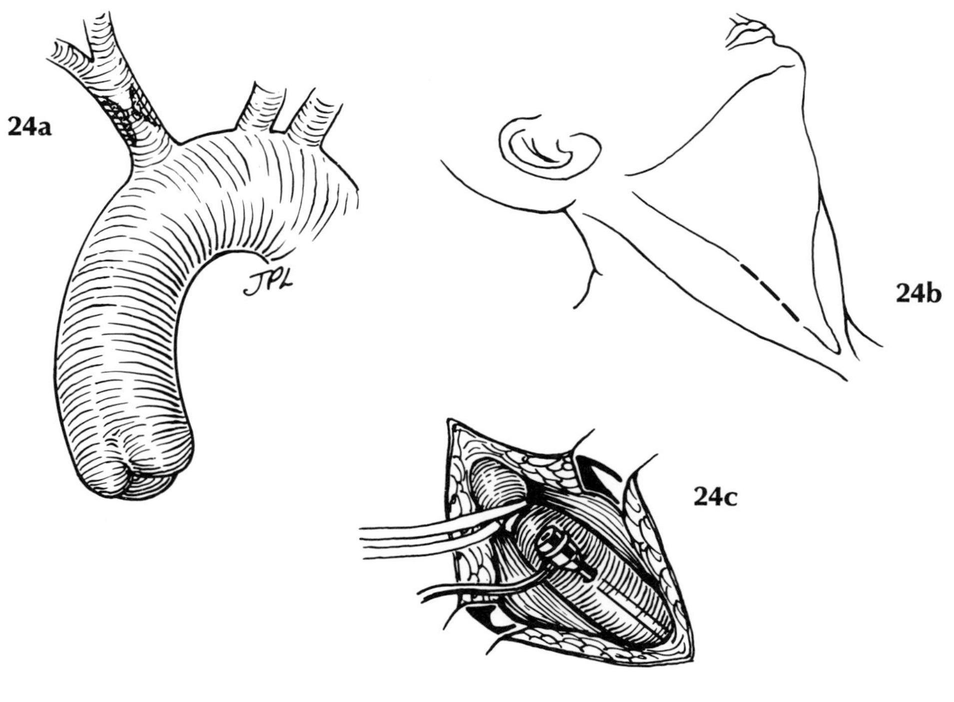

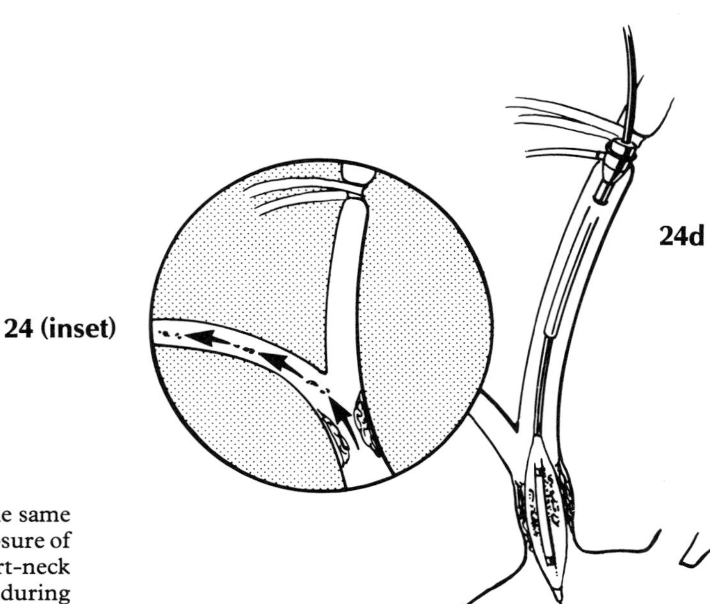

24a, b, c & d

Innominate artery lesions (*a*) may also be treated by the same method. Our preferred technique involves limited exposure of the proximal common carotid artery through a short-neck incision, and vascular control with flow interruption during angioplasty/stenting (*b, c*). By so doing, the proximal common carotid artery becomes a static fluid column, with flow continuing through the subclavian artery only. Should embolization occur, the potential for serious consequences is clearly diminished (*d, inset*).

Problems and troubleshooting

25a, b & c

Heavily calcified lesions, with intraluminal spicules and rough edges may pose a serious problem if the balloon is pierced halfway through inflation (*a, inset*), leaving an incompletely expanded stent (*b*). The device is fortunately often anchored enough, albeit precariously, as to allow exchange for a new balloon which will – hopefully – complete deployment (*c*). On occasion, it is possible to forcibly inflate the balloon for full expansion in spite of the leak. Use of the angiography power injector may also be a useful manoeuvre to effect full inflation of the ruptured balloon.

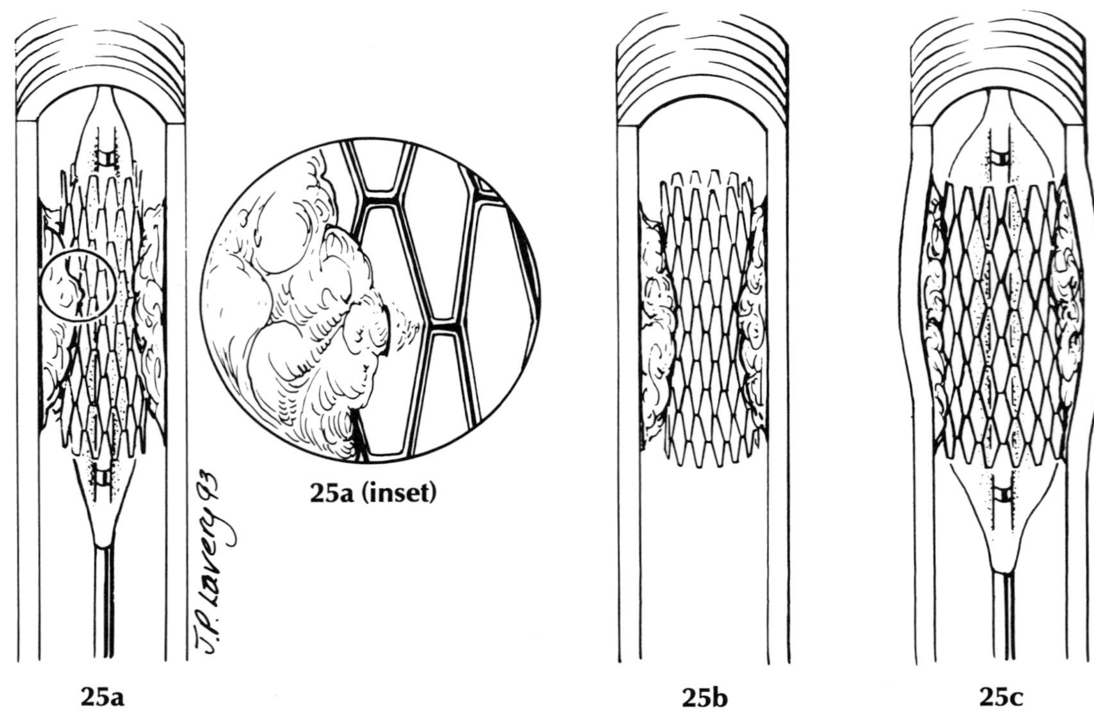

25a **25a (inset)** **25b** **25c**

26

26 (inset)

26

It has happened that the stent becomes detached from the balloon during initial transluminal navigation. Retrieval involves withdrawal of the balloon, and insertion of a smaller angioplasty catheter, perhaps of the coronary type. Such balloon should be able to re-enter the stent, and after being inflated a little, achieve better attachment of the stent which can now be carried upstream on the balloon (*inset*). Partial deployment is effected with this small balloon at the desired location, and then a larger balloon will complete full expansion. The other alternative, which may have prevented such incident in the first place, involves the introduction of a long sheath as shown in *Illustration 19a*. Once the stent is within it, they can both be extracted together.

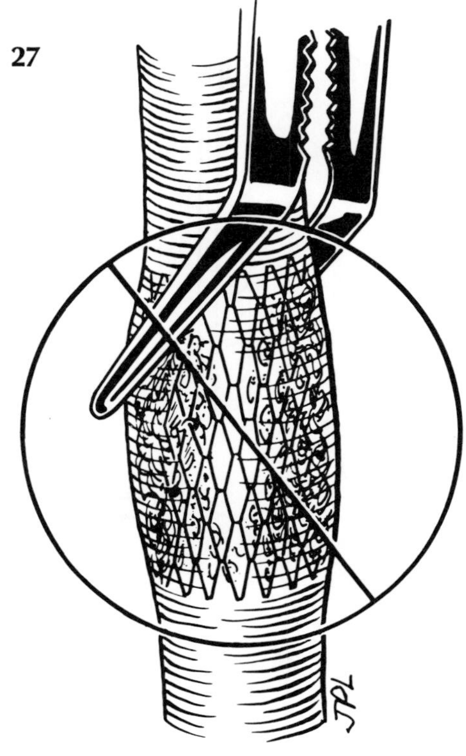

27

27

Finally, it must be realized that a previously stented vessel segment cannot be clamped or repaired directly. If surgical reconstruction is necessary, exclusion/bypass or replacement are the better alternatives.

Endovascular grafting

28 & 29

The use of stents to attach endoluminal fabric grafts is an evolving new horizon for this technology (*28*). Its most immediate and exciting application is to achieve transluminal exclusion of aortic aneurysms as championed by Parodi. Configuration of the stent-graft device is as illustrated (*29*). The entire delivery sheath with its assembled stent-graft mounted on a balloon catheter is tracked over the wire via retrograde transluminal approach after introduction through a femoral arteriotomy. The size and relative rigidity of the device (18 French presently) is an important limitation in cases of small and tortuous iliac arteries.

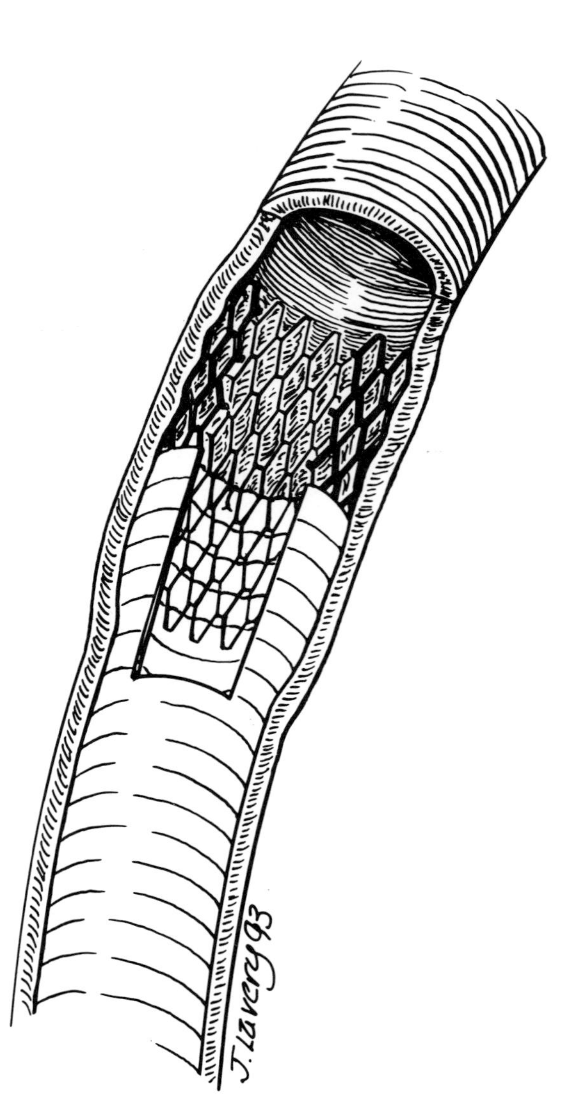

28

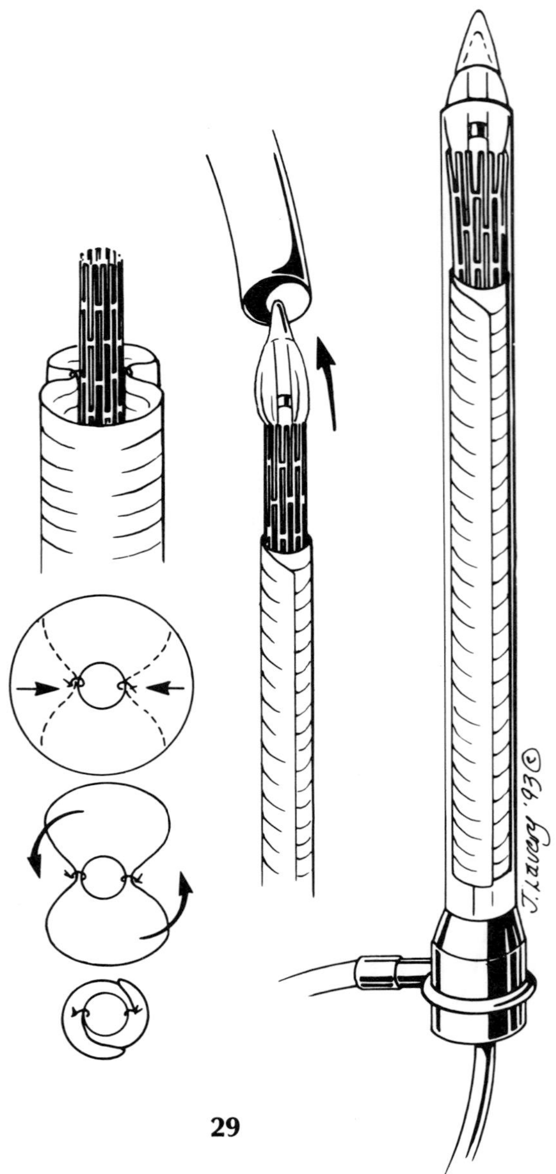

29

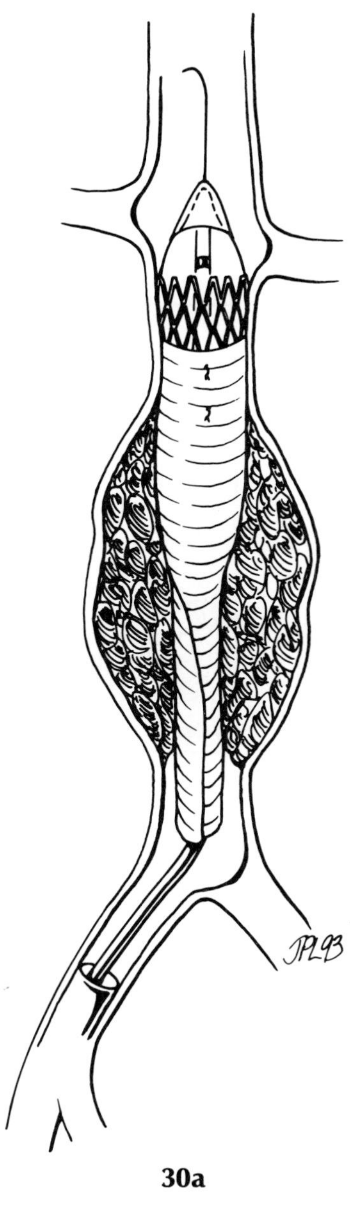

30a

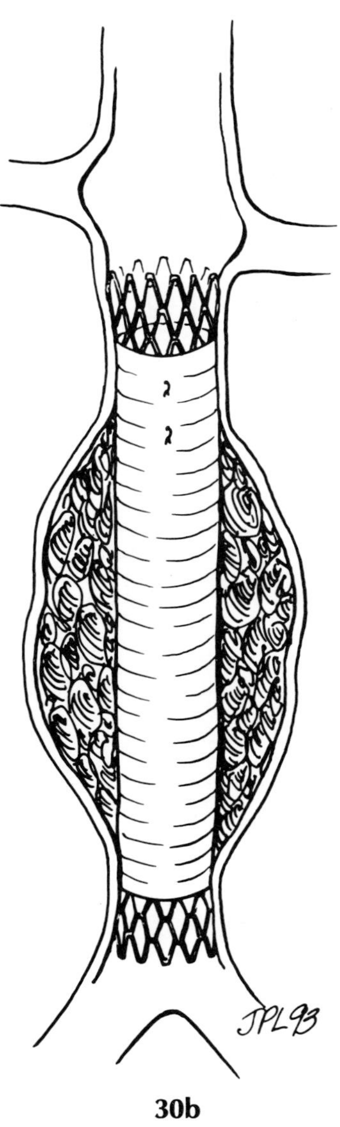

30b

30a & b, 31

The final endoluminal graft configuration is either aorto-aortic (*30a,b*) or aorto-iliac unilateral utilizing a tapered prosthesis, and then a cross-over femoral-femoral bypass. Contralateral exclusion of the iliac system is necessary in the latter, either by surgical interruption or transluminally detached balloons (*31*). Endovascular grafting with this and other devices will have important future applications beyond aneurysm exclusion: internal (transluminal) bypass, obliteration of arterio-venous communications, aortic dissections and others. To date, more than 100 endovascular grafting procedures have been performed by various investigators around the world.

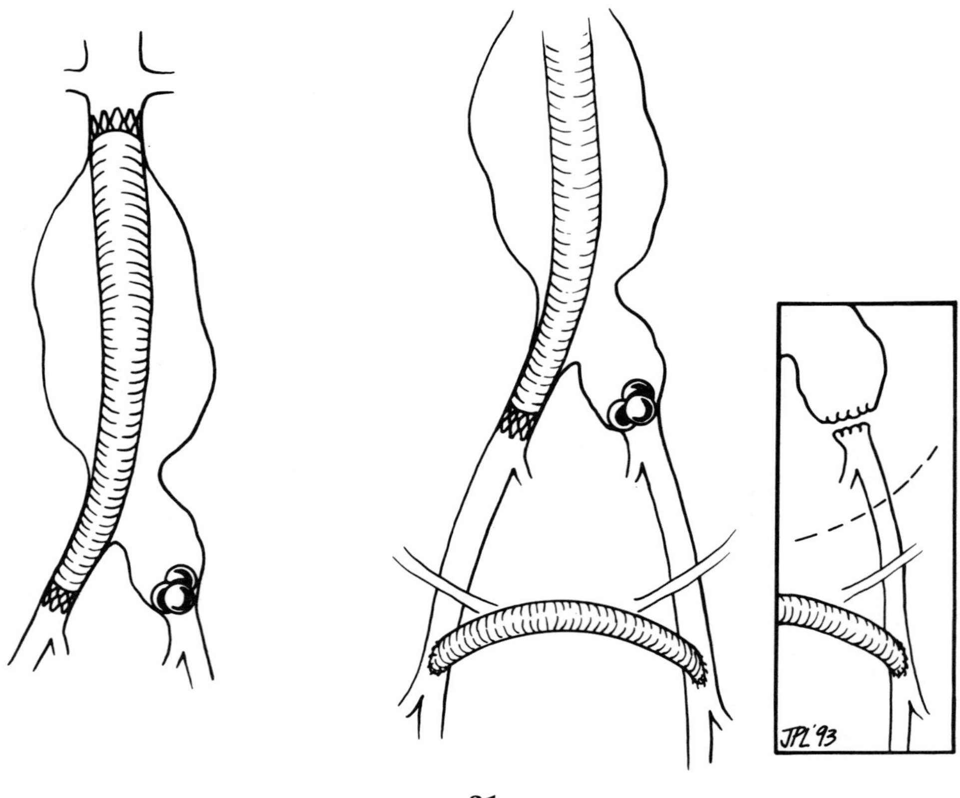

31

Acknowledgement

We would like to thank Joyce P. Lavery, MFA for all the fine drawings in this chapter.

References

Criado, F. J., Queral, L. A., Patten, P. *et al.* (1993). The role of endovascular therapy in lower extremity revascularization: lessons learned and current strategies. *International Angiography* **12**, 221.

Dotter, C. T. and Judkins, M. P. (1964). Transluminal treatment of arteriosclerotic obstruction: description of a new technique and a preliminary report of its application. *Circulation* **30**, 654.

Gruntzig, A. and Hopff, H. (1974). Perkutane rekanalixation chronischer arterieller: verschlusse miteinem nellen dilatation—skatheter modification der dotterechnik. *Dtsch Med Wochenscher* **9**, 2502.

Johnston, K. W. (1992) Factors that influence the outcome of aortoiliac and femoropopliteal percutaneous transluminal angioplasty. *Surgical Clinics of North America* **72**, 843.

Parodi, J. C., Criado, F. J., Barone, H. D. *et al.* (1994). Endoluminal aortic aneurysm repair utilizing the Parodi balloon-expandable stent-graft device: a progress report. *Annals of Vascular Surgery* (in press).

Palmaz, J. C., Laborde, J. C., Rivera, F. J. *et al.* (1992). Stenting of the iliac arteries with the palmaz stent: experience from a multicenter trial. *Cardiovascular Interventional Radiology* **15**, 291.

Weller, B. F. (1989). "Crackers, breakers, stretchers, drillers, scrapers, shavers, burners, welders, and melters"—the future treatment of atherosclerotic coronary artery disease? A clinical–morphologic assessment. *Journal of the American College of Cardiologists* **13**, 969.

Transfemoral intraluminal graft implantation for abdominal aortic aneurysms

JUAN C. PARODI MD

Chief, Department of Vascular Surgery, Instituto Cardiovascular de Buenos Aires, Buenos Aires, Argentina and Adjunct Associate Professor of Surgery, Bowman Gray School of Medicine, Wake Forest University, Winston–Salem, North Carolina, USA

Introduction

Dacron replacement of abdominal aortic aneurysm has followed an established technique since Dubost's first operation with homograft in 1952. The procedure involves a generous incision and related hospital stay. Improvements in materials, anaesthetic and surgical techniques have led to a fairly safe procedure today. Nonetheless, in some cases where the aneurysm is large and there are associated morbid conditions the attendant risks of surgical intervention are prohibitive. Alternative treatment in these cases includes the exclusion technique followed by extra-anatomical bypass (Blaisdell, Hall and Thomas, 1965). Others have combined this approach with catheter occlusion techniques. These alternatives have neither eliminated the risk of rupture nor decreased the incidence of mortality (Schemzer, Papa and Miller, 1985; Kwamm and Dahl, 1984).

Rapid development of endovascular techniques and instrumentation have given rise to the development of a transluminal graft technique in the treatment of an abdominal aortic aneurysm in patients who are poor surgical risks.

Principles and justification

Indications

The sole indication for this procedure is confined to those patients for whom conventional open surgical intervention represents an excessive risk. With increasing experience and extended follow-up demonstrating the safety and patency of these grafts, the procedure may also be extended to patients who are considered for elective replacement of an abdominal aortic aneurysm.

Certain anatomical conditions should be present to make the procedure technically feasible, these are: (1) a proximal and distal neck (or cuff) of more than 2 cm; (2) a suitable iliac axis and at least one patent iliac artery. The iliac artery should be more than 7 mm in diameter with a straight or nearly straight axis.

Preoperative

Assessment

In addition to routine studies to evaluate patients for aortic surgery, all patients require infusion computed tomographic (CT) scanning and complete arteriography. For precision diameter measurement the CT scan slices should be set at 5 mm intervals. Three-dimensional reconstruction, particularly with the spiral CT scanning method, will help to evaluate the diameter and length of both the neck and distal aorta. Arteriography will identify accurately the neck of the aneurysm and its proximity to orifices of the renal artery and the actual length of the aorta measured from the renal arteries to the aortic bifurcation. The status of the visceral artery, the presence of a meandering mesenteric artery or dual renal artery, and the patency of the inferior mesenteric artery arc also best assessed by arteriography. Arteriography also gives vital information about the status of the iliac artery and its patency.

Instrumentation

The device consists of a graft-stent combination. This technique is based on the concept that stents may be used in place of sutures to fix the proximal and distal ends of a fabric graft along the length of the aneurysm. Experimental studies have shown that stents could replace surgical sutures and could act as a friction seal to fix the ends of a graft to the vessel wall. These friction seals were developed by creating a transluminal graft-stent combination, by suturing a modified Palmaz balloon expandable stent on the particle overlapping ends of a tubular, knitted Dacron graft. This was done so that stent expansion would press the graft against the aortic wall, creating a watertight seal.

1

The assembly comprises a balloon expandable stent, 5.5 mm in diameter and 3.5 cm in length. These are stainless steel, modified Palmaz stents. A specially made, thin-walled, crimped knitted Dacron graft (Barone Industries, Buenos Aires, Argentina) is sutured to the stents, overlapping half of the length of the stent.

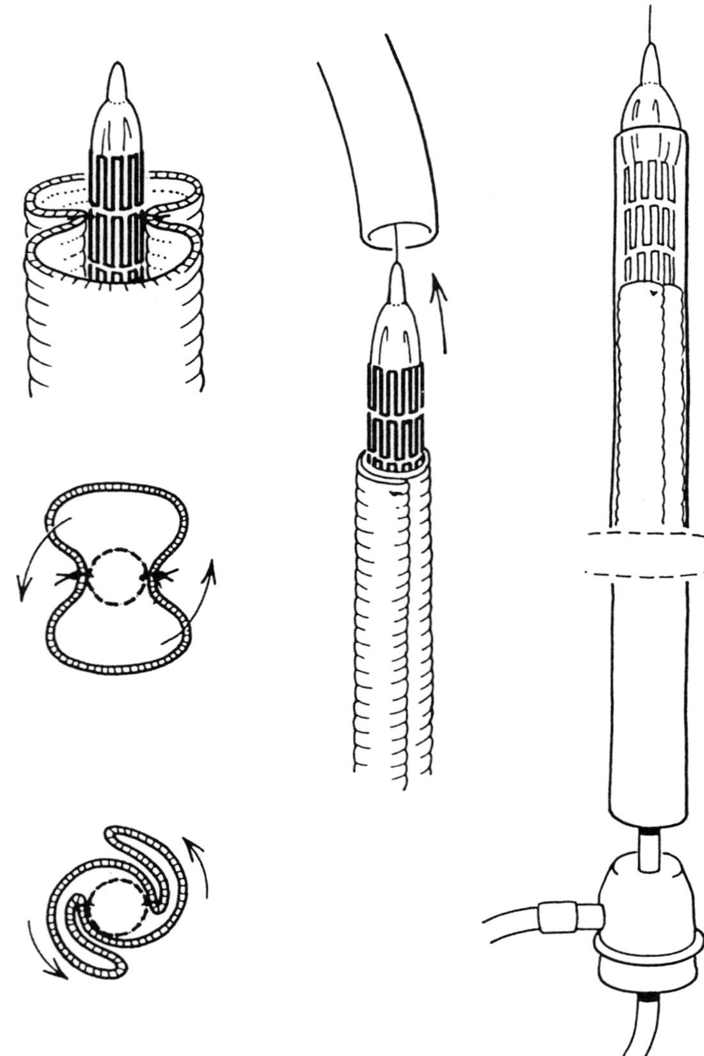

1

Patient preparation

The procedure should be performed in an operating room equipped with fluoroscopic equipment. A mobile C-Arm image intensifier providing real-time digital subtraction with instantaneous replay of each digital exposure and roadmapping is ideal. The patient should be prepared and draped as for aortic surgery. The anaesthesia team should be alerted about the possibility of immediate surgical intervention.

Operation

2

Incision

Under local anaesthesia, the common femoral artery is exposed through a standard groin incision. In general, the common femoral artery is chosen on the side of the iliac artery with a straighter course and with fewer atherosclerotic changes.

Once 5000 i.v. units of heparin has been given, an 18-gauge Cournand needle is introduced and manoeuvred cephalad into the common femoral artery. A soft-tip (0.38 inch) guidewire is advanced through the needle into the distal thoracic aorta, and a 5-French pigtail catheter is introduced over the guidewire. When the catheter is positioned in the visceral segment of the abdominal aorta, the guidewire is withdrawn and preoperative arteriography performed. The pigtail catheter has radio-opaque calibrations at 20 mm intervals. In order to obtain measurements from the arteriogram, a radio-opaque rule is placed behind the patient parallel to the axis of the aorta.

When the intraoperative measurements have been compared with those determined properatively, an endoluminal device of suitable size is selected. The graft overlaps the proximal stent by one-half and is attached to it using braided, synthetic suture material.

After the stent has been mounted over the balloon, the graft is folded (as shown in *Illustration 1*) and the entire assembly is introduced into an 18-French polytetrafluoroethylene sheath through a transverse arteriotomy.

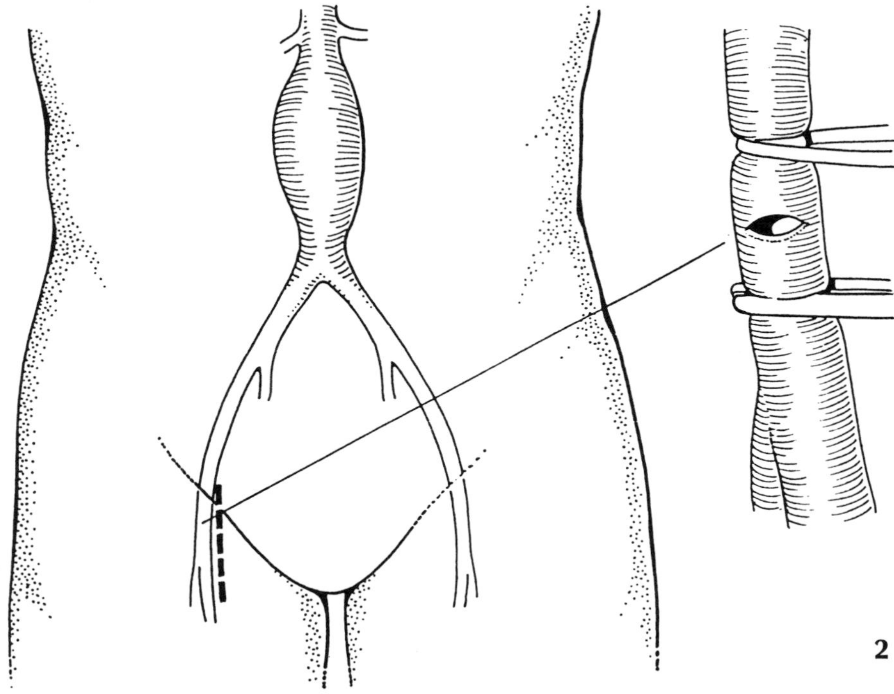

2

3a, b & c

A guidewire is reintroduced, the pigtail catheter is removed, and the wire is replaced with a super-stiff wire. The sheath containing the device is advanced over the wire to the level of the proximal neck of the aneurysm. The sheath is then removed, leaving the graft, stent and balloon in the aortic lumen. Attention is now paid to lowering blood pressure. The author prefers to keep mean blood pressure below 80 mmHg by intravenous infusion of glyceryl trinitrate. When blood pressure is stable at this value, the proximal balloon is inflated for less than 1 min to a volume necessary to achieve an appropriate diameter for that particular patient. In order to create a perfectly cylindrical stent, the balloon can be reinflated at both ends of the stent. Occasionally, the stent shape must be adapted to an irregular aneurysm neck by repeated low pressure inflations along the entire length of the stent.

After the proximal stent has been deployed, the balloon is inflated along the shaft of the graft to distend it under low pressure. Provided all previous measurements were correct, the distal radio-opaque calibrations on the graft should be level with the aortic bifurcation. A second stent is then applied to the distal end to establish a seal preventing reflux around the graft. A completion aortogram is then obtained by introducing an arteriographic catheter over the guidewire. Arteriography confirms the success of the procedure and patency of the renal arteries. The guidewire and overlying catheter are removed and the arteriotomy is then closed with 6/0 polypropylene suture. Extreme care is taken to ensure complete haemostasis.

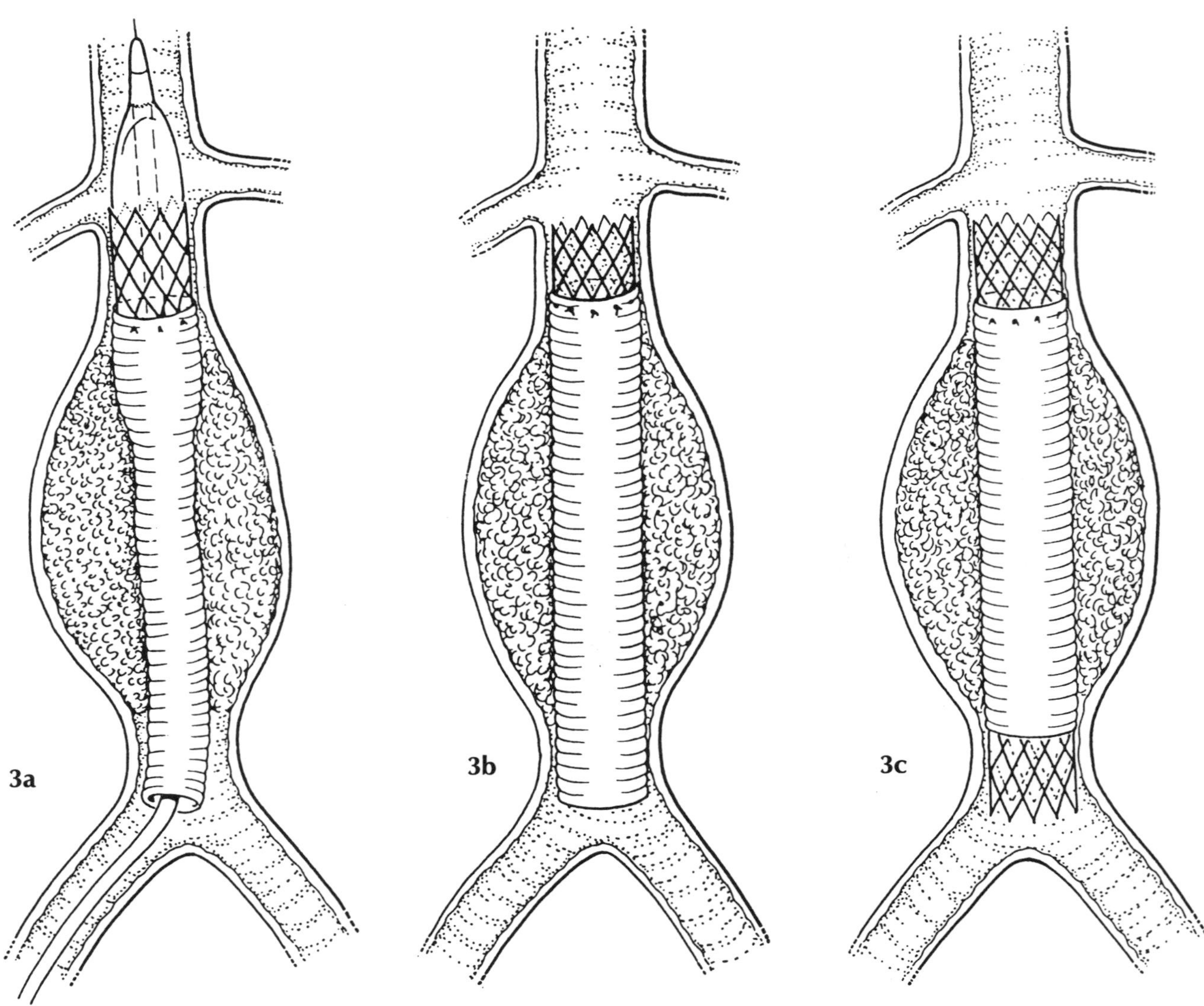

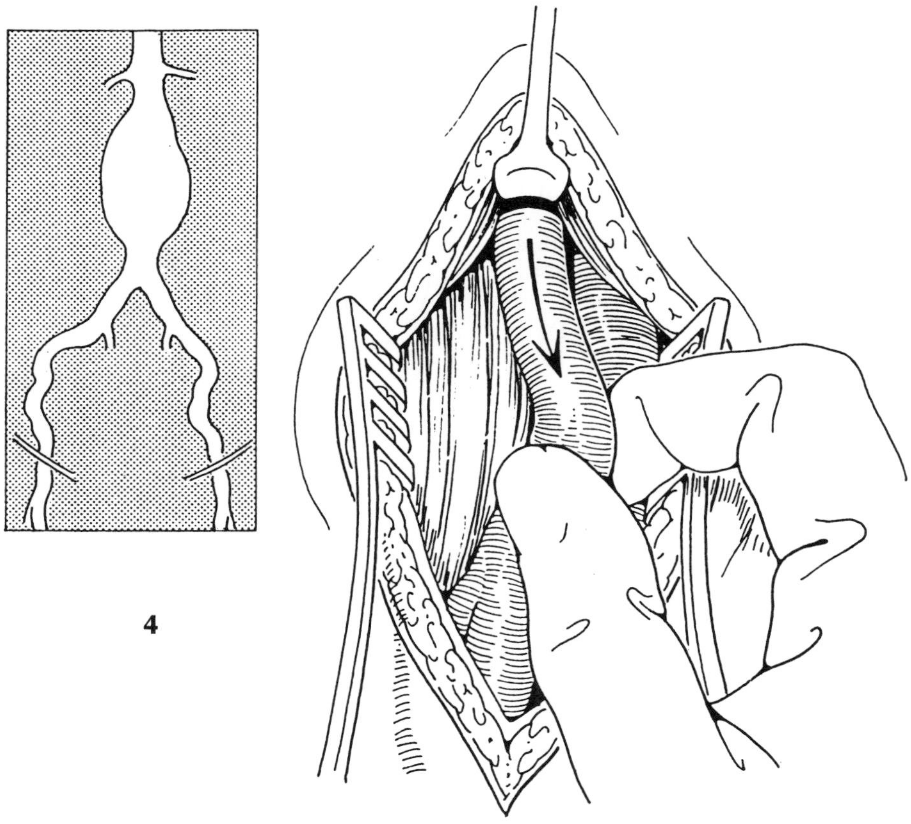

4

4

When both iliac arteries are very tortuous, a 'pull-down manoeuvre' can be employed. This involves circumferential dissection of the common femoral artery. By ligating some of the small branches, the external artery is then dissected bluntly. By this means the external iliac artery can be freed of the surrounding tissue and a gentle pull caudad will straighten the course of the artery and ease instrumentation.

5a, b

If the above manoeuvre fails to allow passage of the device to the aorta, the alternative would be a separate incision above the tortuous area. A transverse incision similar to that required for kidney transplantation will expose the common iliac artery. A Dacron graft is then anastomosed end-to-side as shown and is tunnelled to the groin area where its distal end is externalized for instrumentation.

The defect in the common iliac artery is repaired with a patch graft subsequent to completion of the aortic procedure.

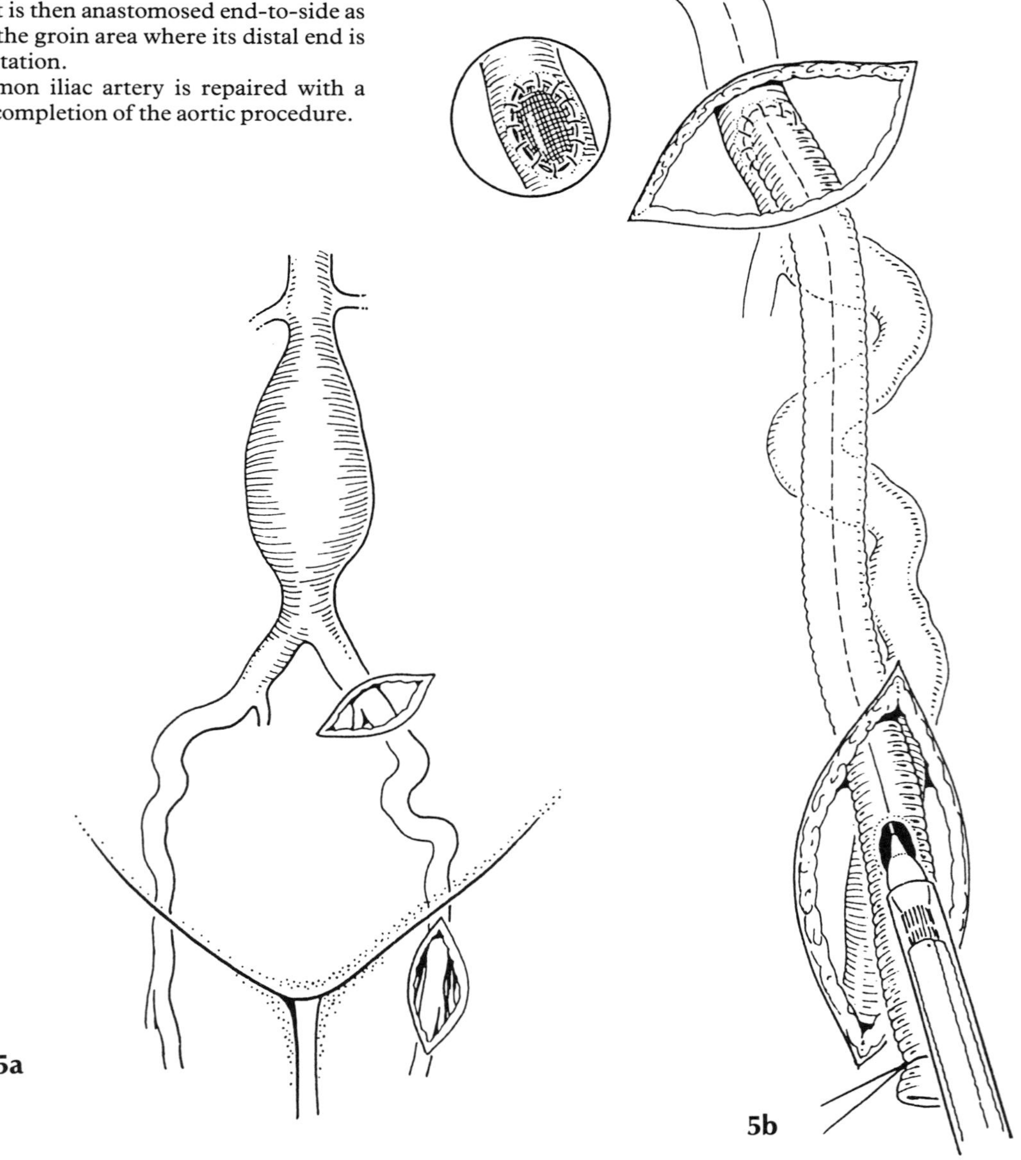

Postoperative

Postoperative care is as for any aortic procedure. Patency of the graft is assessed by measuring ankle pressure. Evidence of microembolization must be sought. Special attention must be paid to urine output because proximity of the device to the renal artery may cause a problem. When the patient walks, an infusion CT scan is obtained to confirm correct placement of the graft. Arteriography, if required can give further information. Patients require close monitoring during the first postoperative year and should undergo repeated CT scanning.

References

Berguer, R., Schneider, J. and Wilner, H. I. (1978). Induced thrombosis of inoperable abdominal aortic aneurysm. *Surgery* **84**, 425.

Blaisdell, F. W., Hall, A. D. and Thomas, A. N. (1965). Ligation treatment of an abdominal aortic aneurysm. *American Journal of Surgery* **109**, 560.

Dubost, C., Allary, M. and Oeconomos, N. (1952). Resection of an aneurysm of the abdominal aorta re-establishment of continuity by preserved human arterial graft with results after 5 months. *Archives of Surgery* **64**, 405.

Kwamm, J. H. M. and Dahl, R. K. (1984). Fatal rupture after successful surgical thrombosis of an abdominal aortic aneurysm. *Surgery* **95**, 235.

Laborde, J. C., Parodi, J. C., Clem, M. F. *et al.* (1992). Intraluminal bypass of abdominal aortic aneurysm: feasibility study. *Radiology* **194**, 185.

Parodi, J. C., Palmaz, J. C., Barone and H. D. (1991). Transfemoral intesluminal graft implantation for abdominal aortic aneurysm. *Annals of Vascular Surgery* **5**, 491.

Schemzer, H., Papa, M. C. and Miller, C. M. (1985). Rupture of surgically thromboses abdominal aortic aneurysm. *Journal of Vascular Surgery* **2**, 278.

Transfemoral endovascular repair of abdominal aortic aneurysm using the endovascular graft system device

WESLEY S. MOORE MD
UCLA Medical Center, Los Angeles, USA

Introduction

Approximately 40 000 patients undergo elective abdominal aortic aneurysm repair in the USA each year. In spite of this, approximately 15 000 patients die from ruptured abdominal aortic aneurysm on an annual basis. This makes ruptured abdominal aortic aneurysm the fourteenth leading cause of death in the USA. Efforts to reduce this continued mortality risk from aneurysm rupture would include the introduction of population screening with ultrasound and the willingness to offer elective aneurysm repair to good risk patients with aneurysms both larger and smaller than the conventional 5.0 cm diameter cut-point.

Currently, elective repair of abdominal aortic aneurysm can be done with a mortality of <3.0% in centres of excellence. However, community-wide studies have shown that mortality for elective abdominal aortic aneurysm repair is probably in the range of 10–14% (Veith *et al.*, 1991). This relatively high mortality rate has an adverse effect on the risk/benefit ratio for operating on small aneurysms.

The introduction of the concept of endovascular repair of abdominal aortic aneurysm may alter the current scepticism concerning repair of small abdominal aortic aneurysm as well as making repair of larger aneurysms simpler and safer.

Through the years, there have been several experimental attempts at endovascular aneurysm repair (Cragg *et al.*, 1993; Balko *et al.*, 1986). With the first documented clinical application of this technique by Parodi in 1991, the concept became a reality (Parodi, Palmaz and Barone, 1991). Parodi has accumulated a wide experience, primarily in Argentina, but also in other centres around the world as his device has been applied on a compassionate use basis.

Several other investigators have developed similar techniques, and the first device to receive Federal Drug Administration (FDA) approval for clinical investigation in the United States was the endovascular graft system (EGS) system introduced by EndoVascular Technologies. A Phase 1 trial was begun in the USA with the first implantation performed at UCLA Medical Center on 10 February 1993. As Phase 1 implant patients rapidly accumulated and were found to be successful, we are now making preparation for Phase 2, which will be a prospective randomized trial comparing conventional repair with endovascular repair.

The objective of this chapter will be to present a detailed description of the technical aspects of implantation.

Patient evaluation

At the present time, the current graft configuration is suitable for those patients whose aneurysm is limited to the infrarenal abdominal aorta and can be repaired with a tube graft implantation. The anatomic requirements include a sufficient length of neck between the lowest renal artery and the beginning of the aneurysm, and a sufficient neck length at the distal extent of the aneurysm, proximal to the iliac bifurcation. The diameter of the proximal and distal neck must not exceed 24 mm, which is the current upper limit of available graft size. It is preferable to have an occluded inferior mesenteric artery. If patent, there should be no evidence that the inferior mesenteric artery provides collateral blood flow to a compromised coeliac or superior mesenteric artery circulation.

Evaluation of a prospective patient includes a computed tomographic (CT) scan. This provides information concerning the presence of proximal and distal aneurysm neck, neck diameter, and aneurysm size. At the present time, the next step involves obtaining a magnetic resonance imaging/magnetic resonance angiography (MRI/MRA) of the abdominal aorta. This provides a good estimate of what an angiogram would show and permits us to make a final decision before committing the patient to an invasive angiogram. If the first two tests demonstrate suitable anatomy, the final step is a contrast angiogram performed with an angiogram catheter that has radio-opaque marks at 1.0 cm intervals in order to achieve an accurate measurement of both the length and diameter of the graft that will be required.

Once it has been determined that the patient has an aneurysm of appropriate anatomic characteristics, preparation is made for operation. Repair of the aneurysm must be performed in an operating room by a team that is prepared to convert the operation to a conventional open repair should this become necessary. General anaesthesia is employed. The patient's abdomen and both groins are prepared and surgically draped for either transfemoral repair or transabdominal conventional repair of abdominal aortic aneurysm. Surgical nurses are scrubbed in the usual manner and instrumentation is available as for conventional operation.

We have not found it necessary to have a specially equipped operating room for these procedures. A Skytron 3100 operating table has been quite satisfactory. The mechanics of this table permit horizontal sliding of the tabletop to its full length in order to provide adequate space beneath the table top for the C-arm of a fluoroscopic unit. We have utilized a portable OEC-Biasonics C-arm that has digital imaging and road-map capability. Since this instrument is portable, it can be used in any operating suite for most purposes, including endovascular graft repair.

1a & b

The common femoral artery is exposed through a vertical incision (*1a*). Selection of either the right or left femoral artery is based upon the size and configuration of the iliac artery and its relationship to the aorta in order to make passage of the catheter system as smooth as possible.

The edge of the inguinal ligament is incised. The circumflex branches are divided in order to provide good mobilization of the common femoral artery.

If there is significant tortuosity or redundancy of the iliac artery, this can be straightened out by bluntly mobilizing the external iliac artery and drawing it into the operative field (*1b*).

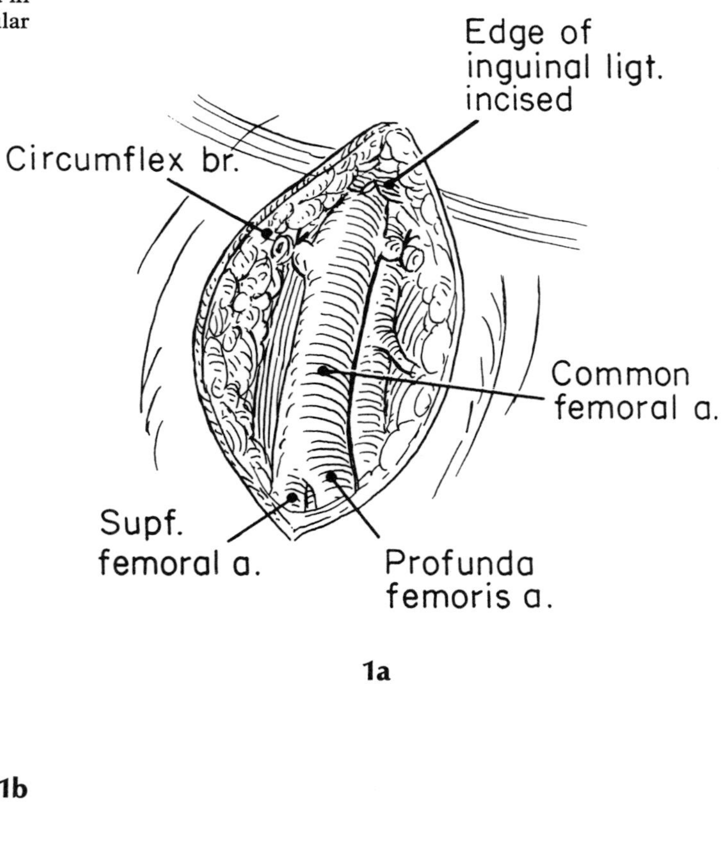

1a

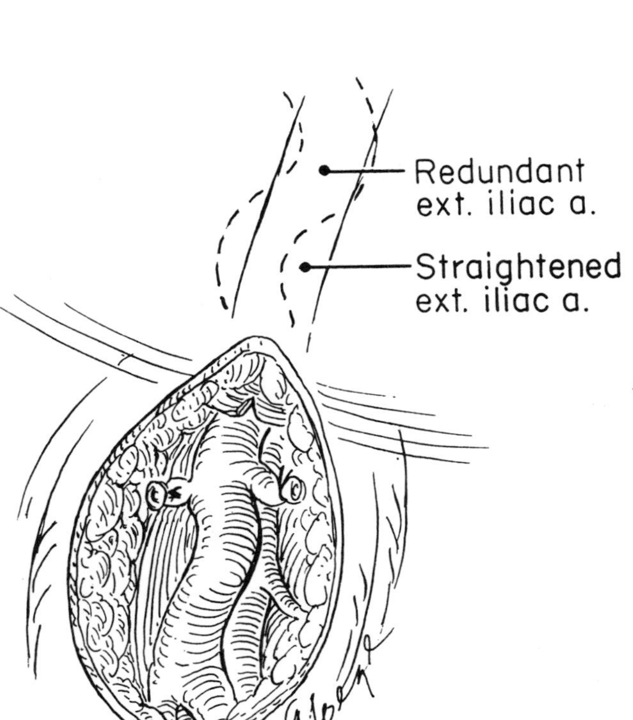

1b

2a & b

The femoral artery is punctured with a 16-gauge needle, and a guidewire is placed through the lumen of the needle (*2a*). The needle is withdrawn, and a 9 French angiogram sheath is passed over the guidewire into the femoral artery and advanced into the external iliac artery under fluoroscopic guidance.

A pigtail angiogram catheter with 1.0 cm radio-opaque marks is then advanced (*2b*) over the guidewire, through the sheath, and into the aorta under fluoroscopic guidance. The catheter tip is manipulated through the aneurysm and positioned in the vicinity of the T12-L1 interspace. A test injection is made with contrast material to determine that the catheter is above the renal arteries. The fluoroscopy tube is appropriately positioned to be certain that the entire extent of the abdominal aorta from renal arteries to iliac bifurcation is centered within the fluoroscopic field of image. An aortogram is then obtained utilizing a pressure injector, and the aortographic image is frozen on the screen using the roadmapping mode.

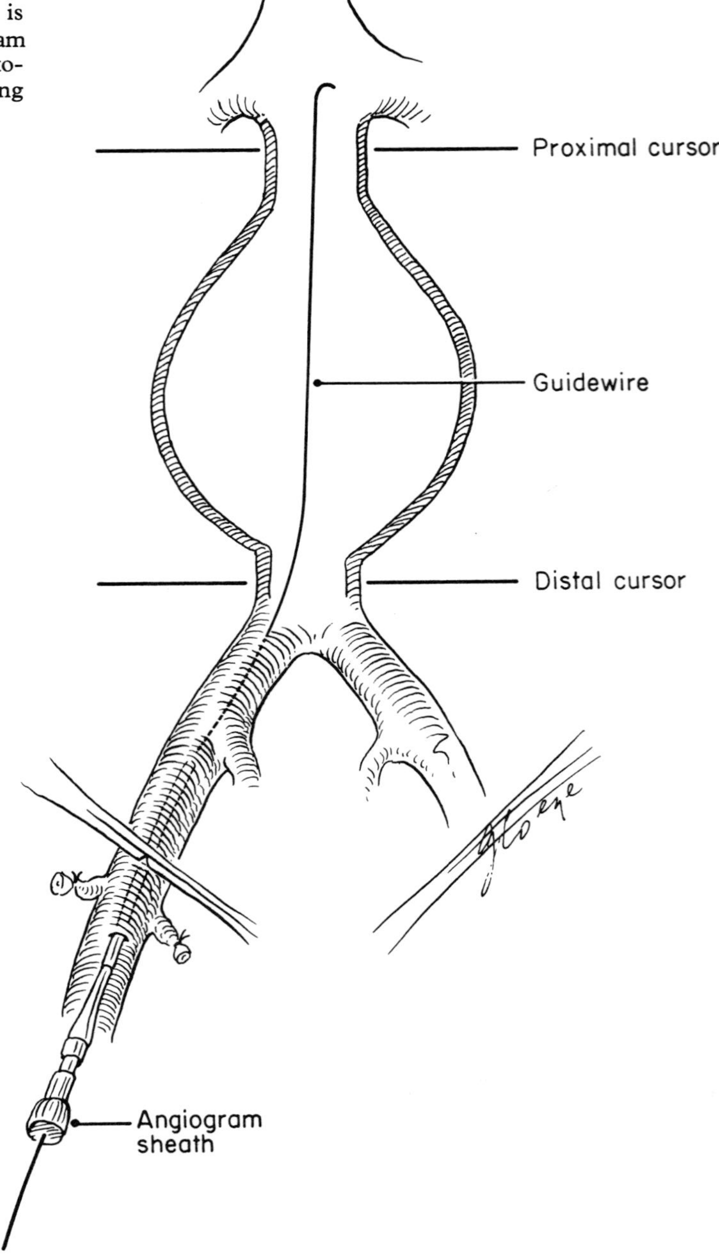

2a

The patient has been positioned on a board that permits the remote movement of horizontal cursor lines that are radio-opaque. The superior line is moved into the optimal point for proximal graft deployment. This should be just below the lowest renal artery. A distal cursor line is positioned in the distal neck of the aneurysm as far proximal from the aortic bifurcation as possible. Ideally, there should be enough length of aorta between the point of distal graft deployment and the aortic bifurcation as possible. This will permit the best positioning of the balloon catheter in order to permit full expansion without encroachment upon the orifice of the iliac artery.

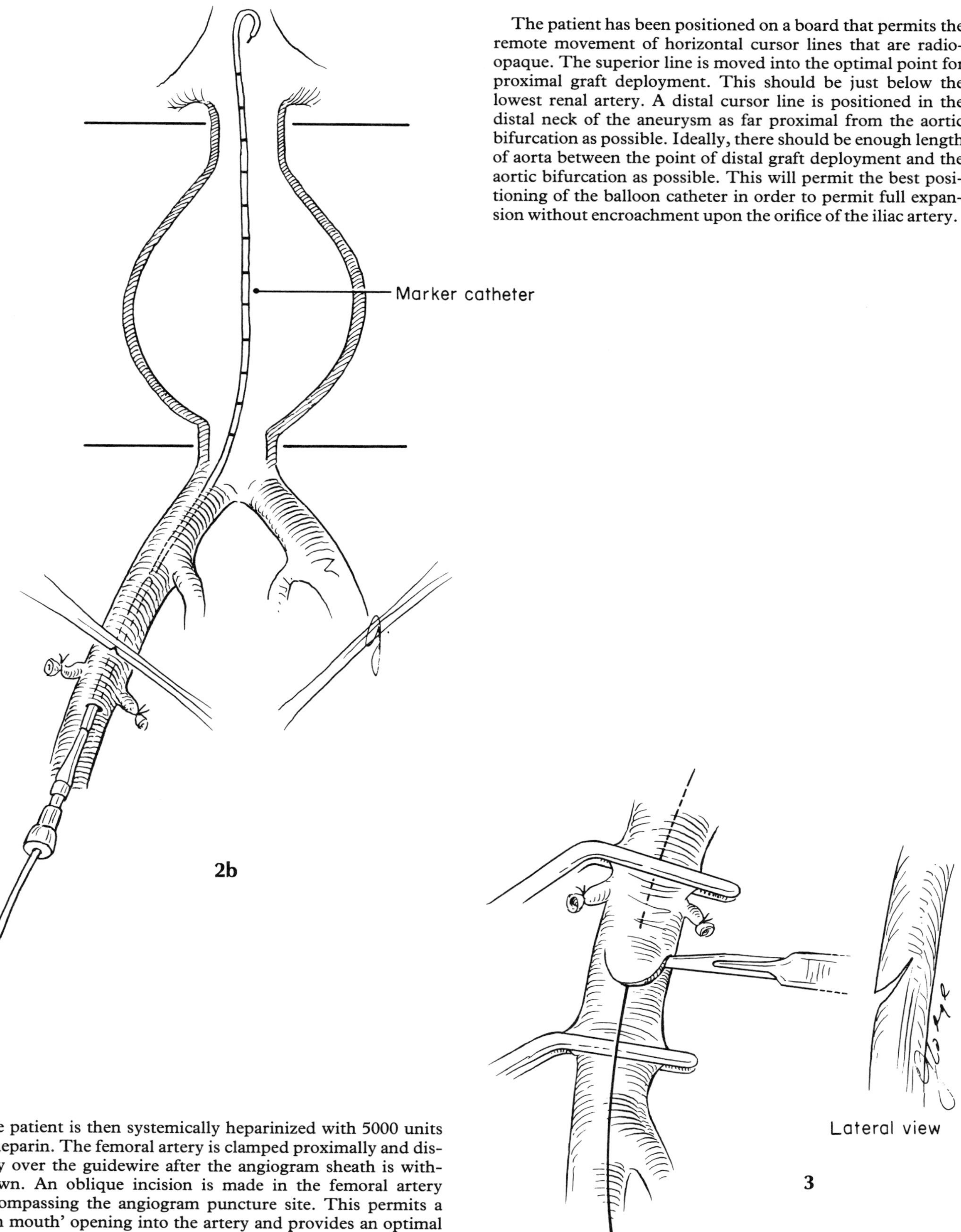

2b

3

3

The patient is then systemically heparinized with 5000 units of heparin. The femoral artery is clamped proximally and distally over the guidewire after the angiogram sheath is withdrawn. An oblique incision is made in the femoral artery encompassing the angiogram puncture site. This permits a 'fish mouth' opening into the artery and provides an optimal aperture for placement of the sheath.

4a & b

A 28F EndoVascular Technologies (EVT) expandable sheath is then passed over the guidewire (*4a*). As the tip of the sheath approaches the femoral artery, the proximal clamp on the femoral artery is removed while maintaining haemostasis by digital compression of the artery. The expandable sheath is then inserted into the femoral artery, over the guidewire, using bi-manual control to minimize blood loss. The sheath is advanced over the guidewire, up the iliac artery, into the aorta, and through the aortic aneurysm approaching the proximal neck.

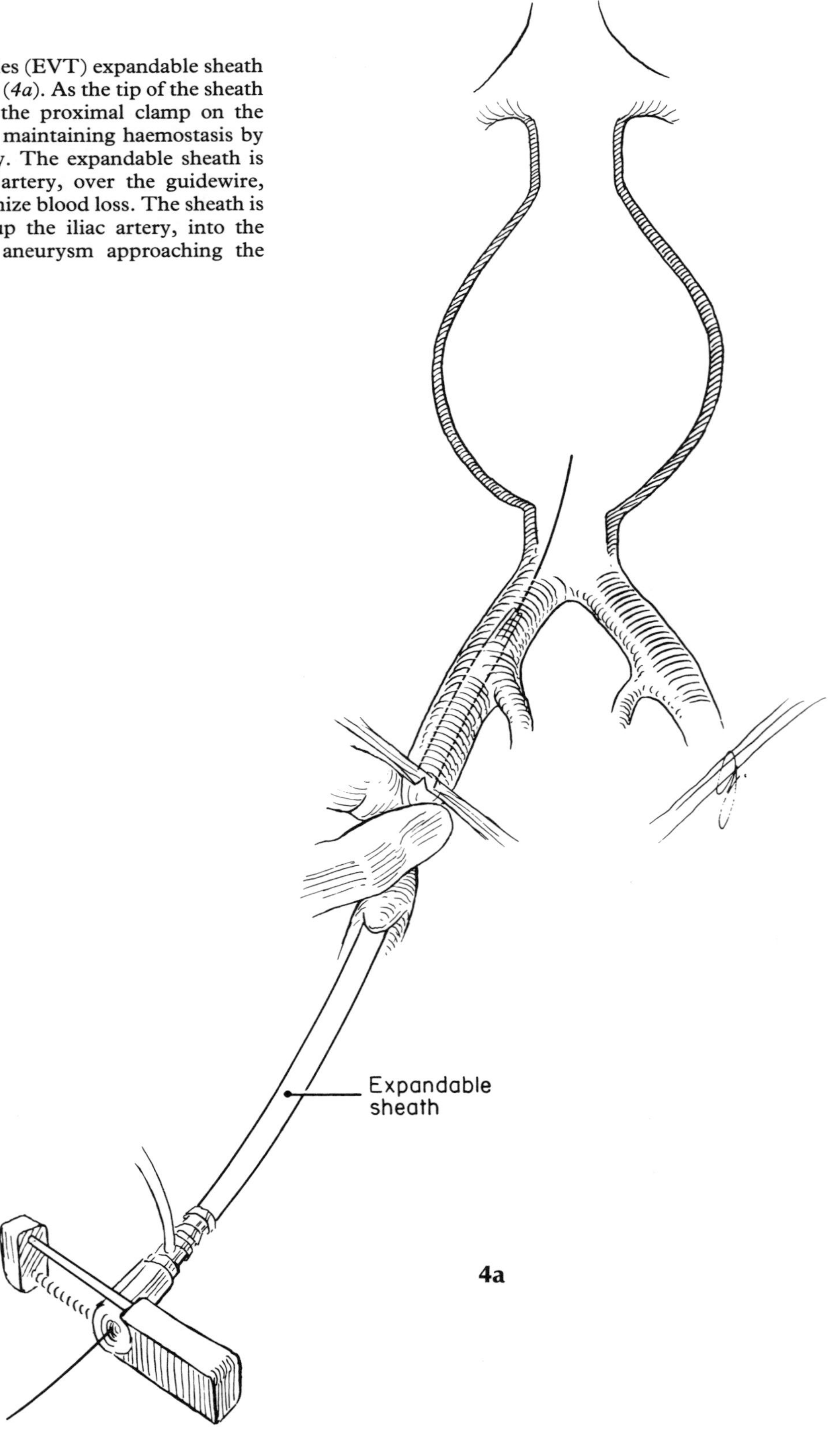

4a

Once the sheath is in place, the obturator within the sheath is fully advanced in order to expand the distal portion of the sheath to its full diameter (*4b*). The obturator and guidewire are then removed from the sheath, and backbleeding through the sheath is controlled with a manually adjustable, iris-type diaphragm.

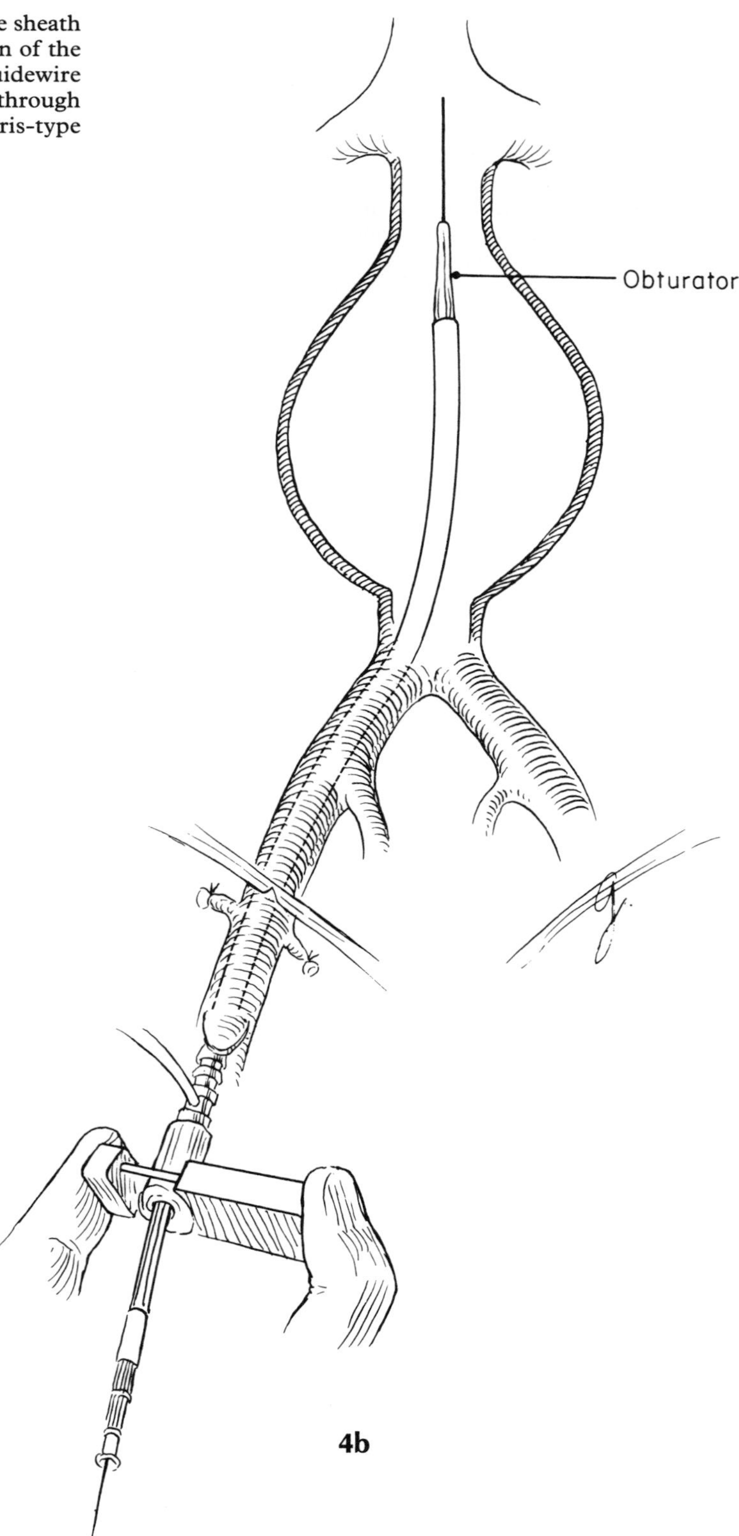

4b

5a & b

Preparation is then made for insertion of the graft deployment catheter system (*5a*). The deployment catheter system has several components, which include a flexible guidewire at its tip, an expandable balloon, and a flexible capsule containing the graft. This co-axial system is then remotely controlled at the handle by the operator. With the assistant pinching the sheath, the iris diaphragm is opened, and the guidewire and co-axial catheter system is inserted into the sheath. As soon as the capsule portion of the catheter delivery system is within the sheath, a haemostatic seal is achieved. The catheter system is then advanced up the sheath under fluoroscopic control.

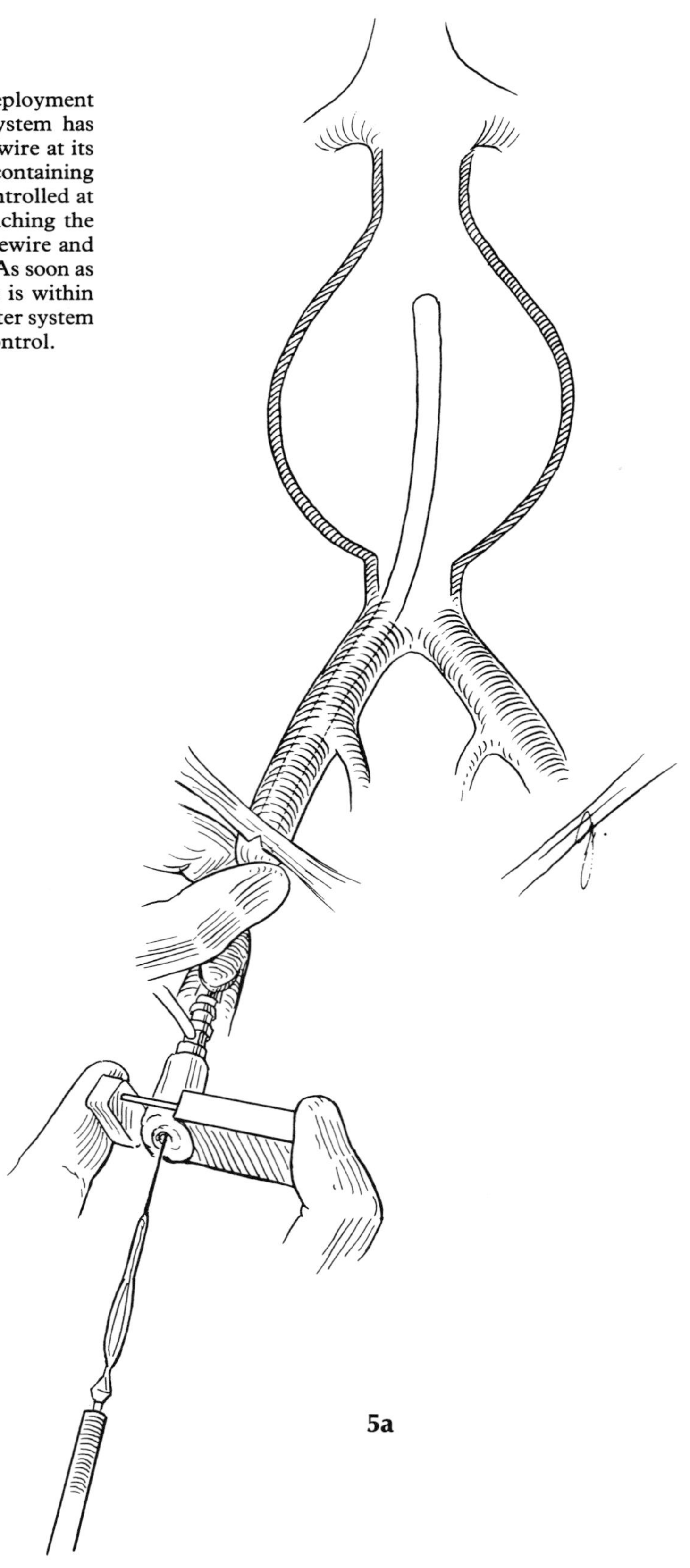

5a

The capsule, which covers the graft, is relatively radiolucent and permits the imaging of the hooks on the proximal and distal stented portion of the graft. The proximal hooks are then positioned opposite the proximal cursor line (*5b*). The distal hooks are then checked for their proximity to the distal cursor line. Final vertical adjustment of graft position takes place at this time in order to be certain that both the proximal and distal points of deployment are optimal.

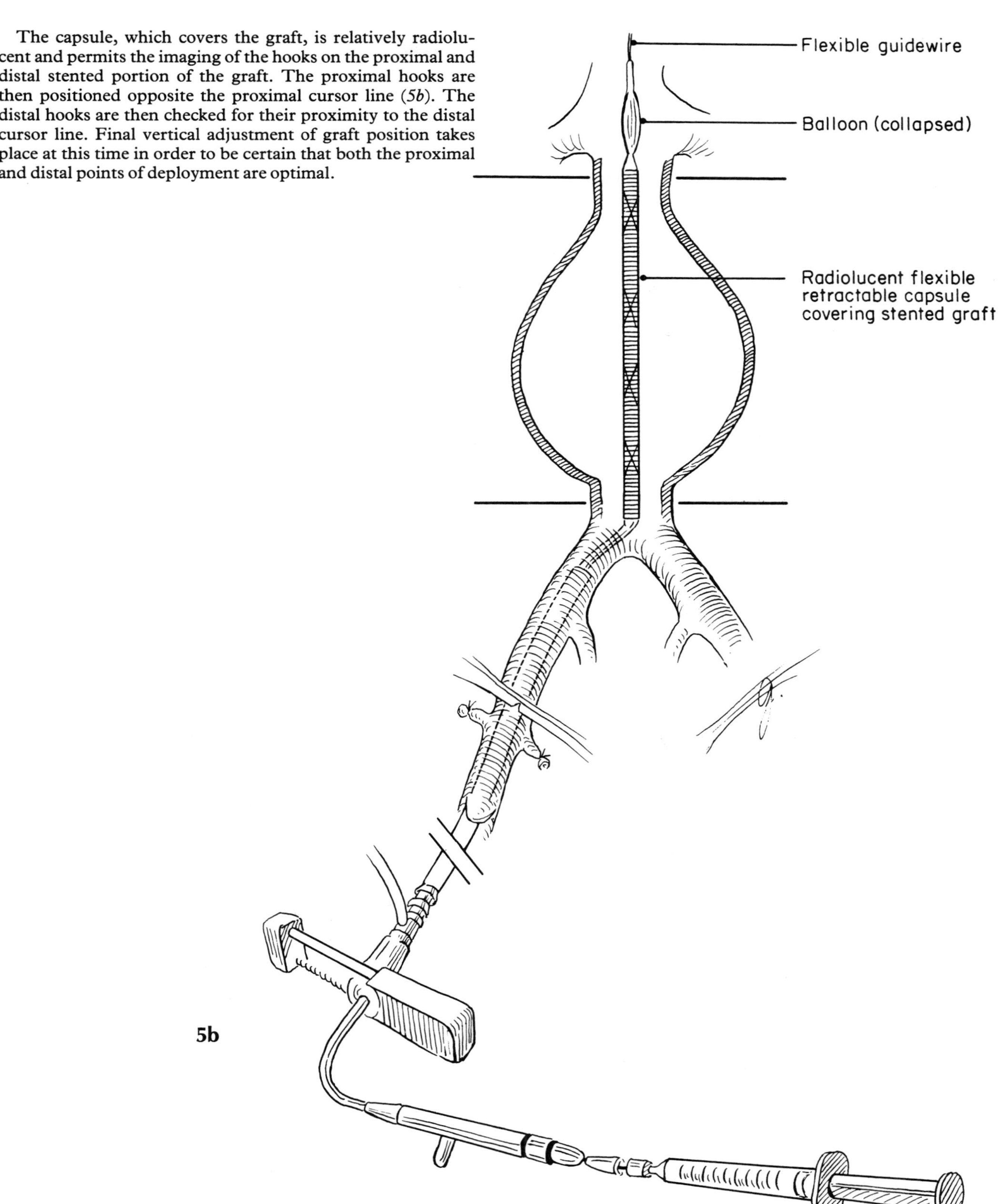

5b

6a & b

The capsule covering the graft is then retracted by turning the knob on the handle of the deployment catheter (*6a*). This is viewed fluoroscopically. Final adjustments are made before the stent on the proximal portion of the graft is allowed to spring open and engage the aorta. Once the operator is certain that the pins on the proximal stent are in the optimal location, final retraction of the sheath takes place, and the graft springs into position.

At this point, the balloon coaxial catheter system is pulled back into position in order to bridge across the proximal stent (*6b*). the balloon is inflated to 2.0 atmospheres of pressure using radio-opaque contrast. The inflation is viewed fluoroscopically within the roadmapped image of the proximal neck of the aorta. The balloon is then deflated, allowing the proximal portion of the graft to fill with pressurized blood. Radio-opaque, longitudinal markers, are then seen to expand along the course of the graft, ensuring that the graft is expanding and that there is no twisting of the prosthesis.

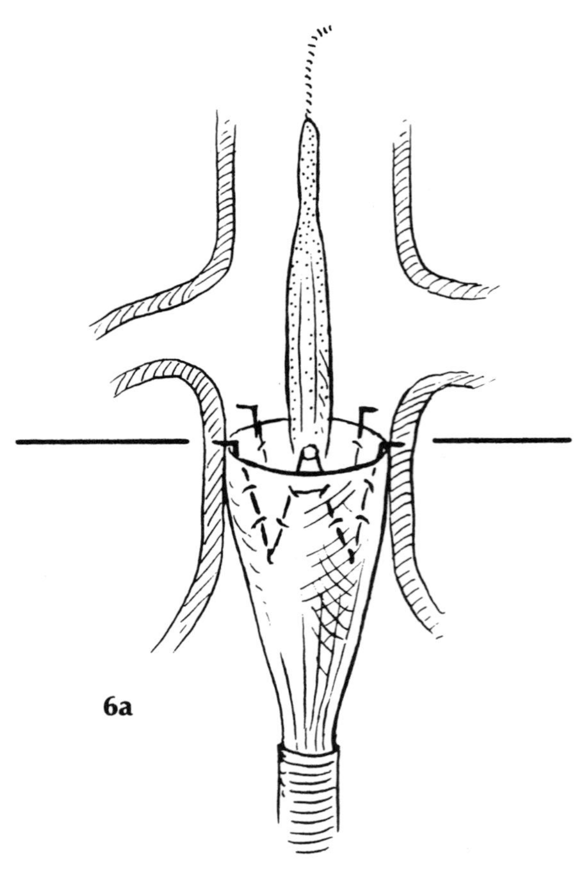

6a

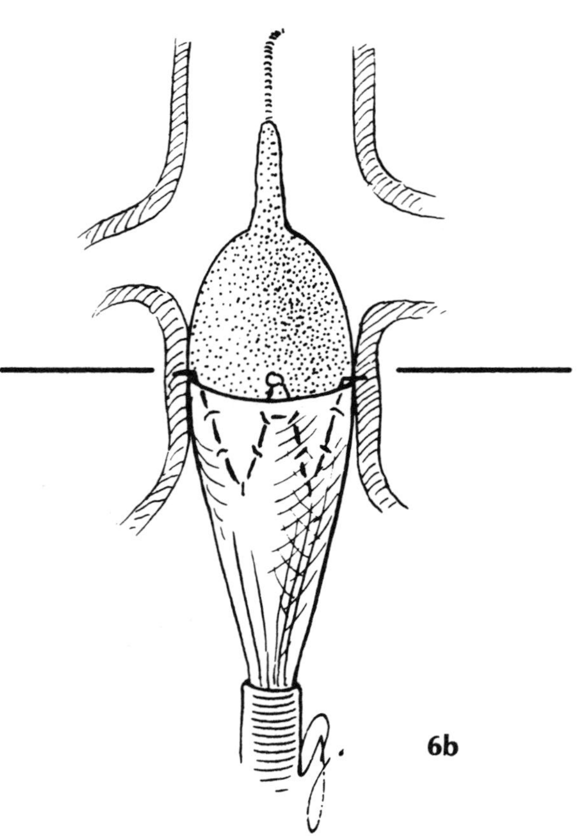

6b

7a & b

Final positioning of the distal stent with respect to the distal cursor line is now possible. If it appears that the hooks of the distal stent are too far distal, an adjustment can be made remotely by the operator. Once optimal positioning is assured, the remaining portion of the capsule is deployed by retracting the catheter delivery system (*7a*). This allows the distal portion of the stented graft to spring into place.

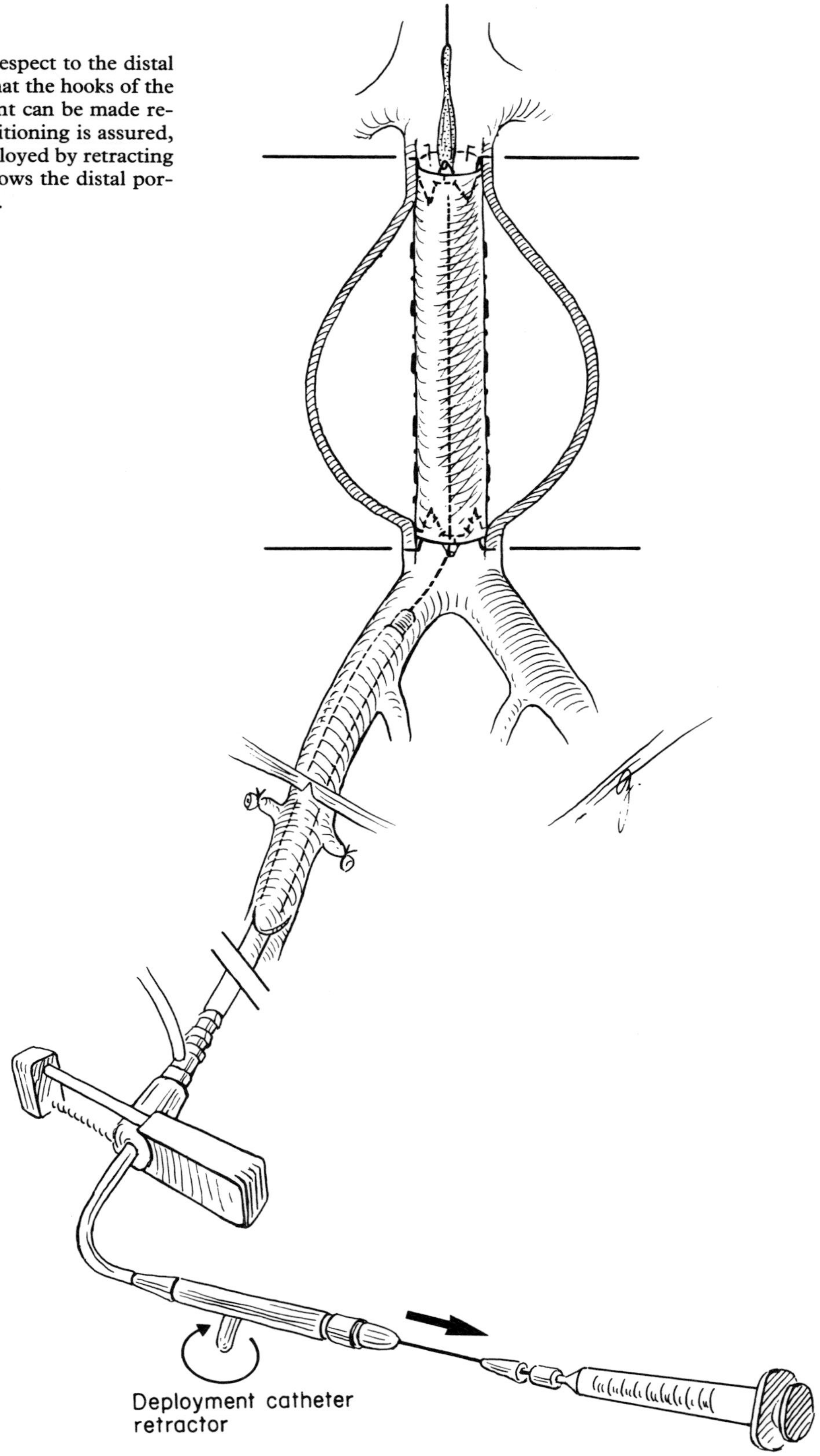

7a

The co-axial balloon catheter system is then drawn into position, and the balloon is inflated in order to seat the pins at the site of distal anastomosis (*7b*).

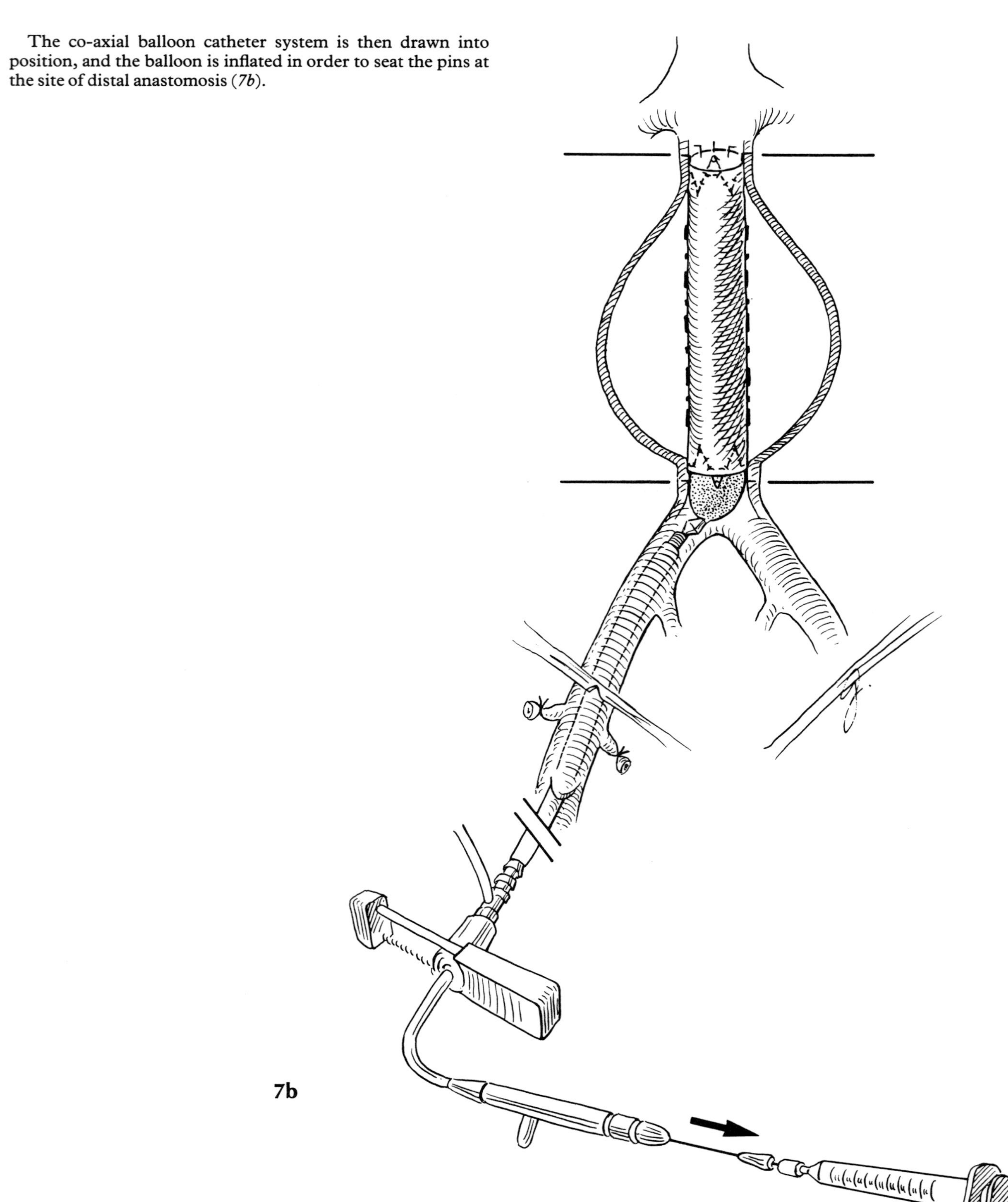

7b

8

The stent deployment catheter is then removed from the sheath.

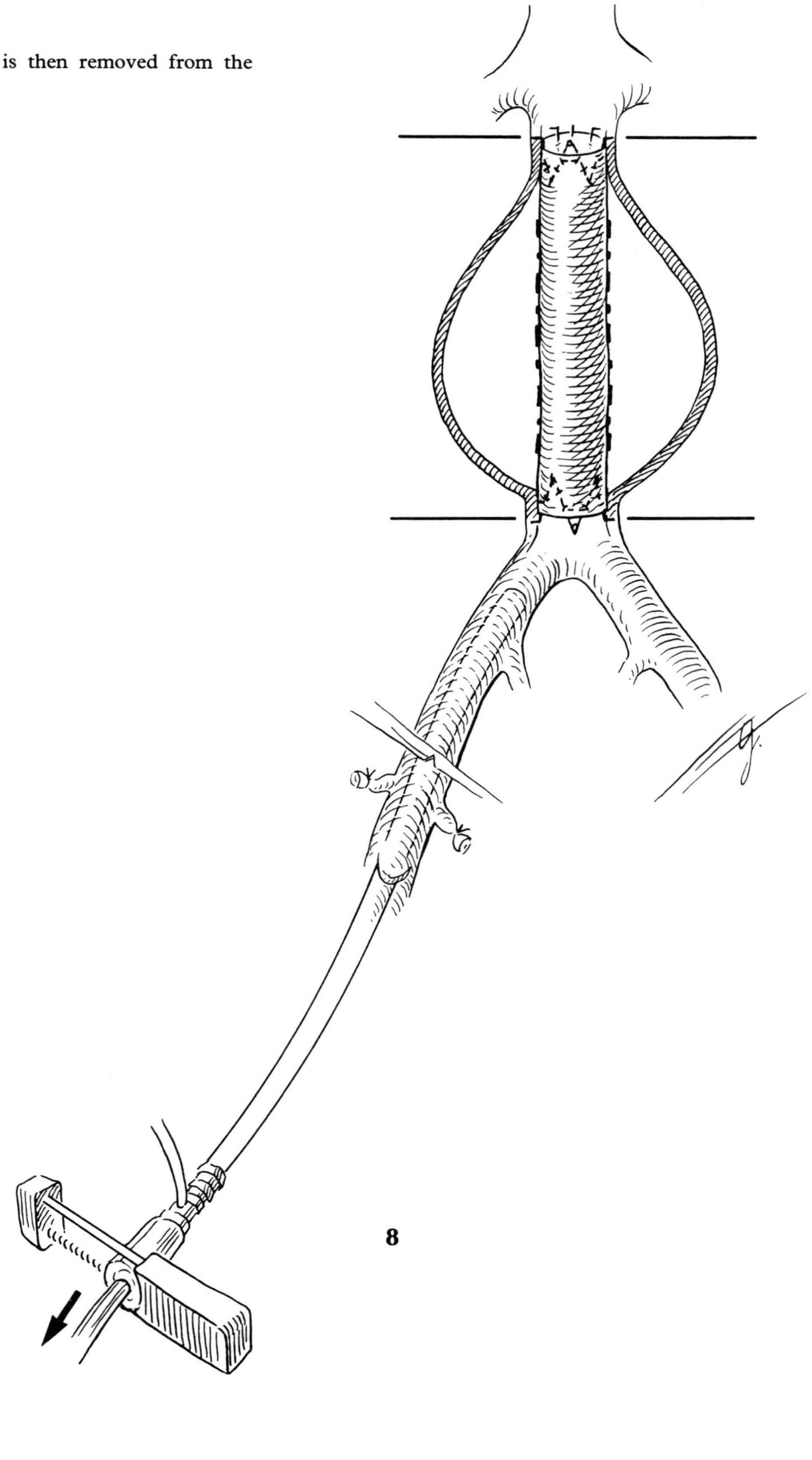

8

9

A pigtail catheter is then inserted over a guidewire into the supra-renal aorta through the graft. A completion angiogram is obtained to verify graft positioning and to be sure that there is no evidence of perigraft leak of contrast into the aneurysm at the anastomotic sites.

9

10

Following removal of the sheath, the arterotomy is closed, and flow to the femoral artery is restored.

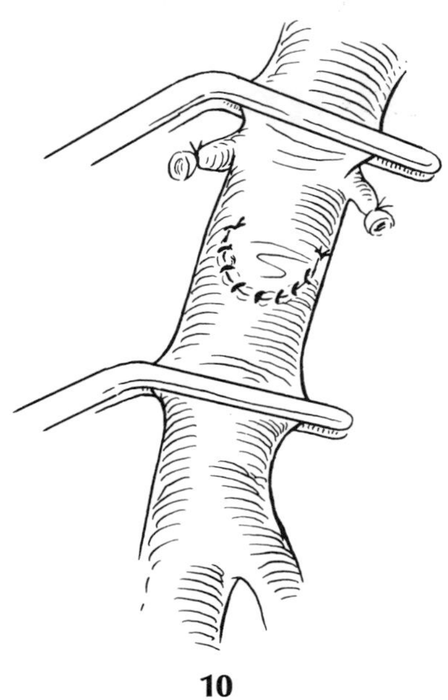

10

Postoperative care

The patient is allowed to wake up in the recovery room, then transferred to regular ward care. An intensive care unit is not necessary. A regular diet is ordered for the evening, and the patient is discharged from the hospital the following day.

Follow-up studies

Prior to discharge, on the first postoperative day, a plain film of the abdomen is obtained for purposes of visualizing the radio-opaque markers along the course of the graft as well as the radio-opaque proximal and distal stents. This then serves as a baseline. A colour-flow duplex scan of the graft is obtained, documenting flow through the graft and determining whether there is evidence of small leak at either the proximal or distal points of fixation in the aorta. Finally, a CT scan is obtained for baseline purposes. These studies are then repeated periodically for the next 2 years as a part of the protocol.

Several questions remain unanswered and can only be documented with continued observation and follow-up. These include the security of fixation. To date, there has been no tendency of any of the prostheses implanted to migrate. It is important that this continue during the life of the patient and the functioning of the graft. Furthermore, it is not known whether the proximal neck of the aorta will continue to expand and possibly pull away from the sites of fixation. Only time will tell. Finally, there is a risk that a patent inferior mesenteric artery, or perhaps even a lumbar artery, may form an important collateral to mesenteric circulation or that the left colon may be dependent upon blood flow through a patent inferior mesenteric artery. The risk of mesenteric ischaemia exists but has not yet been seen. Finally, it is clear that special training must be obtained before a surgical team can begin implantation. The deployment device is relatively complex, and the series of steps that are necessary for implantation are new and unique in the experience of most surgeons. It may well be desirable for the surgeon to work with an interventional radiologist as a team in the placement of these grafts. However, because of the surgical nature of the procedure, including not only the exposure of the femoral artery but the possible need to immediately convert to an open repair of an abdominal aortic aneurysm, the procedure must be done in the operating room with the surgeon in charge of the team.

References

Balko, A., Piosecki, G. J., Shaw, B. M. *et al.* (1986). Transfemoral placement of intralumenal polyurethane prosthesis for abdominal aortic aneurysm. *Journal of Surgical Research* **40**, 305.

Cragg, A., Lund, G., Rysavy, J. *et al.* (1993). Nonsurgical placement of arterial endoprosthesis: A new technique using nitinol wire. *Radiology* **147**, 261.

Parodi, J. C., Palmaz, J. C. and Barone, H. D. (1991). Transfemoral infralumenal graft implantation for abdominal aortic aneurysms. *Annals of Vascular Surgery* **5**, 491.

Veith, F. J., Goldsmith, J., Leather, R. P. and Hannan, E. L. (1991). The need for quality assurance in vascular surgery. *Journal of Vascular Surgery* **13**, 523.

Bifurcated endovascular graft insertion for abdominal aortic aneurysm

TIM CHUTER

College of Physicians and Surgeons of Columbia University, New York, New York, USA

Patient selection

All these procedures are currently performed as part of clinical trials, which adhere to rigid selection criteria. Only patients who would normally be candidates for conventional repair are included. High risk patients and those with small aneurysms are specifically excluded. All patients who satisfy the (CT) computerized tomography and clinical criteria for inclusion in the study have multi-plane arteriography with intra-aortic injection of contrast to assess aortic and iliac arterial anatomy. Anatomic exclusion criteria are: 1. Proximal neck shorter than 20 mm; 2. Iliac artery diameter wider than 20 mm; 3. Iliac artery stenosis with diameter of less than 6 mm; 4. Signs that the inferior mesenteric artery (IMA) is indispensable. These include angiographic visualization of a large IMA, filling of superior mesenteric artery (SMA) via collaterals, stenosis of coeliac or SMA on oblique views.

An additional requirement for insertion of a straight graft is the presence of a distal cuff longer than 15 mm. The rarity of this anatomic feature excludes the vast majority of patients from straight graft repair. Indeed, we have yet to perform a straight graft insertion.

General points

The procedure is performed in the operating room under local anaesthesia, with an anaesthesiologist in attendance. The patient is positioned on a radiolucent operating table to permit fluoroscopic examination of the entire abdomen and groins. A radioopaque ruler under the patient provides a useful frame of reference for fluoroscopy. A high resolution digital imaging system is required to guide placement. Desirable features of the imaging system include last image hold, digital subtraction, roadmapping and hard copy output. Grafts may be inserted from either femoral artery. The main factor that determines the side of insertion is tortuosity or stenosis of the iliac arteries on preoperative angiography.

Bifurcated graft insertion

The lower chest, abdomen and both groins are prepared and draped in the usual sterile fashion. Both common femoral arteries are exposed and dissected free from surrounding structures using standard surgical techniques. A soft, disease free portion of the anterior common femoral artery is selected for arteriotomy on each side. Double looped tapes are used to encircle the common femoral (or distal external iliac artery) at two points proximal to the site of the arteriotomy. Heparin (100 units/kg) is administered by intravenous injection 3 minutes prior to tightening the loops proximally and applying non-crushing vascular clamps distally. A short transverse femoral arteriotomy is used as a means of access to the distal arterial tree on each side. A slightly larger aperture is needed on the side selected for insertion of the delivery system. Following femoral arteriotomy, the steps in bifurcated graft insertion are as follows:

1

Placement of a cross-femoral catheter, using a stone retrieval basket. A guidewire is passed, under fluoroscopic guidance, up the iliac arteries into the aneurysm. A sheath is then inserted over the guidewire. The guidewire is then replaced with a stone retrieval basket. The basket is opened in the aneurysm and pulled back to the orifice of the iliac artery. The cross-femoral catheter is passed over a second guidewire up the contralateral iliac artery into the waiting basket, which is closed and withdrawn. This occasionally requires preliminary manipulation of the guidewire into the basket using curved (visceral) angiographic catheters.

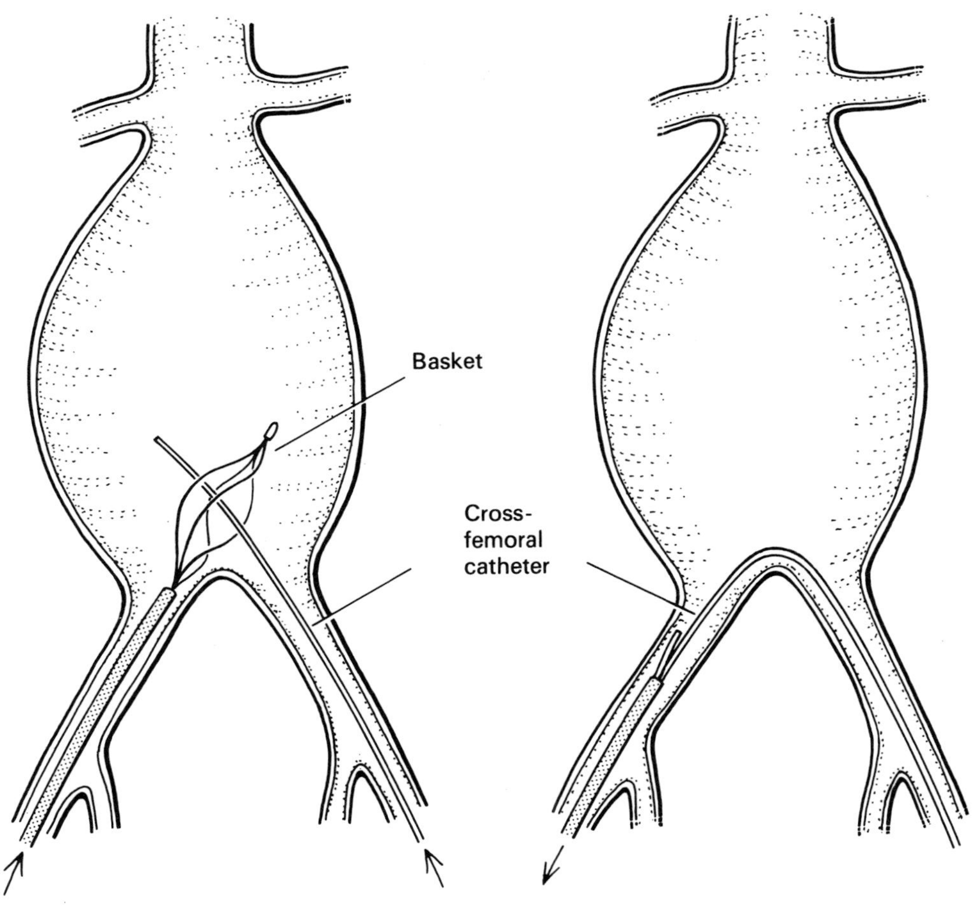

1

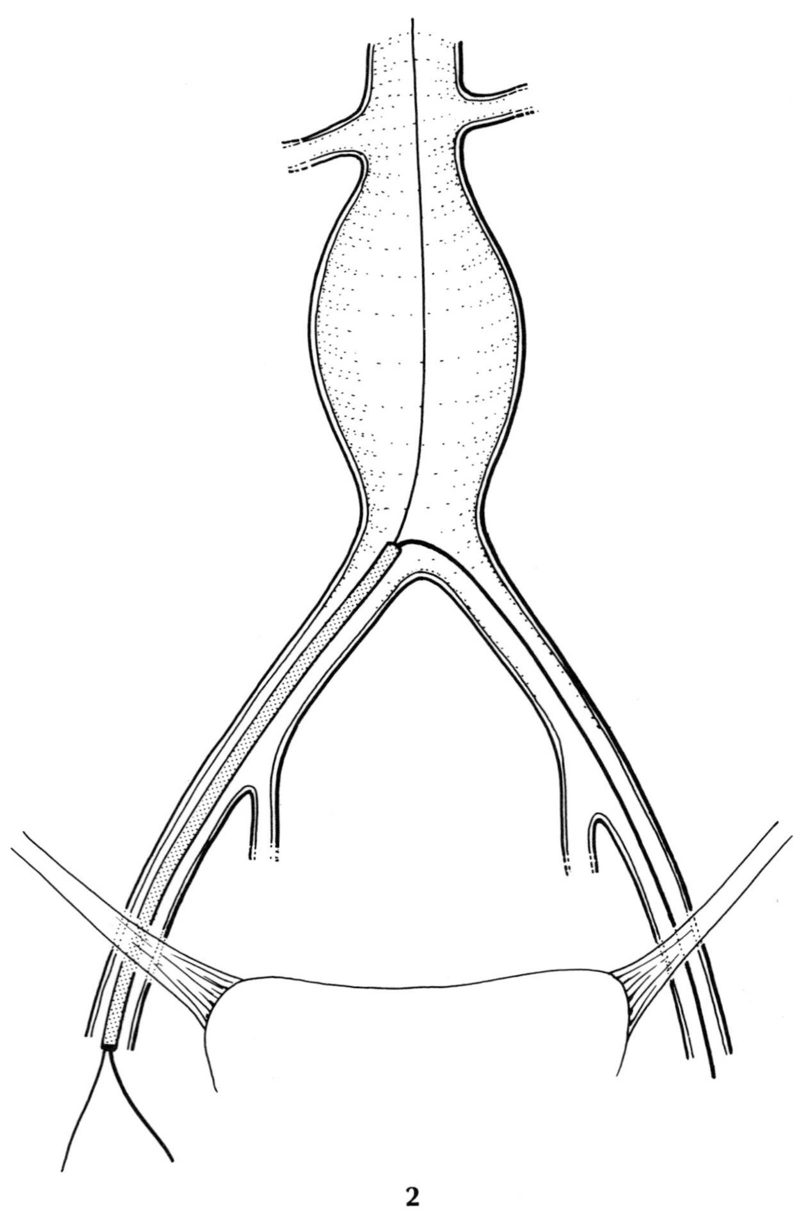

2

2

A double lumen catheter is used to separate the cross-femoral catheter from an angiographic guidewire. This prevents twisting of the catheter and the guidewire, that would later be reflected as twisting of the graft limbs. An angiographic catheter is inserted over the guidewire.

Aortography is used to locate the renal and iliac arteries. These are marked on the video screen, together with markings of the ruler, as a guide to stent/graft placement. Alternatively the angiogram can be stored as a 'road map', to be superimposed on subsequent fluoroscopy. Whatever technique is used, correct positioning of the prosthesis depends on a constant relationship between the imaging system and the patient. If it is necessary to move either the C-arm or the patient, their relative positions can be restored by reference to the markings of the ruler.

The angiographic catheter is exchanged for the delivery system over a stiff guidewire. Markings on the delivery system are used to ensure proper orientation of the graft. The delivery system can be rolled back and forth a little to facilitate introduction, but it should not be rotated continually in the same direction. The delivery system is advanced to bring the proximal stent to its desired location.

3 & 4

The outer sheath of the delivery system is released from the central carrier by advancing the locking ring towards the cranial end of the device (*Illustration 3*).

The graft is extruded by withdrawing the sheath slowly over the carrier. The position of the graft is maintained during graft extrusion by manipulation of the central carrier. Precise control is enhanced by bracing the carrier against the patient's thigh with one hand while the other pulls back the sheath (*Illustration 4*).

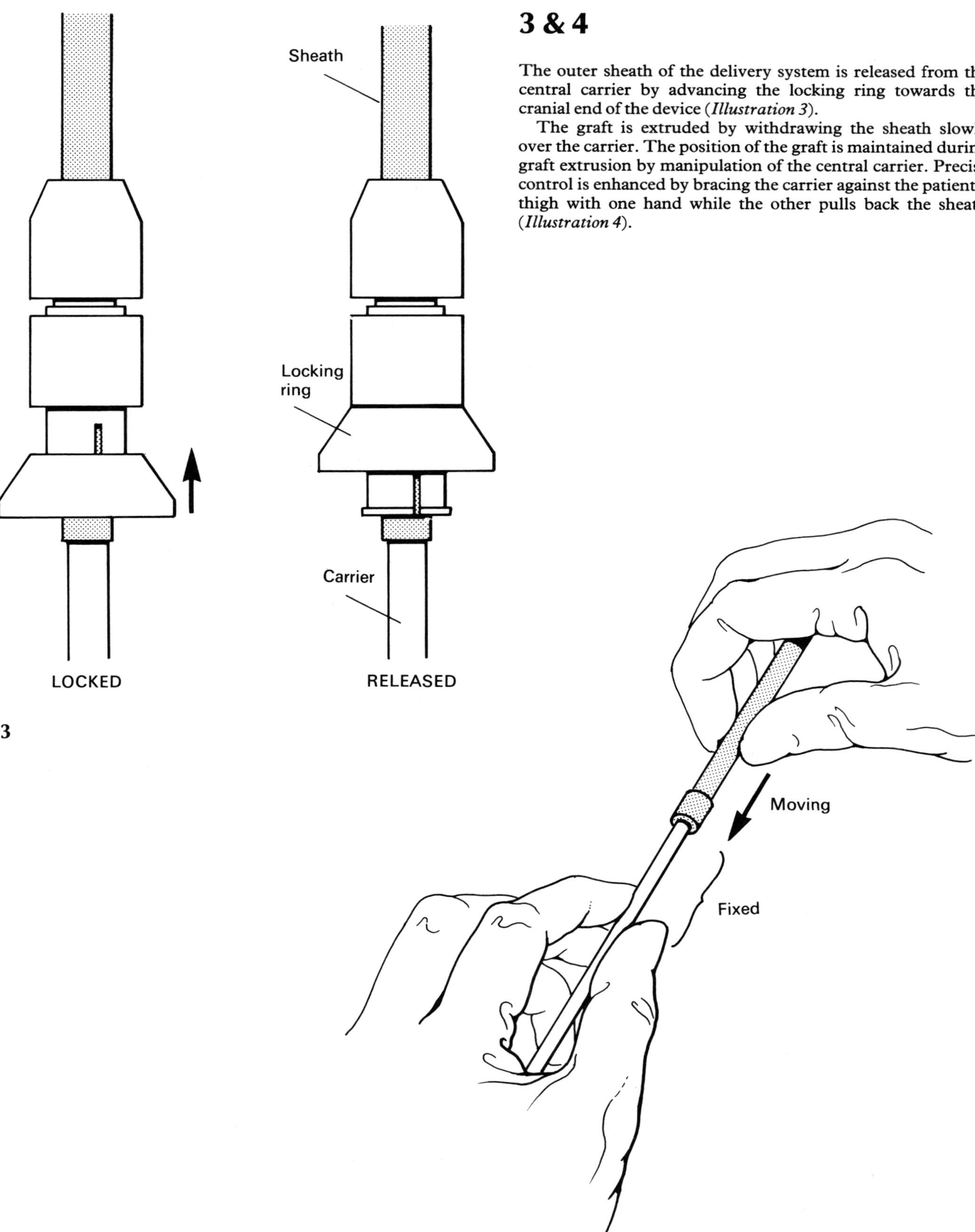

3

4

5 & 6

The small catheter, that extends from the graft limb alongside the carrier (*Illustration 5*), is sutured to the cross-femoral catheter (*Illustration 6*). Placement of sutures in the cross-femoral catheter is after the fashion of a tendon repair.

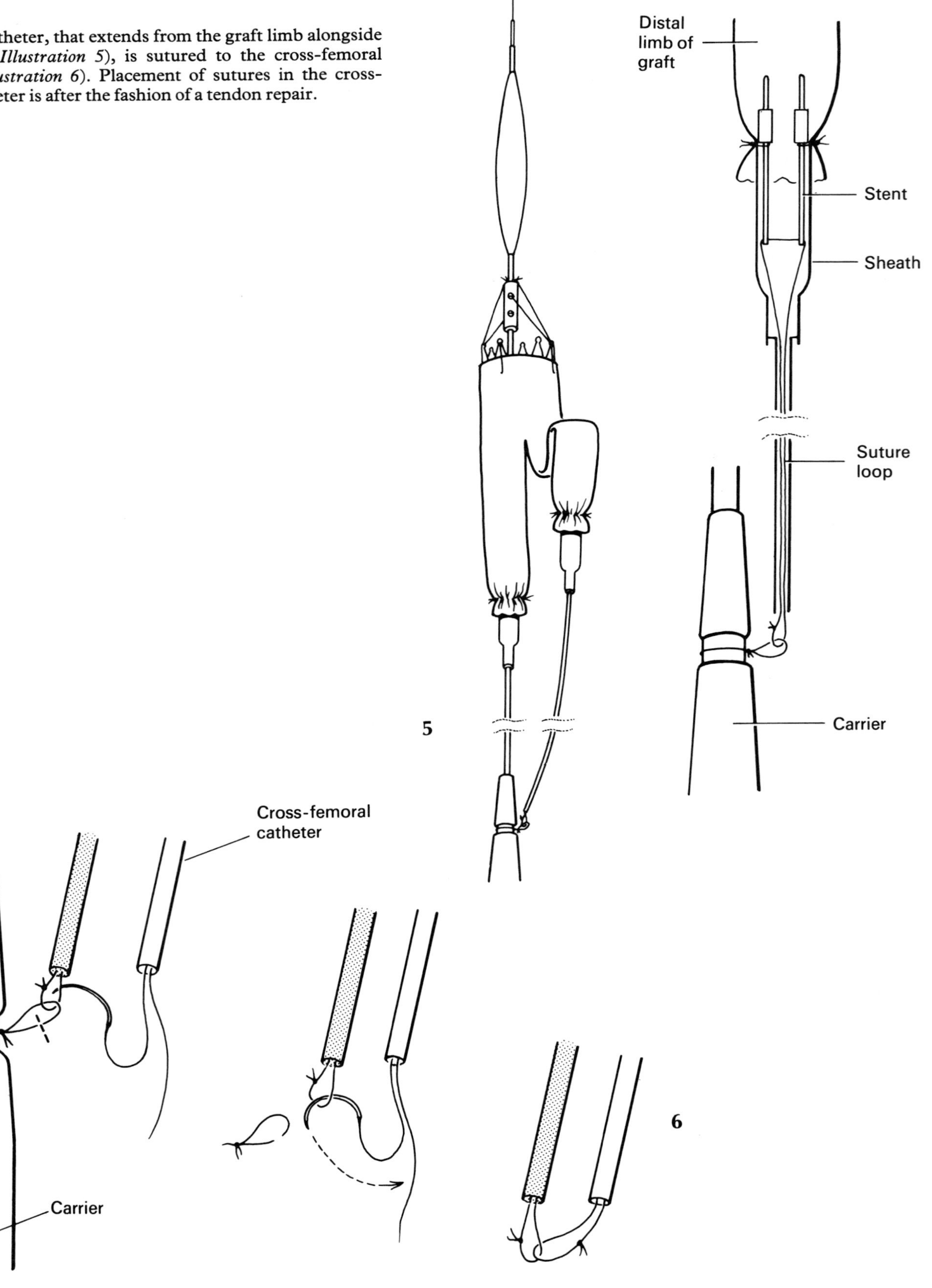

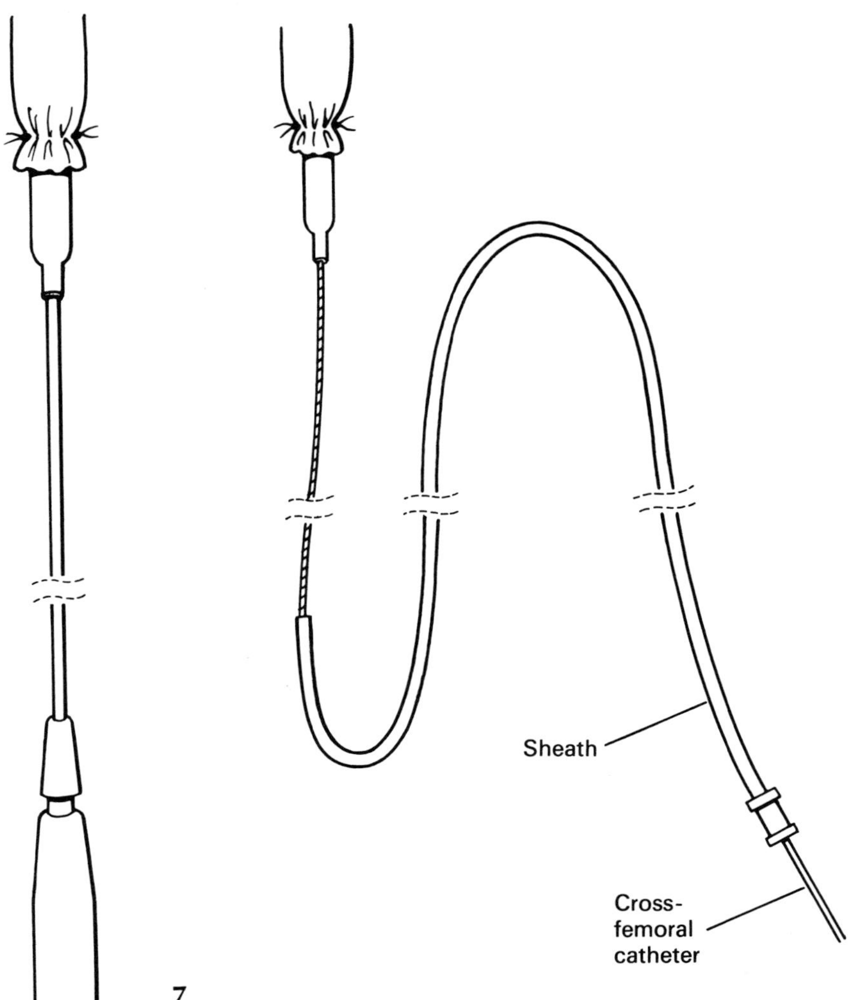

7

A sheath is advanced over the cross-femoral catheter onto the small catheter, thereby covering the sutured joint.

8

Traction on the cross-femoral catheter pulls the graft limb into position.

9

The small catheter is cut while under a little tension. This also cuts the suture within and releases the distal stent.

The haemostatic bands around the femoral artery must be relaxed a little to permit the atraumatic removal of the small sheath and attached catheter. When this has been done two cut ends of suture protrude from the arteriotomy. These are still looped around the stent. They can remain, as a means of manipulating that graft limb, until the procedure is complete.

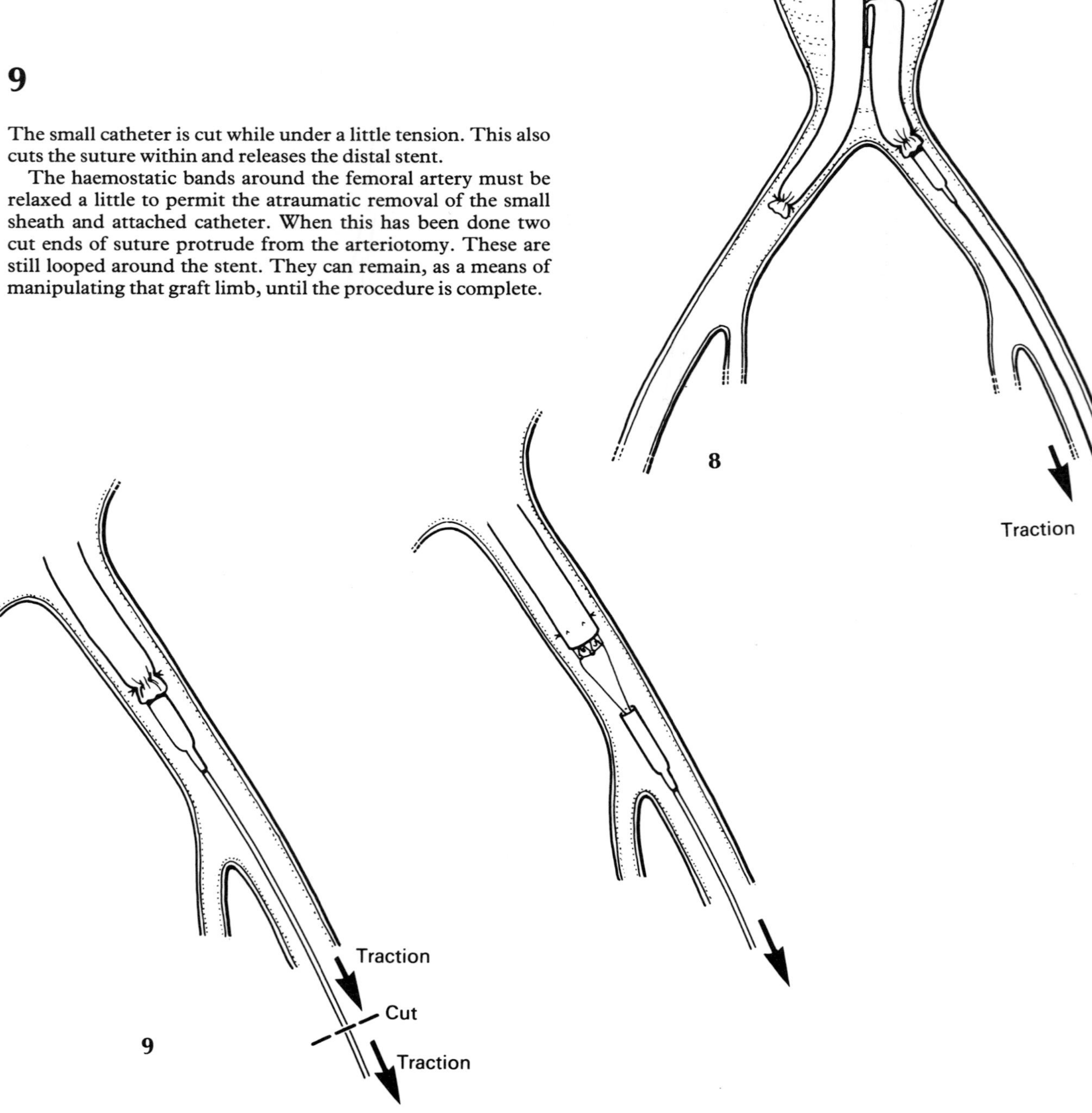

8

9

10

Release of a Luer® lock mechanism permits removal of the inner catheter, which detaches the graft from the delivery system. Removal of the delivery is accompanied by removal of the last distal stent sheath and expansion of the third stent. The guidewire is reinserted before the tip of the delivery system is entirely out of the graft to facilitate replacement of the angiographic catheter.

Completion angiograms are obtained mainly to check for renal artery flow. High resolution digital subtraction systems will also provide angiographic information on any flow limiting kinks or twists in the graft limbs and possible perigraft leakage. Both femoral arteries are flushed to remove particulate matter. The femoral arteriotomies and the wounds are closed in the standard fashion.

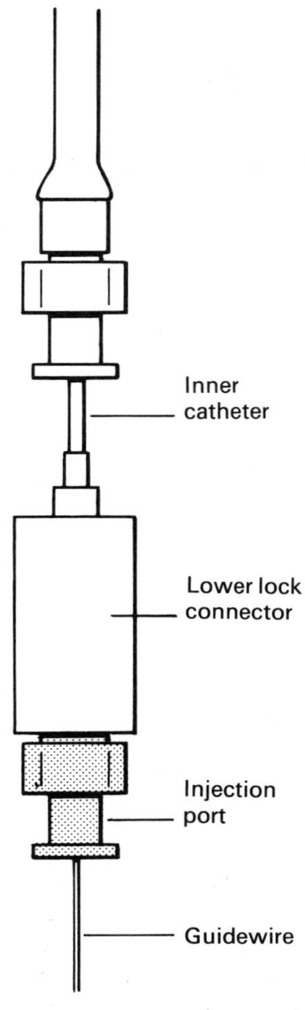

10

Follow-up

The patients are followed by serial colour flow duplex ultrasound examinations and abdominal radiographs. In some institutions we also perform postoperative magnetic resonance angiograms and three-dimensionally reconstructed spiral CT scans.

Endoluminal stented graft aorto-bifemoral reconstruction

MICHAEL L. MARIN MD, *Assistant Professor of Surgery*
FRANK J. VEITH MD, *Professor of Surgery*
Division of Vascular Surgery, Montefiore Medical Center–Albert Einstein College of Medicine, New York, New York, USA

Introduction

Aorto-bifemoral bypass has been the operation of choice for extensive aorto-iliac occlusive disease (Brewster and Darling, 1978). In some instances, local stenotic or occlusive lesions of the iliac arteries can be managed by percutaneous techniques including balloon angioplasty (PTA) and intravascular stenting (Palmaz *et al.*, 1992). In appropriately selected patients, both of these therapies have achieved excellent long-term results for the treatment of clinically significant iliac disease. Despite good results with these techniques in selected patients, there are recognized complications and limitations to both approaches. Aorto-iliac surgical reconstruction may be associated with perioperative complications including, bleeding, infection, impotence and cardiac ischaemia. Similarly, results of catheter based techniques such as PTA and stenting may be compromised by early and late failures, bleeding at the site of percutaneous entry, and in some instances, distal embolization.

Another technique which blends surgical- and catheter-based technologies for treating aorto-iliac occlusive disease is a stented graft endoluminal reconstruction (Parodi, Palmaz and Barone, 1991; Marin *et al.*, 1993; Cragg and Drake, 1993). While this technique is currently novel, it shows promise for minimally invasive management of long segment aorto-iliac and femoral artery occlusive disease. It is a procedure that is feasible to perform under general, regional or local anaesthesia and it can be performed safely in patients who have serious co-morbid medical illnesses.

Procedure

1

Suitable diagnostic arteriography must be performed before the initiation of a stented graft aorto-iliac reconstruction. When total aortic occlusions are encountered, this study can be effectively performed through a translumbar aortic or brachial artery puncture. Visualization must include the proximal and distal abdominal aorta, as well as all the outflow vessels into both lower extremities. When a total aortic occlusion is present below the renal arteries, it may be necessary to perform an aortic arch contrast injection to provide visualization, via collateral vessels, of the femoral and popliteal arteries. Once diagnostic arteriography has been completed, a determination can be made of the best site for access into the vascular system. A transvascular endoluminal graft can be inserted through a stenotic or totally occluded vessel. A total occlusion is approached via an open arteriotomy in the reconstituted femoral artery just distal to the external iliac occlusion. A 7 French introducer catheter is inserted into the lumen of the reconstituted artery distal to the occlusion. Through this introducer catheter, controlled arterial recanalization can be performed.

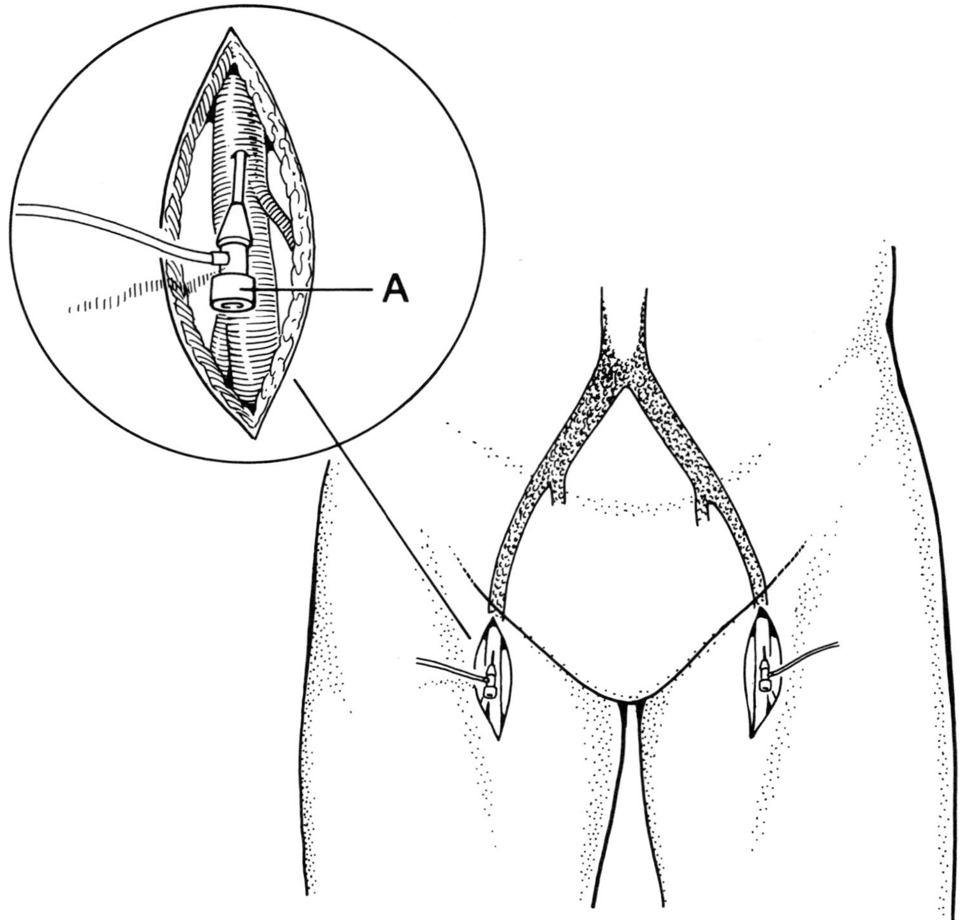

1

2

Through the introducer catheters, a recanalization wire and a directional catheter are inserted. We use 105° curved tip Berenstein catheter (CR BARD, Inc., Billerica, Massachusetts) for this function. An effort is made to direct the recanalzation wire and catheter totally within the intra-intimal layer of the occluded artery. A variety of recanalization wires are used depending on the anatomic situation and composition of the occlusion. The most commonly employed recanalization wire is a hydrophilic 0.035 inch stiff glide wire (Meditech, Corporation, Watertown, Massachusetts). Once the recanalization wire and catheter have been successfully directed through the occluded segment into the lumen of the proximal patent vessels the same procedure is repeated on the contralateral side. Satisfactory proximal intraluminal position is confirmed fluoroscopically by injection of dye through the catheter.

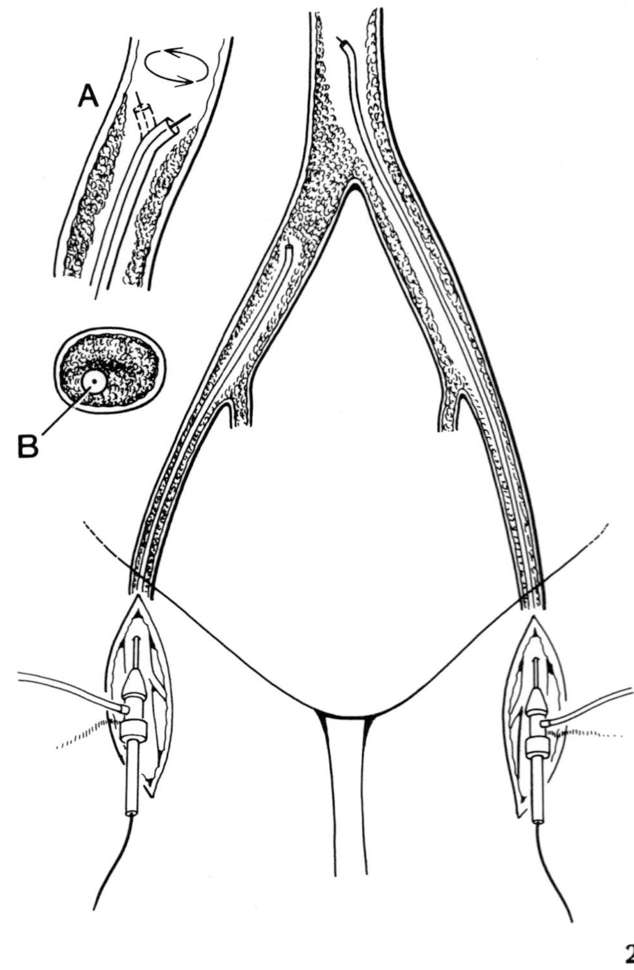

2

3

Using the Seldinger Technique, the directional catheter is removed leaving the wire in place, and a balloon angioplasty catheter is inserted over the wire through the introducer catheters into both iliac arteries. We use 8 mm balloon dilatation catheters for the majority of iliac artery dilatations in preparation for placement of stented grafts. The iliac artery is dilated over its entire length down to the level of the arterial entrance site of the introducer catheter.

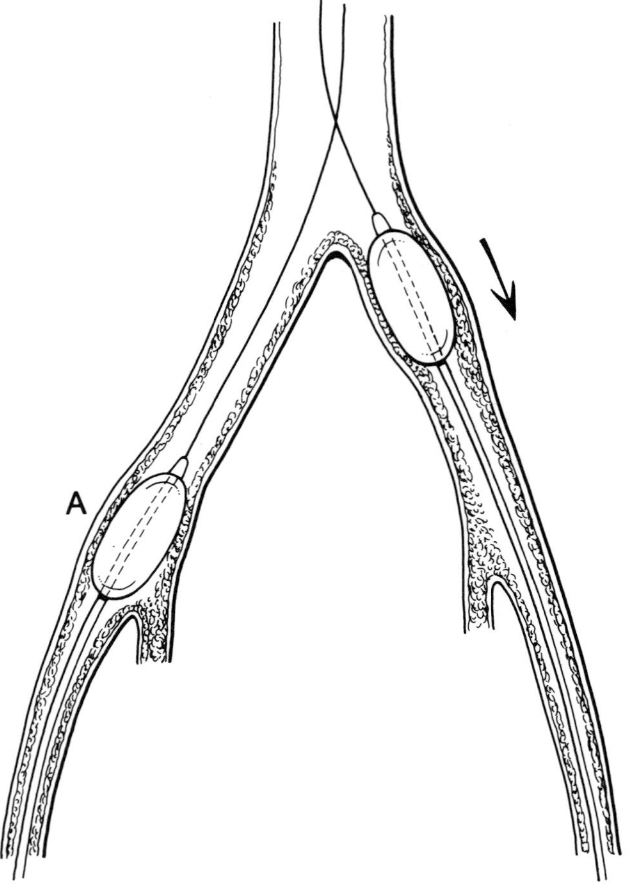

3

4

Recanalization wires in both iliac arteries are held in a stable position, and the introducer catheters are removed bilaterally. A new (14 French) introducer catheter preloaded with a folded 6 mm polytetrafluoroethylene (PTFE) graft and Palmaz stent is inserted. The Palmaz stent is sutured to the proximal end of the PTFE graft using four PTFE stabilizing sutures (Goretex, Flagstaff, AZ). Using fluoroscopic control, the two stent-graft devices and their radiopaque Palmaz stents are positioned at a preselected site in each iliac artery creating an aortic bifurcation. The balloons underlying the two Palmaz stents in each common iliac artery are simultaneously inflated to synchronously deploy both stents. Two dilatations are performed of each stent to ensure firm fixation of the stent to the arterial wall. The balloon catheters are then used to gently dilate the PTFE grafts in a serial descending segmental fashion as each balloon is withdrawn. The introducer catheters and balloons are then removed. At the completion of this step, free ends of both PTFE grafts are visible within the vessel arteriotomy site. Completion arteriograms are performed by retrograde injection to inspect for technical problems or possible arterial recoil. If extrinsic compression is noted, balloon dilatation is carried out through the PTFE graft.

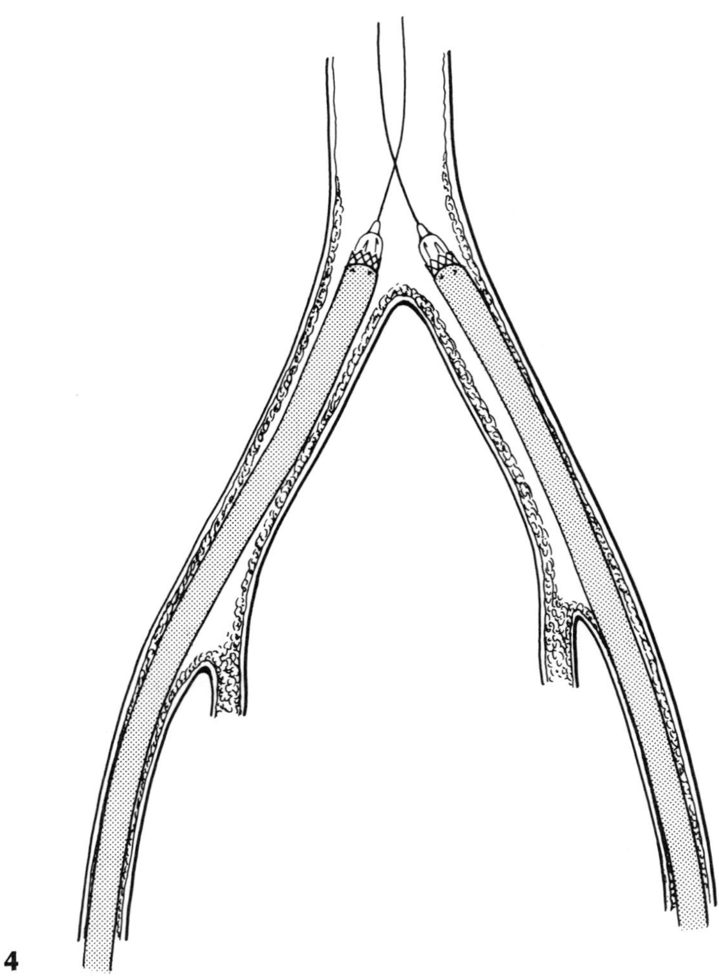

4

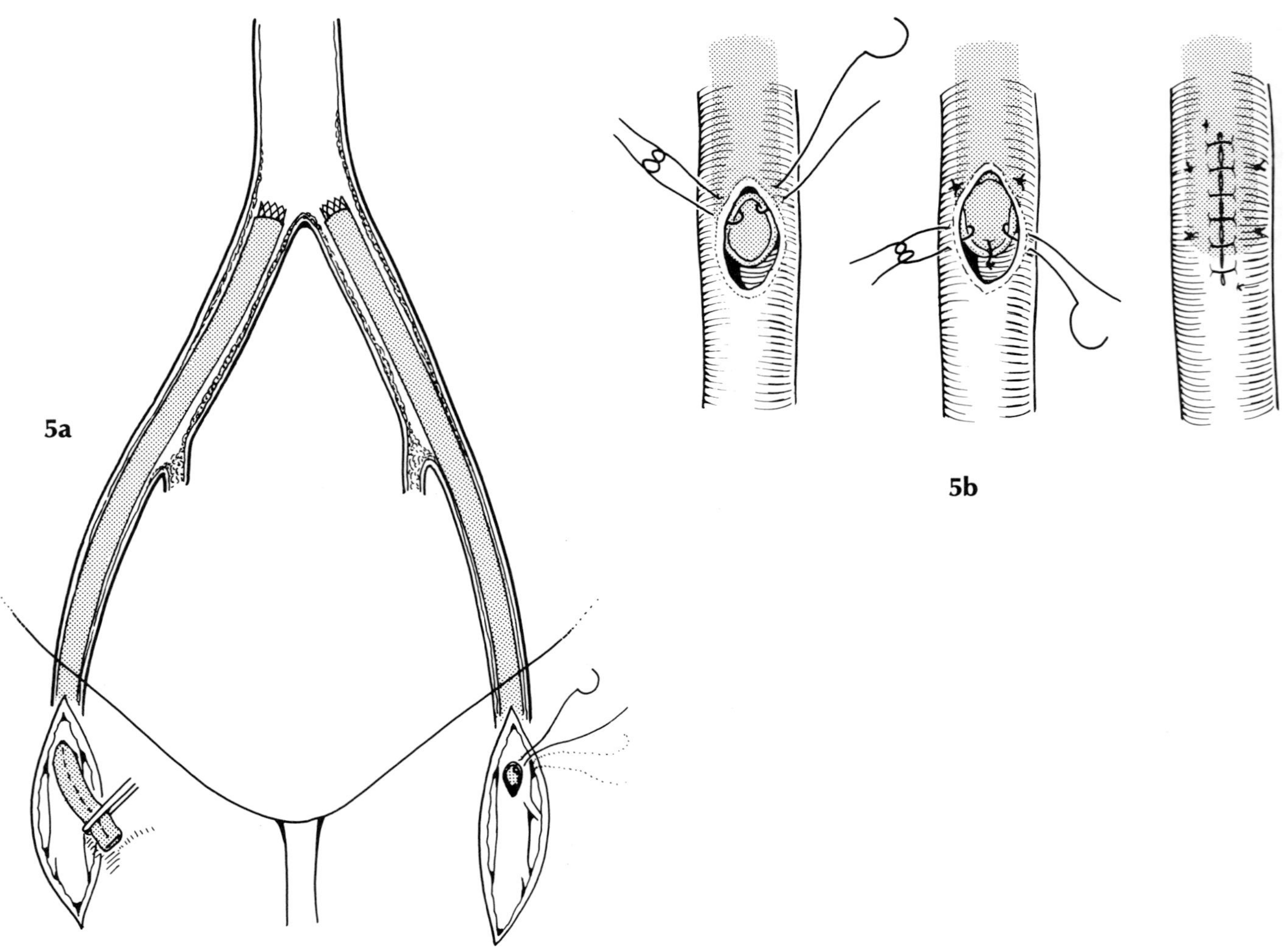

5a & b

The distal free end of the PTFE graft is then sutured to the inside of the patent segment of the common femoral artery in an endoluminal fashion with a series of interrupted polypropylene sutures placed from within. This technique is similar to that used for tacking a distal intimal flap at the time of an endarterectomy. After careful inspection of the entire completed anastomosis, each graft is carefully flushed of possible thrombotic material prior to the placement of a running suture closure of the arteriotomy. After careful inspection for adequate haemostasis, each groin wound site is closed in layers using an absorbable suture. Postoperative care and assessment of an endoluminal graft is identical to that for a standard arterial reconstruction. Physical examination and non-invasive laboratory testing including duplex ultrasonography are useful techniques for detecting technical defects and the failing state. If defects or diminished flow are detected, arteriography and appropriate correction should be performed using catheter-guidewire (balloon/stent) or surgical techniques.

Acknowledgements

This paper was supported in parts by grants from the James Hilton Manning and Emma Austin Manning Foundation, The Anna S. Brown Trust, and the New York Institute for Vascular Studies.

References

Brewster, D. C. and Darling, R. C. (1978). Optimal methods of aorto-iliac reconstruction. *Surgery* **84**, 739.

Cragg, A. H. and Dake, M. D. (1993). Percutaneous femoropopliteal graft placement. *Radiology* **187**, 643.

Marin, M. L., Veith, F. J., Panetta, T. P. *et al.* (1993). Transfemoral stented graft treatment of occlusive arterial disease for limb salvage: A preliminary report. *Circulation* **88**(4), 1.

Palmaz, J. C., Laborde, J. C., Rivera, F. J. *et al.* (1992). Stenting of the iliac arteries with the Palmaz stent: Experience from a multicenter trial. *Cardiovascular Interventional Radiology*, **15**, 291.

Parodi, J. C., Palmaz, J. C. and Barone, H. D. (1991). Transfemoral intraluminal graft implantation for abdominal aortic aneurysms. *Annals of Vascular Surgery* **5**, 491.

Direct reconstruction of intrathoracic great vessels

E. KIEFFER
C. PETITJEAN
Y. BENSAÏD
J. NATALI
Service de Chirurgie Vasculaire, Groupe Hospitalier Pitié-Salpétrière, Paris, France

Introduction

Direct surgical management of intrathoracic great vessel disease was used exclusively in the first years following the pioneering work of Bahnson, Spencer and Quattlebaum (1959) and Davis, Grove and Julian (1956). Reconstruction of the innominate artery, left common carotid artery or multiple lesions was performed through a median sternotomy, and a posterolateral thoracotomy was used for left subclavian artery procedures. However, owing to the magnitude of these operations in poor-risk patients, operative mortality remained high (Crawford *et al.*, 1969), leading to a progressive decrease in indications for intrathoracic procedures and the introduction of extrathoracic reconstructions. By far the most popular of these has been the carotid-subclavian bypass (Dietrich *et al.*, 1967), but other operations have been developed including direct reimplantation of subclavian artery into the common carotid artery (Edwards and Wright, 1972) and various types of cross-over cervical bypasses (Finkelstein, Byer and Rush, 1972; Sethi, Scott and Takaro, 1975; Manart and Kempczinski, 1980).

The cervical procedures facilitate surgical management of most isolated lesions of the intrathoracic great vessels. Their low operative risk and clinical effectiveness certainly make their use valid and logical in the management of isolated subclavian or common carotid lesions, particularly left subclavian artery lesions, which are the most commonly found and whose direct surgical management is possible only through left thoracotomy. However, it is our opinion that most cases of innominate artery and multiple lesions are best treated using direct reconstruction through a median sternotomy.

The purpose of this chapter is to describe the most commonly performed procedures in our 10-year experience including 142 patients treated by direct intrathoracic procedures.

Patterns of intrathoracic arterial lesions

A knowledge of arterial pathology is important as it governs the type of reconstructive procedure to be used.

Most occlusive lesions are atherosclerotic in origin. They are usually very localized, although sometimes multiple.

Atherosclerotic involvement of the aortic arch, leading to ostial stenosis, is the most frequently encountered lesion. Each of the three intrathoracic great vessels – the innominate artery, the left common carotid artery (LCCA) and the left subclavian artery (LSCA) – may be involved. Different combinations of these lesions are possible, but when all three are involved it is called the 'aortic arch syndrome'. Lesions of the middle part of the innominate artery or the LSCA, not involving the aortic origin of these vessels, are much rarer, as are localized lesions of the bifurcation of the innominate artery, extending in various degrees to the right subclavian artery (RSCA) and/or to the right common carotid artery (RCCA).

Ulcerated atherosclerotic lesions, especially in the innominate artery, may lead to embolization in the brain, eye or upper extremity. Haemodynamic consequences are to be expected only in the presence of tightly stenosing and/or completely occluding lesions, especially when multiple. Innominate artery and LSCA occlusions are usually segmental, sparing the bifurcation of the artery or remaining proximal to the origin of the left vertebral artery (VA). In such cases some form of reversed flow in the VA and RCCA is present. Occlusion of the LCCA always extends at least up to the carotid bifurcation. The presence of a significant stenotic lesion at this level usually leads to an extensive occlusion including the whole length of the internal carotid artery (ICA), sparing the external carotid artery (ECA), whose distal part is revascularized by numerous collateral branches coming from the ipsilateral SCA and contralateral ECA. In the presence of a normal carotid bifurcation, LCCA occlusion is usually only segmental, with the ICA remaining patent, often with a reversed flow to the ECA.

Takayasu's arteritis is usually localized to the middle or distal part of the common carotid and/or subclavian arteries (Kieffer and Natali, 1983). Involvement of the intrathoracic great vessels is less frequent but, when present, it is commonly associated with severe involvement of the aortic arch, leading to a complete form of 'aortoarteritis'.

Traumatic lesions are uncommon. They may be observed following penetrating or blunt deceleration injuries. The latter usually results in avulsion of the artery at its origin on the aortic arch (Kieffer *et al.*, 1977) but rupture of the middle part of the intrathoracic segment is possible. Acute lesions leading to emergency operations are beyond the scope of this chapter. Chronic sequelae include occlusions, false aneurysms and arteriovenous (AV) fistulae.

Congential lesions of the intrathoracic great vessels may be associated with the left or right aortic arch. A retro-oesophageal subclavian artery is present in 0.5% of the normal population but surgery is only indicated in the occasional symptomatic case. Isolation of the innominate or left subclavian artery is much less common. These abnormalities are usually found in association with intracardiac and/or aortic congenital lesions but may be completely isolated.

Although anatomically frequent, especially in the innominate artery, kinking is usually not haemodynamically significant and should lead to surgery only on very rare occasions. Spontaneous aneurysms are atherosclerotic or luetic in origin but remain much rarer than occlusive lesions.

Special preoperative preparation

The intrathoracic nature of the procedure obviously necessitates a precise assessment of the patient's cardiopulmonary status and medical treatment of all treatable abnormalities whenever possible. Pulmonary function should be assessed precisely. Preoperative pulmonary physiotherapy is often indicated in this middle-aged smoking population. Cardiac abnormalities should be looked for carefully through history and a standard ECG. Coronary angiography and cardiac catheterization should have broad indications even in the presence of stable angina, since coronary artery bypass, if indicated, should be performed in the same operative session. Arterial hypertension should be treated preoperatively in order to allow for safe lateral clamping of the aorta and prevent cardiac and cerebral complications. A CT scan should be obtained in the presence of any permanent neurological symptoms.

Although non-invasive ultrasonic techniques are of great value and should be obtained routinely, angiography is necessary for a precise assessment of the cerebral circulation. Arch aortography should visualize not only the intrathoracic vessels but also the carotid bifurcations and vertebral arteries. Distal arteries may be difficult to visualize in the presence of multiple extensive occlusions. In rare cases we used to begin the operation with surgical exploration of one or both of the carotid bifurcations. More recently, most of these problems have been overcome using non-invasive techniques and intra-arterial digitalized subtraction angiography.

Special intraoperative monitoring for these procedures

Much of this is as described in the chapter on 'Operative planning'. Blood pressure is recorded through an intra-arterial line placed either in the radial artery opposite the artery to be revascularized or in either of the femoral arteries in the presence of multiple lesions. Cardiac function assessment by a Swan-Ganz catheter should be routinely used since intraoperative lowering of the blood pressure using halothane or preferably sodium nitroprusside or trinitrin is often necessary to allow for precise and safe lateral clamping of the aorta. Multiple venous lines are also used, avoiding the cervical and left brachial regions because the left innominate vein may have to be transected in order to obtain adequate access to the lesions.

We use no special intraoperative cerebral monitoring such as EEG or pressure measurements. The only routine cerebral protective measures taken are: (1) systemic heparinization during arterial clamping (0.5 mg/kg, with neutralization by protamine sulphate at the end of the procedure); (2) avoidance of hypotension during arterial clamping and of hypertension in the postoperative period; and (3) sequential declamping of the arteries, beginning with the non-cerebral arteries (ECA or distal SCA). In the presence of multiple proximal lesions, revascularization should begin with the most stenotic lesion(s). Similarly, tandem intrathoracic and cervical lesions should be treated sequentially, beginning with the more proximal one.

The use of cardiopulmonary bypass (CPB) may be necessary in a few selected situations, the most frequent of these being simultaneous coronary revascularization. Circulatory arrest using deep hypothermia has been used in a few cases to perform transaortic endarterectomy of multiple proximal lesions of the great vessels (Thevenet, Chaptal and Negre, 1968). However, although this technique seems logical and appealing, reasonable clinical and angiographic indications remain rare and the whole procedure may seem unnecessarily complicated.

Shunting devices such as Gott (Murray, Brawley and Gott, 1971) or Javid shunts inserted into the ascending aorta have no routine indication but may be used in very selected cases in order to avoid a prosthetic bypass if endarterectomy or reimplantation necessitates simultaneous clamping of both the innominate artery and LCCA.

The operations

Incisions and approaches to the great vessels

Anterolateral thoracotomy through the second or third intercostal space has been advised by some surgeons (Crawford *et al.*, 1969). However, this approach only allows for the proximal implantation of a bypass. In addition, tunnelling through the thoracic inlet seems to be a rather blind procedure, carrying the risk of venous trauma. We have used this approach only for very selected indications for subclavian artery reconstruction such as failure or infection of a cervical

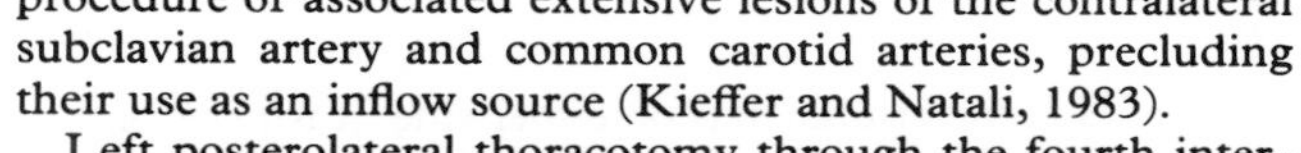

procedure or associated extensive lesions of the contralateral subclavian artery and common carotid arteries, precluding their use as an inflow source (Kieffer and Natali, 1983).

Left posterolateral thoracotomy through the fourth intercostal space is unique in providing direct access to the whole length of the intrathoracic portion of the LSCA. However, it has several drawbacks that explain its declining use in recent years: distal exposure is limited to the origin of the VA; associated surgery is not possible: and above all respiratory complications are more frequent than with a median sternotomy. Except for aneurysmal lesions, this route involves an unduly extensive technique for isolated lesions of the LSCA, since they may be managed easily through a much simpler cervical approach.

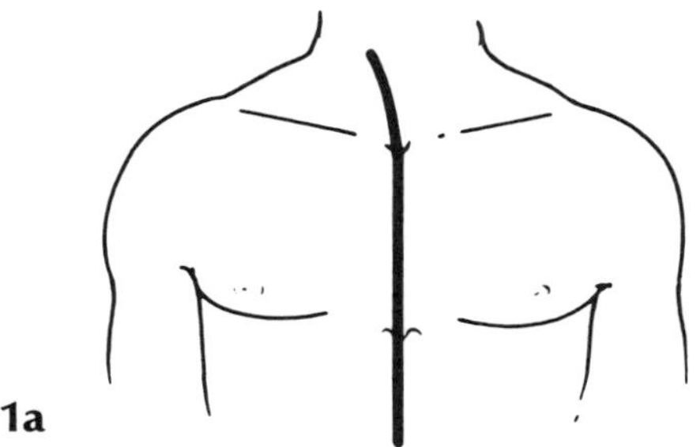

1a

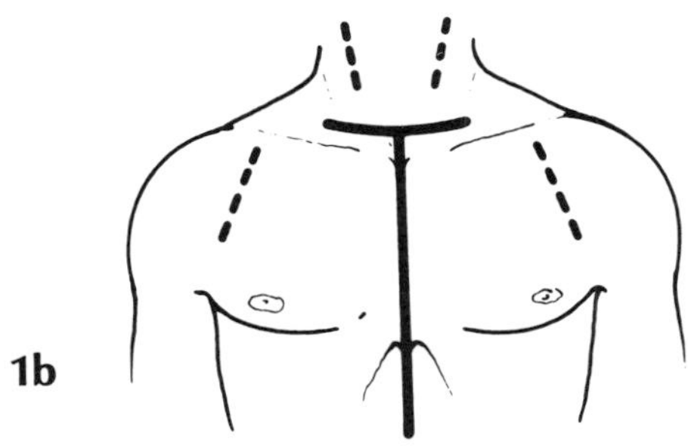

1b

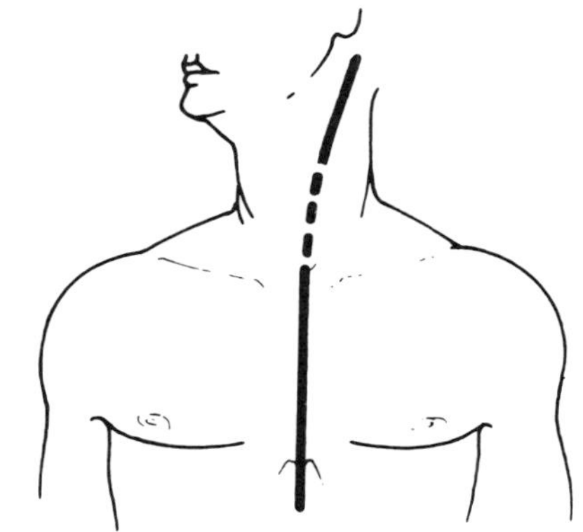

1c

1a, b & c

The standard approach is through a median sternotomy. Aside from its simplicity, well-known advantages of this route include (1) low rate of respiratory complications (as evidenced by cardiac surgery in the aged patient); (2) possibility of extension to all supra-aortic vessels, either intrathoracic (except perhaps the origin of the LSCA) or cervical, as well as to the abdomen (sternolaparotomy); and (3) possibility of associated cardiac surgery.

One or more complementary cervical incisions are usually necessary, according to the vessel(s) to be revascularized. The innominate and left common carotid arteries are approached by a short presternomastoid incision at the base of the neck, permitting a very easy direct approach (*a*). The proximal subclavian arteries are approached through the same incision, which is sufficient to give access to the subclavian artery medial to the internal jugular vein and to permit its dissection up to the scalenus muscles, beyond the origin of the VA. On the left side, the proximal subclavian artery is reputedly difficult if not impossible to approach through sternotomy. In fact this is possible after section of the vertebral vein and thoracic duct, although this does not allow for safe clamping of the aortic arch at the origin of the artery. The approach to the distal subclavian artery necessitates a complementary supraclavicular incision on either side (*b*), with section of the sternomastoid and scalenus muscles and reclination of the phrenic nerve. The entire aortic arch and its proximal branches may be approached through a low horizontal cervicotomy without sectioning of the sternomastoid muscles, provided the approach to the subclavian arteries does not have to go beyond the scalenus muscles (*b*). The carotid bifurcation is approached by presternomastoid incision either by extending the sternotomy, especially if the neck is short, or by a separate approach (*c*). The axillary arteries are easily reached by deltopectoral incisions (*b*). The transection or removal of the clavicle does not offer any additional advantage. Multiple great vessel lesions can be approached by combining these cervical incisions, particularly if the low horizontal cervicotomy is completed by one or more separate distal approaches to the carotid and/or axillary arteries. For all distal revascularizations (axillary artery or carotid bifurcation), complementary cervicotomies are done at the beginning of the operation in order to confirm the possibility of revascularization suggested by angiography.

2

To approach the arterial axis on either side, it is necessary to transect the subhyoid muscles and the thymic remnants. The left innominate vein hides the aortic arch and the proximal part of the great vessels. It does not have to be isolated for distal revascularization (axillary artery and carotid bifurcation). When revascularizing a proximal artery it is usually sufficient to mobilize the vein by complete dissection and division of its lower (thymic) and upper (thyroid) branches. Detachment of the jugular-subclavian venous confluence from the posterior part of the sternal manubrium is useful to allow for a broad sternal opening without undue tension on the vein. However, it may be divided without hesitation, especially if a wide approach to the aortic arch is required and surgery on the proximal LSCA in anticipated. Transection of the left innominate vein usually has no long lasting effect except for a transient oedema of the left upper extremity, possibly followed by the development of prethoracic collateral circulation. The latter may be an uncosmetic sequela in young female patients. We do not usually reconstruct the vein at the end of the operation, although this presents no particular difficulty. At the end of the procedure, the thymic remnants and subhyoid muscles are sutured in front of the intrathoracic portion of the reconstruction. If entered, the pericardium is left partially opened. Closure is made according to routine techniques, following pericardial, mediastinal and cervical drainage.

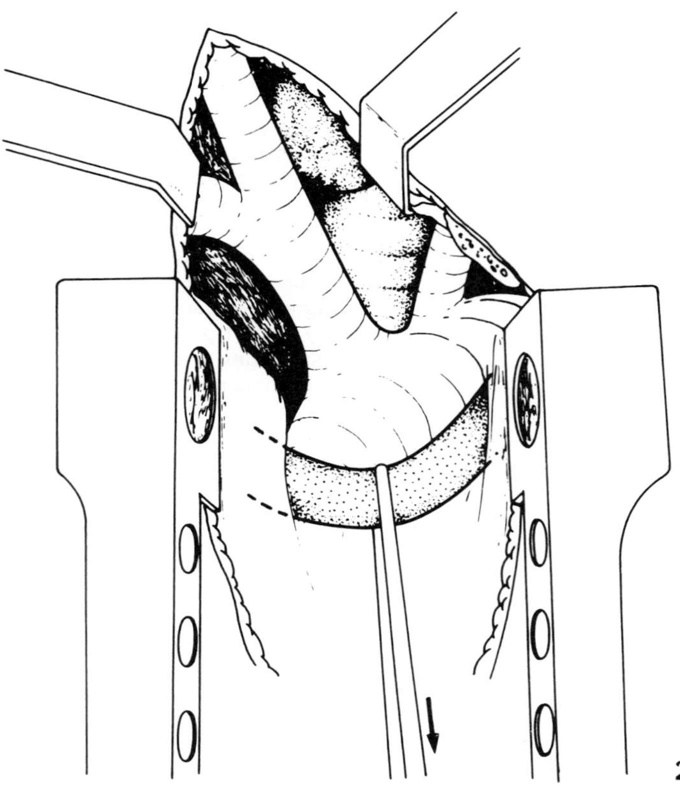

2

Innominate artery reconstruction

Among isolated lesions of the intrathoracic great vessels, those involving the innominate artery present the most logical indications for direct intrathoracic surgery (Kieffer, 1975). In our opinion, cervical bypasses are justified only in very occasional poor-risk patients. Cross-over subclavian-subclavian or axilloaxillary bypasses using the LSCA as an inflow source should be avoided since the artery is the most likely to be or become diseased.

Two reconstructive techniques will be described in detail: endarterectomy and bypass.

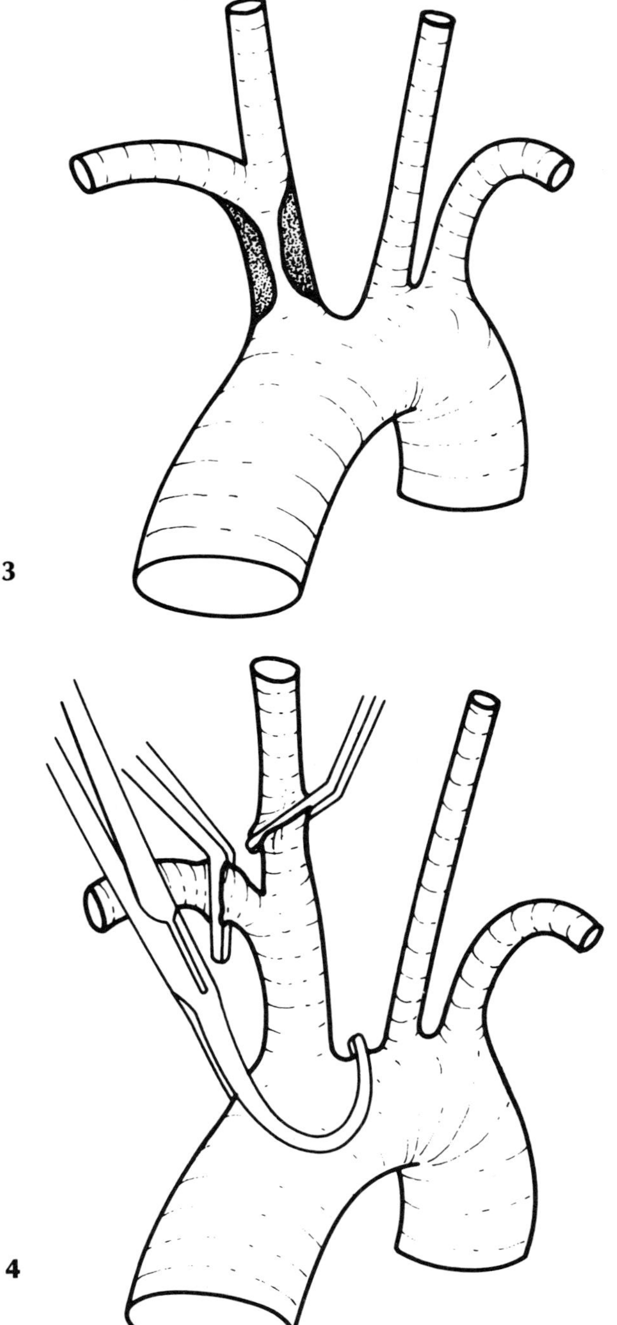

3

4

Innominate endarterectomy

This technique is applicable only in selected cases of atherosclerotic occlusive disease. Exposure of the entire length of the innominate artery, proximal parts of the LCCA, RCCA and RSCA, as well as the upper aspect of the aortic arch is necessary (*see Illustrations 1a* and *2*). The left innominate vein is retracted towards the lower part of the incision. The pericardium is usually not opened.

3

The first step is to make sure that wide lateral clamping of the aortic arch is possible safely. The following two conditions must be fulfilled (Kieffer, 1975).

First, sufficient space must be present in the upper aspect of the aortic arch between the origins of the innominate artery and the LCCA. Inadvertent partial clamping of the LCCA may be complicated by left cerebral embolism due to trauma of an associated non-significant lesion frequently involving the proximal part of the artery. Simultaneous complete clamping of both vessels, such as may be necessary in the presence of a common trunk between the innominate artery and the LCCA, will usually be followed by cerebral ischaemia of variable magnitude. In most of these cases aortoinnominate bypass seems preferable. However, endarterectomy remains possible if a shunting device is inserted between the ascending aorta and one of the common carotid arteries.

Secondly, involvement of the upper aspect of the aortic arch by the pathological process must be minimal if endarterectomy is to be performed with complete security. In our opinion, extensive indications for conventional endarterectomy (Carlson *et al.*, 1977) carry the risk of intra- or postoperative haemorrhage or dissection and for this reason should be discouraged. If endarterectomy must be performed despite the risks, CPB with deep hypothermia and circulatory arrest should be used in order to perform a transaortic operation (Thevenet, Chaptal and Negre, 1968), but this somewhat complex technique seems unwarranted for an isolated innominate artery lesion.

4

When the two above-mentioned conditions are fulfilled, one may proceed to innominate endarterectomy. Under controlled hypotension and with the patient systemically heparinized the aortic arch is widely clamped around the origin of the innominate artery using a specially designed J clamp.

5

The RCCA and RSCA are then clamped separately using right-angle clamps, whatever the distal extension of the innominate artery lesion may be. A longitudinal arteriotomy of the innominate artery is made, extending proximally to the aorta in order to obtain adequate visualization of the origin of the innominate artery and aortic lumen.

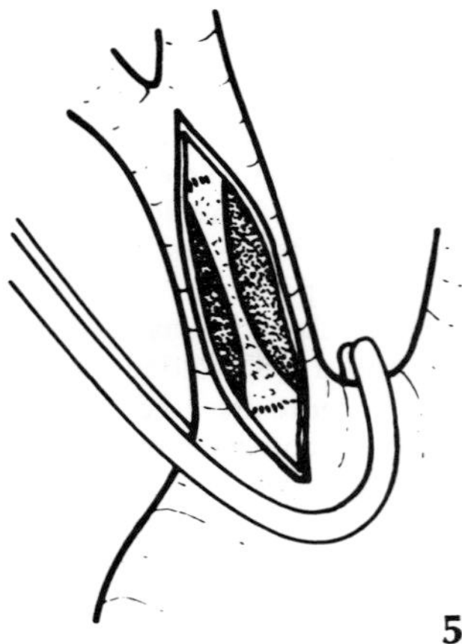

5

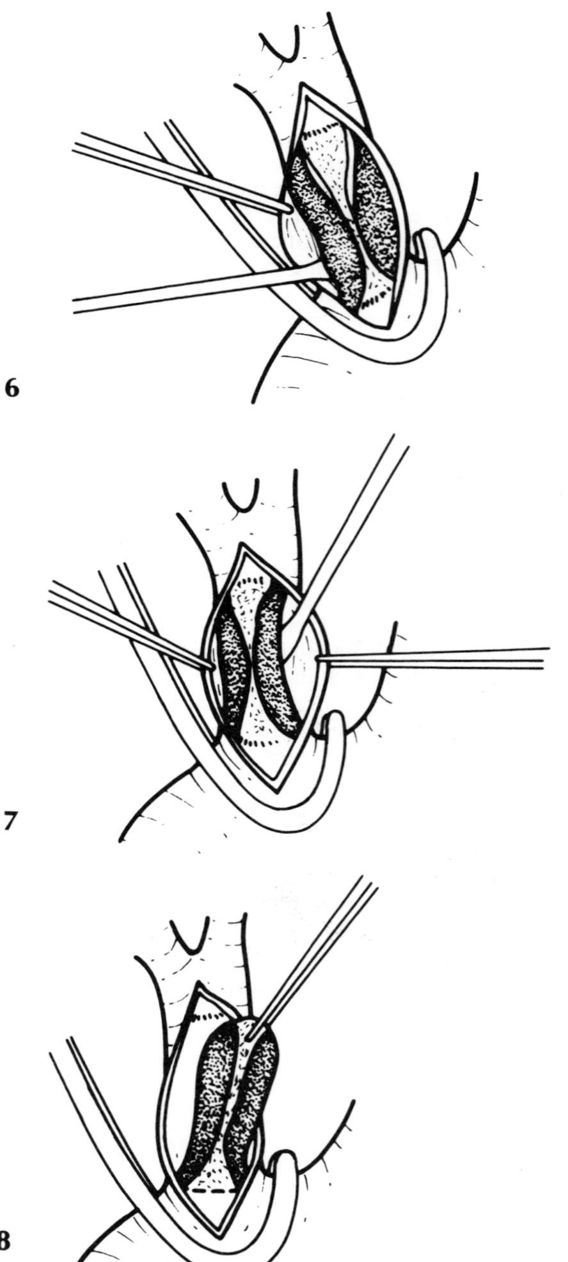

6

7

8

6, 7 & 8

Using an adequate spatula, endarterectomy is begun at the middle part of the innominate artery. The plane of cleavage should not be too external, especially in the proximal part of the artery, if the hazards of aortic dissection, rupture or secondary dilatation of the artery are to be avoided.

The distal limit of the endarterectomy is usually very clear and no intimal fixation is necessary in these circumstances.

9

However, when the distal intima remains thick and easy to mobilize, one should not hesitate to tack it with a few 6/0 monofilament sutures. The proximal intima must usually be transected with scissors at the origin of the vessel, and its posterior aspect tacked using one or two 5/0 monofilament sutures.

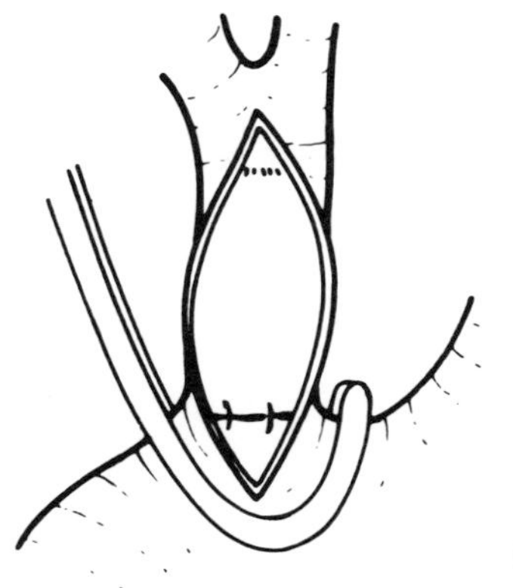

9

10a & b

Closure of the arteriotomy is usually performed using a 5/0 monofilament continuous suture (*a*). Patch angioplasty (*b*) is used in rare cases such as in a small innominate artery or when post-stenotic dilatation would result in relative stenosis of the proximal part of the artery. We prefer to use a knitted Dacron velour patch since a vein patch may lead to late dilatation.

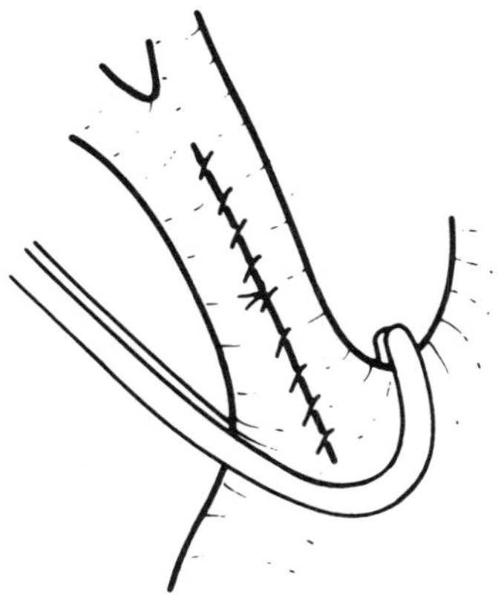

10a

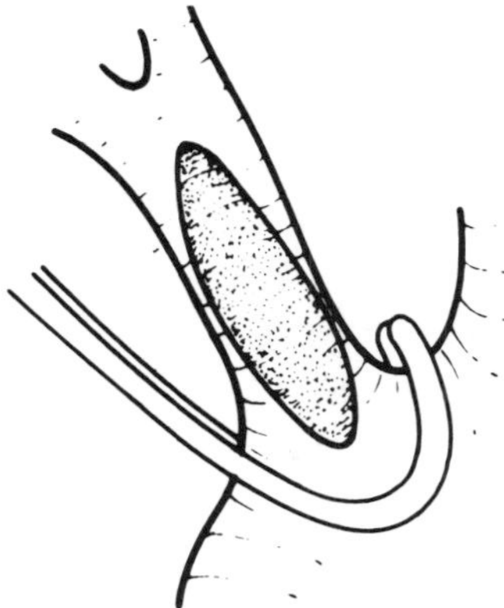

10b

11 & 12

Whichever form of closure is used, declamping is done sequentially, first towards the RSCA and then towards the RCCA.

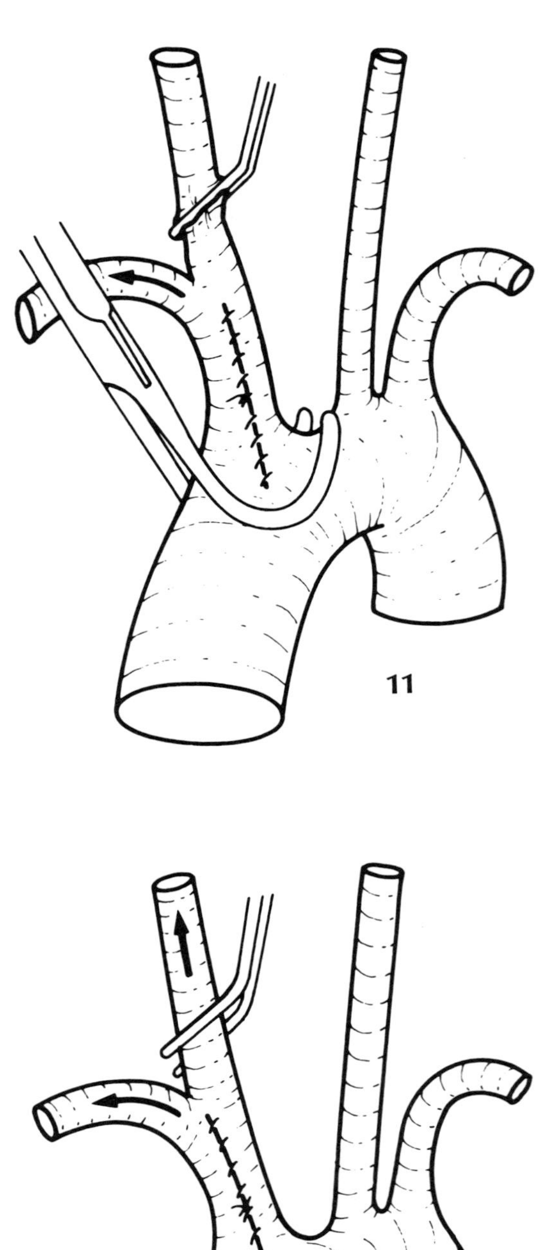

13

Distal extension of the lesion may necessitate associated endarterectomy of the RSCA and/or RCCA. However, this extended procedure should not be performed in the presence of SCA lesions extending distal to the origin of the VA. Separate clamping of RCCA, distal RSCA and VA is applied distally and the innominate arteriotomy is extended up to the level of the right VA. In most cases lesions stop proximal to the VA and endarterectomy of the proximal SCA is performed easily under direct vision.

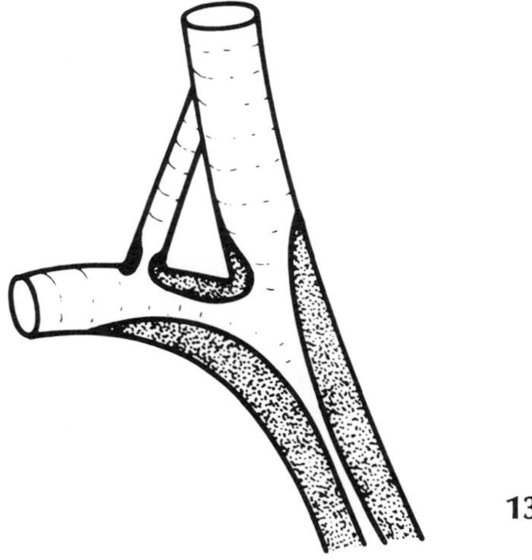

13

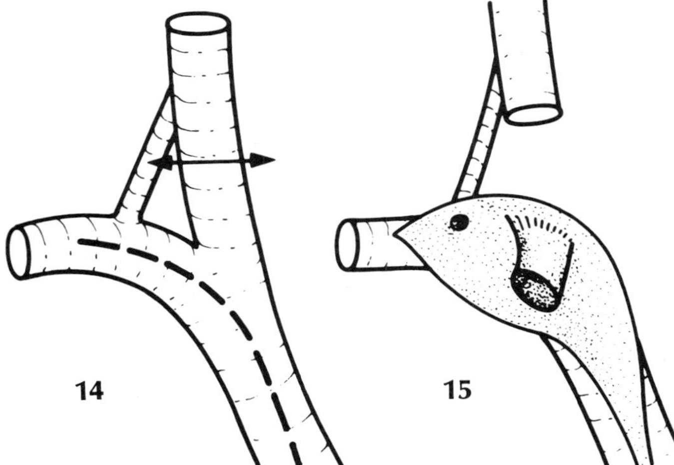

14 15

14 & 15

Associated stenosis of the VA may be treated by trans-subclavian endarterectomy. On rare occasions tacking the distal intima of the SCA may be indicated. The RCCA is completely transected 1 or 2cm above its origin and endarterectomy of the proximal part of the artery is done using an eversion technique. In the presence of extensive lesions of the RCCA and carotid bifurcation, a conventional endarterectomy of the birfurcation is performed. The middle and distal parts of the RCCA are then endarterectomized using an eversion technique through the distal arteriotomy.

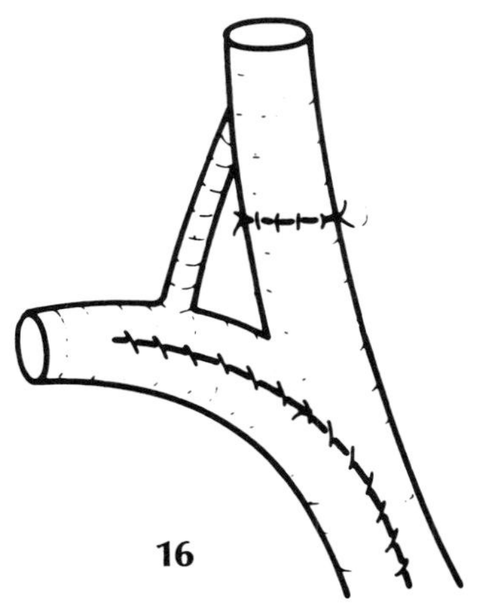

16

16

The two segments of the RCCA are then anastomosed using a 5/0 monofilament continuous suture and the longitudinal innominate-subclavian arteriotomy is closed using either a continuous suture (as shown) or a Dacron patch angioplasty.

Aortoinnominate artery bypass

17

The incision used is shown in *Illustration 1b*. This technique has much broader indications than endarterectomy, since it is nearly always possible. Once the innominate artery and its bifurcation have been freed, the upper part of the pericardium is opened longitudinally and its edges suspended from those of the sternal incision in order to expose the ascending aorta. Palpation of the latter will rarely lead to the unexpected discovery of extensive and/or heavily calcified lesions which preclude use of the procedure. In such exceptional cases, an alternative technique would be to extend the incision to the upper part of the abdomen and to use the supraceliac aorta as an inflow source (Kieffer and Natali, 1983). Although complete transection may be necessary, extensive dissection usually facilitates the appropriate mobilization of the left innominate vein.

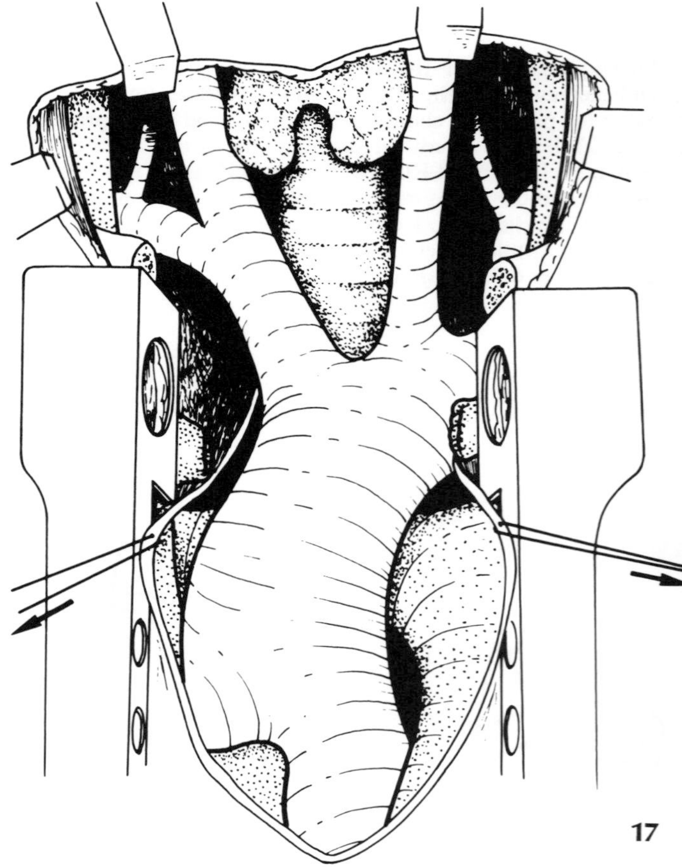

17

18

A knitted Dacron prosthetic graft of suitable size (8, 10, or sometimes 12 mm) is preclotted. When the chosen calibre is 10 mm or more, a tube graft is used. If the calibre is less than 10 mm, we prefer to use a bifurcated graft, only one of its branches and the adjacent part of its body being used. This permits the performance of a wide proximal anastomosis using large bites without any risk of inadvertent anastomotic stenosis.

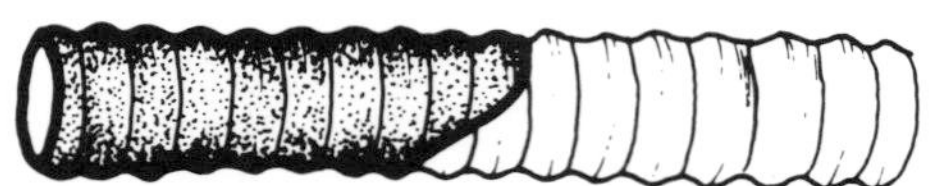

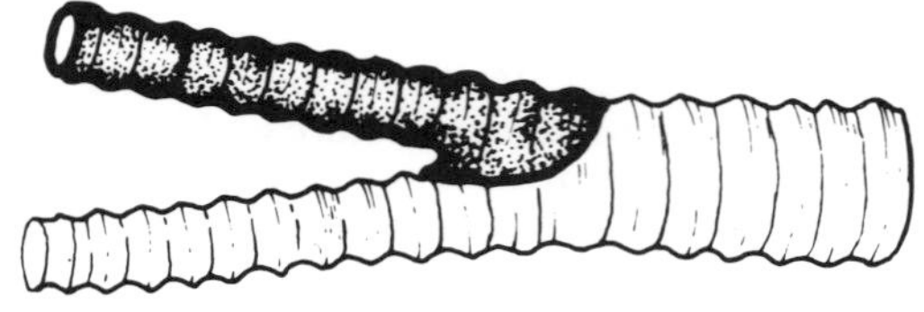

18

19

Palpation of the ascending aorta is performed very carefully in order to avoid either incomplete clamping with its associated risk of uncontrolled haemorrhage or a complete but traumatic clamping with the risk of fracture and/or dissection of the aorta. Heparin is not yet administered. The middle part of the right anterolateral aspect of the ascending aorta is widely clamped using a J clamp. Lowering the blood pressure to around 100 mmHg has the distinct advantages of avoiding aortic clamp trauma and allowing precise placement of the clamp. Indeed, the anterior aspect of the aorta should be avoided since placement of a graft in this position carries the risk of postoperative compression by the sternum. A 2–3 cm longitudinal aortotomy is performed. If the ascending aorta is too thick and rigid a quadrangular or oval-shaped segment has to be excised in order to avoid proximal anastomotic stenosis.

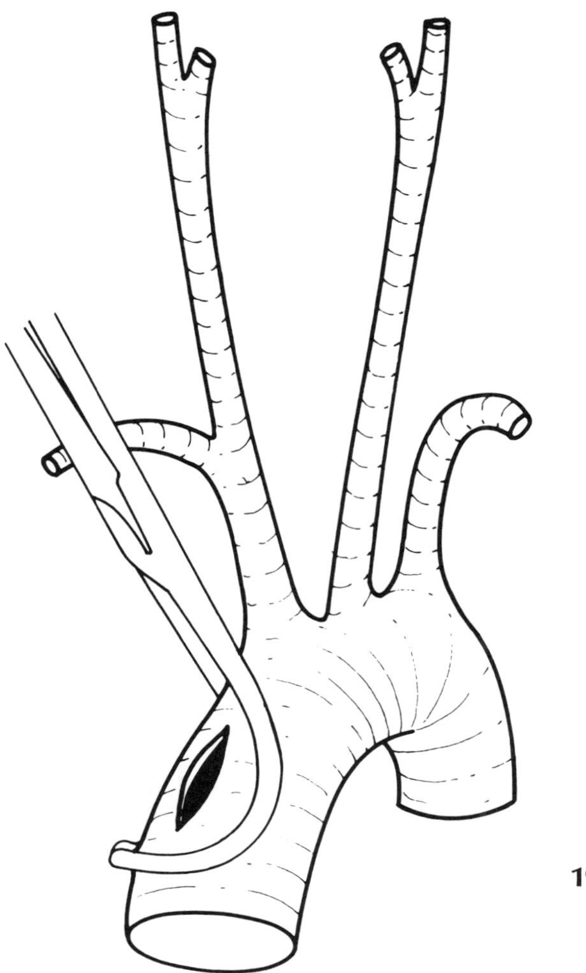

19

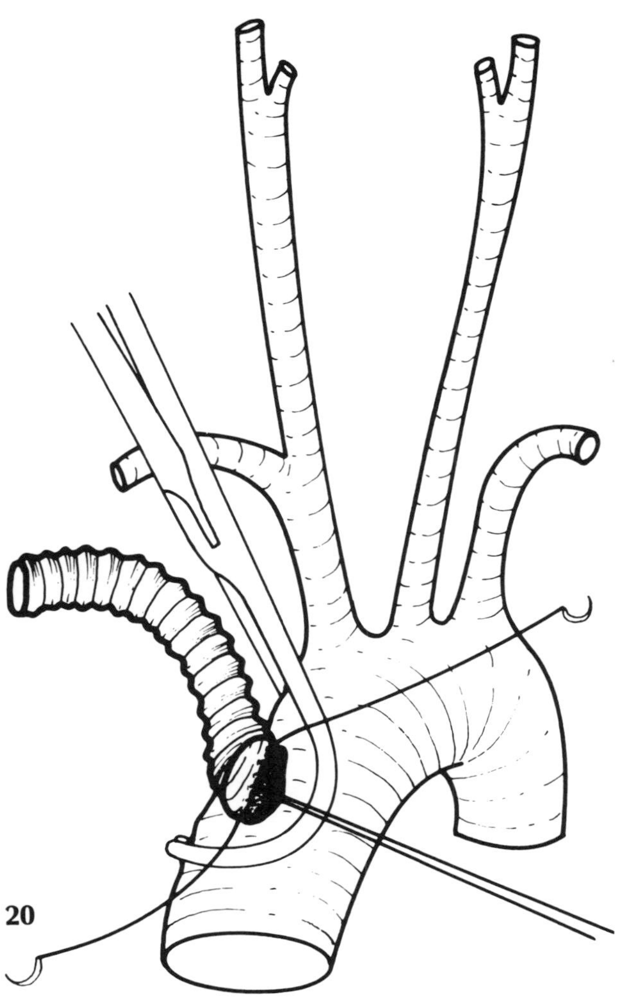

20

20

The graft is bevelled and anastomosed to the aorta using a 3/0 or 4/0 monofilament continuous suture taking large bites through the aortic wall. After slow removal of the clamp, the anastomosis is gently compressed in order to avoid any aortic wall haematoma. The anastomosis is then checked and should any complementary suture be necessary, this is made after reclamping the aorta. Preclotting of the graft is completed as necessary. The precise length necessary to reach the distal innominate artery is calculated with pressure in the graft. The graft is then reclamped close to its origin and any intraluminal clots are carefully removed by aspiration and lavage with non-heparinized saline solution. Any thrombus left on the wall of the graft might cause cerebral embolism when the bypass is made functional.

21 & 22

Heparin is then administered systemically and the blood pressure is allowed to return to normal levels. The origin of the innominate artery and both its branches are clamped using a straight aortic clamp and two right-angle clamps respectively. If its bifurcation appears normal, the distal part of the innominate artery is completely transected and anastomosed to the graft in an end-to-end fashion using 4/0 or 5/0 monofilament continuous suture.

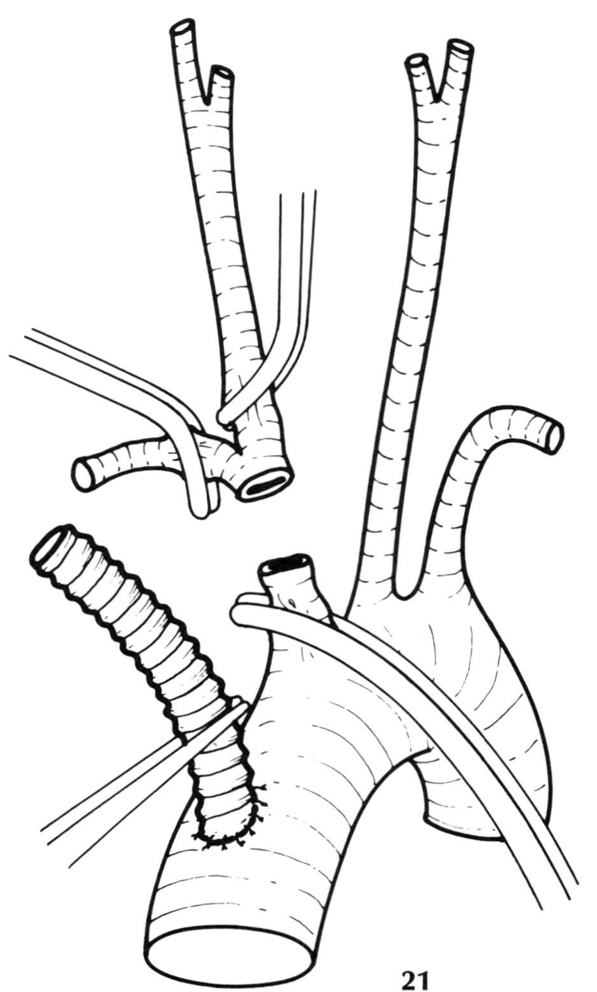

21

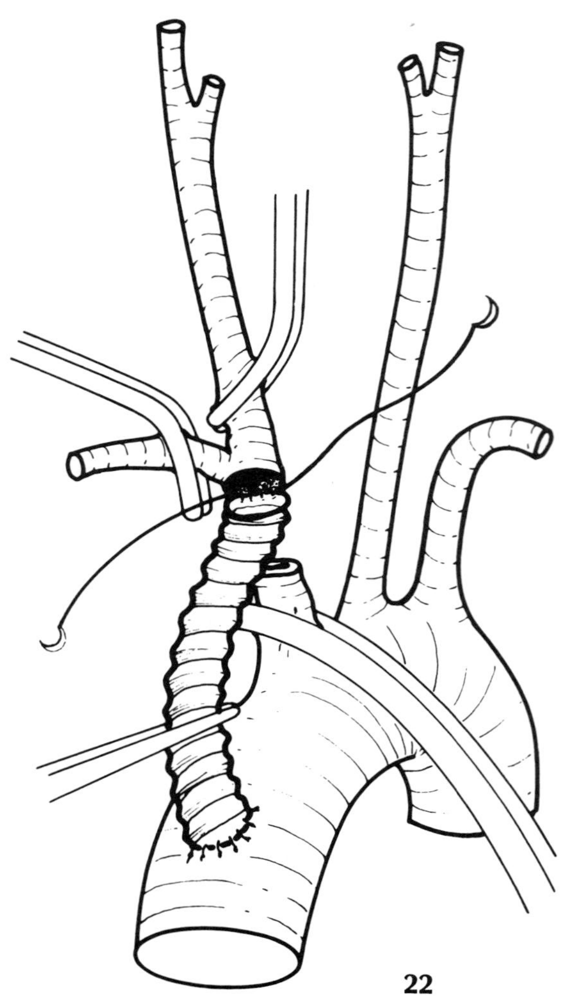

22

In the presence of associated lesions of one or both of the distal branches of the innominate artery, blind distal endarterectomy should be avoided and modifications of the distal anastomosis become necessary.

23 & 24

When one of the branches is stenosed by a smooth localized plaque, a longitudinal incision is made and the graft may be anastomosed in a spatulated end-to-end fashion.

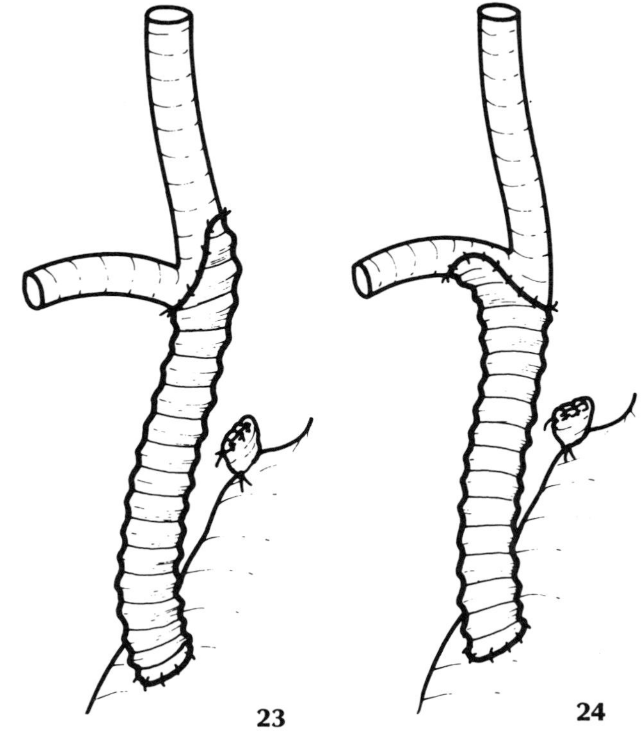

23 **24**

25 & 26

Otherwise, we prefer to transect the two branches distal to the stenotic lesion (Edwards and Wright, 1972) and perform a short sequential bypass.

25 **26**

27 & 28

With both methods declamping is done in the usual manner.

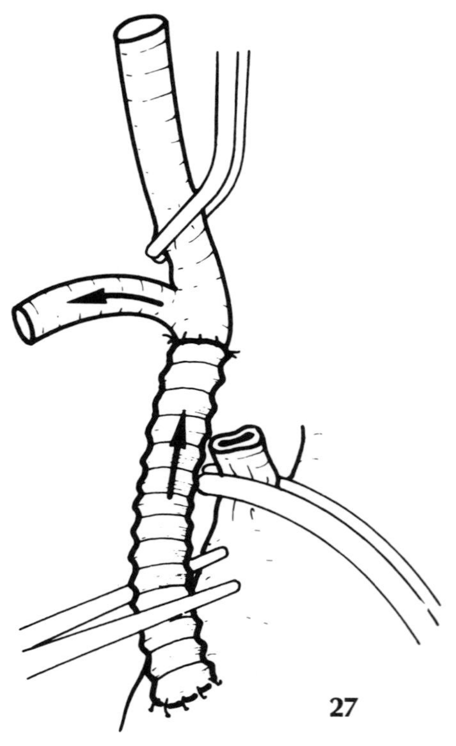

27

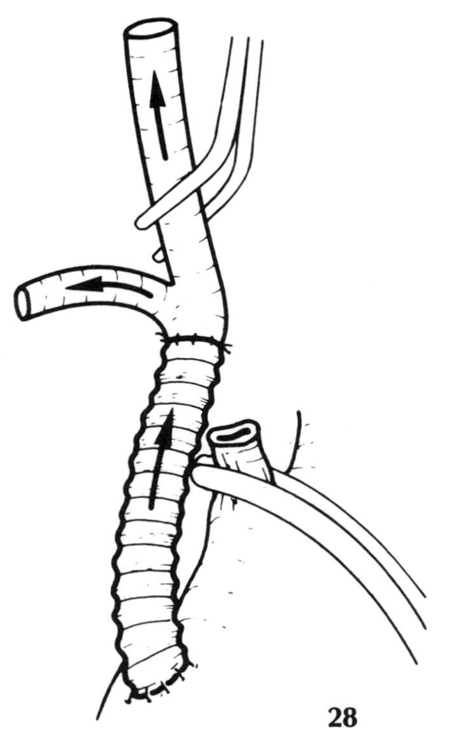

28

29 & 30

The proximal stump of the innominate artery is then closed using a continuous over-and-over 2/0 braided Dacron or 3/0 monofilament suture, the choice depending on the presence of heavily calcified lesions in the proximal part of the artery.

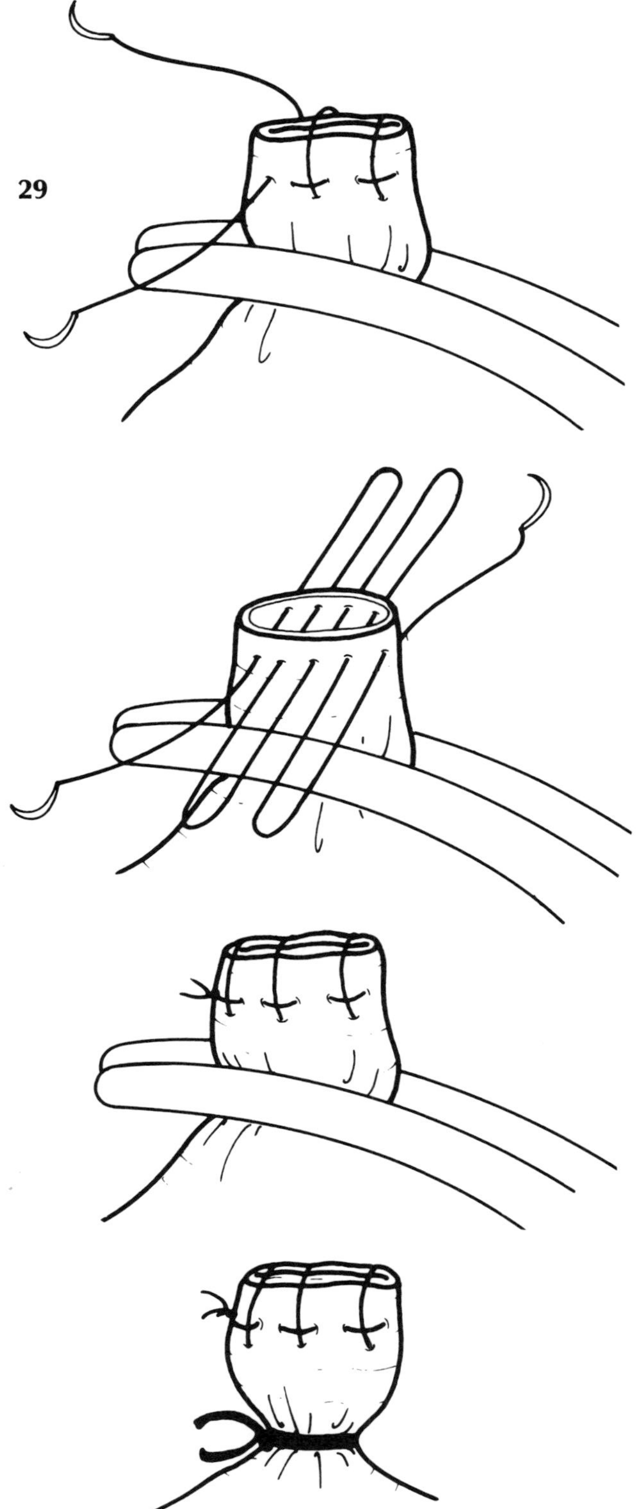
29

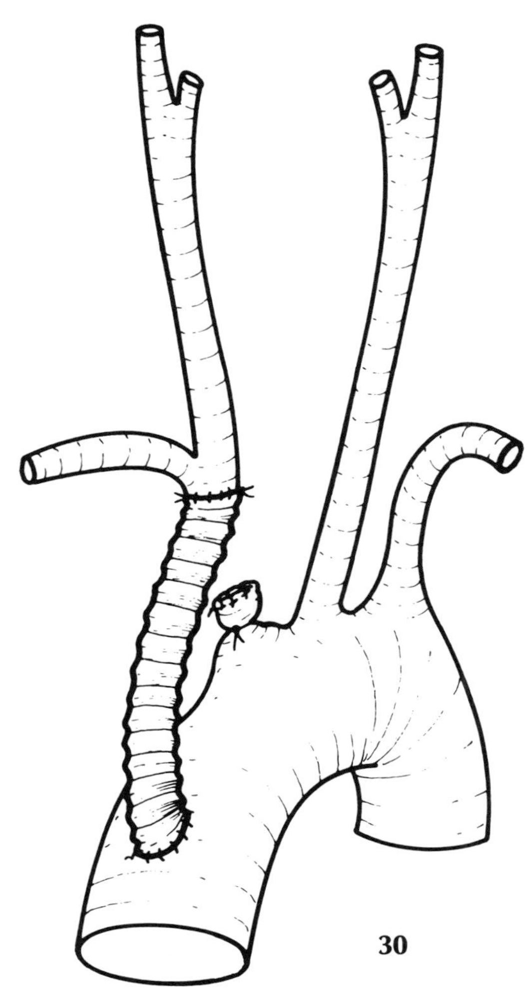
30

Alternative techniques

These are used on rare occasions. Resection and grafting may be done in the presence of aneurysmal or traumatic lesions without involvement of the origin of the artery or in the rare case of intraoperative failure of endarterectomy.

Resection followed by end-to-end anastomosis is the logical technique for managing the very rare cases of kinking in which surgical correction is necessary.

Isolated patch angioplasty may be applicable in a few selected cases of proximal non-ulcerated atherosclerotic lesion, when endarterectomy seems impractical.

Left common carotid artery reconstruction

In many cases an isolated lesion of the LCCA is a good indication for extrathoracic reconstruction using a subclavian-carotid bypass (Dietrich *et al.*, 1967). This is particularly true in poor-risk patients, where the cervical procedure is simpler and much safer. However, the LSCA may already be diseased at the time of initial evaluation or may become diseased afterwards. Conversely, its use as an inflow source seems to be unwarranted in younger patients, leading to consideration of intrathoracic reconstruction.

Endarterectomy is usually impractical because of the difficulty or impossibility of clamping the aortic arch between the innominate artery and the LSCA. Reimplantation into a neighbouring artery is sometimes performed in order to avoid the placement of a prosthetic graft. However, reimplantation into the intrathoracic part of the LSCA is illogical for reasons already mentioned and in any case can be performed through a simpler cervical approach. Reimplantation into the innominate artery is more attractive but necessitates simultaneous clamping of both arteries.

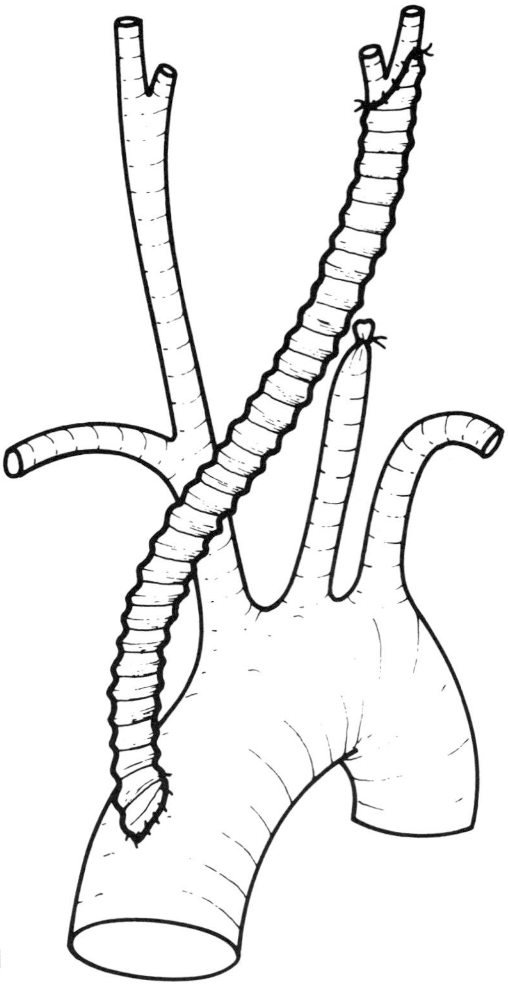

31

31

Aortocarotid bypass thus appears to be the logical procedure in these cases. A 6-, 7- or 8-mm knitted Dacron graft is selected, using part of a bifurcated graft. Alternatively, a saphenous vein graft may be used in young patients with small arteries, as may be encountered in Takayasu's arteritis (Kieffer and Natali, 1983). The technical steps of the procedure are the same as in the previously described aortoinnominate bypass. The length of the graft must be evaluated after temporary closure of the sternal retractor, in order to avoid overestimation with its attendant hazard of kinking. Although the distal anastomosis may be intrathoracic, in most cases it has to be performed to the carotid bifurcation.

Left subclavian artery reconstruction

Isolated lesions of the LSCA are almost always an indication for a cervical approach using either carotid-subclavian bypass (Dietrich *et al.*, 1967) or, preferably, direct reimplantation of the LSCA into the LCCA (Edwards and Wright, 1972). A direct approach using a posterolateral thoracotomy is rarely indicated except for aneurysm or trauma. However, to avoid a cross-over cervical bypass in good-risk patients, atherosclerotic occlusive disease may be best treated through a thoracic incision when the LCCA appears impractical as a source of inflow. Endarterectomy of aortosubclavian bypass may be used. Anatomical indications and technical steps are similar to those described for management of innominate artery lesions.

Management of multiple occlusive lesions

General principles

Whatever their aetiology, multiple lesions constitute a logical indication for intrathoracic procedures (Kieffer, 1975; Thevenet, 1979; Crawford, Stowe and Powers, 1983). A one-stage complete revascularization, including the LSCA, if diseased, is always preferable, since secondary reconstruction of the initially untreated lesion would prove difficult or even necessitate a left thoracotomy.

Multiple revascularizations are usually performed using the bypass principle, according to the following guidelines:

1. Multiple grafts are possible only if the ascending aorta is not too short, too small and/or too thick. This technique is particularly suitable if vein grafts are being used. Multiple prosthetic grafts are more likely to cause compression of the veins and airway in the thoracic inlet, especially in young female patients, and should be avoided.
2. Bifurcated grafts are simpler, but even when small sizes are used (16/8 or preferably 14/7) and the length of the body graft is tailored to be as short as possible, they may be a major cause of compression in the thoracic inlet, leading to serious complications such as venous and tracheoesophageal compression and, at a later stage, stenosis or even occlusion of one or more of the grafts.
3. Sequential grafts are to be preferred in most cases. One large prosthetic tube graft (10–12 mm) is selected to revascularize the largest vessel, usually the innominate artery. The proximal anastomosis is performed first and the graft is sequentially anastomosed to the arteries to be reconstructed, either directly or using an intermediate smaller tube graft (6–8 mm).

Application of these principles to the many possible anatomical combinations is determined mainly by the surgeon's imagination and ingenuity.

References

Bahnson, H. T., Spencer, F. C. and Quattlebaum, K. (1959). Surgical treatment of occlusive disease of the carotid artery. *Annals of Surgery* **149**, 711.

Carlson, R. E., Ehrenfeld, W. K., Stoney, R. J. and Wylie, E. J. (1977). Innominate artery endarterectomy. *Archives of Surgery* **112**, 1389.

Crawford, E. S., DeBakey, M. E., Morris, G. C., Jr and Howell, J. F. (1969). Surgical treatment of occlusion of the innominate, common carotid, and subclavian arteries. *Surgery* **65**, 17.

Crawford, E. S., Stowe, C. L., and Powers, R. W., Jr (1983). Occlusion of the innominate, common carotid, and subclavian arteries: Long-term results of surgical treatment. *Surgery* **94**, 781.

Davis, J. B., Grove, W. J. and Julian, O. C. (1956). Thrombotic occlusion of the branches of the aortic arch. *Annals of Surgery* **144**, 124.

Dietrich, E. B., Garrett, H. E., Ameriso, J., Crawford, E. S., El Bayar, M. and DeBakey, M. E. (1967). Occlusive disease of the common carotid and subclavian arteries treated by carotid subclavian bypass. *American Journal of Surgery* **111**, 800.

Edwards, W. H. and Wright, R. S. (1972). Current concepts in the management of arteriosclerotic lesions of the subclavian and vertebral arteries. *Annals of Surgery* **175**, 975.

Ehrenfeld, W. K., Wilbur, B. G., Olcott, C. N. and Stoney, R. J. (1979). Autogenous tissue reconstruction in the management of infected prosthetic grafts. *Surgery* **85**, 81.

Finkelstein, N. M., Byer, A. and Rush, B. F. (1972). Subclavian-subclavian bypass for the subclavian steal syndrome. *Surgery* **71**, 142.

Kieffer, E. (1975). Stenoses et occlusions atheromateuses du tronc arteriel brachio céphalique. *Journal de Chirurgie* **110**, 493.

Kieffer, E. and Natali, J. (1982). Ascending aorto-abdominal aorta by-pass. Technical considerations, indications and report of 15 cases. In *Extra-anatomic and Secondary Arterial Reconstruction.* Greenhalgh, R. M., ed. London: Pitman, pp. 313–333.

Kieffer, E. and Natali, J. (1983). Supra-aortic trunk lesions in Takayasu's arteritis. In *Cerebrovascular Insufficiency*. Bergan, J. J., Yao, J. S. T., eds. New York: Grune and Stratton, pp. 395–415.

Kieffer, E., Tricot, J. F., Cousin, M. T., Dauptain, J. and Natali, J. (1977). Desinsertions traumatiques du tronc arteriel brachio-céphalique. *Annales de Chirurgie Thoracique et Cardiovasculaire* **16**, 323.

Manart, F. D. and Kempczinski, R. F. (1980). The carotid-carotid bypass graft. *Archives in Surgery* **115**, 669.

Murray, G. F., Brawley, R. K. and Gott, V. L. (1971). Reconstruction of the innominate artery by means of a temporary heparin-coated shunt bypass. *Journal of Thoracic and Cardiovascular Surgery* **62**, 34.

Ochsner, J. L. and Mills, N. L. (1979). Profound hypothermia and circulatory arrest in control and repair of infected aortic prosthesis. *Journal of Cardiovascular Surgery* **20**, 1.

Selle, J. G., Cook, J. W., Elliott, C. M. Robicsek, F., Daugherty, H. K. and Hess, P. J. (1982). Simultaneous revascularization for complex brachiocephalic and coronary artery diseases. *Surgery* **90**, 97.

Sethi, G. K., Scott, S. M. and Takaro, T. (1975). Extrathoracic bypass for stenosis of innominate artery. *Journal of Thoracic and Cardiovascular Surgery* **69**, 213.

Stolf, N. A. G., Bittencourt, D., Verginelli, G. and Zerbini, E. J. (1983). Surgical treatment of ruptured aneurysms of the innominate artery. *American Journal of Thoracic Surgery* **35**, 394.

Thevenet, A., Chaptal, P. A. and Negre, E. (1968). L'arrêt circulatoire en hyppothermie profonde dans la chirurgie des branches de la crosse de l'aorte. *Annals de Chirurgie Thoracique et Cardiovasculaire* **7**, 69.

Thevenet, A. (1979). Surgical management of atheroma of the aortic dome and origin of supra aortic trunks. *World Journal of Surgery* **3**, 187.

Carotid endarterectomy

JESSE E. THOMPSON MD, FACS

Attending Surgeon, Former Chief of Surgery and Vascular Surgery, Baylor Medical Center, Dallas, Texas, USA; Clinical Professor of Surgery, University of Texas Southwestern Medical School, Dallas, Texas, USA

Introduction

Carotid endarterectomy is the procedure most frequently employed in the operative treatment of cerebral ischaemic syndromes due to atherosclerotic disease. Clinical considerations determine the indications and contraindications for operation. These are listed in detail in Table 1. The principal indication is transient cerebral ischaemia since strokes can be prevented and troublesome episodes of ischaemia are largely abolished. Indication for operation is also based on a critical evaluation of operative risk, since a high proportion of these patients have hypertension and generalized atherosclerosis, especially coronary disease.

Table 1
Indications for carotid endarterectomy in cerebrovascular insufficiency

Indications
1. Transient cerebral ischaemia
2. Stable strokes (selected)
3. Asymptomatic stenoses (selected)
4. Chronic cerebral ischaemia (selected)

Contraindications
1. Acute profound strokes
2. Progressing strokes
3. Severe intracranial disease
4. Other severe generalized disorders (e.g. cancer)

Table 2 summarizes the appropriate timing of operation for the various clinical categories. There is considerable difference of opinion regarding operation for acute carotid thrombosis following arteriography or endarterectomy. If operation can be performed immediately (1–2 h), it is probably a justifiable and worthwhile procedure. Controversy has also developed over the advisability of performing emergency endarterectomy on patients with unstable or fluctuating deficits and with crescendo transient ischaemic attacks. Management of these patients is fraught with difficulty. Although CT and MRI scans are helpful, in the absence of totally reliable methods for distinguishing between cerebral infarction and reversible ischaemia without infarction, the results of therapy, whether surgical or medical, are unpredictable. In general, if the deficit is mild and the lesion severe, emergency operation is justified. Patients with significant bilateral lesions should have bilateral endarterectomies, but in separate stages at least 1–2 weeks apart or even longer.

Table 2
Timing of carotid endarterectomy for cerebrovascular insufficiency

Elective operation
1. Stable stroke, recent or old
2. Transient cerebral ischaemia
3. Asymptomatic stenosis
4. Chronic cerebral ischaemia (rare)

Delayed operation (days to weeks)
1. Mild stroke
2. Fluctuating stroke

Emergency operation (rarely necessary)
1. Frank stroke
   - disappearance of bruit
   - slowly worsening
   - fluctuating, unstable
2. Transient cerebral ischaemia
   - severe stenosis, especially if bilateral
   - disappearance of bruit
   - crescendo TIAs
3. Carotid thrombosis immediately following arteriography or endarterectomy.

Technique of carotid endarterectomy

Technical considerations are of the utmost importance in carotid endarterectomy, since the limits of tolerance to temporary occlusion of the blood supply to the brain may be quite narrow. Safety factors must be employed which will eliminate in most instances the occurrence or aggravation of neurological deficits. Any method of carotid endarterectomy should carry low mortality, few complications, satisfactory immediate and long-term anatomical results, and good functional results relative to cerebrovascular insufficiency. The technique to be described has evolved over a period of 36 years and has proved safe and reliable. It involves the routine use of a temporary inlying bypass shunt.

1

Operation is performed under light general anaesthesia. The head is turned away from the side to be operated upon and placed on a rubber ring. The shoulders are elevated slightly using a folded sheet but there should be no undue extension of the neck. An oblique incision is made along the anterior border of the sternocleidomastoid muscle, curving medialward at its lower end, centred over the bifurcation of the common carotid artery, and curved slightly inferior to the lobe of the ear at the upper end.

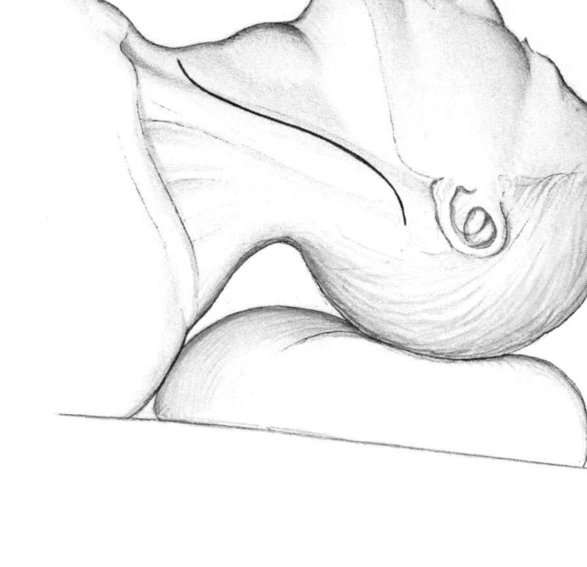

1

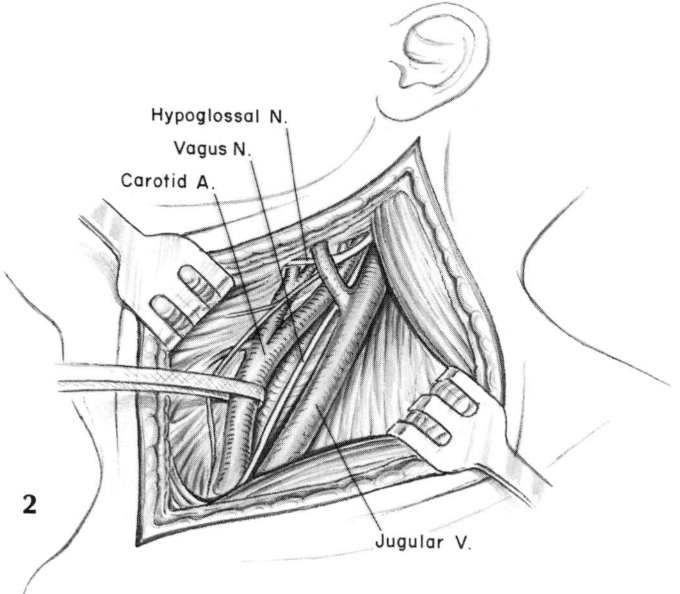

2

2

Adequate exposure of the common carotid and of the internal and external carotid divisions is essential. The carotid sinus area is infiltrated with 1% lidocaine to prevent hypotension and bradycardia. The artery is freed completely including division of the carotid sinus plexus if necessary.

One must avoid injury to the mandibular branch of the facial nerve and the vagus, hypoglossal and superior laryngeal nerves. A small branch of the external carotid artery, supplying the sternocleidomastoid muscle, usually passes over the hypoglossal nerve holding it down as a sling. This small artery should be ligated and divided to free the hypoglossal nerve off the external and internal carotid divisions. Though rarely necessary, the superior thyroid artery may be ligated and divided to facilitate dissection and exposure. An umbilical tape is first placed around the external carotid artery. Umbilical tapes are then placed around the common and internal carotid arteries and segments of #16 French rubber catheters are threaded over the tapes to act as tourniquets.

3

The occluding plaque is usually located at the bifurcation of the common carotid and extends only a short distance into the internal carotid. The distal internal carotid is ordinarily soft and thin-walled and is freed up for at least 1 cm beyond the palpable distal end of the plaque. Utmost gentleness is used throughout manipulation and the artery is simply palpated, never squeezed, since platelets, thrombi or athero-sclerotic debris may break off and embolize intracranially.

When satisfactory exposure is obtained, systemic herariniz-ation is affected with 3500–5000 u of heparin. The external carotid is occluded with a bulldog clamp and heparinized locally with 10 ml of a solution containing 100 u of heparin per ml. The common carotid is then clamped proximally with an angled vascular clamp. The distal internal carotid is occluded with a soft bulldog clamp and a linear arteriotomy is made from the common carotid into the internal carotid beyond the distal extent of the plaque. It is important that the internal carotid be opened beyond the plaque and that the entire extent of plaque be visualized in order to facilitate the succeeding steps of the operation.

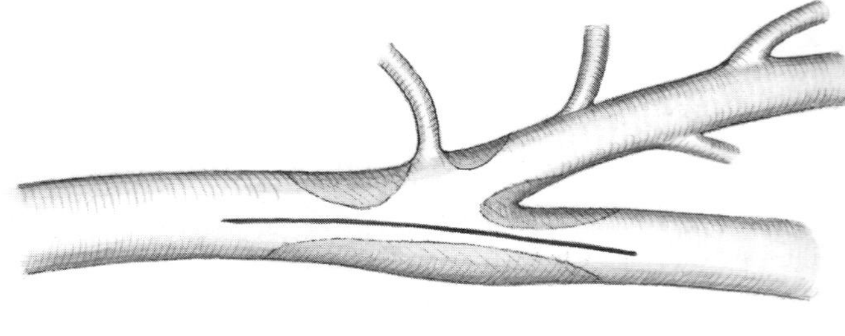

3

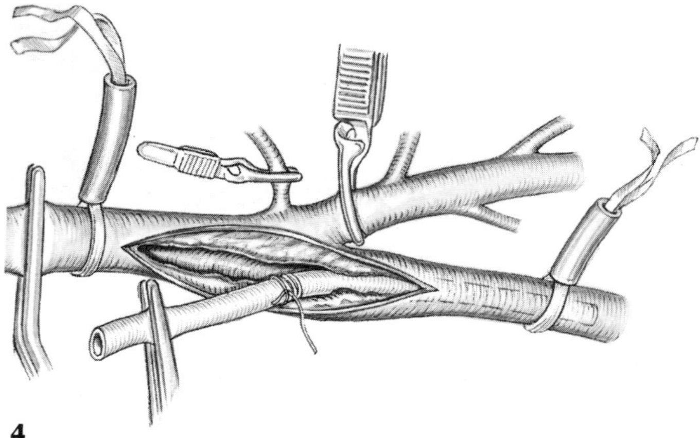

4

4

A plastic catheter shunt is then inserted into the distal internal carotid and the artery allowed to backflow.

5

The proximal end of the plastic shunt is then placed into the common carotid lumen and the umbilical tapes with rubber tourniquets are made snug.

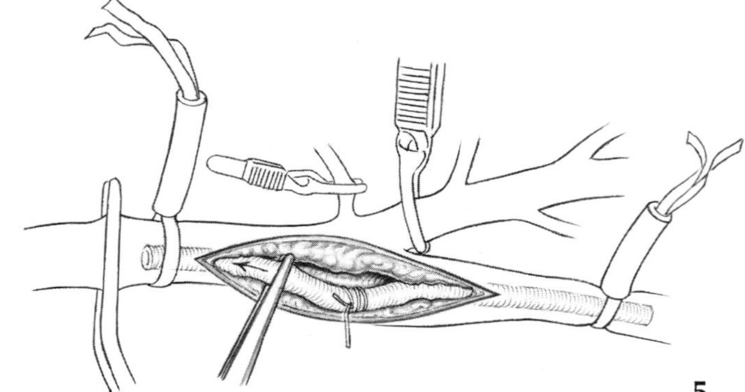

5

6

Cerebral blood flow is thus restored through the shunt. This step of the operation requires 45–90 s.

The average size shunt which fits the distal internal carotid is a #10 French plastic catheter about 9 cm in length. A #8 or #12 catheter may be used as a shunt if the artery is smaller or larger than usual. The internal diameter of the #10 catheter used is 2.5 mm. With normal levels of blood pressure this shunt carries approximately 125 ml of blood per min. Experience has shown that this is an adequate flow during the period required for endarterectomy.

6

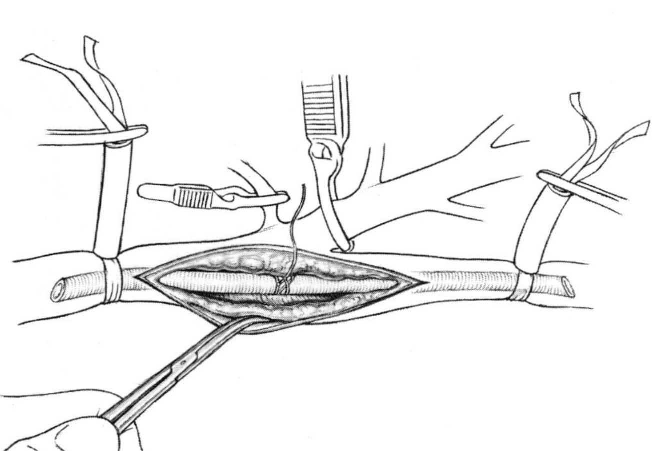

7

7

With the intraluminal shunt in place one may endarterectomize the vessel without undue haste. The appropriate plane is entered with a fine pointed clamp or other dissector and the plaque dissected from the common carotid, the bifurcation, first portion of the external carotid and that portion of the internal carotid containing the plaque.

8

The distal end of the plaque in the internal carotid usually feathers off quite smoothly leaving only thin intima above, which should not be disturbed. Small bits of debris may be lifted out with forceps or flushed out with saline. It is of the utmost importance that the distant extent of the endarterectomy be visualized so that no large pieces of intima be left to dissect distalward and produce a postoperative occlusion.

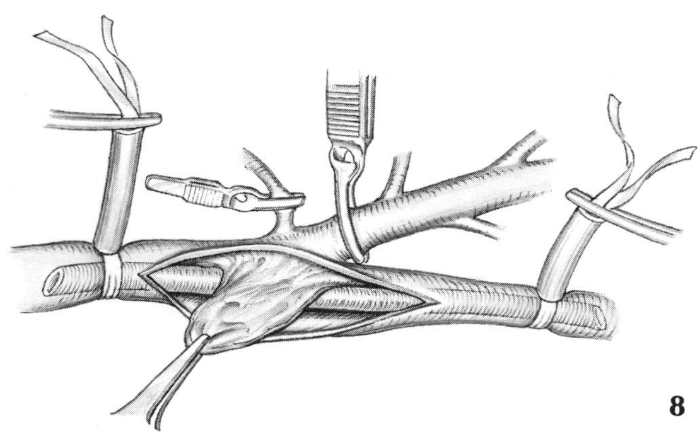

8

9

Occasionally, it is advisable to secure the distal intima with a few interrupted stitches to prevent dissection. Some 6/0 polyester sutures serve well to tack down the intima as well as to close the arteriotomy. It is also important to endarterectomize carefully the origin of the external carotid, since this artery is an important source of blood supply to the brain.

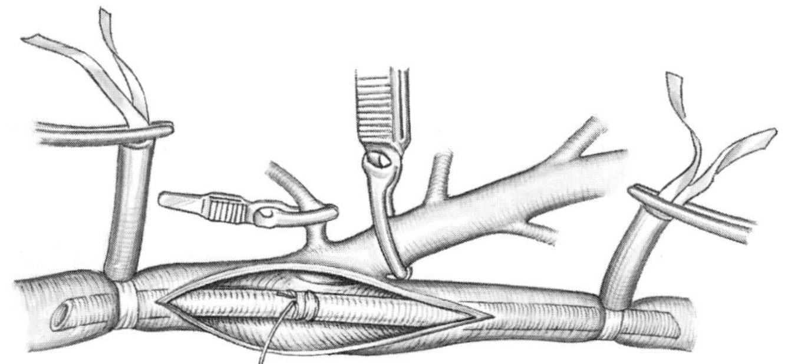

9

10

The arteriotomy is then closed with running sutures of 6/0 polyester beginning at each end. Immediately prior to placing the final three or four sutures the common carotid and internal carotid are clamped and the shunt removed. The vessels are then flushed. The final sutures are quickly placed and tied. At this point the internal carotid is allowed to backflow and is then reclamped.

Clamps are removed from the external carotid and common carotid arteries and flow restored into the external carotid allowing any debris or air to be flushed into it rather than into the internal carotid. The clamp is then removed from the internal carotid and flow restored to the brain. The occlusion time during this final step is 1–2 min. The heparin is then reversed with protamine, if necessary.

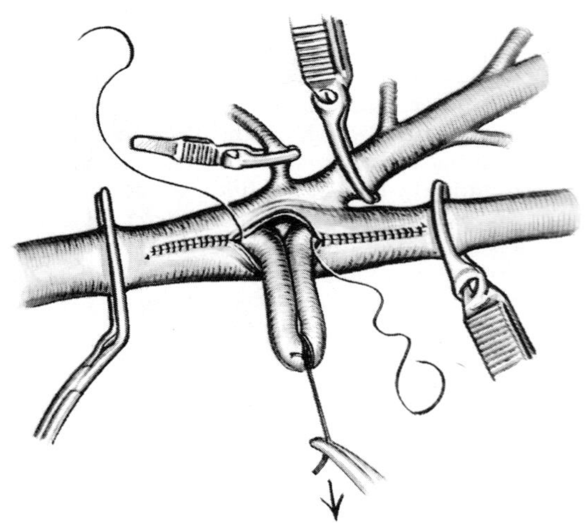

10

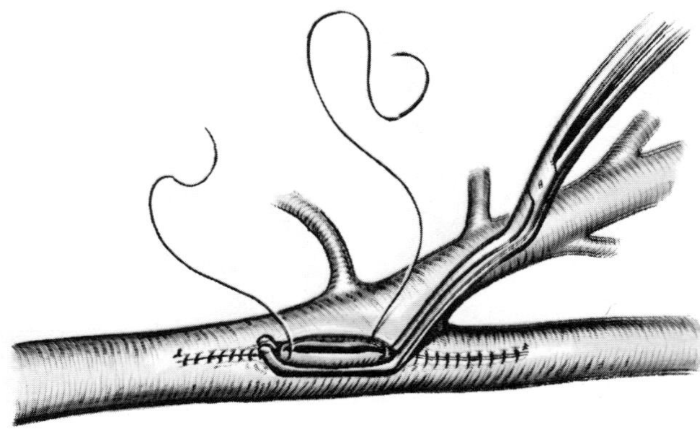

11

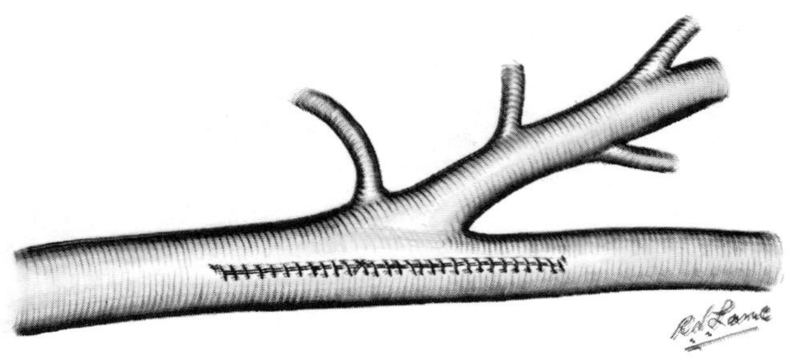

12

11 & 12

One may vary the technique of arteriotomy closure by using a thin-blade, partially occluding clamp to include the unfinished portion of the suture line after the shunt is removed. In this way cerebral blood flow is quickly re-established and the suture line is then completed.

If one is concerned about completeness of endarterectomy or the quality of pulsation in the internal carotid following restoration of flow, arteriograms may be performed on the operating table. Some surgeons perform this step routinely, but the author has not found its routine use necessary. A sterile Doppler probe to check the signals in the internal carotid is useful at this point.

It is rarely necessary to use a patch graft for closure of the arteriotomy, but if the artery is quite small, a patch graft of autologous vein or prosthetic material may be used. The wound in the neck is then closed anatomically in two layers with interrupted sutures of fine cotton. A small rubber drain is brought out of the lower end of the wound and is removed 24 h post operatively. Bilateral operations when necessary are done in separate stages about 1 week apart to avoid complications of laryngeal oedema, transient hypoglossal paresis, and cerebral oedema.

It is important that adequate levels of blood pressure be maintained during the operation and in the immediate postoperative period. The most satisfactory way to achieve this is to administer 500–1000 ml of lactated Ringer's solution during the operation and postoperatively. Vasopressors are occasionally necessary even when adequate fluids have been given. Routine postoperative heparinization is not used. Aspirin is administered postoperatively.

The technique may vary depending upon variation in pathology. If the plaque is a long one and extends quite far distally, a longer arteriotomy is necessary as is a longer shunt. At times it is prudent to close the distal portion of the arteriotomy and move the shunt proximalward before completing the endarterectomy at the common carotid bifurcation. Occasionally, one finds a plaque in the common carotid 1 cm or so proximal to the bifurcation. In this case, the arteriotomy may be extended proximally, as it is important to remove this plaque as well.

Rarely does one encounter patients with bilaterally occluded internal carotid arteries which cannot be opened by operation. Under these circumstances it is important that patency of the external carotid arteries be maintained, and endarterectomy of the orifices of these arteries may be necessary to improve collateral cerebral blood flow. The shunt technique is easily adapted to endarterectomy of the external carotid arteries.

The technique as described depicts carotid endarterectomy with the aid of a temporary inlying shunt, which is the most reliable method for cerebral support. Some surgeons use the shunt routinely in all partially occlusive lesions, some use it selectively based on an assessment of cerebral collateral circulation, while a few rarely if ever use it. Those who advocate selective shunting rely on one of several criteria of inadequacy of cerebral collateral circulation. Some test the patient under local anaesthesia and use a shunt if temporary clamping cannot be tolerated. Others, using general anaesthesia, insert a shunt if internal carotid artery stump pressure is below 50–55 mmHg or if EEG changes occur upon carotid clamping. In the hands of experienced operators, comparable results may be obtained using selective shunting.

Acknowledgements

I would like to thank Little, Brown for Permission to reproduce *Illustrations 1, 2, 4, 5, 6, 7,* and *9* from Thompson (1984), and J. B. Lippincott for permission to reproduce *Illustrations, 3, 8, 10, 11* and *12* from Thompson (1988).

References

Thompson, J. E. (1984). Carotid endarterectomy with shunt. In *Mastery of Surgery*. Nyhus, L. M. and Baker, R. J. eds. Boston: Little, Brown.

Thompson, J. E. (1988). Thrombo-obliterative disease of the vessels of the aortic arch. In *Hardy's Textbook of Surgery*, 2nd ed. Hardy, J. D., ed. Philadelphia: J. B. Lippincott.

Thompson, J. E. (1993). Standard carotid endarterectomy. In *Surgery for Stroke*, Greenhalgh, R. and Hollier, L. H. eds. London: W. B. Saunders Co., pp. 149–156.

Selective shunting during carotid endarterectomy

ROGER M. GREENHALGH MA, MD, MChir, FRCS
Professor and Chairman, Department of Surgery, Charing Cross & Westminster Medical School, London, UK

Introduction

The previous chapter by Dr Thompson fully discusses indications and his personal incision and mandatory shunting technique for carotid endarterectomy. Here, a curved incision is described which is preferred by some surgeons for cosmetic reasons; arguably this approach allows equivalent access to the carotid artery. The use of an intraluminal shunt for every procedure is not my practice because its very use carries a morbidity from dislodging artereal debris which can embolise to the brain.

The operation

Position of patient and anaesthesia

1

The skin is prepared and the towels are placed so that the whole neck area and the earlobe can be seen. The intended skin incision is marked in ink with cross-stripping marks to show the correct apposition points for the eventual skin closure. It is convenient to secure the towels and maintain sterility by using a plastic drape after the skin has been marked. The skin incision is placed as shown in relation to the anterior border of the sternomastoid muscle. Many surgeons prefer a longitudinal incision down the anterior border of the sternomastoid but this is less cosmetic and does not provide better exposure. The skin crease incision is preferable and care should be taken to ensure that it is at least two fingers' breadth away from the angle of the jaw for fear of damage to the cervical branch of the facial nerve. The great auricular and other cutaneous nerves are shown and these must be avoided as the incision is deepened through the platysma muscle to locate the anterior border of the sternomastoid. This is the vital landmark to find, because the rest of the dissection is continued along the plane of the anterior border of this important muscle.

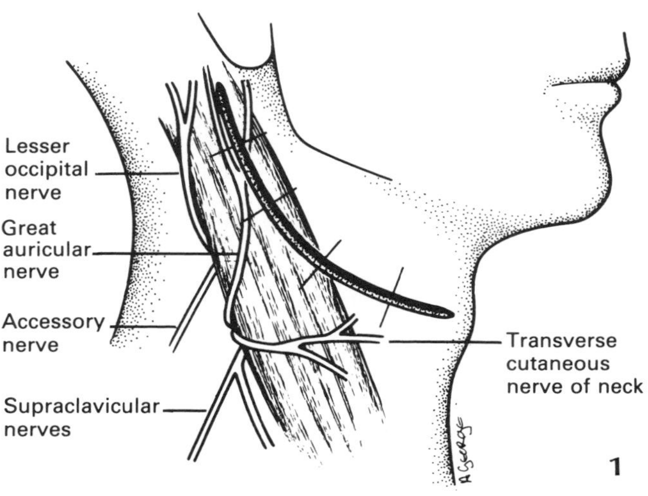

1

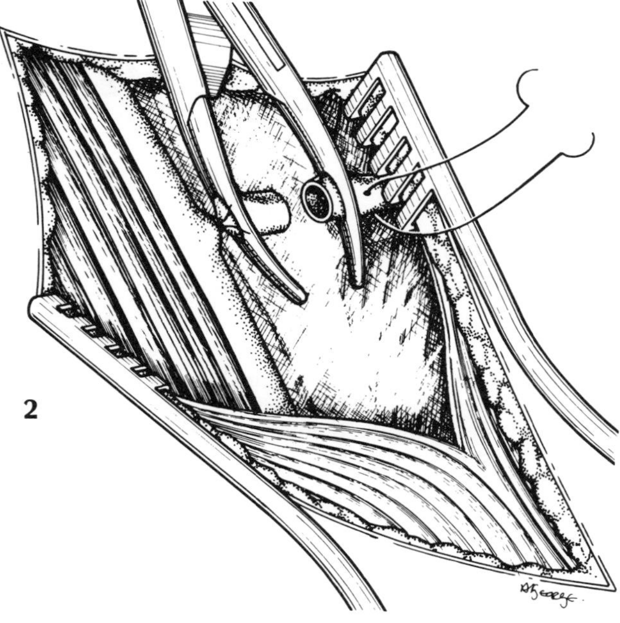

2

2

The carotid sheath is approached by dividing and transfixing the common facial vein. A simple ligature for this vein is frequently inadequate as tremendous pressures are achieved during extubation and when coughing occurs. The dissection then continues as described in the previous chapter.

Selective intraluminal shunting

3 & 4

The subsequent figures concentrate on the carotid vessel itself. The patient is given heparin 5000 u intravenously and after 3 min a clamp is placed across the external carotid artery. A needle attached to a monitoring line is placed in the external carotid artery as this avoids risk of embolization to the brain. Pressure in this artery is measured using the monitoring equipment. When the pressure is displayed on the monitoring system the common carotid is cross-clamped using a very soft clamp such as the Fogarty clamp with Silastic implants. This provides a 'back pressure' or 'stump pressure' reading.

At this stage the internal carotid artery is behaving as a side arm to the circle of Willis and this pressure is an estimate of the pressure in that circle. Those surgeons who, like the author, take notice of this reading will, in practice, find that one of two things happens the moment the common carotid artery is clamped: either the pressure falls slightly but stays at around 90 mmHg mean pressure with a pulsatile waveform, or the pressure suddenly falls and the waveform goes flat. As soon as the pressure falls to below 50 mmHg the author waits no longer but inserts an intraluminal shunt. If the pressure is above 50 mmHg and the waveform is pulsatile, no shunting is performed. Others use different methods for deciding whether to use a shunt, such as monitoring with the electro-encephalogram.

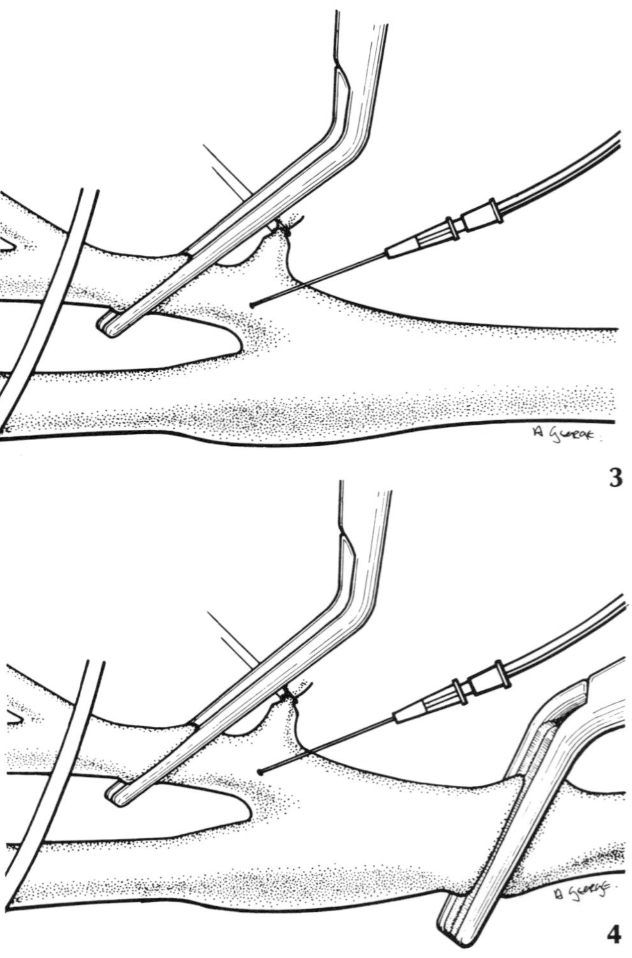

3

4

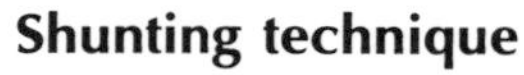

Shunting technique

5

When it is decided that an intraluminal shunt should be used, the author's preference is for the Javid shunt. This is a plastic shunt which fits comfortably into the common carotid below and the internal carotid above. Special ring clamps can be used to hold it in place as shown. As soon as the use of an intraluminal shunt for cerebral protection is indicated, an artery clip is placed across the Javid shunt, the larger end of the shunt is introduced into the common carotid artery below the atheroma and the ring clamp is made secure.

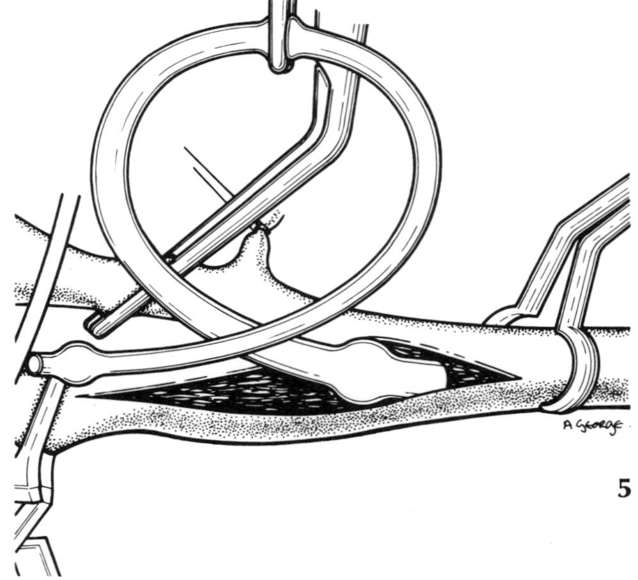

5

6

The artery clip is then momentarily removed to allow forward squirt to occur onto a swab. This clears both the shunt and the common carotid artery of any debris, minimizing the risk of embolization to the brain, and indicates that a good flow can be delivered to the brain.

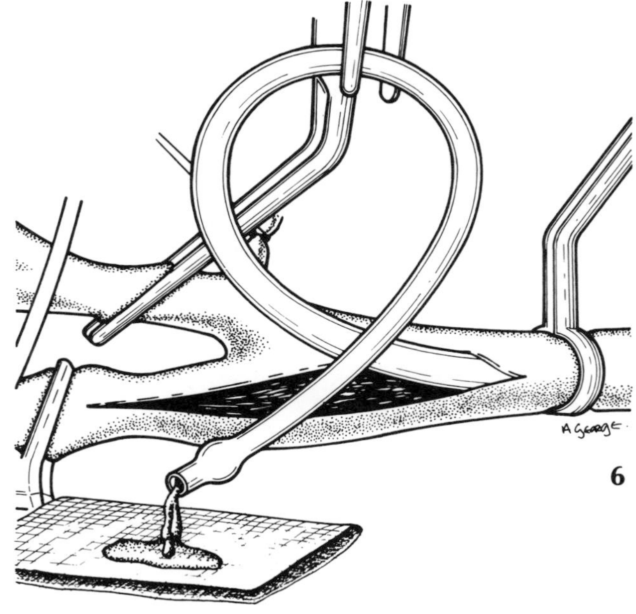

6

7

The artery clip is replaced on the Javid shunt and the bulldog clamp is removed from the internal carotid artery, allowing backbleeding to occur, which removes any debris from this vessel. The shunt is then gently manipulated into the internal carotid artery well above the diseased bifurcation.

7

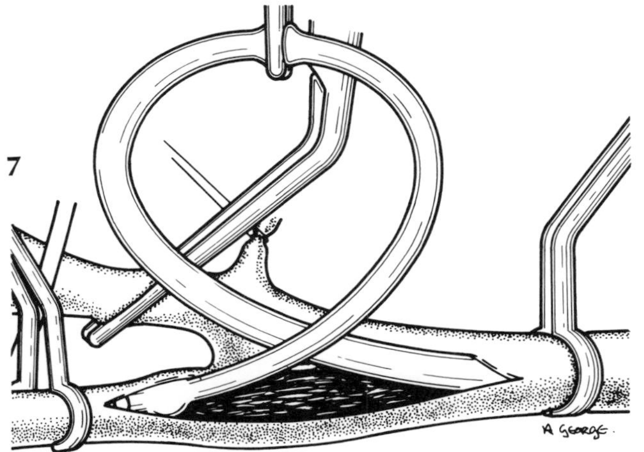

8

The smaller ring clamp is now secured and the artery clip is taken off the shunt. This allows blood flow to pass through the shunt from the common carotid to the internal carotid artery so that endarterectomy can be performed without any hurry.

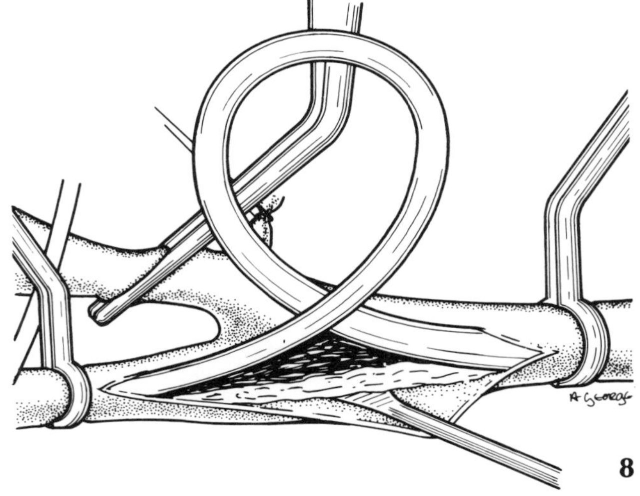

8

9

Suturing is performed as before. The shunt is no hindrance; in fact, it acts as a stent and can be a very useful aid to performing a good suture line. When no more suturing can be performed, the shunt is one again clamped with an artery clip and the ring clamps are removed; the former arterial clamps are then replaced and the shunt is removed. The arteriotomy is closed, the sutures tied and the unclamping procedure is exactly as described previously.

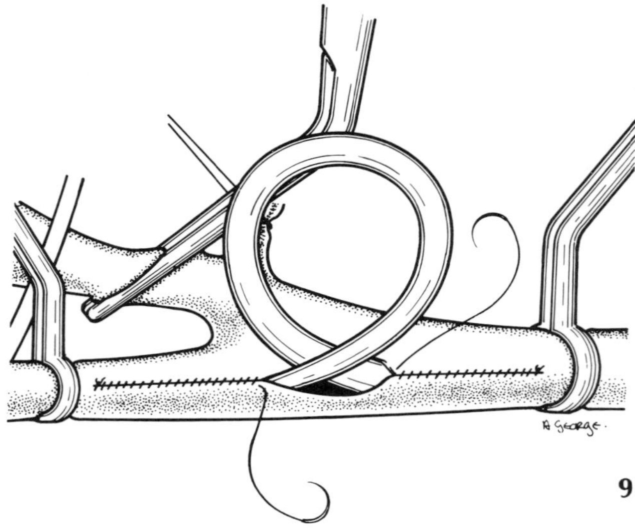

9

Approach to the internal carotid artery at the skull base

WILHELM SANDMANN

Department for Vascular Surgery and Kidney Transplantation, Chirurgische Universitätsklinik Düsseldorf, Düsseldorf, Germany

Introduction

In contrast to the rather uniform and frequent appearance of atherosclerosis at the carotid bifurcation, the lesions of the internal carotid artery at the skull base show a much more variable morphology and remain a challenge even for the experienced vascular surgeon. In our experience, with 60 reconstructions over 10 years, stenotic lesions have outweighted aneurysms by 2:1. Fibromuscular dysplasia appeared in 31%, chronic trauma in 26% atherosclerosis in 21%, spontaneous dissection in 10% and other diseases in 12%. Embolism from local thrombus formation was the major cause of preoperative transitory ischaemic attacks or strokes. Therefore, the distal segment of the internal carotid artery is not only difficult to approach for anatomical reasons but delicate to repair. Manipulation at the diseased vessel wall before clamping inevitably causes cerebral embolism. Sometimes the reconstruction has to be performed with a weakened arterial wall. Although indications for reconstruction of the internal carotid artery at the skull base are rather rare and amount to only 0.5% of all carotid operations at our institution, the approach to the skull base and technical details for reconstruction are described in this chapter.

Like other reconstructions in areas difficult to approach, surgery at the skull base requires excellent diagnostic work-up. Large skull-base aneurysms can be palpated through the nasopharynx and may be measured by CT-scanning of the neck. Doppler studies are helpful to detect flow-restricting lesions, but neither extra- or transcranial Doppler examination nor angiography can predict if longer time periods of clamping will be tolerated. The majority of these patients are much younger than the typical atherosclerotic patient. Therefore, collateral flow is not restricted by generalized occlusive disease and the risk of clamping ischaemia is very low. At least in our experience, recurrent or new postoperative deficits could not be attributed to temporary interruption of cerebral blood flow.

Superselective catheterization using conventional techniques or intra-arterial DSA in at least two planes is mandatory to determine the aetiology, anatomical extension and emboligenic potential of the disease and to visualize intracranial circulation.

Applied surgical anatomy

The extracranial portion of the internal carotid artery can be divided into three segments. The first extends from the bifurcation, where the hypoglossal nerve crosses the internal carotid artery at the level of the third vertebra. At the beginning of the second segment the hypoglossal nerve joins the sheath of the vagus nerve. At this level the architecture of the arterial wall changes from the elastic to the muscular type. Spontaneous dissections usually originate from this transition zone. The second segment reaches up to the body of C2, which is about the tip of the styloid process, where the superior laryngeal nerve leaves the vagus nerve in a dorsomedial direction. The internal jugular vein and the vagus nerve accompany the internal carotid artery within the same sheath. At the bifurcation the position of nerve and vein is lateral and not very close to the internal carotid artery, whereas at the skull base both are in a more dorsal position and the vein becomes rather close to the artery. The third segment extends from the tip of the styloid process to the carotid canal, which is entered obliquely. The view into the canal is hampered both caudally and laterally by a squamous portion of the temporal bone, which is located between the styloid process and the petrotympanica fissure below the acoustic canal.

1

The patient is placed in a supine position on the operating table with the head slightly elevated and turned towards the opposite side. The skin is incised vertically along the anterior border of the sternocleidomastoid muscle just behind the ear lobe.

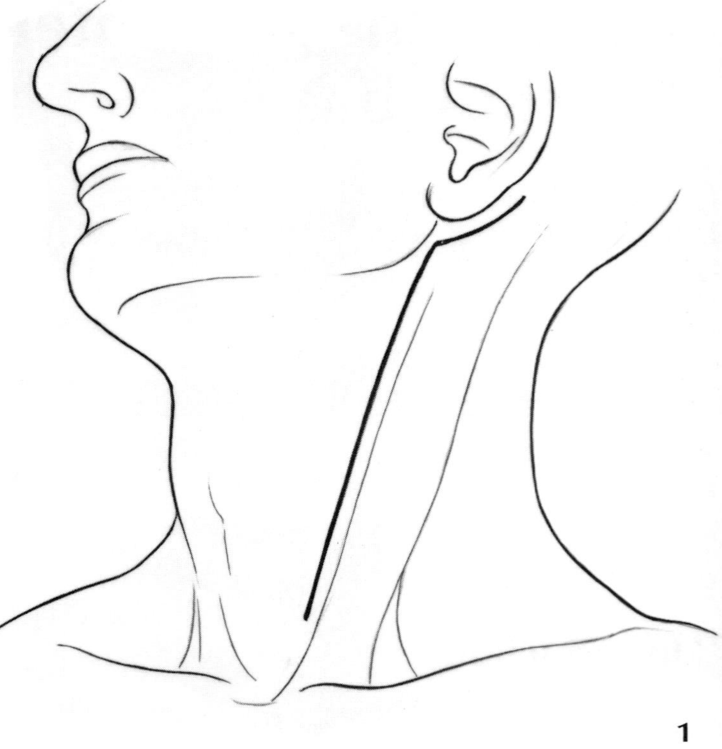

1

2

After transection of the platysma, the posterior facial vein and the posterior belly of the digastric muscle can be seen in front of the carotid artery.

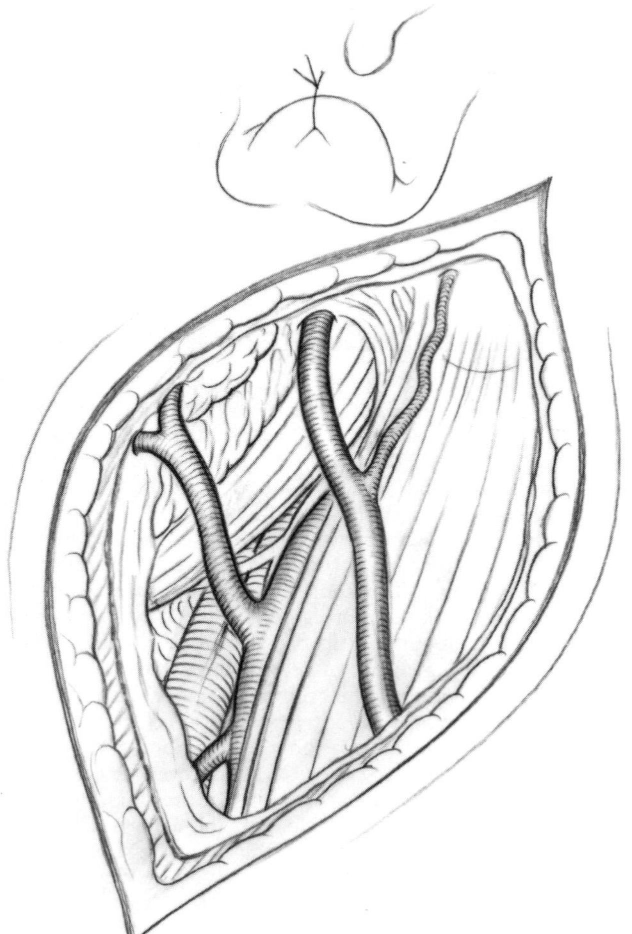

2

3

The internal carotid artery is exposed stepwise. The descendens hypoglossi is seen passing down from the hypoglossal nerve and may be divided if it helps the exposure. Any vessels lying in front of the hypoglossal nerve are divided.

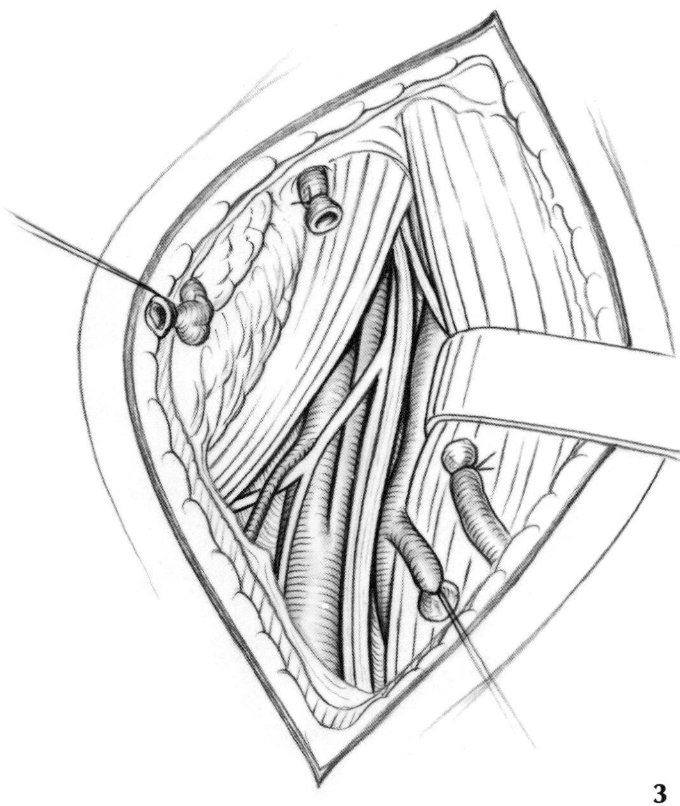

3

4

The digastric muscle is divided using electrocautery. The occipital artery or a major branch, usually located behind the digastric muscle, is ligated to avoid postoperative bleeding. Most of the skull-base arterial lesions begin at about this level.

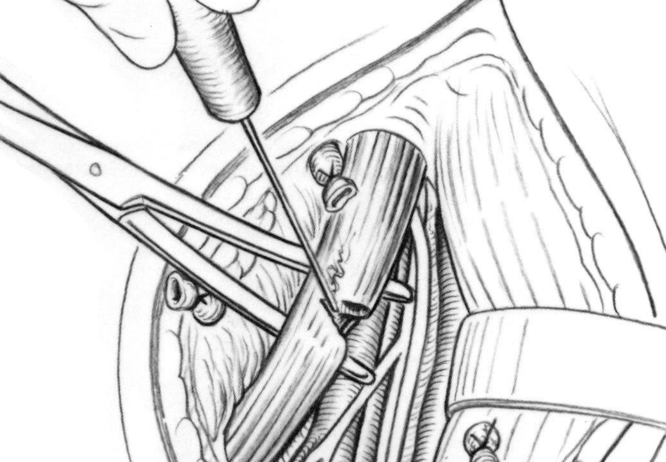

4

5

Before exposure of the diseased segment, the patient is fully heparinized and the internal carotid artery is clamped near the bifurcation. A long but shallow retractor is placed against the styloid process, which usually breaks at its base. The retractor is pulled towards the skull base and a second retractor is placed more laterally, so that a tunnel is created around the diseased internal carotid artery. The glossopharyngeal nerve and the rami pharyngei are identified and mobilized using a silicon vessel loop.

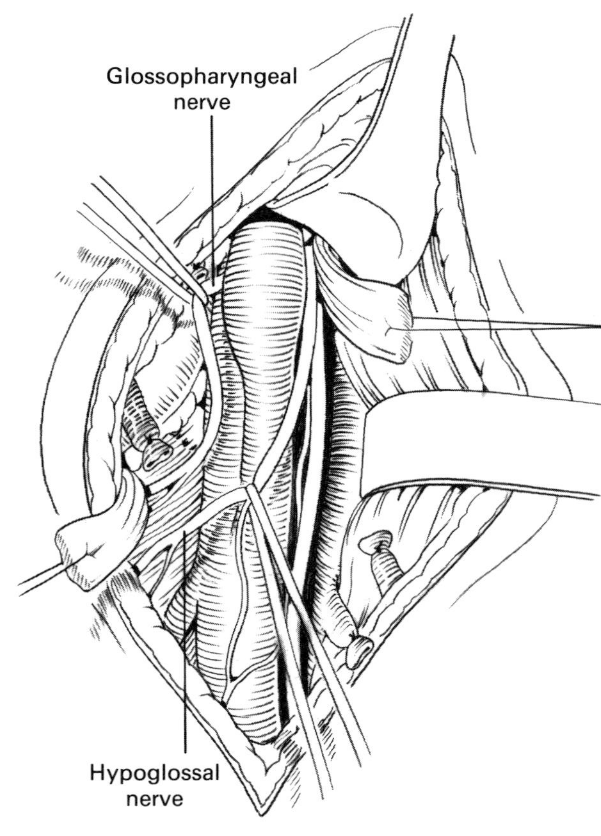

5

6

At this point the internal carotid artery is cross-clamped below the lesion and divided.

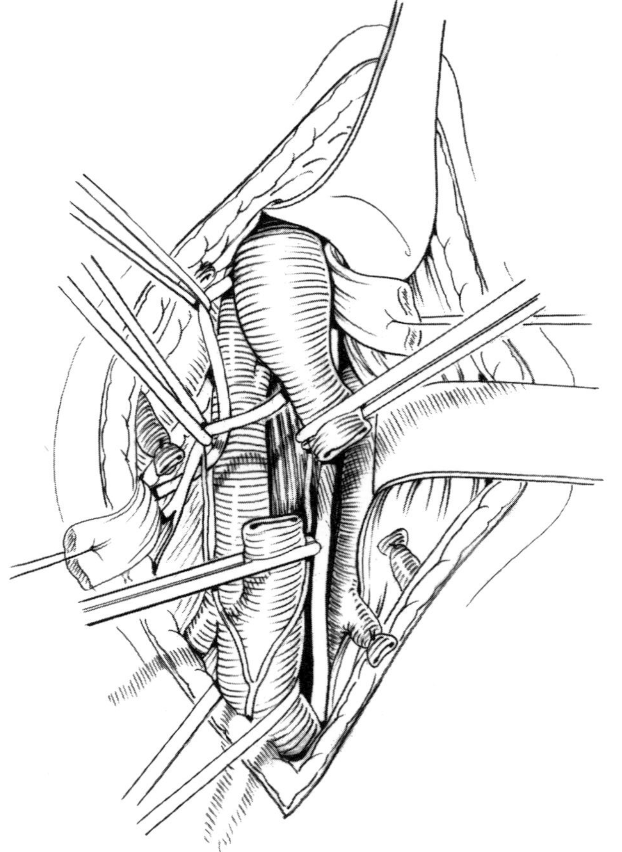

6

7

A suitable segment of harvested saphenous vein is pulled over a 3F balloon catheter. The internal carotid artery is opened and backbleeding is controlled by the balloon catheter.

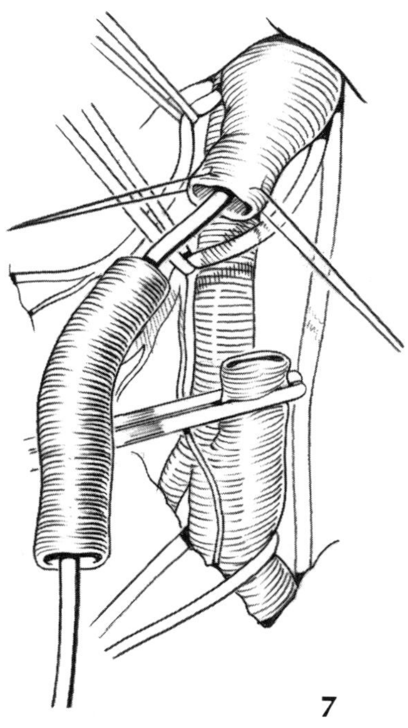

7

8

In patients with aneurysms, the aneurysmal sac is partially resected and the graft is anastomosed from the inside (the graft inclusion technique) with absorbable suture material using interrupted sutures to avoid stenosis of the anastomosis.

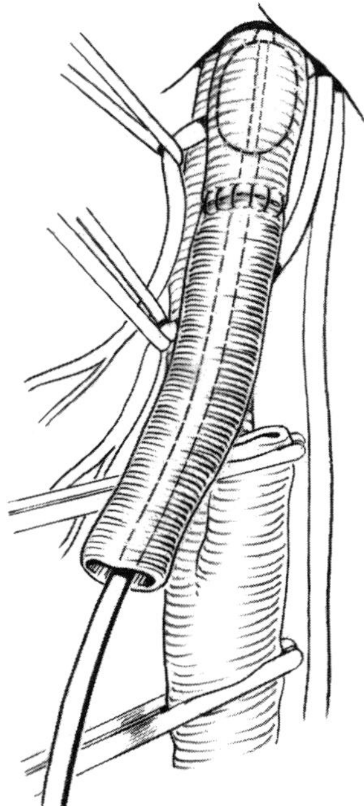

8

9

After the distal anastomosis has been performed, the vein graft is pulled through beneath the glossopharyngeal and hypoglossal nerves.

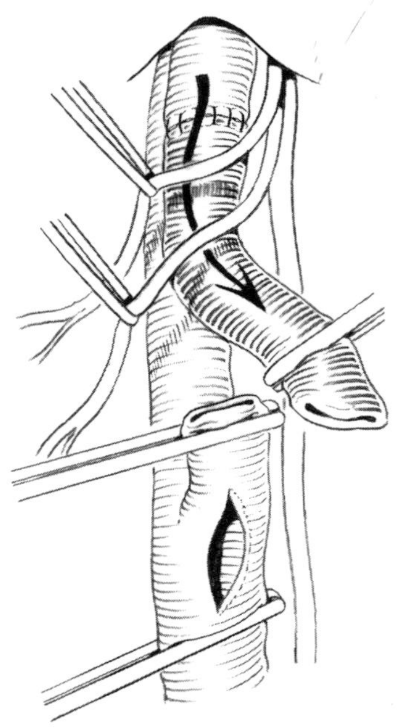

9

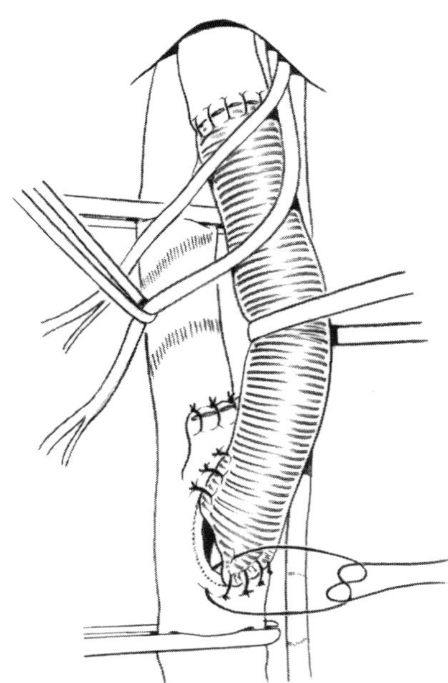

10

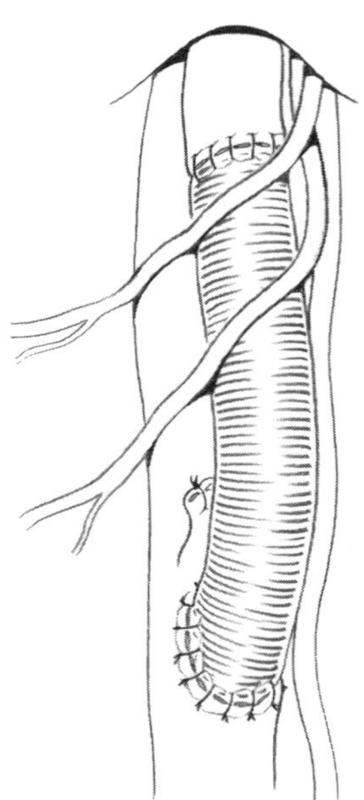

11

10 & 11

The common and external carotid arteries are cross-clamped and the common carotid artery is incised. The stump of the internal carotid artery is oversewn and the graft is anastomosed further proximally. The graft has to be anastomosed with a certain tension, because the neck is over-extended and turned through almost 90°. Before the proximal anastomosis is performed, the optimal length of the graft is determined by turning the head into the normal position.

After the anastomosis, arteriography is performed on the operating table because on occasion a very distal anastomosis cannot otherwise be checked. During cross-clamping, the patient is ventilated with 100% oxygen and anaesthesia is maintained by intravenous methods.

In patients with lesions extending just to the entrance of the carotid canal the lateral wall can be removed using a chisel. It is possible to perform the distal anastomosis 1 cm within the carotid canal. However, at this point, the operation becomes complicated and the surgeon needs to have had great experience of such reconstructions. Early proximal clamping during the dissection avoids embolization. The interrupted suture technique using monofilamentous absorbable suture material avoids stenosis of the anastomosis at the skull base. A shunt cannot be used in extremely high lesions, though through-graft balloon catheter blockage is very helpful. Although I prefer operative angiography, electromagnetic flow measurement is an alternative to detect critical stenoses or distal occlusions during the procedure. Heparinization is necessary throughout clamping to avoid distal thrombosis. Graft length must be checked in the normal head position at the end of the procedure to ensure that kinking and twisting will not occur.

Excision of carotid body chemodectoma

AVERIL O. MANSFIELD ChM, FRCS

Professor of Surgery, St Mary's Hospital, London;
Honorary Senior Lecturer in Vascular Surgery, Royal Postgraduate Medical School, London, UK

Introduction

1

Paraganglia are widely disseminated organs with sensory and perhaps local neurosecretory function. Those APUD cells with an affinity for chrome salts are known as chromaffin paraganglia and their tumours are phaeochromocytomas. Those without chrome salt affinity are the non-chromaffin paraganglia; their most common tumour affects the carotid body. The most common sites of non-chromaffin paraganglion tumours are illustrated. In the author's experience the second most common paraganglioma in the neck is of vagal origin. On angiography this is seen as a vascular tumour which does not splay the internal and external carotids apart. When vocal cord paralysis also exists the preoperative diagnosis is complete.

Histological distinction between benign and malignant tumours is not possible and only the development of metastases can determine malignancy. This is fortunately uncommon.

There has been much discussion about whether it is necessary to remove these usually benign tumours, but in the author's experience the tumour can be removed safely with little or no risk of recurrence and it is usually easier to deal with this tumour while it is small, rather than to wait until it is an advanced tumour involving local cranial nerves.

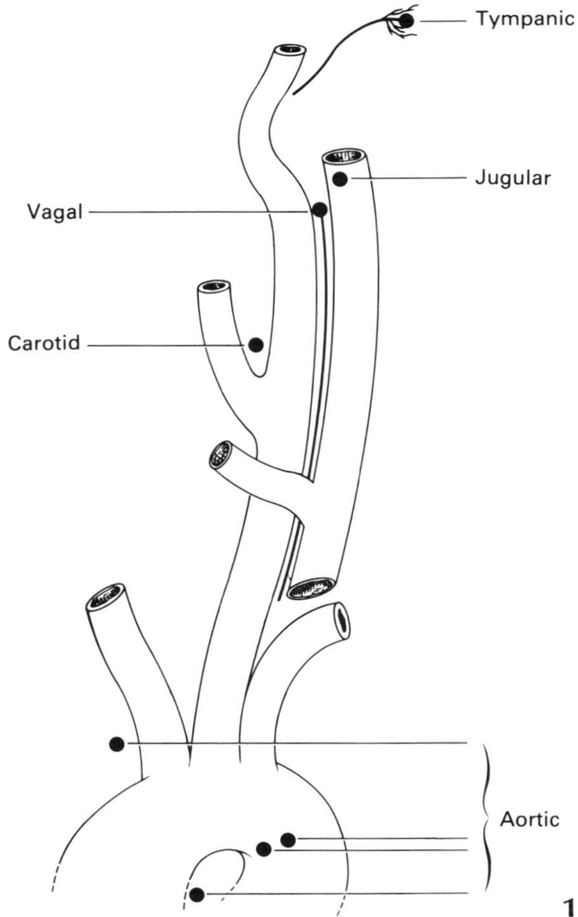

Investigations

The important and diagnostic investigation is the angiogram. Normally, this consists of a selective carotid injection and views in two planes. Intravenous digital subtraction angiography, where available, avoids the risk of a carotid injection and when doubt exists about the presence of a tumour this technique is a valuable first investigation and may be all that is required.

Duplex Doppler scanning may also be a useful non-invasive test.

The cranial nerves must be examined with care and indirect laryngoscopy must be a routine preliminary examination. The oropharynx should be inspected.

Carotid body tumours are rarely secretory but the routine examination for vanillylmandelic acid should prevent unexpected problems.

Large and particularly vascular tumours should be considered for preoperative embolization to reduce the technical problems in excising them. However, the evidence that this helps is anecdotal and the procedure carries some risk.

Position of patient

The patient is placed supine with the head of the table slightly elevated. A pad is placed longitudinally between the scapulae (a litre bag of i.v. fluid is suitable). The head, supported in a head ring, is extended and turned towards the opposite side. A bladder catheter may be inserted if a large tumour is to be removed.

Preoperative preparation

The usual preparations for major vascular surgery are undertaken and the blood pressure should be maintained at normal levels. Although hypotensive anaesthesia is an attractive theoretical prospect, it may increase the risk of stroke occurring during carotid manipulation. In addition to normal diathermy, the provision of a bipolar coagulator is valuable. A nerve stimulator may sometimes be helpful.

It is often helpful to palpate the oropharynx before starting the operation to assess the size of the tumour.

Nasal intubation in a high tumour may increase access.

The operation

Incision

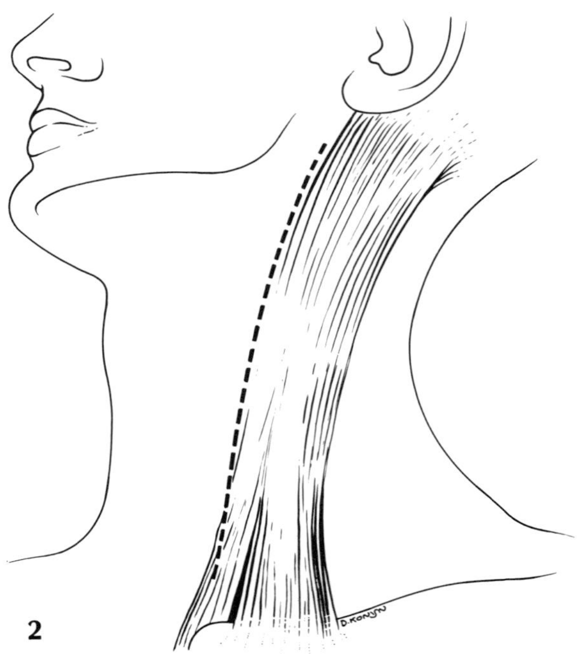

2

2

The incision can be made exactly as in the previous chapter but the author prefers to make it along the anterior border of the sternomastoid muscle from the mastoid process to the lower part of the neck. The exact position depends on the level of the tumour.

3

If the upper part of the tumour extends well above the angle of the mandible, the upper part of the incision may usefully be extended around the ear and anterior to the external auditory meatus, as in the routine approach to the parotid gland.

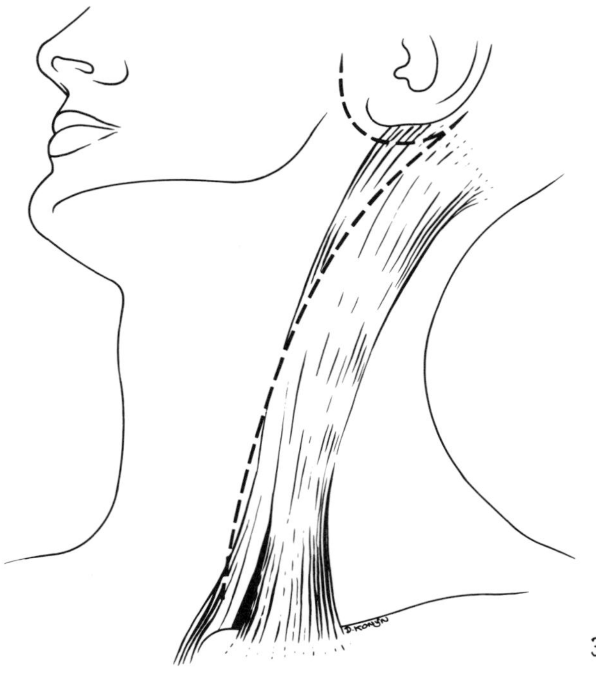

3

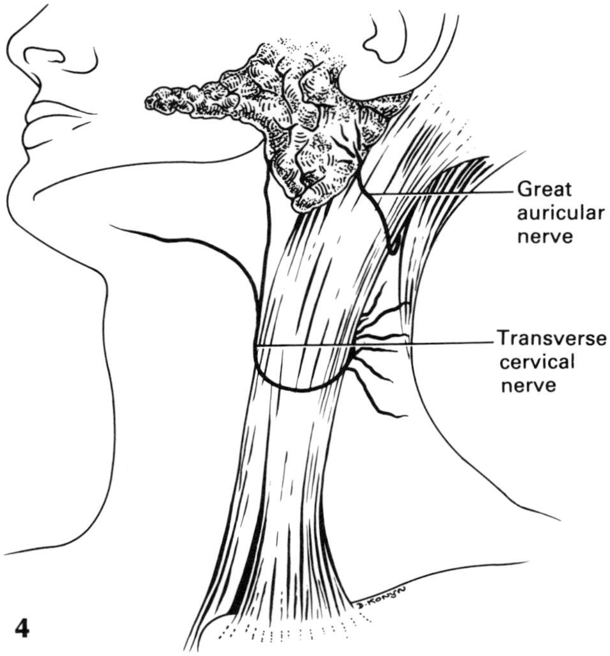

Great auricular nerve

Transverse cervical nerve

4

4

Cutaneous nerves cross the incision and are divided but the great auricular nerve is preserved.

The platysma is divided and the anterior border of the sternomastoid is exposed. Exposure is developed from the mastoid process to the lower limit of the wound by 'walking over' the muscle until the internal jugular vein comes into view. The muscle can then be mobilized and retracted with a self-retaining Travers retractor.

Internal jugular vein

5

The internal jugular vein is now dissected from the artery throughout its visible course, taking care not to injure the adjacent vagus nerve in the groove between artery and vein. The common facial vein and any other anterior tributaries are ligated and divided. The Travers retractor with its rounded 'teeth' can safely be used to retract the vein.

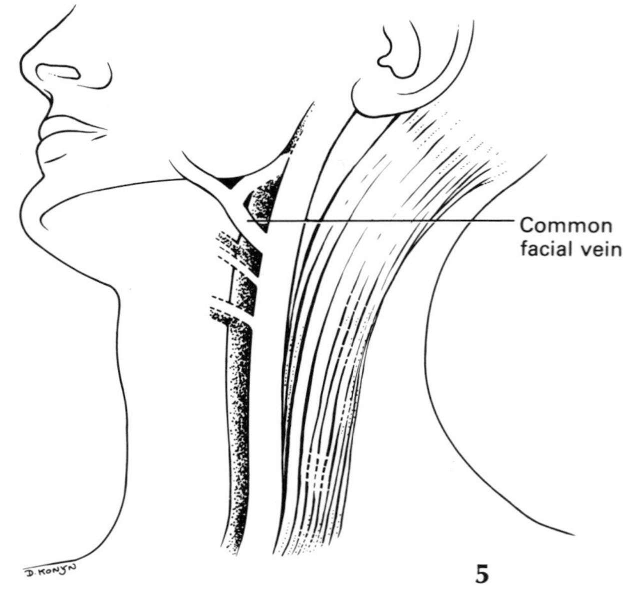

5

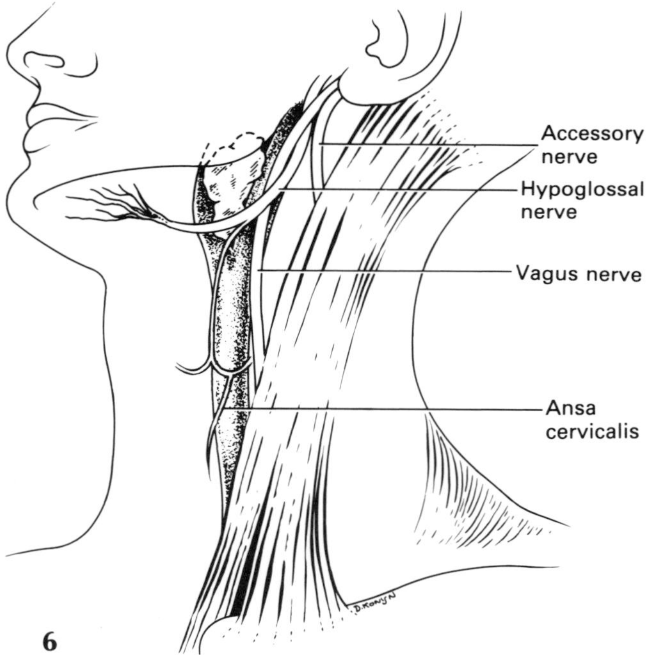

6

6

The vagus nerve is carefully identified throughout its course in the neck. The hypoglossal nerve can usually be identified and preserved but sometimes its course is within the tumour and it can only be dissected out at a later stage. The ansa cervicalis is usually visible and, if possible, is preserved.

7

Carotid arteries

In the common form of chemodectoma, the carotid body tumour, the tumour begins at the level of the carotid bifurcation and the internal and external carotids are splayed apart by it. In the simplest form the carotid vessels are clearly identifiable throughout, but in more complex tumours the arteries may be embedded in and surrounded by the tumour.

The internal and external carotids will come closer together again above the tumour and it is important to identify the internal carotid at that level, i.e. beyond the upper limits of the tumour, before commencing the dissection, in order to ensure its safety.

From then on the operation consists of the safe and meticulous dissection of the carotid vessels from the tumour. As most of the blood supply is derived from the external carotid the dissection is begun with that vessel.

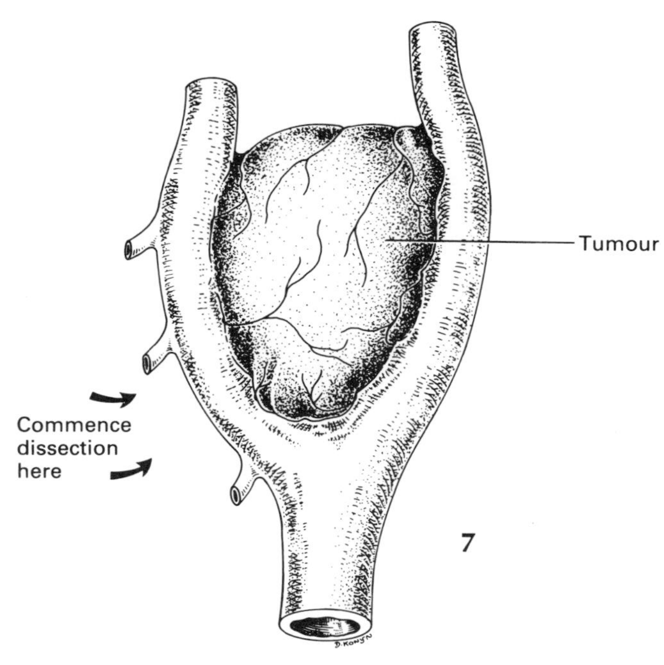

7

The upper end of the dissection

When the carotid body tumour is confined to within the bifurcation which is at or below the angle of the mandible there is no need for this upper part of the operation. However, in the high and extensive tumours this is the most important and the most difficult part of the operation and these routine steps undertaken before exposure of the tumour will facilitate the excision.

8

First the facial nerve is identified by following up the sternomastoid until the posterior belly of the digastric is displayed and then dissection is carried out in the angle above this and between the posterior belly of the digastric and the mastoid process. There is usually no difficulty in recognizing the facial nerve but if any doubt exists the nerve stimulator can be valuable. The reason for displaying the facial nerve is simply to ensure its safety during the remainder of the dissection.

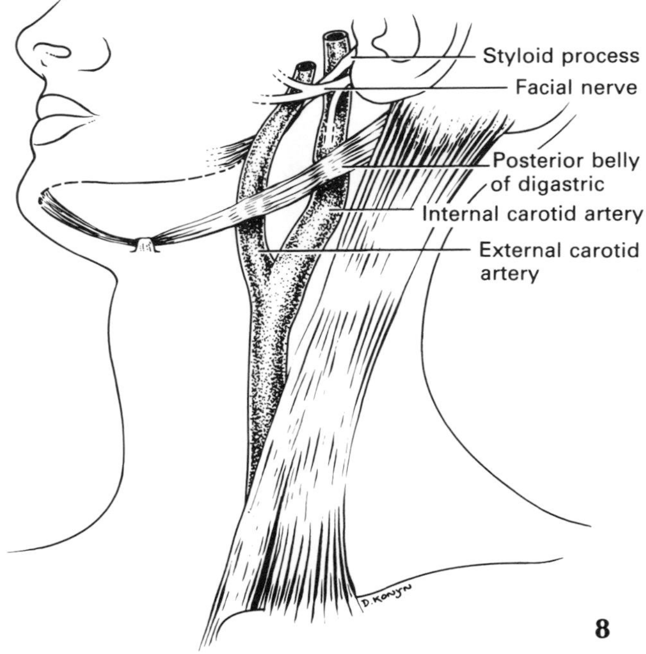

8

9

The posterior belly of the digastric can then be divided along with the stylohyoid. The occipital artery may have to be divided because it runs backwards along the inferior edge of the stylohyoid. The transverse process of the atlas can be palpated. It must remembered that deep to these muscles are the accessory nerve, the internal jugular vein and the carotid arteries. The styloid process is palpated in the depths between the mastoid process and the mandible. The styloid can then, if necessary, be fractured, allowing the space to open up further. Using this approach the author has never found it necessary to employ the alternative methods of anterior dislocation of the temporomandibular joint or osteotomy of the ramus of the mandible.

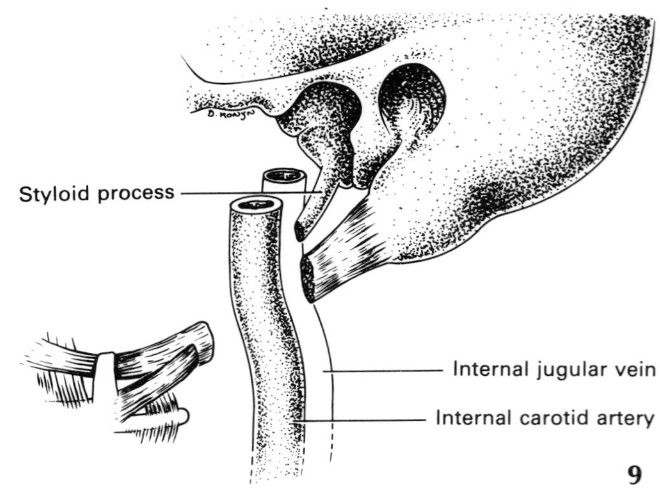

9

The dissection

10

Beginning with the external carotid side of the tumour, the plane between the tumour and vessel wall is identified and developed. The so-called white line of Gordon-Taylor in the adventitia can often be identified (as illustrated), but in other cases, when the tumour is particularly vascular, this is not apparent. Numerous small vessels will course between the vessel and the tumour and the diathermy is invaluable. The bipolar coagulator is very helpful for the numerous tiny vessels encountered. Larger feeding vessels are ligated and divided. Each such division renders the tumour less vascular but the vessels cannot be sought for and ligation must wait until the tumour is peeled off the carotid and they are exposed in the course of the dissection.

If the tumour completely surrounds the vessels it is usually necessary to divide the tumour in order to reach the correct plane of dissection. Again, any such dissection is best carried out on the external carotid side of the lesion. The dissection will then proceed over the external carotid to its anterior surface and similarly to its posterior surface. It is very important to avoid twisting the tumour, and hence the vessels, as this may result in cessation of flow up the internal carotid.

The lumen is most easily entered during the final stages of separation from the vessels in the 'crutch' between internal and external carotids. This is because the exact configuration of the vessels is unknown and because traction may be exerted on the tumour at this stage.

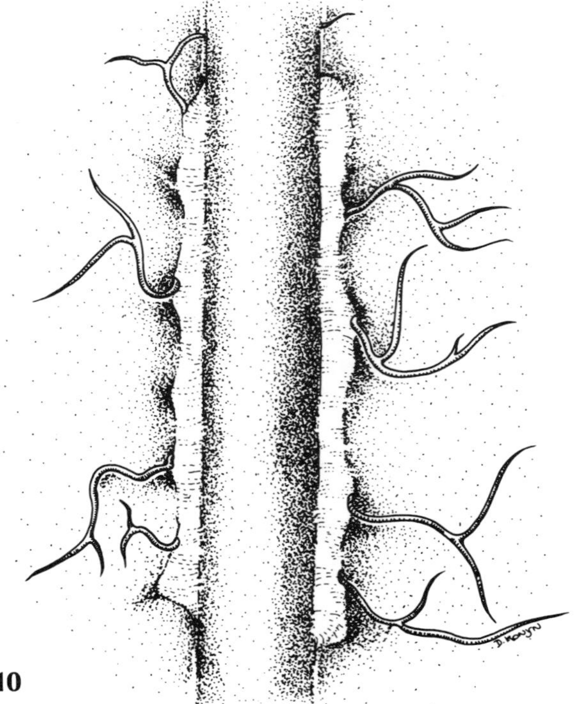

10

11

When the posterior surface of the tumour is being separated from the deep tissues it is very important to avoid injury to the glossopharyngeal nerve, which is in an immediate posterior relation in most moderate-sized tumours. It is not easy to identify and must be assumed to be in danger.

When the tumour has finally been separated from the vessels it will appear smaller and firmer. Most of the bleeding ceases at this stage although an occasional vessel in the tumour bed is diathermied using bipolar coagulation, ensuring first that the cranial nerves are not close by. The author employs suction drainage routinely.

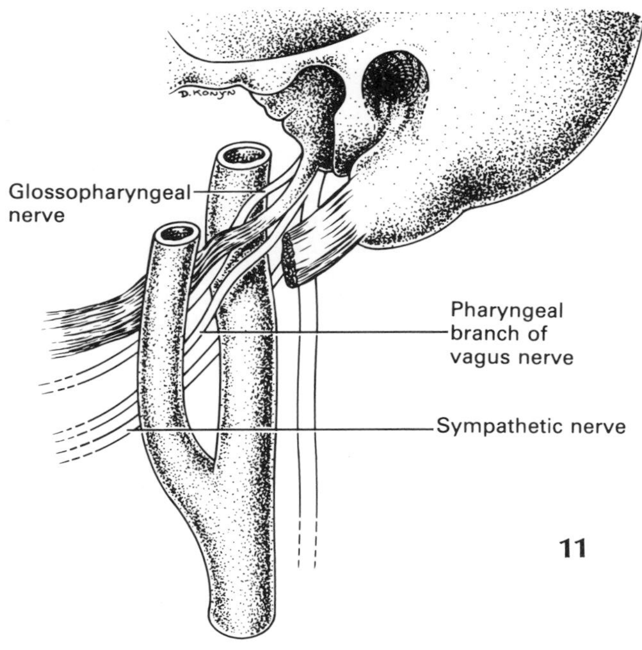

11

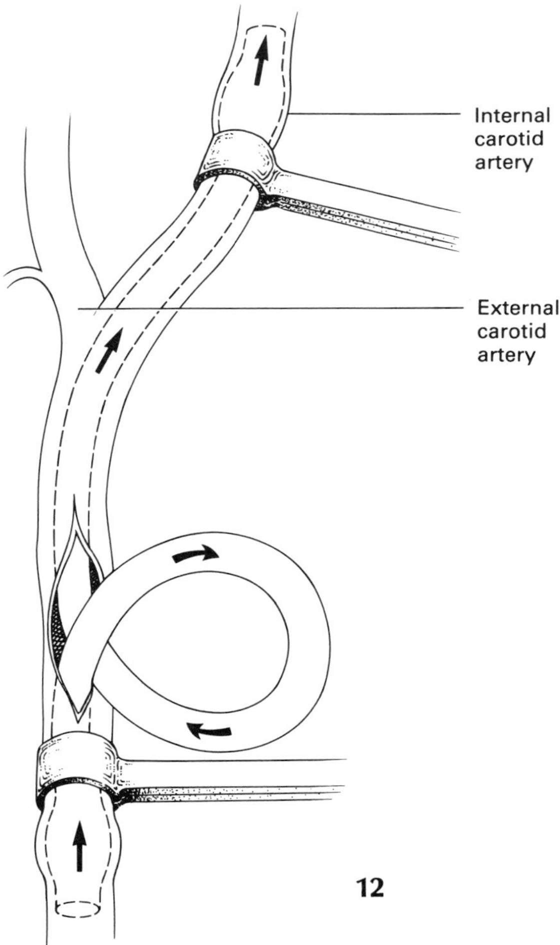

12

Shunt

A shunt, such as the Javid or Brenner shunt, should be available, so that if unexpected carotid injury occurs it can be inserted when prolonged clamping is envisaged.

12

Use of the shunt in order to reduce blood loss has also been advocated, although the author has no experience of this method. The shunt is inserted from the common carotid to the internal carotid, cutting off the orifice of the external carotid and hence the supply to the tumour. Consequently, the tumour is less vascular and the vessels safer.

Ligation of the external carotid to aid haemostasis has been suggested. However, the ligation would have to be at the origin of the external carotid and if this can be dissected out the operation is half completed; little would seem to be gained from ligation at that stage.

Complications

Stroke

Stroke is potentially the most worrying risk of the operation, but the author has had no experience of this. Reports would suggest two possible causes: injury to the internal carotid, and thrombosis as the result of stasis, which may be caused by twisting the vessels or by a haematoma in the vessel wall. In the older age group there is always the possibility of atheroma at the bifurcation and its embolization as the result of manipulation.

Cranial nerve injury

Three cranial nerves are anatomically closely related. Preoperative examination is essential as they may already be affected by tumour. The vagus nerve, except in chemodectomas arising from the vagus, can usually be easily identified and preserved. The hypoglossal is always seen crossing or entering the tumour and should be preserved, provided this does not prejudice the safety or completeness of the excision. The glossopharyngeal is the most difficult to identify and its injury can have serious effects on swallowing.

Arterial injury

If the vessel wall is entered accidentally it can usually be repaired with a 6/0 polypropylene suture. Arterial clamps must always be available. Invasion of the arterial wall by the tumour is rare, but when encountered it will require resection of the artery and vein graft replacement.

Haemorrhage

This can be steady and prolonged but rarely becomes a problem under the conditions of wide exposure, as advocated. Haemorrhage is only a serious problem when the tumour is an unexpected finding at attempted biopsy of a lump in the neck.

Haematoma

As there is a large dead space, suction drainage is necessary.

Conclusion

Carotid body tumours are slow growing and usually benign. They can be bilateral and may be associated with other tumours of APUD cells. Small tumours are easily removed, provided a preoperative diagnosis is made by angiography so that adequate wide exposure can be made. The necessary instruments for arterial repair should always be available but will rarely be required. A carotid shunt should also be available but the author has rarely used one and its use should not be regarded as routine.

Careful identification and preservation of the cranial nerves is a necesary part of the operation, but occastionally one or more of these nerves will already be involved in the tumour and have to be sacrificed.

Transperitoneal approaches to the abdominal aorta and its branches

TAMMY K. RAMOS MD
RONALD J. STONEY MD
Vascular Division, Department of Surgery, University of California at San Francisco, San Francisco, California, USA

Introduction

In 1951 Charles Dubost performed the first abdominal aortic aneurysm repair using a left subthoracic retroperitoneal approach (Dubost, Allary and Oeconomos, 1952). Since that time, multiple approaches to the abdominal aorta and its branches have been described and compared. Although there are many differences among the various approaches, they differ primarily by location of the incision (abdominal vs flank), anatomic route to the aorta (transperitoneal vs extra-peritoneal) and the number of body cavities involved (abdominal vs thoracoabdominal). The controversy over which approach is superior has been focused on perioperative morbidity. During the past decade, the left flank-extra-peritoneal approach has been revitalized. Several studies (Johnson *et al.*, 1986; Peck *et al.*, 1986; Sicard *et al.*, 1987; Leather *et al.*, 1989; Gregory *et al.*, 1989) have suggested that it is less morbid than the traditional midline-transperitoneal approach. The only prospective study (Cabria *et al.*, 1990) did not substantiate these findings. Although perioperative morbidity is a major consideration when selecting an approach to the abdominal aorta and its branches, the overriding consideration should be which approach provides the required exposure to perform the optimal repair of the aortic disease.

Adequate exposure of any arterial bed is determined by the distribution and extent of pathology in the artery wall, the surgical objective, and the anticipated reconstructive technique. Atherosclerosis is the most common disease involving the abdominal aorta and its branches and it may result in obstruction to blood flow, thromboembolism, and aneurysmal degeneration. Therefore, the therapeutic objectives of treatment are reperfusion of distal arterial beds, removal or exclusion of embolic sources, and replacement of unstable arterial walls. These objectives can be accomplished by two fundamental cular reconstructive techniques: endarterectomy and grafting (replacement; bypass—with or—without exclusion). Endarterectomy and replacement grafting require unrestricted exposure of the aorta and its branches. Bypass grafting can usually be accomplished with limited exposure of the inflow and outflow vessels.

After the necessary exposure is determined, then the best approach to achieve it can be selected. This chapter will present our methods for achieving and maintaining optimal exposure of the abdominal aorta and its branches. Our current practice is to employ a full-length midline abdominal incision and one of three transperitoneal approaches, the infracolic approach, the transcrural approach, or the medial visceral rotation approach.

Optimal exposure of the abdominal aorta and its branches requires that the area of interest be brought into view and that unobstructed access to the area be maintained throughout the reconstruction. The retroperitoneal location of the aorta, its fixation to the spine by the diaphram, its proximity to major venous structures and its coverage by abdominal viscera present a challenge for exposing this area. The superficial wound margins must be widely *retracted* throughout the procedure; the soft tissue and viscera must be mobilized, displaced and *retained* for long periods of time. The use of self-retaining retractors has helped to overcome the challenge of aortic exposure. We use the Omni-Tract vascular retractor system (Omni-Tract Surgical, A Division of Minnesota Scientific, Inc., St. Paul, Minnesota), which is a table-mounted, self-retaining mechanical retractor that provides extended exposure or simultaneous multi-site exposure for an indefinite period of time.

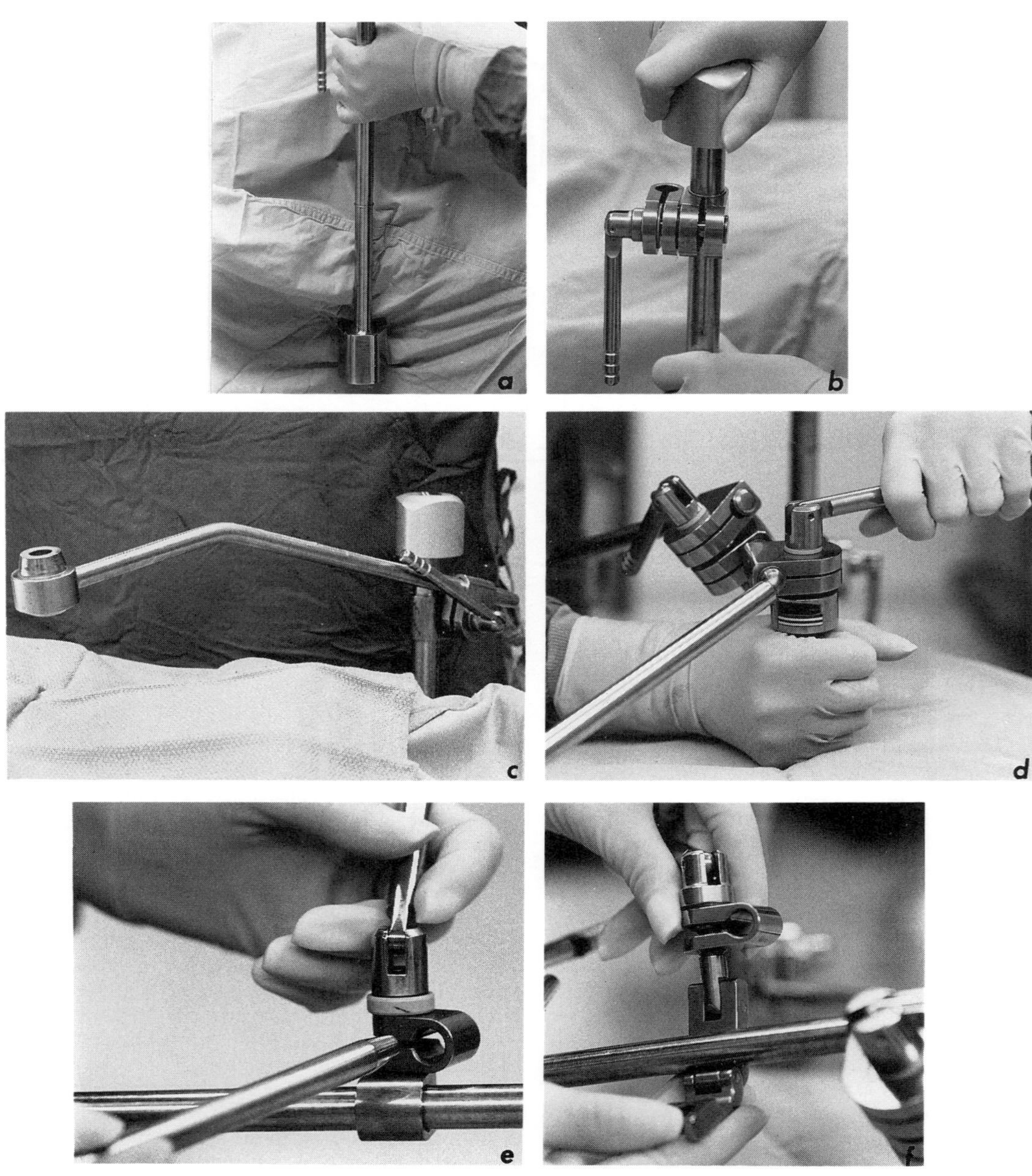

1a, b, c, d, e & f

This retractor system can be rapidly set-up and dismantled. The Omni-Clamp sterile field post is placed on the operating table rail over the sterile drapes (*a*) and secured by rotating the top knob (*b*). An adjustable wishbone support arm slides into the clamp on the Omni-Clamp sterile field post and the handle is tightened (*c*). The adjustable wishbone frame is placed on the support arm and positioned around the surgical field as desired; all of the handles are firmly tightened to secure it (*d*). Retractors and blades are used by first sliding the appropriate number of circle clamps onto the arms of the wishbone frame and then placing the shaft of the retractor through the circle clamp before engaging the abdominal wall or viscera with the retractor blade (*e*). Quick clamps open up and can be placed and can be placed directly on the arms of the frame (*f*); they can be used later in the procedure when retractors are added for retention of deeper structures. The single attachment of this retractor system to the operating table and the adjustability of the support arm and wishbone frame provides a low profile over the patient so that there is minimal spatial interference with the surgeon and the assistant (*Illustration 2*). The combination of joints, and swivelling and non-swivelling retractors allows for retraction at any depth, angle, or tension. These characteristics are particularly helpful when using a self retaining retractor to achieve and maintain optimal exposure of the abdominal aorta and its branches by the three approaches described below.

Infracolic approach

2

The abdominal cavity is entered through a full-length midline incision extending from the xiphoid process to the symphysis pubis. After exploration, the Omni-Tract vascular retractor system is assembled as described previously. When this incision is used, the primary joint of the wishbone frame should be positioned so that it sets one hand-breadth cephalad to the incision and one hand-breadth above the lower sternum (*Illustration 1d*). The wound edges are retracted laterally from the mid-portion of the incision using the Mayo swivel retractors. Special care is always taken to protect the soft tissue and viscera by using moistened sponges beneath the retractor blades. The stomach is decompressed with a nasogastric tube. The transverse colon and omentum are wrapped in a moist sponge and reflected cephalad over the wound edges where they are retained with splanchnic retractors. The small bowel is placed in an intestinal bag, displaced to the right, and retained with the corral malleable disposable retractor.

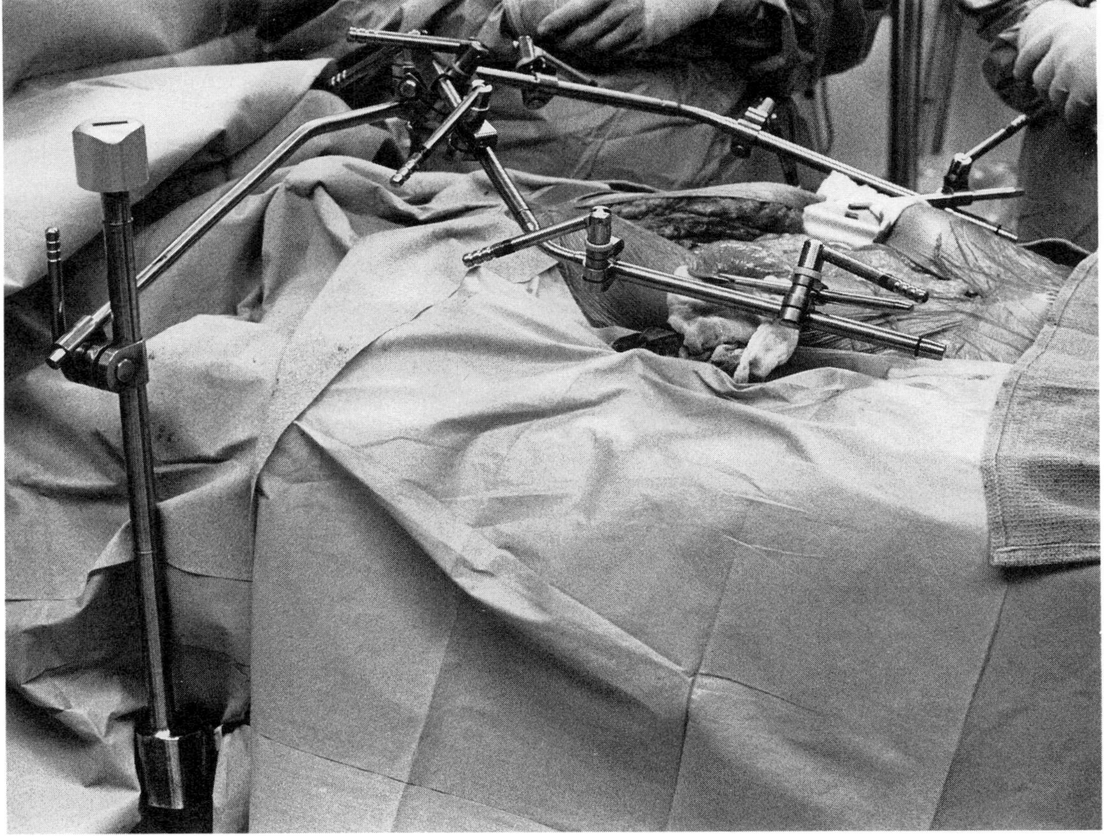

2

3

These manoeuvres bring the midline retroperitoneum into view. The infrarenal aorta is exposed by incising the posterior peritoneum just to the right of the midline from the aortic bifurcation to the base of the transverse colon mesentery. Proximally the periaortic tissue is divided and the left renal vein is identified and circumferentially mobilized.

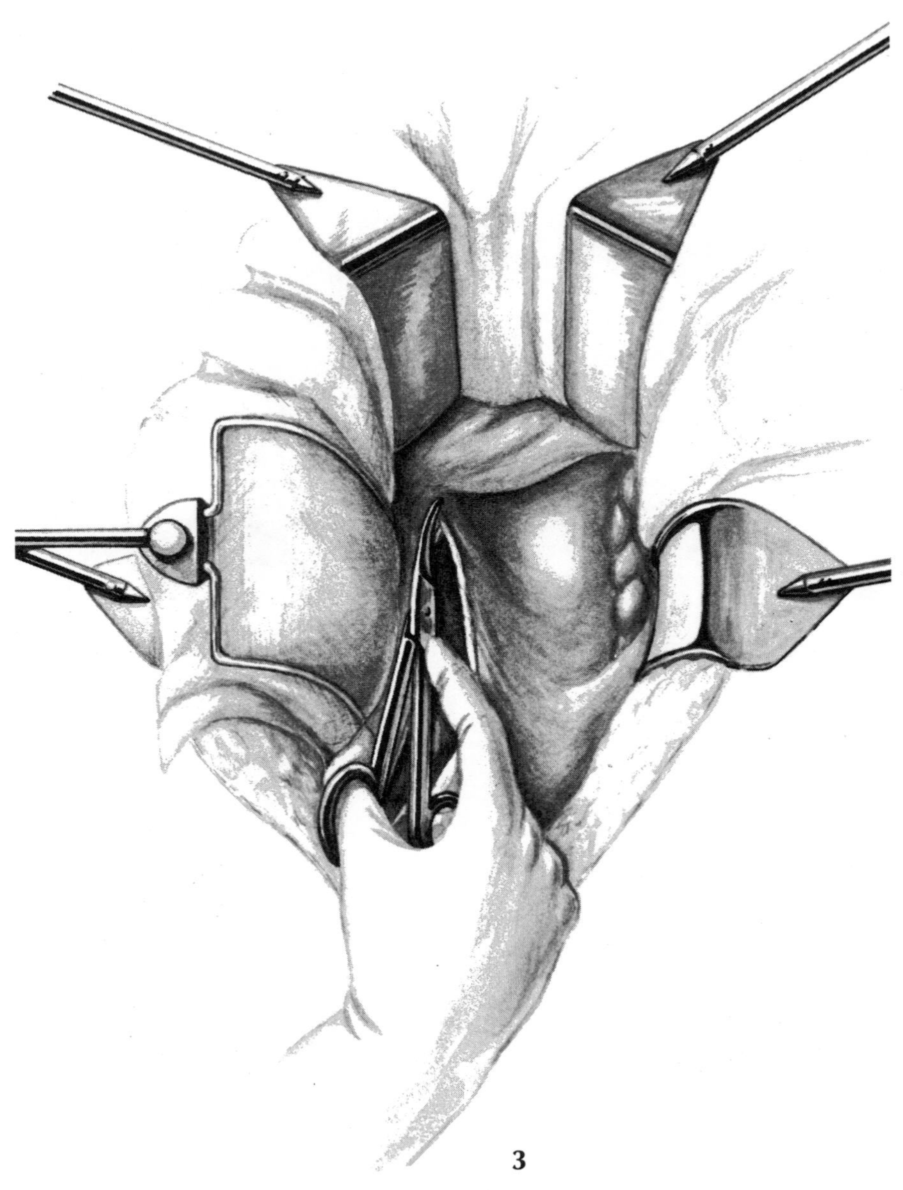

3

4

Visualization of the juxtarenal aorta is facilitated by displacing the left renal vein cephalad using the renal vein retractor. Depending on the number of retractors and circle clamps already deployed, a quick clamp may need to be placed on the wishbone frame to attach the renal vein retractor. Now mobilization of the proximal infrarenal aorta can be safely accomplished by dissecting in the plane of Leriche.

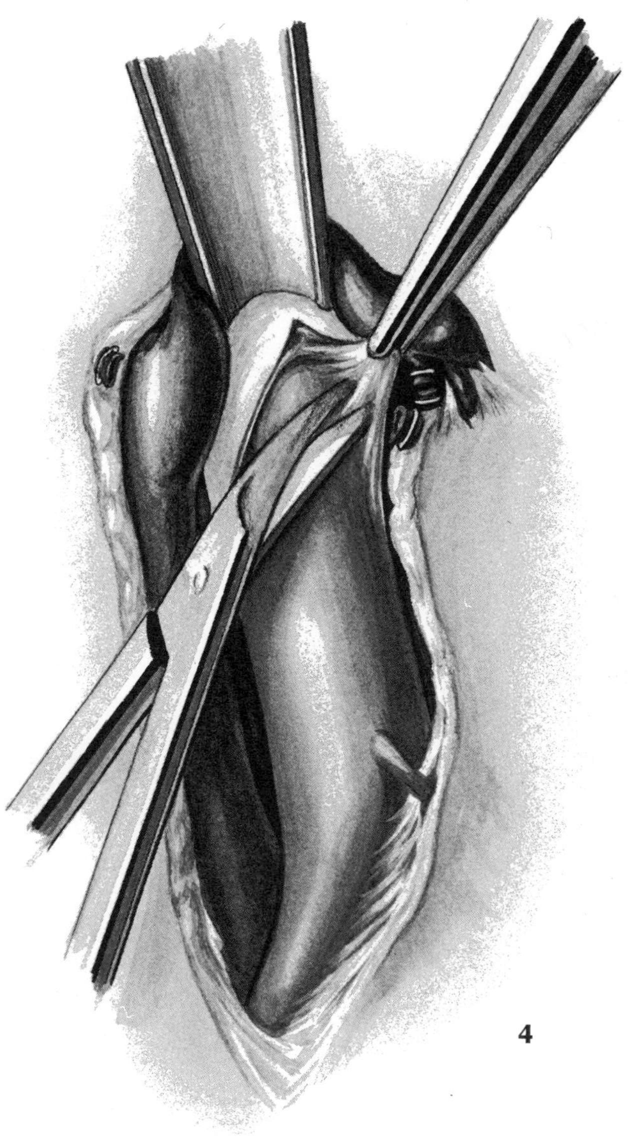

4

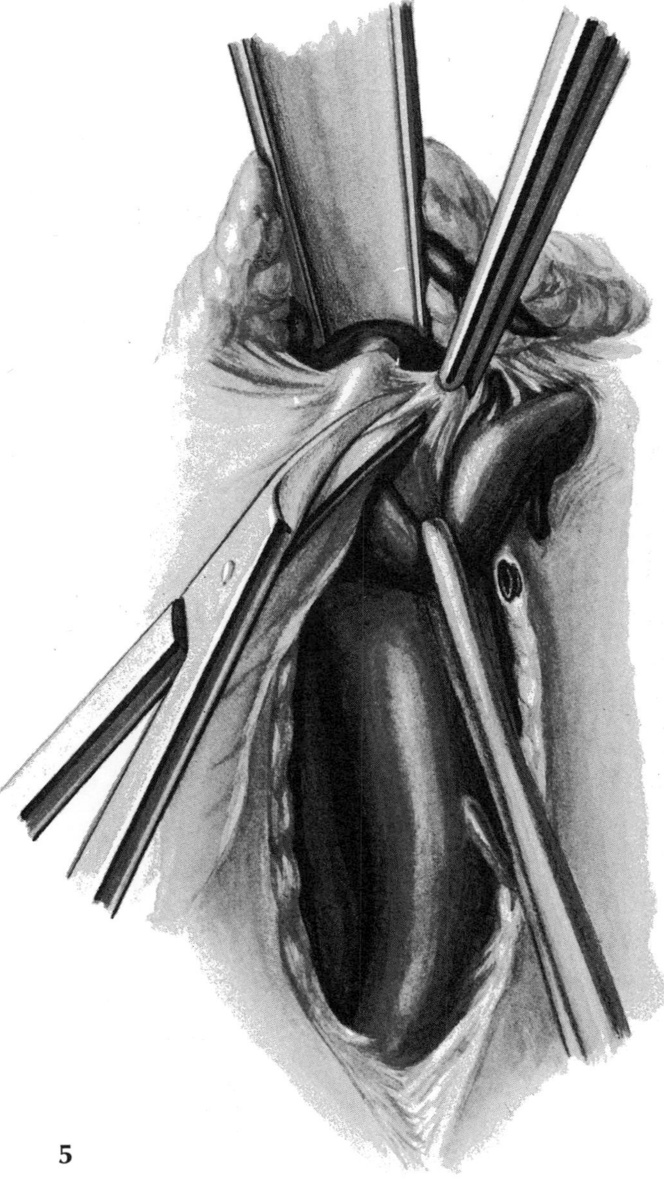

5

5

Exposure of the pararenal aorta requires that the left renal vein be circumferentially dissected to its junction with the inferior vena cava. Approximately 2 cm of the inferior vena cava is freed adjacent to this junction to ensure adequate mobility. Flexible tubing placed around the left renal vein serves as an atraumatic mobile retractor. The autonomic ganglian tissue is dissected from the anterior surface of the aorta until the origin of the superior mesenteric artery is identified. This may require cephalad, then caudad retraction of the left renal vein. The renal vein retractor is then placed to retain the left renal vein and pancreas cephalad and the splanchnic retractors are repositioned deeper in the wound so that the dissected periarterial tissue is pulled laterally away from the aorta.

6

Division of the musculotendinous crura of the diaphragm opens up the confined space cephalad to the renal arteries and greatly facilitates mobilization of the suprarenal aorta and renal arteries.

The entire infrarenal aorta and the inferior mesenteric artery can be exposed by carrying the dissection caudally along the anterior surface of the aorta. When exposing the common iliac arteries, the incision in the posterior peritoneum must be extended distally over the right common iliac artery. This avoids the autonomic nerves crossing over the left common iliac artery.

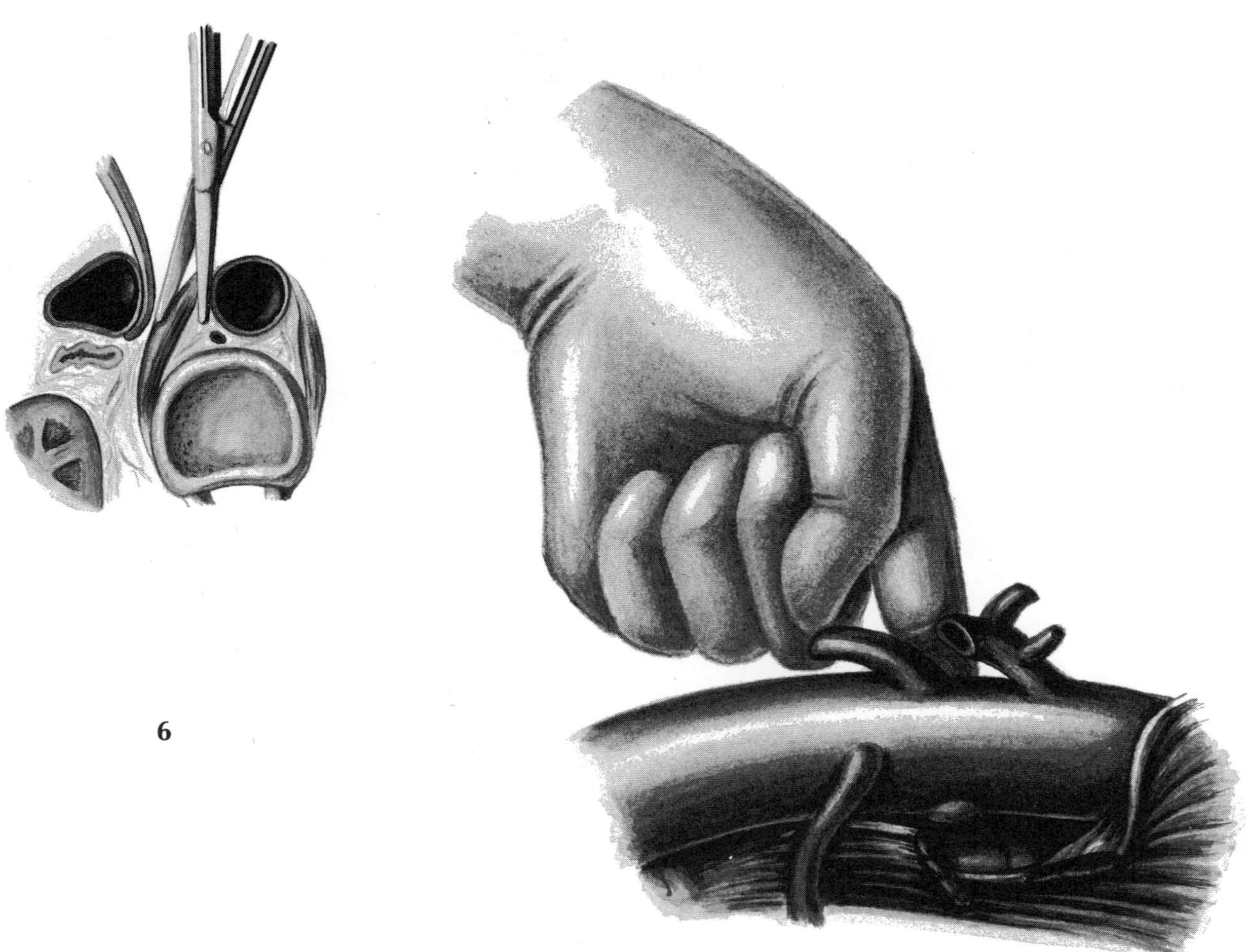

6

Transcrural approach

7

The abdominal cavity is entered through an upper midline abdominal incision extending from above the xiphoid to below the umbilicus. The self-retaining retractor system is assembled and the wound edges are retracted laterally as described above. Resection of the xiphoid process facilitates upper abdominal exposure. The left triangular ligament is divided, the left lobe of the liver is folded on itself and retained to the right using the malleable slotted swivel blade. The lessor sac is entered through a vertical incision in the gastrohepatic ligament and the oesophagus and stomach are displaced to the left and held with a splanchnic retractor. The midline posterior peritoneum is incised. The muscle fibres of the diaphragm are separated, uncovering the median arcuate ligament lying immediately cephalad to the origin of the coeliac axis. Division of the median arcuate ligament exposes the distal thoracic and supracoeliac abdominal aorta. Dissection of the autonomic ganglion tissue along the left anteriolateral surface of the aorta allows the coeliac axis and the paramesenteric aorta to be mobilized. The crura of the diaphragm and freed periaortic tissue can now be displaced away from the sides of the aorta using the renal vein retractors. Dissection in the plane of Leriche is carried caudally to mobilize the proximal superior mesenteric artery behind the pancreas.

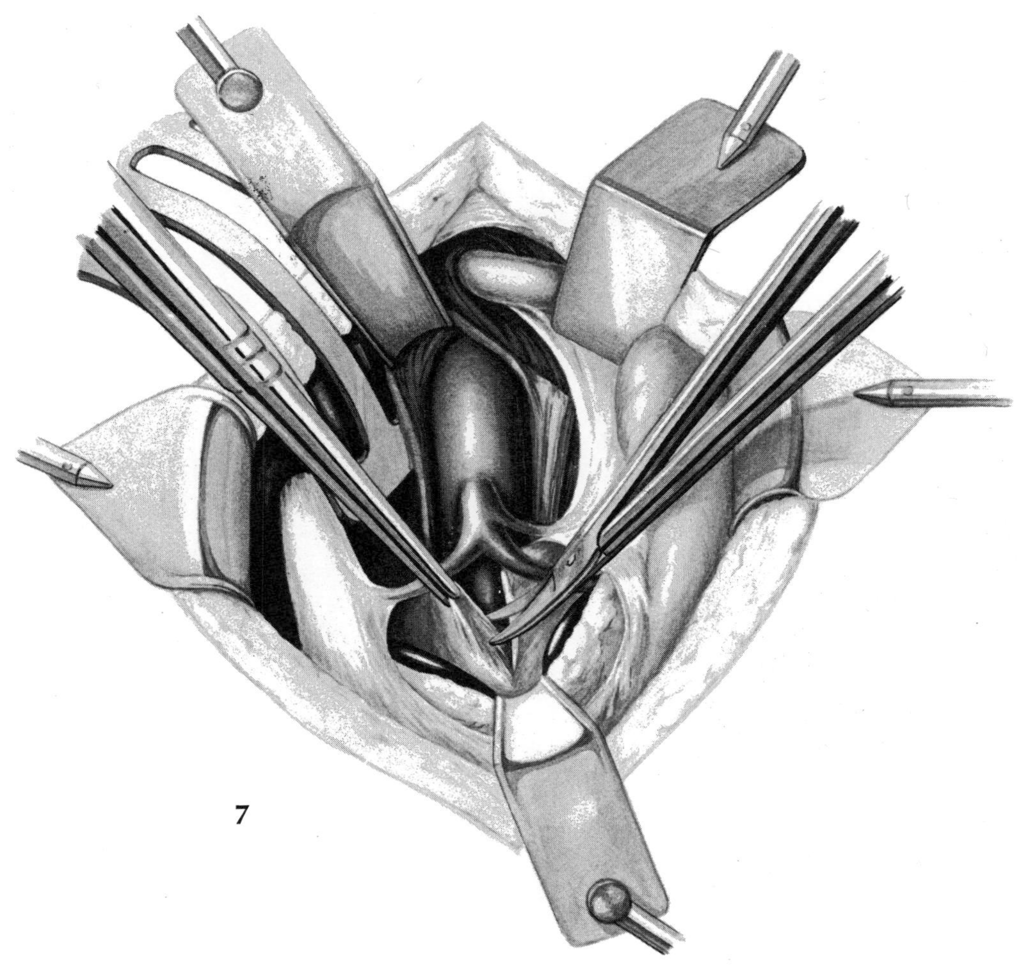

Medial visceral rotation approach

8

The abdominal cavity is entered through a full length midline incision that is carried above the xiphoid. The wound edges are retracted laterally and the small bowel is placed in an intestinal bag and retained to the right as described for the infracolic approach. The large mayo swivel retractor is used to retract the left costal margin cephalad and lateral to better exposure the left colic gutter.

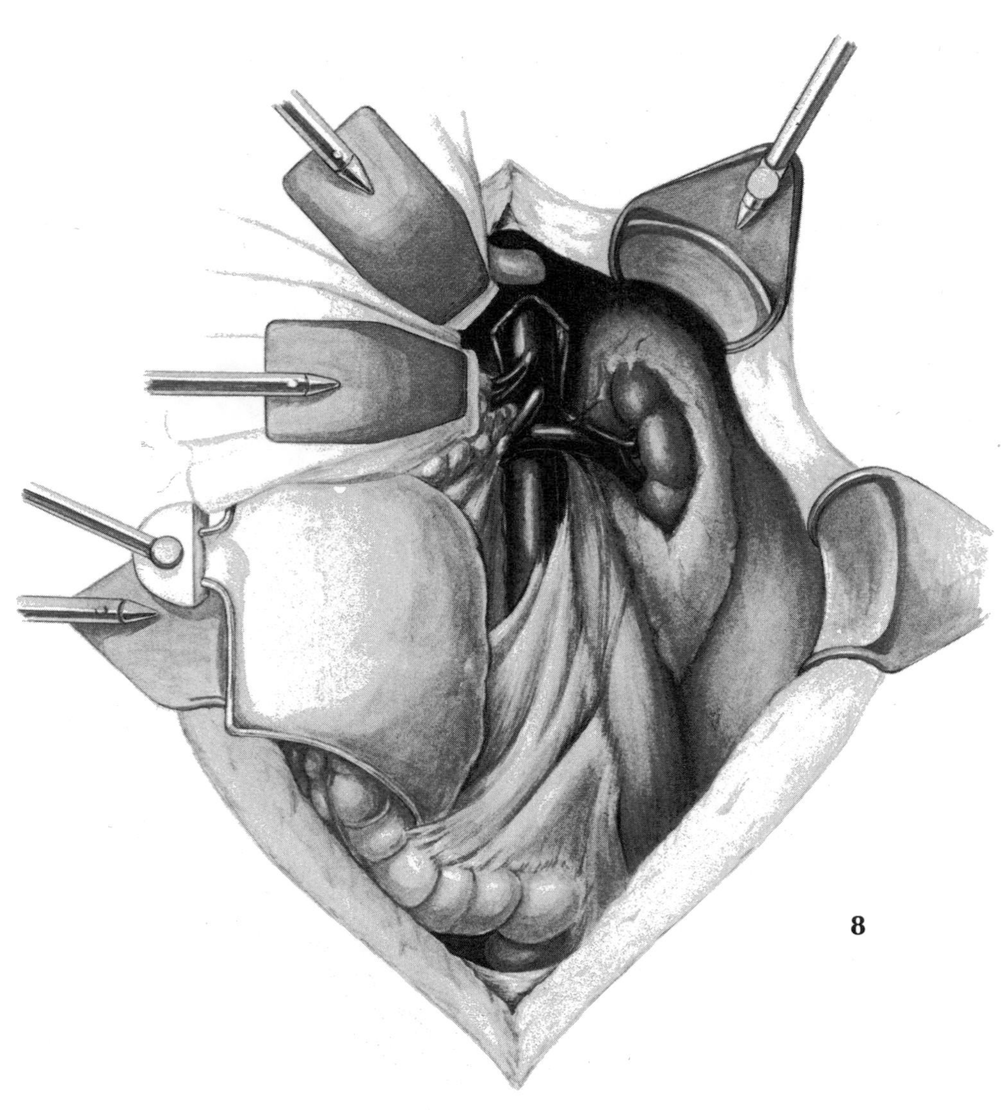

8

9

Mobilization of the sigmoid and descending colon is begun in the standard manner by incising the lateral peritoneal reflection. This peritoneal incision is carried cephalad through the phrenocolic and lienorenal ligaments. Using gentle blunt and occasional sharp dissection, a plane is developed between the pancreas and Gerota's fascia. The descending colon, pancreas, spleen, and stomach are then rotated anteriorly and medially, leaving the gonadal vein, ureter, left kidney and adrenal gland *in situ*.

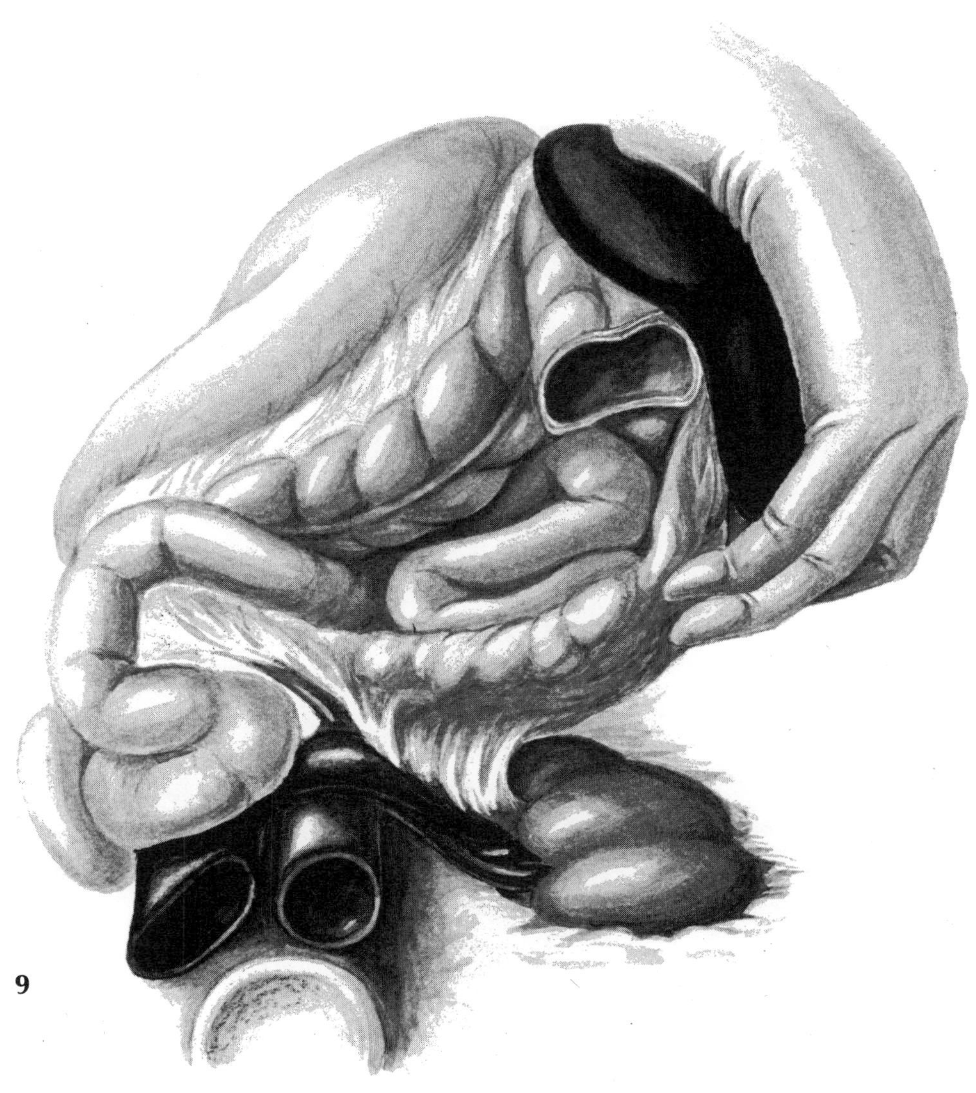

9

10

The spleen and pancreas are protected with moistened sponges and retained with splanchnic retractors. The remainder of the anteriorly mobilized viscera is retained to the right by repositioning the corral malleable disposable retractor. The viscera are visible through the corral malleable disposable retractor and can be continuously surveyed for ischaemia throughout the procedure. In addition, to ensure adequate perfusion of the displaced viscera, the retractors are periodically released and repositioned. The peritoneum is reflected from the left crus of the diaphragm. The triangular ligament is incised and the left lobe of the liver is folded on itself and held to the right by repositioning the more cephalad splanchnic retractor. The aorta is now clearly in view, crossed only by the left renal vein, the autonomic ganglia tissue and the muscle of the left crus of the diaphragm.

Exposure of the upper abdominal aorta also requires circumferential dissection of the left renal vein to its entry into the inferior vena cava. Flexible tubing placed around the left renal vein allows it to be widely retracted. Caudal retraction of the left renal vein exposes the origin of the renal arteries. The left renal artery can easily be freed from its origin to the renal hilum. Right lateral retraction of the inferior vena cava brings the proximal 2–3 cm of the right renal artery into view. The dense autonomic ganglia on the left anteriolateral surface of the aorta is resected and the musculotendinous left crus of the diaphragm is divided to mobilize the supraceliac aorta and to expose the major visceral branches. Transection of the median arcuate ligament and separation of the muscle fibres of the diaphragm exposes the distal thoracic aorta within the mediastinum. The crura of the diaphragm and freed periarterial tissue can now be displaced using the renal vein retractors as described with the transcrural approach.

Mobilization of the lower abdominal aorta proceeds by incising the loose areaolar tissue along its left lateral surface. Reflection of this tissue to the right reveals the origin of the inferior mesenteric artery with the course of this vessel now vertical as a result of the colon displacement. In addition to the aortic bifurcation and the common iliac arteries, the entire length of the left internal and external iliac arteries are easily accessible for mobilization.

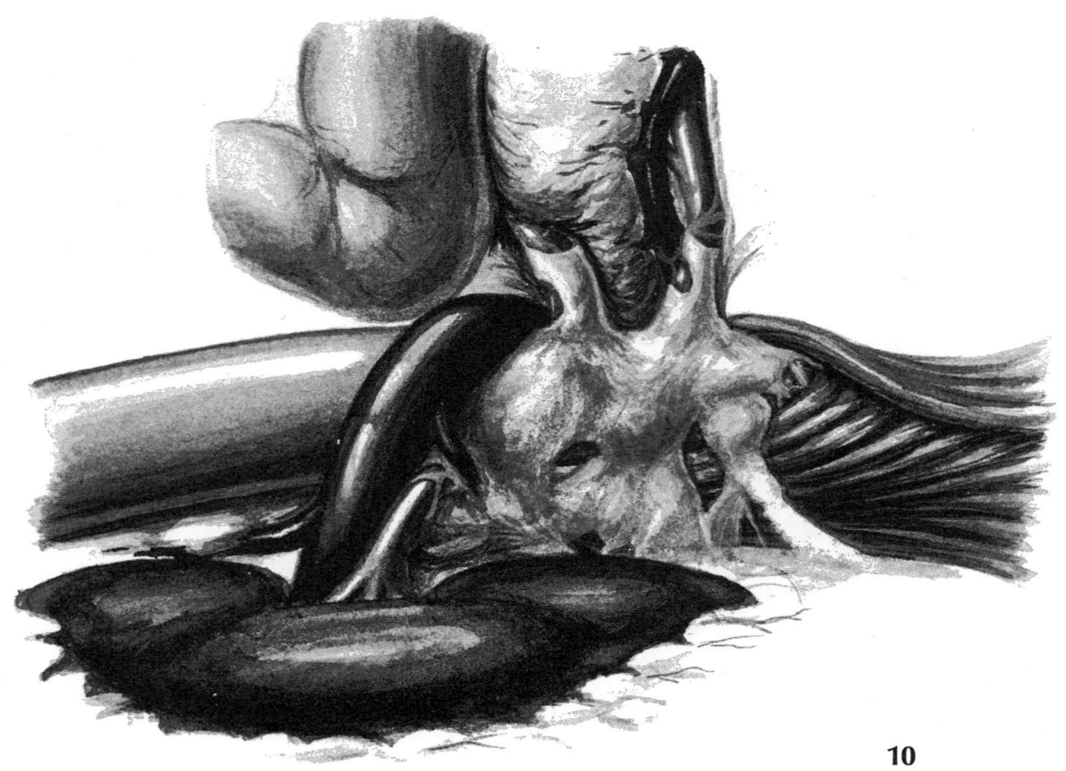

10

Summary

Table 1 summarizes the three approaches described above. The infracolic approach is simple. In most cases, it provides adequate exposure of the diseased para- and infrarenal abdominal aorta. Access to the upper abdominal aorta is limited with the infracolic approach; therefore, in some cases of pararenal aneurysmal disease, the exposure is inadequate. When the proximal extent of the aneurysm is juxtaposed to the origin of the superior mesenteric artery, some prefer to combine the infracolic approach with the transcrural approach to achieve safe proximal aortic control. However, this provides discontinuous aortic exposure separated by the transverse colon and pancreas, which prevent both segments of the aorta from being viewed simultaneously. The medial visceral rotation approach may be a superior option in this situation since it provides continuous exposure of the upper abdominal aorta.

The transcrural approach provides very limited access to the upper abdominal aorta and its branches. However, it is a direct approach to the supracoeliac aorta that provides rapid and effective proximal aortic control for the treatment of more distal aortic disease or for the treatment of visceral occlusive disease with aortovisceral bypass.

Although the medial visceral rotation approach to the aorta is indirect and more complex to establish than the above two approaches, it provides unrestricted, continuous exposure of the distal thoracic aorta and the entire abdominal aorta and its branches. Virtually all aortic disease can be treated when it is exposed using the medial visceral rotation approach. This approach maximizes the reconstructive options available to the surgeon and allows for flexibility in handling unanticipated problems.

Table 1.
Comparison of approaches to the abdominal wall aorta and its branches

Approach	*Exposure*	*Limitations*	*Advantages*	*Disadvantages*
Infracolic	Para- and infrarenal aorta and branches	Supracoeliac and paravisceral aorta and branches	Simple, Often adequate	Restricted
Transcrural	Supracoeliac and proximal paravisceral aorta and branches	Para- and infrarenal aorta and branches	Direct, Effective control	Restricted, Limited options
Medial visceral rotation	Entire abdominal aorta and branches	Right paramesenteric aorta, Right renal hilum, Right iliac artery bifurcation	Unrestricted, Maximum options	Complex, Indirect

Acknowledgement

This paper was supported in part by the Pacific Vascular Research Foundation, San Francisco, California. Illustrations by Eileen S. Natuzzi MS, MD.

References

Cabria, R. P., Brewster, D. C., Abbott, W. M., Freehan, M., Megerman, J., LaMuraglia, G., Wilson, R., Wilson, D., Teplick, R. and Davison, J. K. (1990). Transperitoneal versus retroperitoneal approach for aortic reconstruction: A randomized prospective study. *Journal of Vascular Surgery* **11**, 314.

Dubost, C., Allary, M. and Oeconomos, N. (1952). Resection of an aneurysm of the abdominal aorta: Reestablishment of the continuity by a preserved human arterial graft, with results after five months. *Archives of Surgery* **64**, 405.

Gregory, R. T., Wheeler, J. R., Snyder, S. O., Gayle, R. G. and Love, L. P. (1989). Retroperitoneal approach to aortic surgery. *Journal of Cardiovascular Surgery* **30**, 185.

Johnson, J. N., McLoughlin, G. A., Wake, P. N. and Helsby, C. R. (1986). Comparison of extraperitoneal and transperitoneal methods of aorto-iliac reconstruction. *Journal of Cardiovascular Surgery* **27**, 561.

Leather, R. P., Shah, D. M., Kaufman, J. L., Fitzgerald, K. M., Chang, B. J. and Feustel, P. J. (1989). Comparative analysis of retroperitoneal and transperitoneal aortic replacement for aneurysm. *Surgery, Gynecology and Obstetrics* **168**, 387.

Peck, J. J., McReynolds, D. G., Baker, D. H. and Eastman, A. B. (1986). Extraperitoneal approach for aortoiliac reconstruction of the abdominal aorta. *American Journal of Surgery* **151**, 620.

Reilly, L. M., Ramos, T. K., Murray, S. P., Cheng, S. W. K. and Stoney, R. J. (1994). Optimal exposure of the proximal abdominal aorta: A critical appraisal of transabdominal medial visceral rotation. *Journal of Vascular Surgery* (in press).

Sicard, G. A., Freeman, M. G., VanderWoude, J. C. and Anderson, C. B. (1987). Comparison between the transabdominal and retroperitoneal approach for reconstruction of the infrarenal aorta. *Journal of Vascular Surgery* **5**, 19.

Management of aortic graft infection

LARRY H. HOLLIER MD, FACS, FACC

Chairman, Department of Surgery and Executive Director of Clinical Affairs, Health Care International, Glasgow, Scotland

Introduction

Aortic graft infection is a complication that is universally dreaded by vascular surgeons since it often represents not only a breakdown in surgical technique but also a potentially lethal problem. The natural history of aortic graft infection can vary from a chronic draining fistula to acute arterial wall necrosis with false aneurysm, sepsis, or exsanguinating haemorrhage. Obviously, the management of graft infection is influenced by multiple factors, the most prominent of which are time of onset in relation to surgery, site of infection, extent of infection, location of the graft, aortoenteric fistula, and run-off vessels.

In general, aortic graft infections that occur shortly after surgery should be considered as diffuse infections that will involve the entire graft, since true tissue incorporation and obliteration of perigraft spaces have not yet occurred. These almost invariably require removal of the entire graft. Infections occurring months or years after graft implantation, however, will often be found to be localized to a specific segment of the graft which may allow extra-anatomic revascularization with salvage of most of the previous graft and excision of only the area infected. This technical discussion relates to this aspect of segmental excision of graft infection with preservation of the uninfected graft segments.

Evaluation

Although the literature is replete with multiple modalities used for identifying graft infection, we find only a few tests of significant value.

The physical examination

The presence of a draining sinus in the groin in a patient who has a previous aortofemoral graft should be sufficient evidence to suggest the diagnosis of graft infection. The only question to be answered subsequently relates to the extent of the infection. In this situation, performance of a sinugram with thin barium or Hypaque is often sufficient to delineate any proximal extension of the infection. A more subtle sign of intra-abdominal graft infection is unilateral lower extremity osteoarthropathy with joint swelling and clubbing of the toes that are indicative of bowel erosion by one limb of an aortic bifurcation graft.

Computerized tomography

Computerized tomography (CT scan) is a valuable tool in the evaluation of patients with suspected aortic graft infection and particularly in the evaluation of upper gastrointestinal bleeding in a patient with previous placement of an aortic graft. A CT scan may uncommonly show inflammatory changes and fluid around an aortic graft, though these do not necessarily indicate graft infection. However, perigraft air that is present more than 3 months after aortic graft placement should be considered diagnostic of graft infection. Although one cannot definitively make a diagnosis of aortoenteric fistula on a CT scan, the presence of a continuous and uninterrupted fat line separating the graft line from the overlying bowel is presumptive of there being no aortoenteric fistula if the CT sections are taken at 0.5-cm intervals.

Endoscopy

Upper gastrointestinal endoscopy should be performed routinely in patients with a prior aortic graft who present with gastrointestinal bleeding. Attempts should be specifically made to examine the entire duodenum since graft erosion commonly occurs in the third or fourth portion of the duodenum. While endoscopy may be helpful if a graft is visualized through the distal duodenal wall, failure to identify a bleeding point does not necessarily exclude the possibility of aortoenteric fistula. Additionally, identification of other bleeding sites, such as gastric erosion or duodenal ulcer, likewise does not exclude aortoenteric fistula but does mandate the need for further evaluation.

Leukocyte scan

Indium-labelled leukocyte may be injected intravenously and used for identification of indolent graft infection. Although this can occasionally provide some false-positive or false-negative findings, if the scan does show a ‘hot spot’ along the course of the graft or one of its limbs, it may be helpful in localizing and identifying the extent of infection.

Angiography

Angiography is generally not useful in determining the presence of graft infection or aortoenteric fistula. None the less, we routinely recommend angiography in patients with graft infection, primarily for full delineation of the status of run-off vessels. We believe that this allows better planning for operative intervention for removal of the graft, assessment of collaterals, and revascularization of the lower extremities.

Management

1a, b & c

Unilateral groin infection

Under general anaesthesia, the draining site in the groin is carefully sealed with an occlusive dressing and the abdomen and lower extremity is prepped with povidone-iodine solution and draped in a sterile fashion. A vertical transabdominal incision is made and the peritoneum over the aortic graft bifurcation is incised transversely. The graft limb to the involved side is dissected proximally just beyond the bifurcation of the graft. Good incorporation of surrounding tissues suggests that the graft in this area is free of infection. Even though some perigraft fluid may be present, if the perigraft space does not obviously connect to the groin and if the perigraft fluid is free of bacteria (as evidenced by Gram stain), we would proceed with proximal graft preservation and distal revascularization through the obturator canal. The involved limb is doubly clamped, transected and oversewn distally. That end of the graft is then pushed distally and the peritoneum overlying it is closed to the retroperitoneal space with running sutures of 3/0 prolene to separate the distal graft limb completely from the proximal graft. An 8-mm thin-wall ringed Gore-Tex graft is then sutured end-to-end to the proximal limb of the bifurcation graft and a separate retroperitoneal tunnel is made down to the obturator foramen. A vertical incision is then made distally on the medial thigh and the popliteal artery at this level is exposed and isolated. Using a long metal tunneller, the Gore-Tex graft is passed through the obturator foramen to lie in the space posterior to the pectineus, adductor longus and adductor brevis, and anterior to the adductor magnus. The graft is then anastomosed to the popliteal artery above the knee and flow is restored through the graft (*b*).

The abdominal incision and medial thigh incisions are then closed in standard fashion and sterile dressings are applied. The patient is then redraped and the infected groin is exposed and again prepared with povidone-iodine solution. The fistulous tract is excised and the graft is exposed. The graft is then disconnected from its anastomosis to the femoral artery and arterial back bleeding is controlled with balloon catheters and three-way stopcocks. Simple running closure of the femoral artery is performed with 3/0 prolene. The graft is then gently dissected proximally and forcefully withdrawn from its retroperitoneal tunnel. The entire area is then irrigated copiously with antibiotic solution (neomycin-bacitracin-polymyxin) and a suction catheter is left in the tract from which the graft was removed. The wound is then loosely reapproximated to cover the femoral vessels and the skin is packed open with iodoform gauze (*c*).

All patients undergoing such reconstruction for graft infection are administered intravenous antibiotics preoperatively which are continued for 4–5 days postoperatively. The suction catheter is generally removed after 24 h and local wound care is continued until healing is complete.

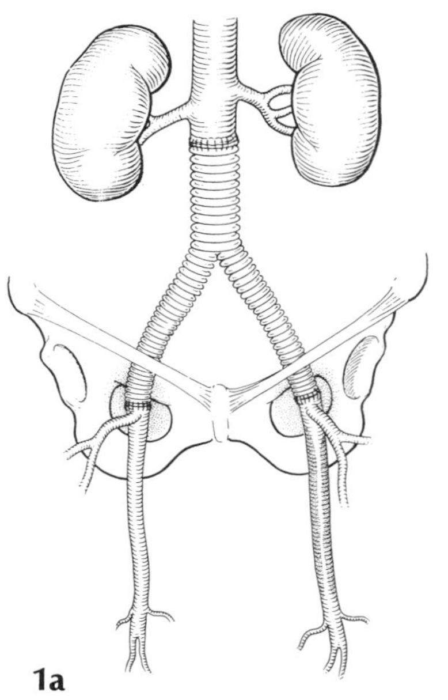

1a

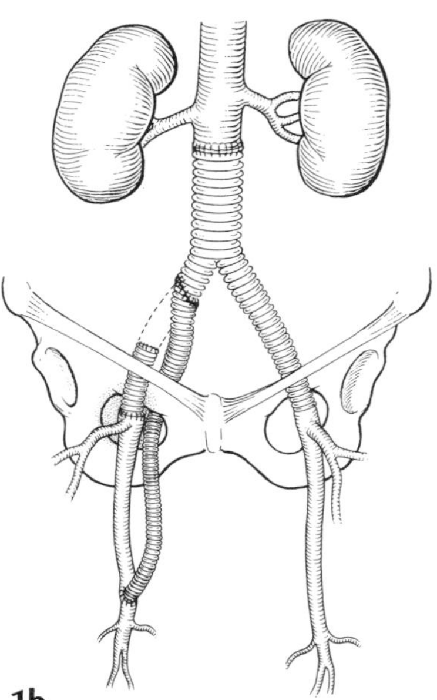

1b

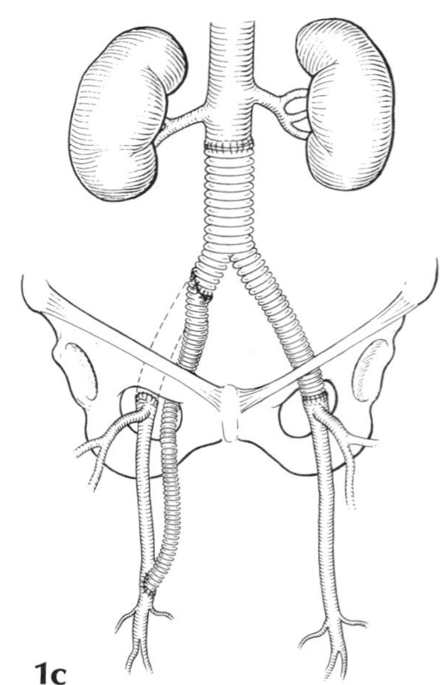

1c

2a, b & c

Isolated bilateral groin infection

The development of bilateral groin infection should strongly suggest that the entire aortic graft is infected. However, if careful evaluation by sinugram, leukocyte indium scan and computerized tomography are all indicative of infections isolated to the groins alone and not the body of the graft, selective proximal graft preservation may be indicated (*a*).

In a fashion similar to the management of unilateral groin infection, the draining sinuses in the groin are carefully sealed, usually by placing a povidone-iodine soaked sponge over the draining sinus and suturing it circumferentially to the skin. The abdomen and lower extremities are then prepared and draped and a midline incision is made in the abdomen. The distal area of the graft bifurcation in each limb is isolated proximally. Again, a Gram stain is made of any perigraft fluid and routine cultures are submitted. The graft is doubly clamped, transected, and the distal portion oversewn. Each limb is then pushed distally into its retroperitoneal tunnel and the distal portion of the tunnel is sealed. Externally supported thin-wall 8-mm Gore-Tex grafts are then sutured end-to-end to the proximal limbs of the bifurcation graft and, as described for unilateral groin infections, the grafts are passed through the obturator tunnel and sutured distally to the popliteal arteries (*b*). The abdominal and thigh incisions are then closed and sterile dressings are applied.

Adhesive drapes are then placed on the patient to completely seal away these previous operative sites. The groin areas are left exposed and the occlusive dressings on the groins are removed. The groins are then prepared with povidone-iodine solution and vertical incisions are made in each groin exposing the infected graft segments. The anastomosis is taken down on each side, with control of bleeding from the femoral vessels obtained by balloon catheters with three-way stopcocks. The femoral arteries are closed primarily with running sutures of 3/0 prolene. The proximal extension of the infected graft segments are then gently mobilized and forcefully removed from their tunnel proximal to the inguinal ligament. The areas of dissection are then copiously irrigated with antibiotic solution and suction catheters are left in each tract and brought out through separate stab incisions in each groin. Deep tissue is closed over the femoral vessels themselves and superficial layers are generally packed open with iodoform gauze. The suction catheters are removed after 24–48 h and the wounds are allowed to heal by secondary intention.

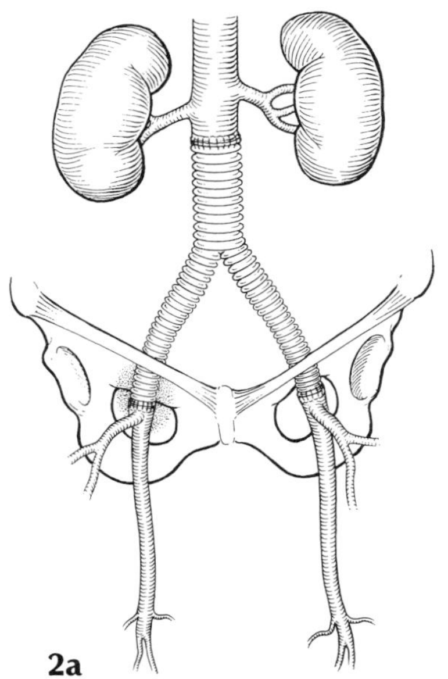
2a

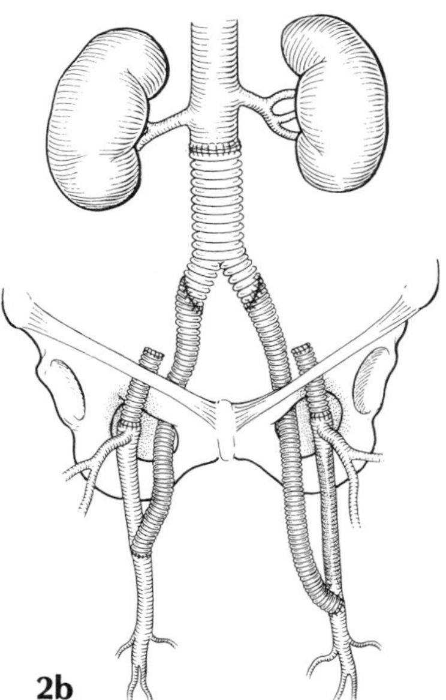
2b

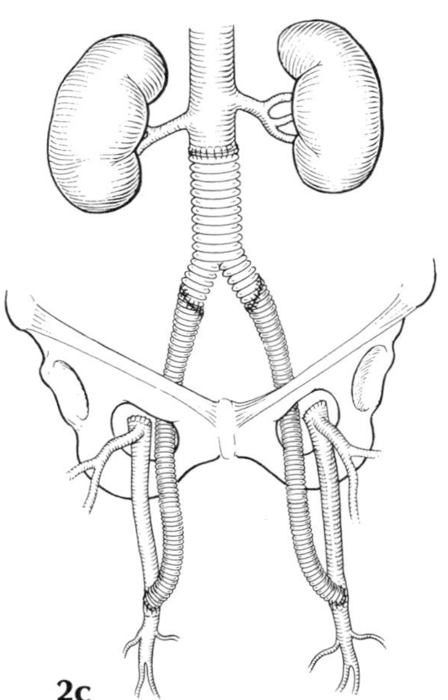
2c

3a, b & c

Proximal graft infection

Aortic graft infection may occur but may be confined to the abdomen if a straight aortic graft has been placed, or if a bifurcation graft has been anastomosed distally to the common iliac or external iliac arteries. In these situations, the groins and the vessels distal to the inguinal ligament are considered to be uninfected *(a)*. Occasionally, patients with aortobifemoral grafts develop isolated proximal graft infections, but with the distal limbs, i.e. the femoral anastomoses, free of infection. This is perhaps most commonly seen in patients who develop aortoenteric fistula from simple graft erosion. Although one might selectively treat some of these patients by removal of the infected graft and direct reimplantation of another Dacron graft, we would generally perform extra-anatomic bypass and complete removal of the infected intra-abdominal graft.

In patients with aortic graft infection isolated to the abdomen, we prefer to do preliminary axillofemoral–cross-femoral bypass as the initial procedure, followed by graft excision either at the same operation or with an interval of 1–2 days, depending upon the stability of the patient. For axillofemoral–cross-femoral bypass, the patient is generally placed under general endotracheal anaesthesia. However, in very high-risk patients, we have performed this procedure under local infiltration anaesthesia for the axillary dissection and epidural anaesthesia for the groin dissection.

The patient is placed on the table in a supine position and prepped from the chin to the knees with povidone-iodine solution. Determination of which axillary artery to use as the donor or inflow vessel is made preoperatively by measuring blood pressure in each arm and selecting the axillary artery with the higher blood pressure. In most cases, the right axillary artery is used. A small roll is placed vertically under the right posterior hemithorax to elevate that side of the chest slightly off of the table and to allow more thorough prepping. The arm is placed outward on an armboard. In these patients, we frequently use a multi-team approach with one surgeon exposing the axillary artery and other surgeons exposing each femoral artery.

The axillary incision is made transversely in the intraclavicular area and the underlying pectoralis major muscle is split in the direction of its fibres. The pectoralis minor muscle is identified and, after dividing the clavipectoral fascia, the insertion of the pectoralis minor on the coracoid process is divided with the electrocautery unit. The underlying axillary artery is thus exposed. The axillary artery at this level must be carefully dissected away from the adjacent nerve trunks. Small bridging veins will sometimes run across the axillary artery in this area and these should be doubly ligated and divided. It is sometimes helpful to divide the artery to the pectoralis major muscle as it arises from the axillary artery. This allows better mobilization of the axillary artery and a more proximal placement of the graft anastomosis can be accomplished. An 8-mm or 10-mm thin-walled externally supported Gore-Tex graft is then sutured end-to-side to the axillary artery. A long metal tunneller is passed cephalad from the right groin without any counter-incision being made in the skin laterally. Every attempt is made to place this tunnel in the mid-axillary line rather than directly anterior over the chest and abdomen. Several rings of the externally supported graft are removed in the proximal-most portion of the femoral incision and a tangential segment of the graft is excised medially. Another segment of externally support 8-mm Gore-Tex graft is then sutured end-to-side to the axillofemoral graft at this level and this side limb is then tunnelled subcutaneously just above the level of the pubis and brought into the opposite groin. Each limb is then sutured end-to-side to the femoral artery and flow can be restored to both lower extremities in this fashion. If the patient has had a previous aortobifemoral graft placed but the femoral portions are free of infection, the previous Dacron graft on each side is simply transected and the proximal portions are oversewn. The proximal graft limbs are then pushed cephalad into their tunnel and are made to lie proximal to the inguinal ligament. The inguinal ligament is then sutured posteriorly to the underlying tissue to separate these tunnels completely from the groin. The axillofemoral–cross femoral limbs can then be sewn directly, end-to-end, to the previous graft just proximal to their femoral anastomoses *(b)*. These wounds are then closed in layers and sterile dressings are applied.

Removal of the infected abdominal graft may be performed either at this time or deferred to a separate operation 24–48 h later. At that time, the abdomen is prepared and draped in the usual fashion and a midline incision is performed. The infected graft is exposed and removed completely *(c)*. Proximally, the aorta is debrided back from the original suture line and closed with interrupted mattress sutures of 3/0 or 0 prolene. A pedicle of omentum is then mobilized and passed through the transverse mesocolon so that it can be carefully wrapped around the aortic stump. If there has been extensive purulence in the peritoneal perigraft space, irrigating and suction catheters may be placed and brought out through separate stab incisions in the flank opposite the axillofemoral–cross-femoral graft *(c)*.

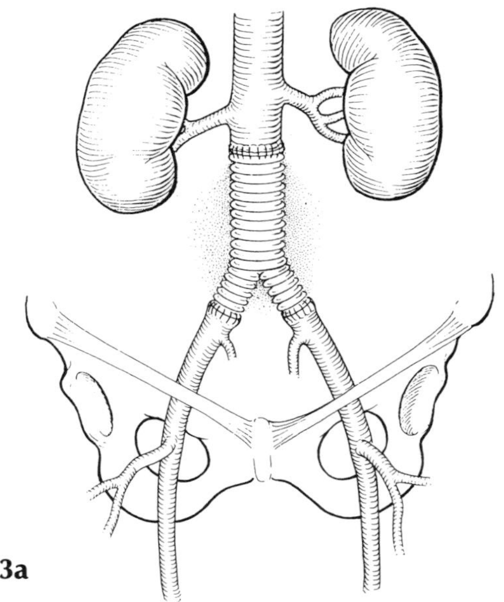

3a

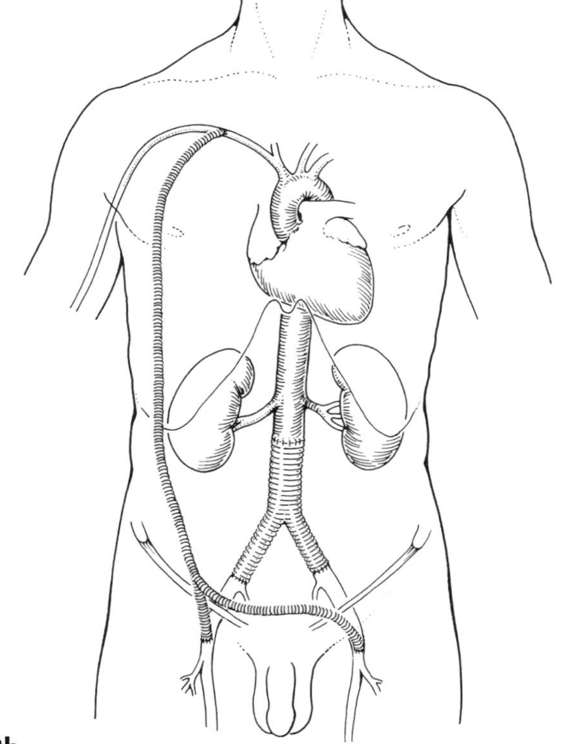

3b

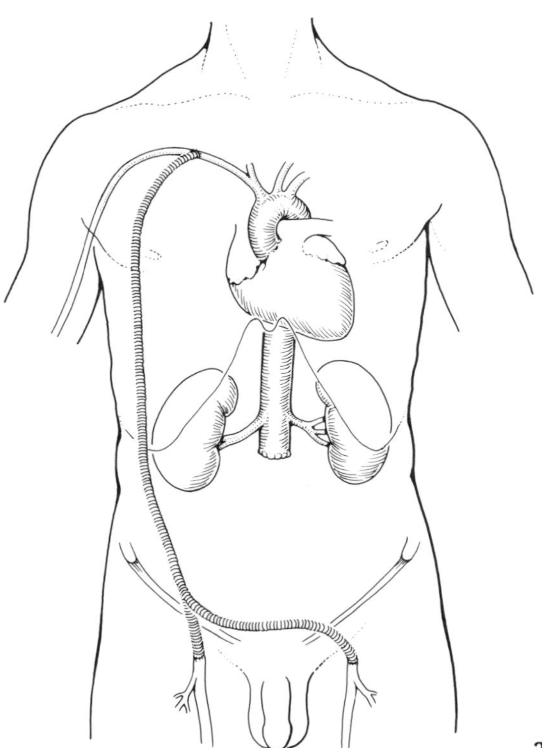

3c

4a, b & c

Aortoenteric fistula

Aortoenteric fistula may present as a sudden, severe, near-exsanguinating haemorrhage or may present as several minor episodes of gastrointestinal bleeding. If the patient has an unequivocal diagnosis and remains relatively stable, we would prefer to do an axillofemoral–cross-femoral bypass as the preliminary step followed by immediate graft removal and repair of the fistula. However, if exsanguinating haemorrhage is the overriding clinical feature, or if the diagnosis is in question, primary laparotomy would be preferred, with revascularization by axillofemoral–cross-femoral graft deferred until after removal of the infected abdominal graft.

For repair of aortoenteric fistula, a transperitoneal approach is made. After entering the abdomen, the peritoneal reflection on the right lateral aspect of the ascending colon is incised and continued medially around the cecum and extended cephalad to mobilize the hepatic flexure of the colon. A Kocher manoeuvre is then performed mobilizing the second portion of the duodenum and the head of the pancreas. This approach allows rapid dissection in previously undissected planes and minimizes the amount of time required to expose the aorta for control. By mobilizing the abdominal viscera to the left, one exposes the inferior vena cava and easily approaches the aorta above the level of the left renal vein where, in most cases, it has been spared the extensive scarring that would be evident in the infrarenal portion. This allows rapid placement of a clamp, suprarenally if necessary (*a*). After proximal control is obtained, the duodenum can be further mobilized and the site of erosion of the duodenum by the graft can be approached in this fashion. Once the aortoenteric fistula is adequately exposed the clamps may be moved to the infrarenal position if adequate infrarenal aorta remains. If not, the aorta may be locally debrided and closed at this point so that the aortic clamp may be removed and flow restored to the renal arteries.

The opening in the duodenum is then gently debrided and the duodenum is closed in two layers. The distal graft is then removed entirely. If the distal anastomoses had been made to the common iliac or external iliac arteries, the anastomotic sites are simply oversewn with 3/0 prolene sutures (*b*).

After closure of the aortic stump and removal of the graft, the right colon is returned to its normal anatomic position. A pedicle of omentum is mobilized and passed through the transverse mesocolon. The omental pedicle is then carefully tacked around the aortic stump to help in the prevention of stump blow-out. Irrigating and suction catheters are then left in the retroperitoneum and brought out through a flank incision opposite to the side of the previous or planned axillofemoral–cross-femoral graft (*c*).

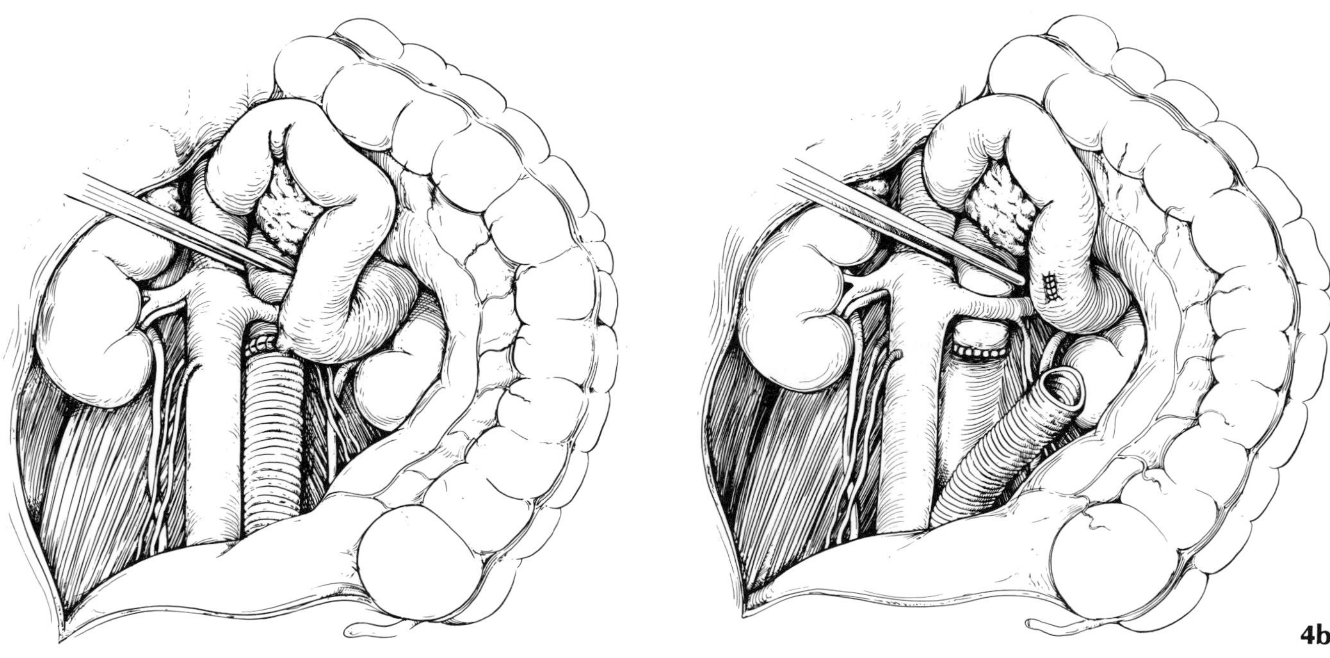

4a

4b

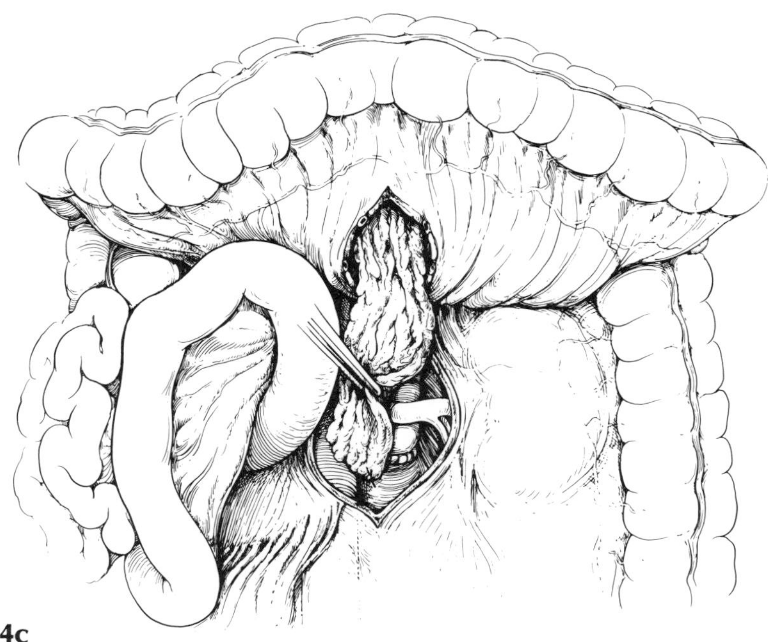

4c

5a & b

Aortofemoral graft infection

When an aortobifemoral graft infection is identified with infection evident both in the groin and intra-abdominally, we generally manage this by bilateral axilloprofunda or axillopopliteal bypasses with subsequent removal of the entire aortobifemoral graft. Any draining sinuses are carefully sealed as previously described and the patient is placed in a supine position with both arms extended laterally on armboards (*a*). The patient is prepped with povidone-iodine solution from the chin to toes so that complete exposure can be facilitated. Since both groins are infected, we avoid any incision in those areas and plan to bring the graft more laterally down to the popliteal artery.

Occasionally, however, if the superficial femoral arteries are patent and the infected graft is placed high on the common femoral artery, one might perform a distal anastomosis to the profunda vessels with expectation of a retrograde filling of the profunda and the superficial femoral artery after ligation of the common femoral artery. If the infected graft is anastomosed to the femoral bifurcation or if the superficial femoral arteries are occluded, the lower extremities are revascularized by bilateral axillopopliteal grafts.

Bilateral infraclavicular incisions are made and the axillary arteries are exposed as previously described. Bilateral incisions are then made laterally just above each knee and the popliteal arteries are exposed and isolated. Because of the distance between the axillary and popliteal incisions, a small counter-incision is usually required to facilitate passage of the graft. This counter-incision is made lateral to the posterior superior iliac spine and a tunnel is made subcutaneously cephalad and caudad from this area. Externally supported 8-mm thin-wall Gore-Tex grafts are then obtained and a graft is sutured to each axillary artery as previously described. Each graft is then passed through the subcutaneous tunnel with the grafts placed along the mid-axillary line and lateral aspect of the thigh. The grafts are then sutured to the popliteal artery above the knee in each thigh and flow is restored to the lower extremities. These incisions are closed and sterile dressings are applied (*b*).

The groins are then opened and the infected grafts are removed from their anastomosis to the femoral vessels. The femoral arteries are closed with prolene and every attempt is made to maintain a patent femoral bifurcation if possible. The abdomen is then opened and the graft is removed as previously described. As always, an attempt is made to provide coverage of the aortic stump by a pedicle of omentum.

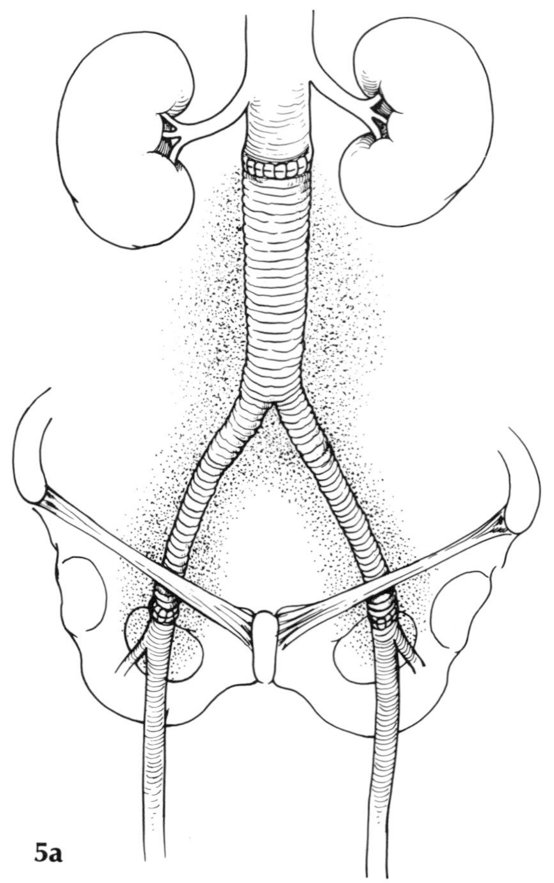

5a

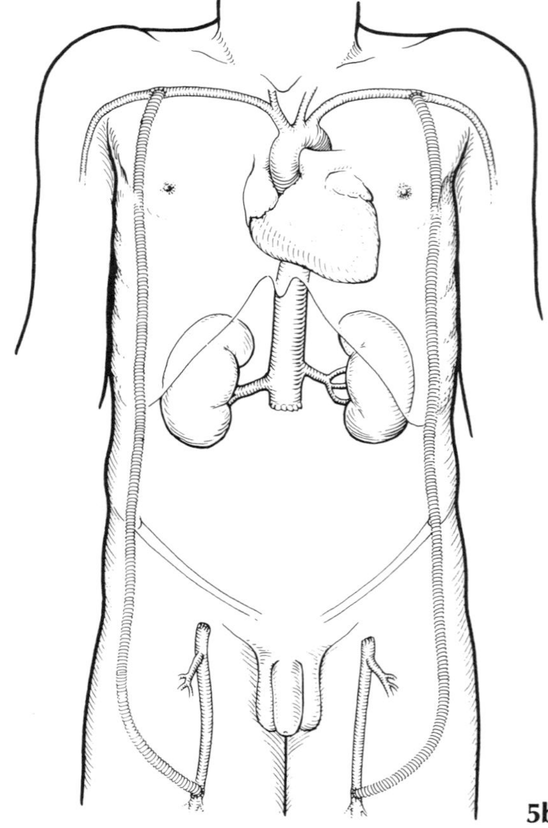

5b

Additional approaches

Obviously, many techniques have been devised for the management of aortic graft infection. These include direct replacement of the infected graft with a new prosthesis, rotation of muscle flaps to cover the infected graft, replacement of infected grafts with autogenous tissue, and graft removal without any revascularization whatsoever. While each of these techniques is occasionally applicable to a specific patient, they are not always feasible. Thus, this discussion has centred primarily on extra-anatomic revascularization and graft removal.

We have inadequate experience with direct replacement of an infected graft by a new prosthesis and are unable to comment about its safety. We have used rotation of muscle flaps to cover grafts in approximately 30 patients, but have been disappointed with the results. Although one can occasionally get healing of a graft that has been exposed by breakdown of overlying tissues, we have found it less helpful in eradicating established graft infection. Similarly, we have used autogenous reconstruction on several patients and found that it is satisfactory for revascularization in contaminated fields, but, unfortunately, blow-out of autogenous tissue may occur when it has been placed in areas of established infection. Because of the high incidence of lower extremity ischaemia following simple removal of an infected aortic graft without revascularization, we have abandoned that technique entirely.

Although specific situations may allow the vascular surgeon to utilize a lesser procedure for the management of graft infection, we believe that most patients with established aortic graft infection are best managed by preliminary revascularization by an extra-anatomic route, followed by removal of all infected graft material.

References

Brown, O. W., Stanson, A. W., Pairolero, P. C. and Hollier, L. H. (1982). Computerized tomography following abdominal aortic surgery. *Surgery* **91**(6), 716.

Cherry, K. J. and Hollier, L. H. (1982). Prophylactic antibiotics in vascular surgery. In *Extra-anatomic and Secondary Arterial Reconstruction*. Greenhalgh, R. M., ed. London: Pitman.

Goldstone, J. and Moore, W. S. (1974). Infection in vascular prostheses. *American Journal of Surgery* **128**, 225.

Paaske, W. P. and Buchart Hansen, J. H. (1985). Graft enteric fistulas and erosions. *Surgery, Gynecology and Obstetrics* **161**, 161.

Perdue, G. D., Smith, R. B., Ansley, J. D. and Constantine, M. J. (1983). Impending aorto-enteric hemorrhage: The effect of early recognition on improved outcome. *Annals of Surgery* **192**, 237.

Shue, W. B., Worosilo, S. C., Donetz, A. P., Trooskin, S. Z., Harvey, R. A. and Greco, R. S. (1988). Prevention of vascular prosthetic infection with an antibiotic-bonded Dacron graft. *Journal of Vascular Surgery* **8**(5), 600.

Szilagyi, D. E., Smith, R. F., Elliot, J. P. and Vrandecic, M. P. (1972). Infection in arterial reconstruction with synthetic grafts. *Annals of Surgery* **176**, 321.

Reilly, L. M., Altman, H., Lusby, R. J., Kersh, R. A., Ehrenfeld, W. K. and Stoney, R. J. (1984). *Journal of Vascular Surgery* **1**, 36.

Reilly, L. M., Stoney, R. J., Goldstone, J. and Ehrenfeld, W. K. (1987). Improved management of aortic graft infection: The influence of operative sequence and staging. *Journal of Vascular Surgery* **5**, 421.

Wilson, S. E., Wang, S. and Gordon, H. E. (1977). Perioperative antibiotic prophylaxis against vascular graft infection. *Southern Medical Journal* **70**, 68.

Surgical management of secondary aorto-enteric fistulae

ROGER N. BAIRD ChM, FRCS
Consultant Surgeon, The Royal Infirmary, Bristol, UK

Introduction

Anaemia from gastrointestinal blood loss, whether of clinically silent onset, or following haematemesis or melaena, in a patient with an intra-abdominal arterial prosthesis, is caused by an aorto-enteric fistula until proved otherwise. This truth is self-evident to all vascular surgeons, but not, it seems, to those whose lack of awareness leads to numerous expensive and usually fruitless investigations, delaying the diagnosis and causing more than necessary blood loss and subsequent replacement (Thomas and Baird, 1986). Upper gastro-intestinal endoscopy detected only two-thirds (8 of 12) of fistulae in a recent series (Tilanus *et al.*, 1988), and arteriography and CT will show extravasation of contrast into the duodenum only if bleeding is brisk when the investigation is being done. The presence of perigraft gas bubbles on CT can clinch the diagnosis of graft infection. The decision to do a laparotomy is usually taken on clinical grounds.

Pathophysiology

1

Most fistulae arise between an aortic/Dacron anastomosis and the fourth part of the duodenum. Occasionally, the abnormal communication is between an iliac/Dacron anastomosis and the small bowel or the appendix or colon, and from the suture line of an aorto-iliac endarterectomy. Isolated examples have been reported in which a length of prosthesis remote from anastomoses erodes through the bowel wall, described as 'cannibalization' (Monson *et al.*, 1985), paraprosthetic-enteric sinus' (Williams, Charlesworth and Jones, 1987), and as graft-enteric erosions.

The overall incidence of aorto-enteric fistulae following Dacron aortic bypass is low (0.7%) and gastrointestinal blood loss occurs without warning 6 months to 5 years or more after the original operation (Bergqvist *et al.*, 1987). The pathogenesis is unknown, but the routine use of antibiotic prophylaxis and the substitution of prolene for silk as the suture material have been associated with fewer reported cases. There is disturbing association between bowel perforation at the primary aortic operation and secondary aorto-enteric fistula. This suggests that Dacron grafting in elective cases should be deferred if the gut is inadvertently opened during operative exposure of the aorta.

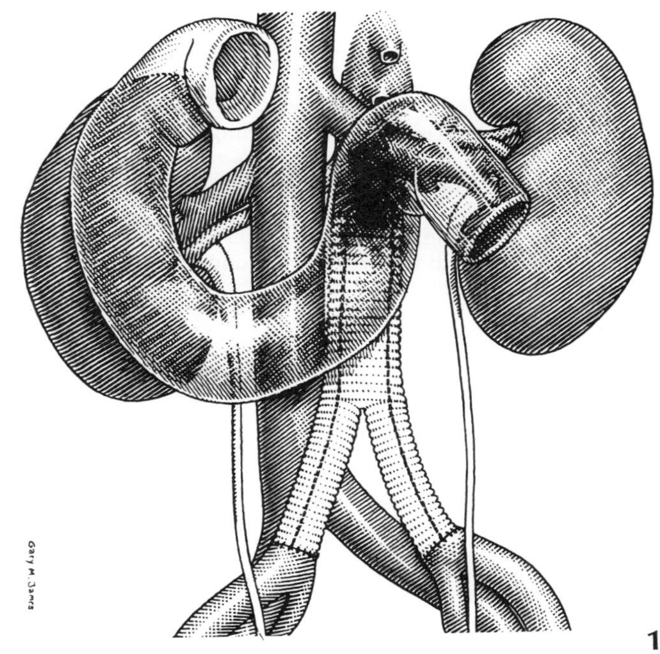

1

2

At laparotomy, three separate categories can be recognized from the operative findings. First, a rupture of a false aneurysm into the bowel and, secondly, a simple fistula between the anastomosis and the duodenum. In both instances, there is no pus around the prosthesis, which remains well incorporated. In the third category, the infective process is advanced and the prosthesis lies slackly and unincorporated in a bed of pus throughout its length.

AORTO-ENTERIC FISTULAE

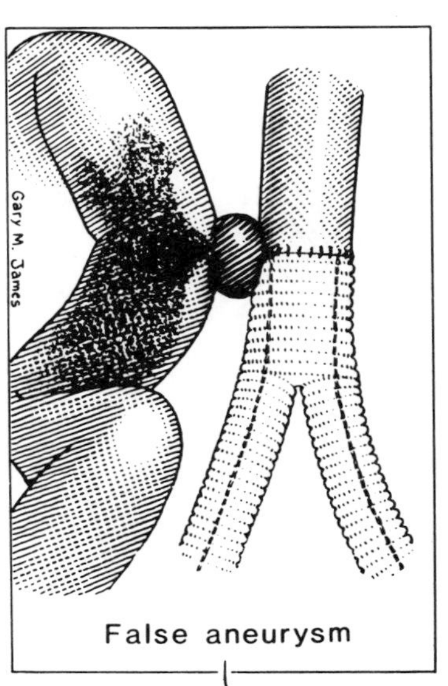

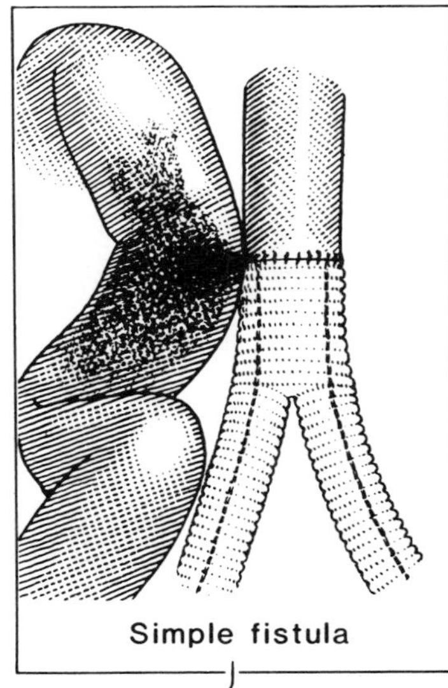

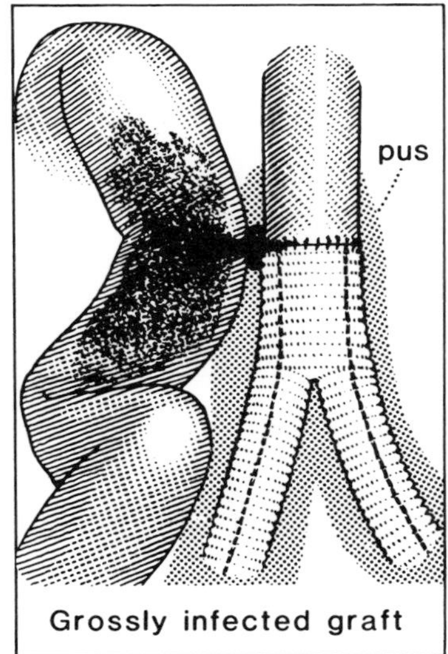

No gross graft sepsis

2

The operation

3

Full cardiovascular monitoring including arterial and central venous lines are mandatory. Wide bore venous access for rapid blood replacement is needed and at least 6 u of blood should be available. The abdomen is opened under antibiotic cover with a combination such as cefuroxine, metronidazole and gentamicin, and the fistula is disconnected.

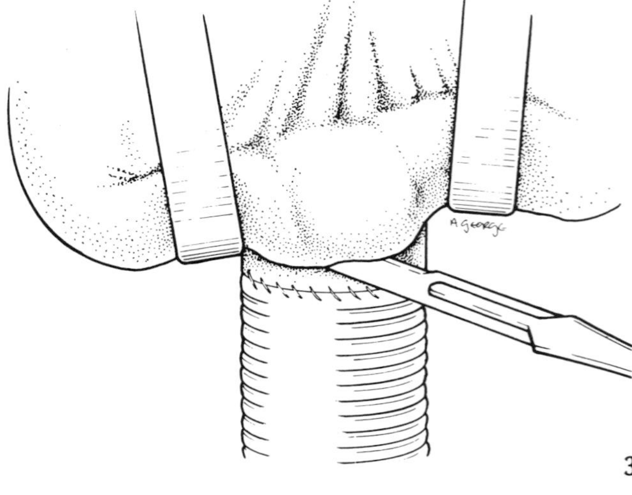

3

4

The duodenal defect is repaired using two layers of catgut or vicryl. Attention is then turned to the aortic prosthesis and suture line. Provided that the aortic wall is not discoloured the prosthesis is well incorporated, and no obvious pus is present, the fistula is likely to be caused by mechanical weakness of the aortic wall.

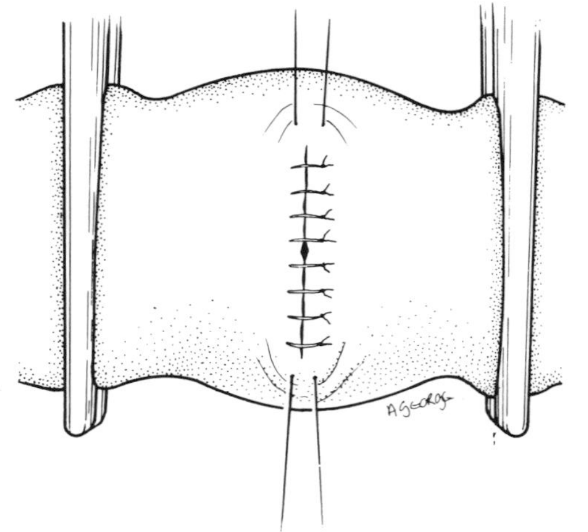

4

5

Consideration is then given to a local repair, either by inserting 2–3 prolene sutures to close the defect, or by inserting a short Dacron tube to link the prosthesis to a more proximal aortic suture line without tension (Robinson and Johansen, 1991; Thomas and Baird, 1986; Eastcott, 1982).

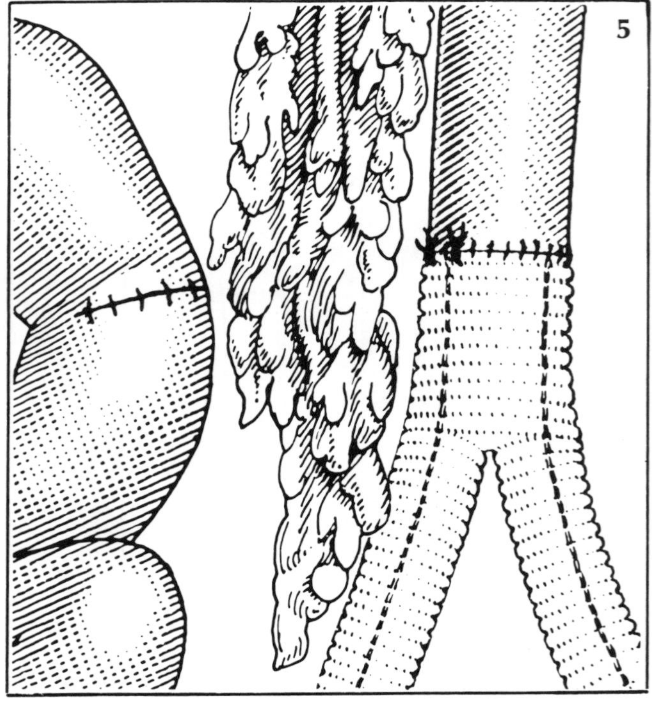

5

6

If, on the other hand, the prosthesis is unincorporated and lies in a bag of pus encased by fibrous tissue, then it should be removed. Usually, the aortic stump is oversewn and an axillobifemoral bypass performed.

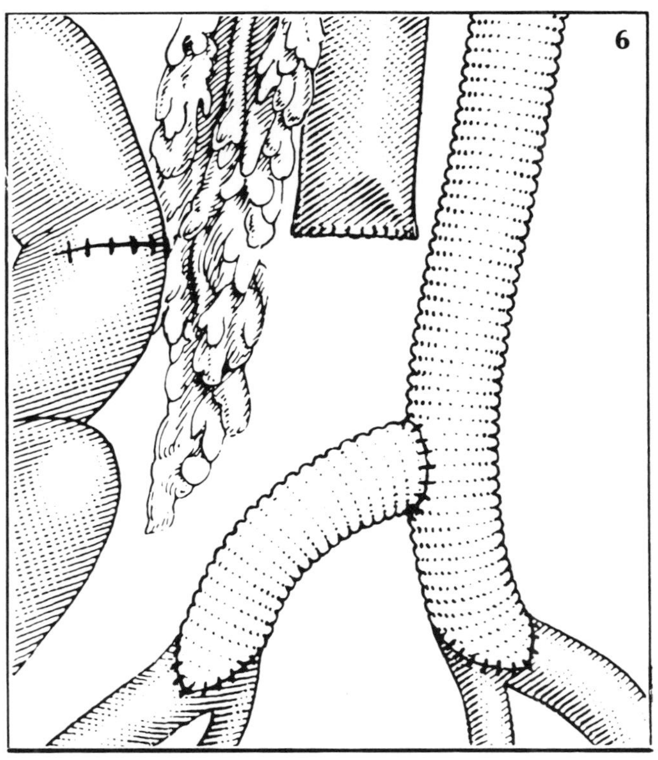

7

Added measures can help to reduce the risk of aortic stump blowout. These include double layers of sutures covering the closure with a flap of the anterior spinous ligament, and covering the omentum. However, Walker *et al.* (1987) have reported an alternative – placing a new prosthesis in the same location by primary exchange similar to the replacement of an infected heart valve. Robinson and Johansen (1991) have reported 11 *in situ* aortic Dacron replacements of five mycotic aneurysms, one secondarily infected aortic aneurysm and five aorto-enteric fistulae (one primary; four secondary). They emphasise the need for aortic debridement to clinically uninvolved tissue, and for omental wrapping of anastomoses.

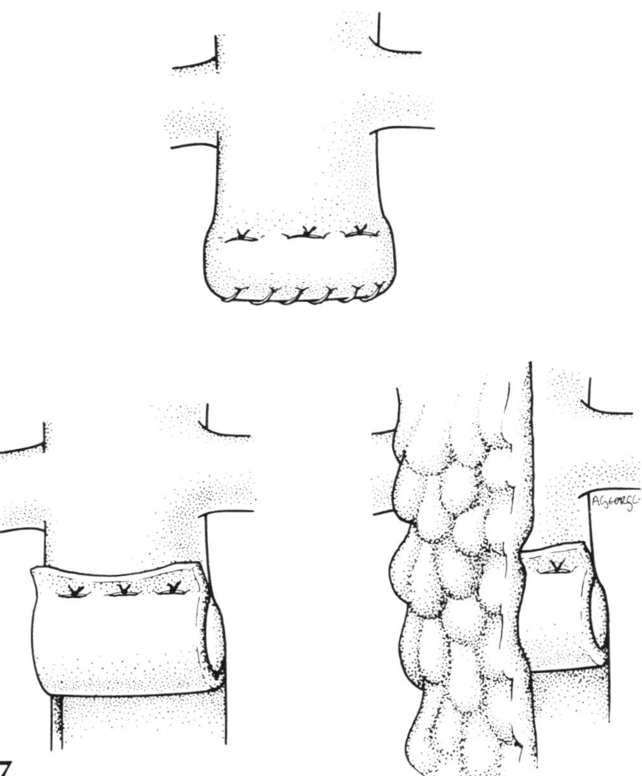

The advocates of extra-anatomical bypass typically acknowledge a high operative mortality of 49% and an amputation rate of 27% resulting from this approach (O'Hara *et al.*, 1986). In an attempt to reduce the magnitude of the undertaking, staged operations for patients not actively bleeding are proposed. The axillobifemoral bypass is inserted first, and the infected prosthesis is removed later (Reilly *et al.*, 1987). The results have gradually improved in the last 20 years (Bouhoutsos *et al.*, 1974; Umpleby, Britton and Turnbull, 1987). Whichever procedure is done, the duodenum and aorta should be separated as far apart as possible to minimize the risk of a further aortoduodenal fistula. The omentum, mobilized if necessary, is used to wrap the aortic anastomosis or stump. In Bergqvist's series of 42 secondary aorto-enteric fistulae, half had further gastrointestinal bleeding postoperatively from the aorto-Dacron anastomosis or from the aortic stump; and few survived for more than 5 years. Such is the anxiety about further gastrointestinal bleeding that there is even a report demonstrating that the duodenum can be transected and relocated in an antecolic position (England and Simms, 1990).

Less frequently, the fistula occurs between the distal anastomosis to the iliac arteries and the small bowel, appendix or colon or the mid-portion of the prosthesis erodes into the gut without anastomotic involvement. In these circumstances a local repair is usually done.

Conclusions

The general risks of treating secondary aorto-enteric fistulae are those of major vascular surgery in arteriopaths rendered weak from blood loss. The likelihood of perioperative death and limb loss is increased if operation is precipitated by a major gastrointestinal bleed or if infection is a problem. Specifically, rupture of the aortic stump and infection of the axillofemoral bypass by cross-contamination are unsolved problems, as is recurrence of the aorto-enteric fistula leading to further haematemesis and malaena. Further thrombosis without premonitory symptoms after months or years is a frequent problem with axillofemoral bypass and the patient should not stray too far from access to skilled hospital care, since urgent embolectomy may be required.

References

Bergqvist, D., Alun, A., Claes, G., Drott, C., Forsberg, O., Larsson, M., Lindhagen, A., Nordström, S., Nybacka, O., Ribbe, E., Spangen, L., Wiklund, B. and Ängquist, K.-A. (1987). Secondary aortoenteric fistulas – An analysis of 42 cases. *European Journal of Vascular Surgery* **1**, 11.

Bouhoutsos, J., Chavatzas, D., Martin, P. and Morris, T. (1974). Infected synthetic arterial grafts. *British Journal of Surgery* **61**, 108.

Busuttil, R. W., Rees, W., Baker, J. D. and Wilson, S. E. (1979). Pathogenesis of aortoduodenal fistula: Experimental and clinical correlates. *Surgery* **85**, 1.

Eastcott, H. H. G. (1982). Aorto-enteric fistula: Possibilities for direct repair. In *Extra-anatomic and Secondary Arterial Reconstruction.* Greenhalgh, R. M. ed. London: Pitman.

England, D. W. and Simms, M. H. (1990). Recurrent aorto-duodenal fistula: a final solution? *European Journal of Vascular Surgery* **4**, 427.

Monson, J. R. T., Courtney, D. G., Jones, N. A. G. and Kester, R. C. (1985). Cannabilization of a Goretex aortohepatic graft by the duodenum. *British Journal of Surgery* **72**, 101.

O'Hara, P. J., Hertzer, N. R. Beven, E. G. and Krajewski, L. P. (1986). Surgical management of infected abdominal aortic grafts: Review of a 25 year experience. *Journal of Vascular Surgery* **3**, 725.

Reilly, L. M., Stoney, R. J., Goldstone, J. and Ehrenfeld, W. K. (1987). Improved management of aortic graft infection: The influence of operation sequence and staging. *Journal of Vascular Surgery* **5**, 421.

Robinson, J. A. and Johansen, K. (1991). Aortic sepsis: Is there a role for *in situ* graft reconstruction? *Journal of Vascular Surgery* **13**, 677.

Thomas, W. E. G. and Baird, R. N. (1986). Secondary aortic-enteric fistulae: Towards a more conservative approach. *British Journal of Surgery* **73**, 875.

Tilanus, H. W., Terpstra, O. T., de Smit, P., van Urk, H. and Veen, H. F. (1988). Diagnosis and management of graft-enteric fistulae. *British Journal of Surgery* **75**, 915.

Umpleby, H. C., Britton, D. C. and Turnbull, A. R. (1987). Secondary arterio-enteric fistulae: A surgical challenge. *British Journal of Surgery* **74**, 256.

Walker, W. E., Cooley, D. A., Duncan, J. M., Hallman, G. L., Ott, D. A. and Reul, G. J. (1987). The management of aortoduodenal fistula by *in situ* replacement of the infected aortic graft. *Annals of Surgery* **205**, 727.

Williams, G. T., Charlesworth, and Jones, D. L. (1987). Enterovosical fistula due to a Dacron aortic graft. *British Journal of Surgery* **74**, 645.

In situ replacement of infected aortic graft

P. FIORANI MD
Professor of Vascular Surgery, University Hospital of Rome, Rome, Italy

F. SPEZIALE MD
L. RIZZO MD
G. F. FADDA MD
Department of Vascular Surgery, University Hospital of Rome, Rome, Italy

Introduction

Aortic graft infection (AGI) can be considered the most serious complication in reconstructive aortic surgery. Although rare (0.8–6%) this continues to be responsible for a high rate of morbidity and mortality and is not influenced by any surgical treatment (Hoffert, 1965; Szilagyi, 1972; Goldstone, 1974; Bunt, 1983; Reilly, 1984; Pons, 1991). Despite improved surgical methods and techniques the poor surgical outcome reported is mostly dependent upon major complication of advanced graft infection including sepsis, suture line disruption and gastrointestinal haemorrhage when aorto-enteric fistula (AEF) or aorto-enteric erosion (AEE) is associated.

The present standard treatment for aortic graft infection is a preliminary revascularization of the lower limbs by axillobifemoral bypass with subsequent graft excision, aortic stump ligation and suture of intestinal lesion when present (O'Hara, 1986; Reilly, 1987). However, a mortality rate of 25–75% can be expected according to a number of reports and the principal complication and cause of death is blow-out of the aortic stump. In addition there is a high risk of lower limb amputation of up to 50% in some reports because of occlusion of the axillobifemoral bypass which is not a durable procedure (Eugene, 1976; Inahara, 1985; Yeager, 1990).

Recently, Walker (1987) and others (Vollmar, 1987; Bandyk, 1991; Robinson, 1991; Jacobs, 1991), reported better early and late results with an '*In situ* replacement of a new aortic graft'. These reports suggest lower operative mortality, limb salvage and documented extended survival with better quality of life, in cases without retroperitoneal abscess or septicaemia, introducing the concept of 'low-grade infection' (Walker, 1987; Bandyk, 1991; Fiorani, 1993). This definition implies, from a clinical point of view, the absence of advanced graft infection symptoms (septicaemia, haemorrhagic shock) and from an anatomical the absence of gross retroperitoneal abscess or dehiscence of aortic anastomosis.

Preoperative management

Preoperative evaluation consists of routine laboratory tests, blood cultures and bacterial cultures of groin sinus secretion when present. Prophylactic therapy with specific antibiotics must be performed in those cases in which the microorganism, potentially responsible, is isolated preoperatively (groin sinus tract or groin abscess needle aspiration). In the other cases prophylaxis is performed by wide spectrum antibiotic therapy with second generation cephalosporins and aminoglycosides at least 72 hours before operation. In patients with preoperative diagnosis of AEF or AEE a total parenteral nutrition is mandatory for at least 3–4 days before surgery

Surgical techniques

Full cardiovascular monitoring including arterial and central vein lines are mandatory. The patient is placed in the supine position and general endotracheal anaesthesia is administered. The abdomen is opened and explored through a midline incision extending from the xiphoid to the pubis. The peritoneum over the aortic graft is incised longitudinally. Aortic control below the proximal anastomosis may be obtained by two principal approaches.

1 & 2

Anterior transperitoneal approach

This approach can be difficult because of frequent retroperitoneal and duodenal adherences around the Ligament of Treitz and left renal vein which can make infrarenal aortic control a problem.

1

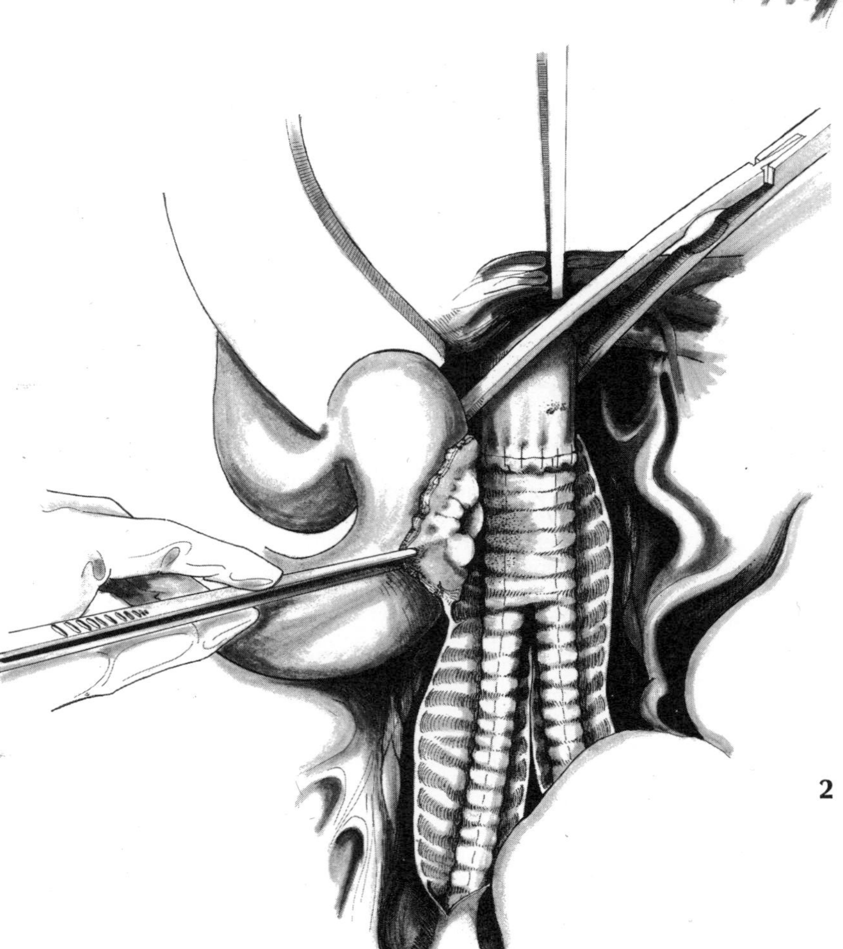

2

3

Right transperitoneal approach

This approach is possible and preferred in the majority of cases with associated AEE or AEF. After peritoneal incision, the peritoneal reflection on the right lateral aspect of the ascending colon is incised and continued medially around the caecum and extended cephalad to mobilize the epatic flexure of the colon. A Kocher manoeuvre is then performed mobilizing the second portion of the duodenum and the head of the pancreas. This approach permits a rapid dissection in previously undissected planes. After mobilization of the abdominal viscera to the left, the inferior vena cava is exposed facilitating aortic control.

3

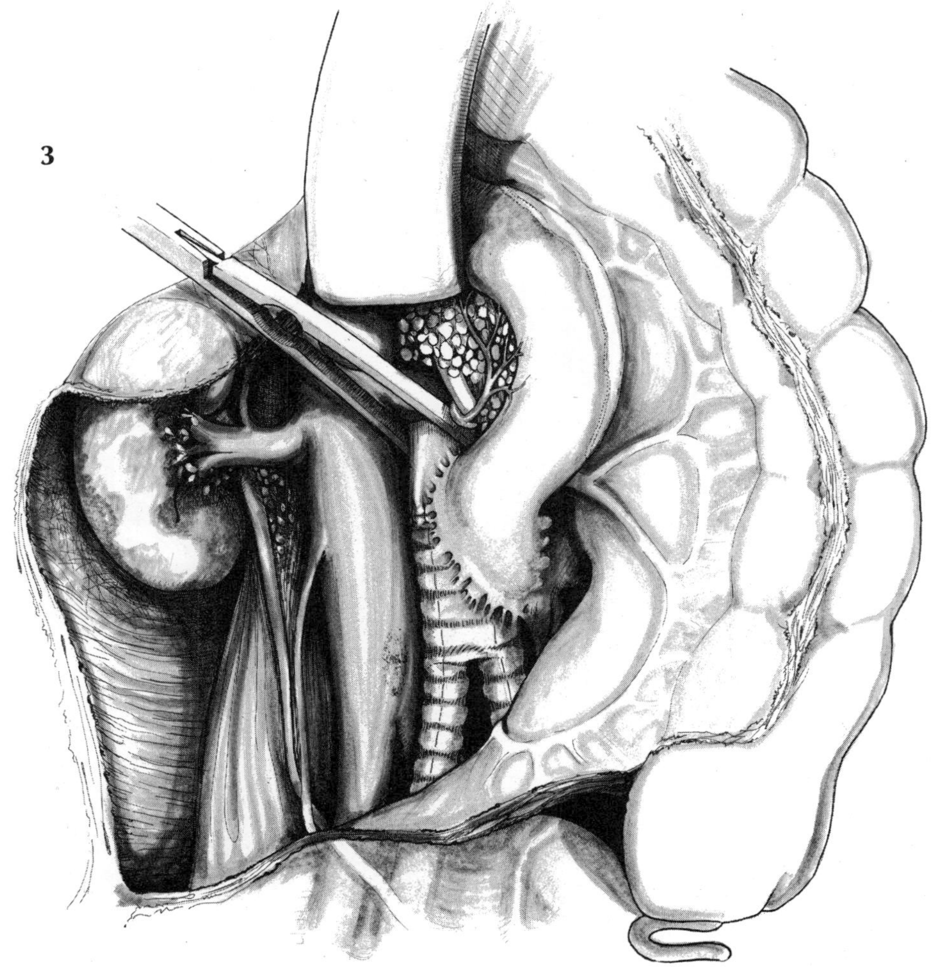

4, 5 & 6

Graft explantation

In the presence of AEF or AEE, the first priority is to perform intestinal repair, by either simple suturing and deepening of the erosion (*4*) or by a segmental duodenal resection with an end to end anastomosis (*5*).

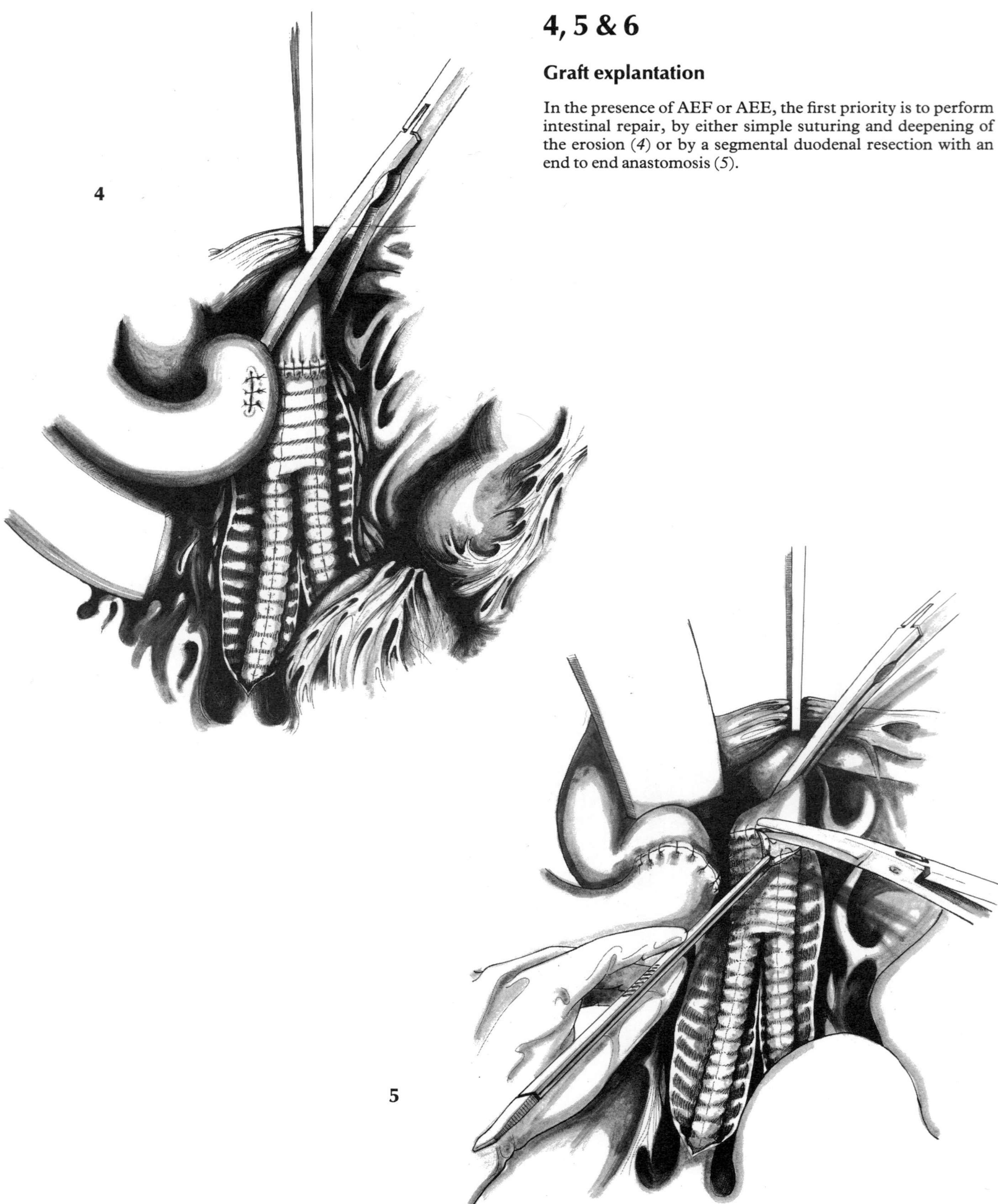

After aortic clamping, the infected aortic graft is removed followed by irrigation of the retroperitoneal area by antiseptic solution of 2% povidone-iodine. Explanted graft material is collected for bacteriological cultures. *Illustration 6* shows completion with an *in situ* new graft replacement. The choice of the type of reimplanted graft is debated. We prefer a PTFE graft, because of the demonstration of suggested higher resistance for those strains more frequently implicated in low-grade infection (Schmitt, 1986; Bandyk, 1991). Other authors report successful reimplantation with Dacron graft or homologous tissue (Kieffer, 1993) and recently with rifampin-soaked Dacron grafts (Torsello, 1993).

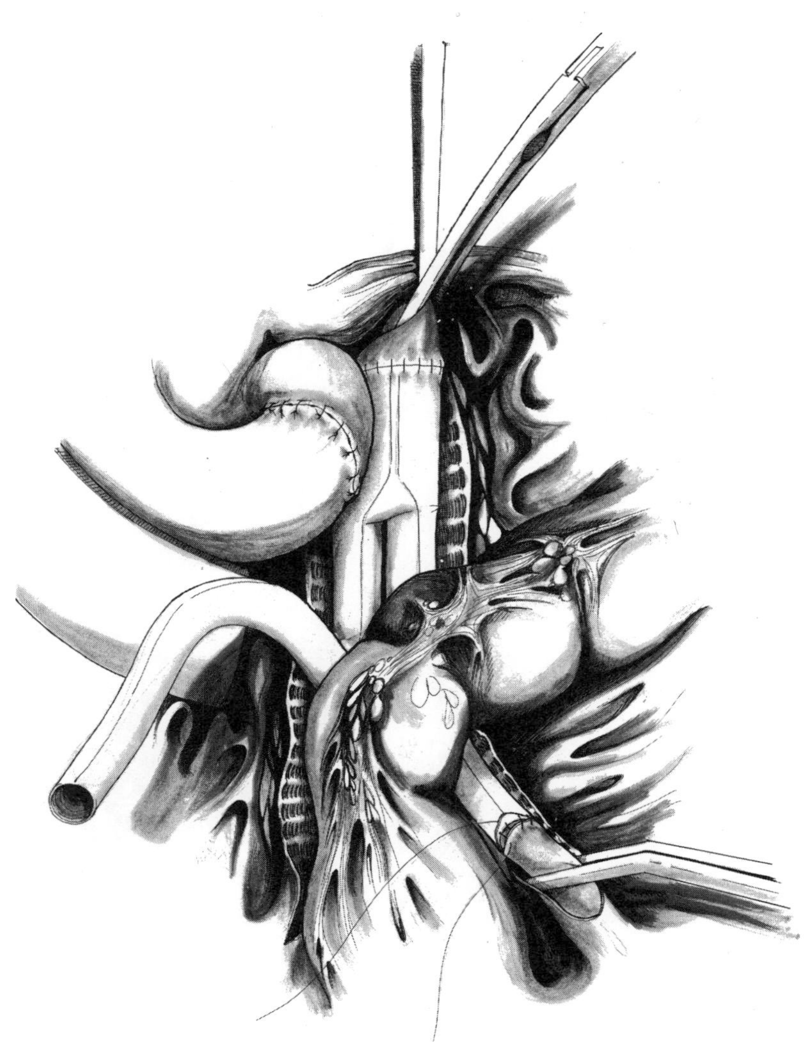

6

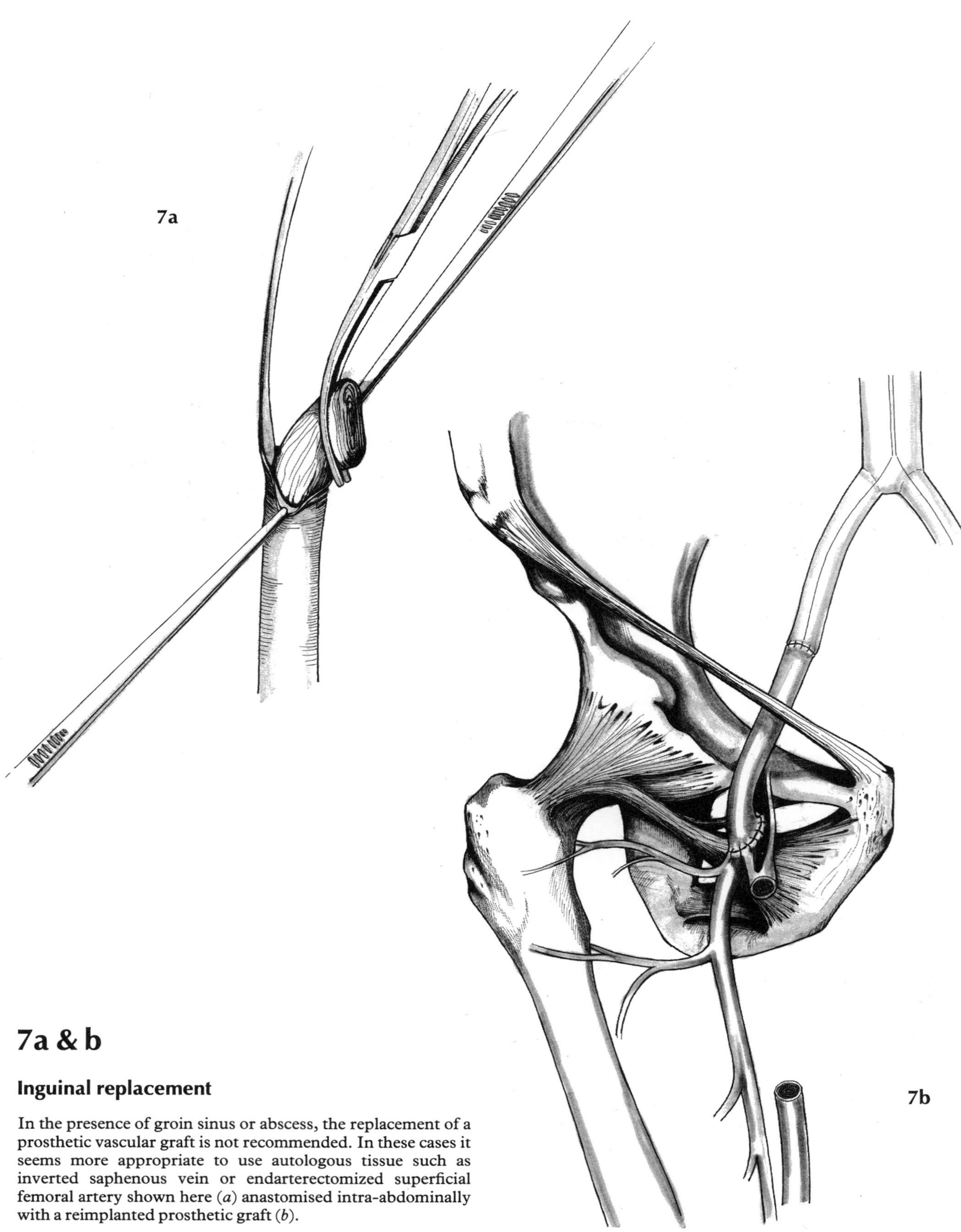

7a & b

Inguinal replacement

In the presence of groin sinus or abscess, the replacement of a prosthetic vascular graft is not recommended. In these cases it seems more appropriate to use autologous tissue such as inverted saphenous vein or endarterectomized superficial femoral artery shown here (*a*) anastomised intra-abdominally with a reimplanted prosthetic graft (*b*).

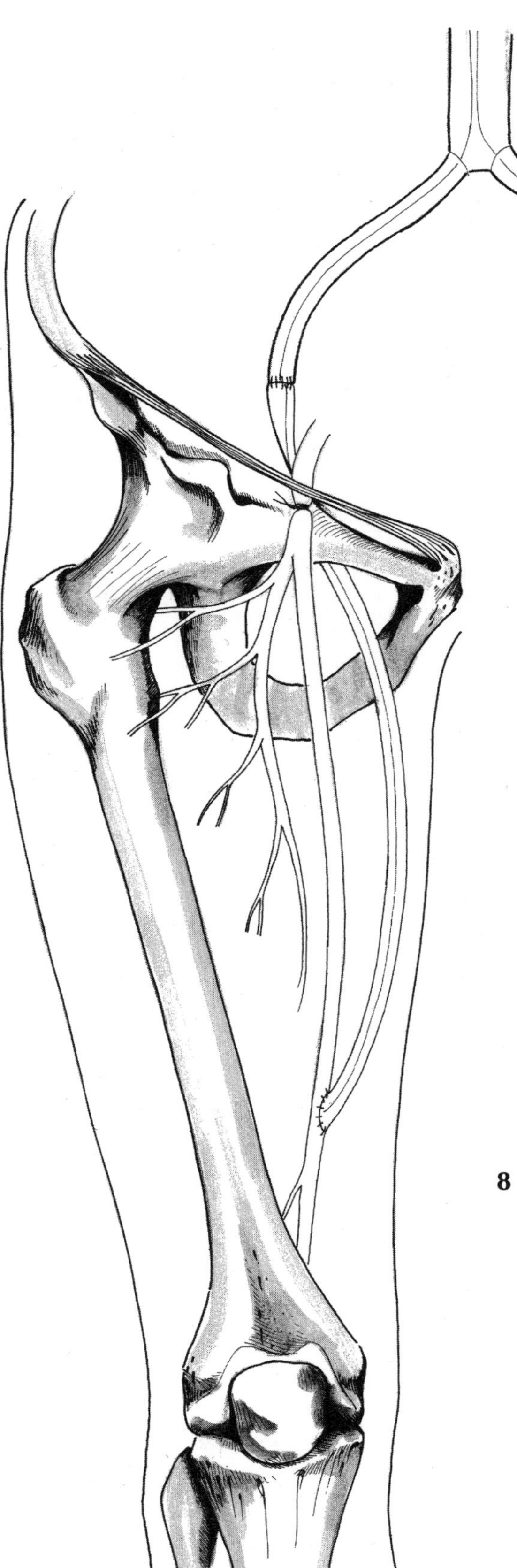

8

8

Another possible alternative to avoid the infected groin is to perform a trans-obturatory bypass to the inferior third of the superficial femoral artery with avoidance of the infected inguinal area.

9

At the end of whatever procedure a pedicle of omentum is mobilized and passed through the transverse mesocolon to cover the new aortic graft and two drainage tubes are positioned to permit postoperative antiseptic irrigation and monitoring of bacterial culture.

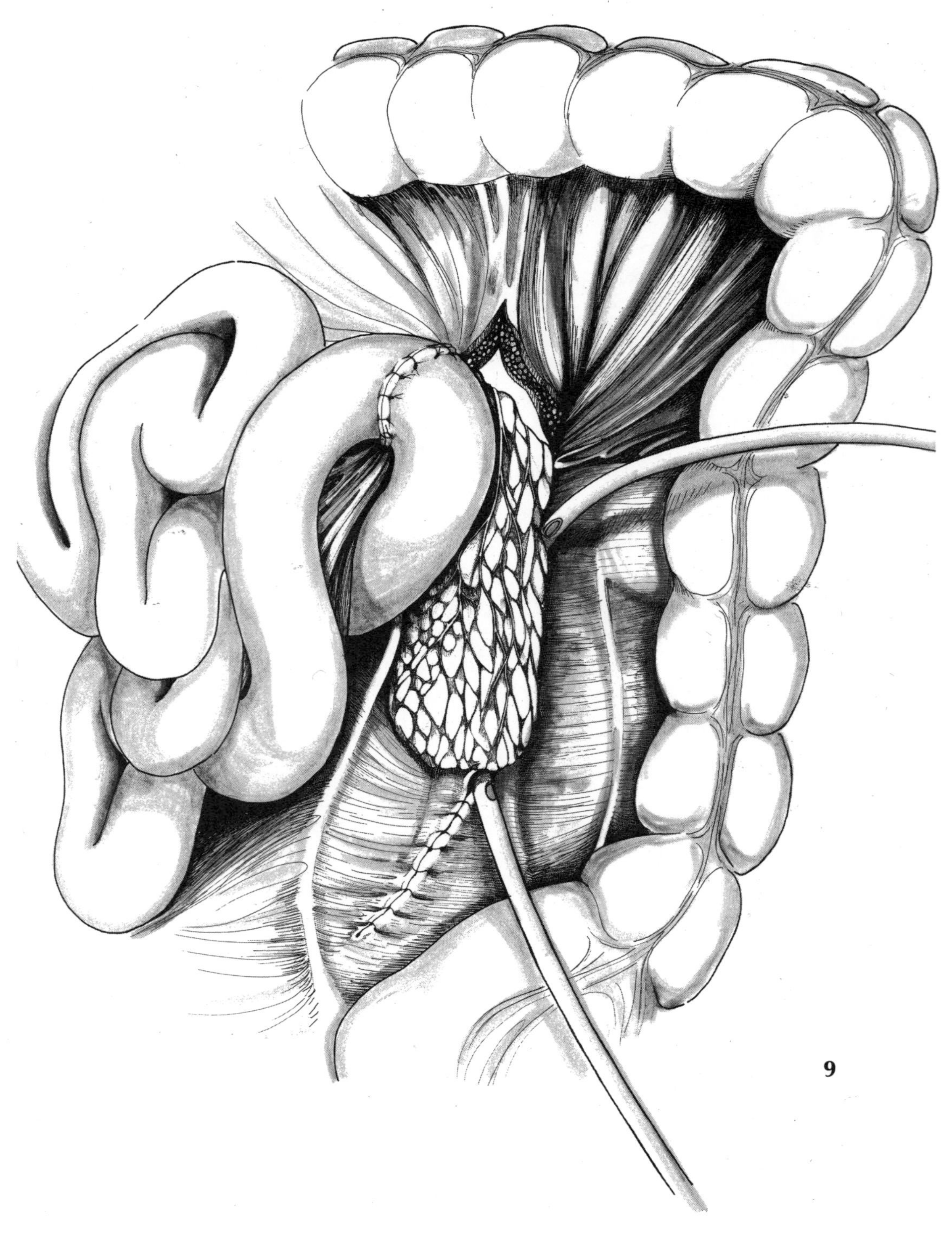

9

Conclusions

Postoperative mortality ranges from 0 to 20% with no amputations. Walker (1987) in a paper dealing with the selection of patients as candidates for an *in situ* replacement showed a significant correlation between the presence of retroperitoneal abscess and mortality; the perioperative mortality following *in situ* replacement in patients with extensive purulent graft infection (retroperitoneal abscess) was 60% vs 22% in patients with low grade infection.

Bandyk (1991), in a more recent experience, recommended *in situ* PTFE replacement for late graft infections in those patients in which no systemic (septicaemia) or local signs (perigraft abscess, dehiscence of the anastomosis) of infection are present. From these experiences the concept of 'grade' of infection should determine the choice of management. Reinfections among survivors are rare.

However for severe and acute onset infections *in situ* replacement seems contraindicated, but in patients with low-grade infection a better prognosis for life and limb is claimed.

References

Bandyk, D. F., Bergamini, T. M., Kinney, E. V., Seabrook, G. R. and Towne, J. B. (1991). *In situ* replacement of vascular prostheses infected by bacterial biofilms. *Journal of Vascular Surgery* **13**, 575.

Bunt, T. J. (1983) Synthetic vascular graft infections: I. Graft infections. *Surgery* **93**, 733.

Eugene, J., Goldstone, J. and Moore, W. S. (1974). Fifteen-year experience with subcutaneous bypass grafts for lower extremity ischemia. *Annals of Surgery* **186**, 177.

Fiorani, P., Speziale, F., Rizzo, L. *et al.* (1993). Detection of aortic graft infection with leukocytes labeled with Technetium 99m hexametazine. *Journal of Vascular Surgery* **17**, 86.

Goldstone, J. and Moore, W. S. (1974). Infection in vascular prostheses: Clinical manifestation and surgical management. *American Journal of Surgery* **128**, 225.

Hoffert, P. W., Gensler, S. and Haimovici, H. (1965). Infection complicating arterial grafts. *Archives of Surgery* **90**, 427.

Inahara, T., Geary, G. L., Mukherjee, D. *et al.* (1985). The contrary position to the non-resective treatment of abdominal aortic aneurysm. *Journal of Vascular Surgery* **4**, 42.

Jacobs, M. J. H. M., Reul, G. J., Gregoric, I. and Cooley, D. A. (1991). *In situ*-replacement and extranatomic bypass for the treatment of infected abdominal aortic grafts. *European Journal of Vascular Surgery* **5**, 83.

Kieffer, E., Bahnini, A., Koskas, F., Ruotolo, C., Le Blevec, D. and Plissionier, D. (1993). *In situ* allograft replacement of infected infrarenal aortic prosthetic graft: Results in forty-three patients. *Journal of Vascular Surgery* **17**, 349.

O'Hara, P. J., Hertzer, N. R., Beven, E. G. and Krajewski, L. P. (1986). Surgical management of infected abdominal aortic grafts: Review of 25-year experience. *Journal of Vascular Surgery* **3**, 725.

Pons, V. G. and Wurtz, R. (1991). Vascular grafts infections: A 25-year experience of 170 cases. *Journal of Vascular Surgery* **5**, 751.

Reilly, L. M., Altman, H. Lusby, R. J., Kersh, R. A., Ehrenfeld, W. K. and Stoney, R. J. (1984). Late results following surgical management of vascular graft infection. *Journal of Vascular Surgery* **1**, 36.

Reilly, L. M., Stoney, R. J., Goldstone, J. and Ehrenfeld, W. K. (1987). Improved management of aortic graft infection: The influence of operative sequence and staging. *Journal of Vascular Surgery* **5**, 421.

Robinson, J. A. and Johansen, K. J. (1991). Aortic sepsis: Is there a role for an *in situ* graft reconstruction? *Journal of Vascular Surgery* **13**, 677.

Schmitt, D. D., Bandyk, D. F., Peuqet, A. J. and Towne, J. B. (1986). Bacterial adherence to vascular prostheses. A determinant of graft infectivity. *Journal of Vascular Surgery* **5**, 732.

Szilagyi, D. E., Smith, R. F., Elliot, J. P. and Vrandecic, M. P. (1972). Infection in arterial reconstruction with synthetic grafts. *Annals of Surgery* **176**, 321.

Torsello, G., Sandmann, W., Gehrt, A. and Jungblut, R. M. (1993). *In situ* replacement of infected vascular prostheses with rifampin-soaked vascular grafts: Early results. *Journal of Vascular Surgery* **17**, 768.

Vollmar, J. F. and Kogel, H. (1987). Aortoenteric fistulas as post-operative complications. *Journal of Cardiovascular Surgery* (Torino) **28**, 479.

Walker, W. E., Cooley, D. A. and Duncan, J. M. (1987). The management of aortoduodenal fistula by *in situ* replacement of the infected abdominal aortic graft. *Annals of Surgery* **205**, 727.

Yeager, R. A., Moneta, G. L., Taylor, L. M., Harris, E. J. Jr, McConnell, D. B. and Porter, J. M. (1990). Improving survival and limb salvage in patients with aortic graft infection. *American Journal of Surgery* **159**, 466.

Surgical techniques for visceral artery revascularization

WILLIAM K. EHRENFELD MD, *Professor of Surgery*
DOUGLAS L. JICHA MD, *Vascular Fellow*
RONALD J. STONEY MD, *Professor of Surgery*
University of California, San Francisco, California, USA

Introduction

Atherosclerotic visceral artery lesions may cause acute or chronic visceral ischaemia. The chronic form is also known as 'abdominal angina' (Dunphy, 1936; Mikkelsen, 1957). Acute occlusion of one or more visceral arteries due to thrombosis of an atherosclerotic artery or embolus from a proximal source may lead to bowel infarction. Bowel infarction is a surgical emergency requiring immediate removal of the affected bowel and possibly the offending clot or the atherosclerotic lesion. This is rarely technically feasible. Chronic mesenteric insufficiency with abdominal angina is a relatively rare condition. Extensive collateral vessels readily develop between the visceral aortic branches – coeliac axis, superior mesenteric artery (SMA), inferior mesenteric artery (IMA) – and the hypogastric (internal iliac) arteries. These collateral pathways may be so efficient that very rarely gradual occlusion of all major aortic branches may actually occur without bowel infarction. Usually, involvement of two or more visceral branches cause symptoms. The main collateral circuits are: (*1*) the gastroduodenal and pancreaticoduodenal arteries between the coeliac axis and the SMA; (*2*) the middle and left colic arteries between the SMA and the IMA ('meandering mesenteric artery', the arc of Riolan); and finally (*3*) the sigmoid and haemorrhoidal vessels between the IMA and the internal iliac arteries. Although at least two of the three major visceral arteries are severely narrowed or occluded in 85% of patients with abdominal angina, the symptoms are related more to the inadequacy of the collateral blood flow than to the actual number of obstructed primary arteries (Wylie, Stoney and Ehrenfeld, 1980). Occlusion of the coeliac axis along with poor collateralization may occasionally cause bowel or organ ischaemia. Chronic occlusion of either the SMA or IMA only does not usually cause ischaemia.

The syndrome most typical of chronic intestinal ischaemia afflicts women between the ages of 50 and 70 years and includes: (*1*) epigastric postprandial cramping pain; (*2*) weight loss due to pain and/or fear of eating; (*3*) bowel motility disturbances (nausea, vomiting, diarrhoea and/or constipation) caused by bowel ischaemia. Malabsorption is seldom present, and there are no specific diagnostic laboratory tests. Evidence of atherosclerotic disease in other peripheral arteries is found in approximately 33% of the affected patients and an epigastric bruit is heard in 70%. The definitive diagnosis depends upon abdominal arteriography using both the anteroposterior projection, which best delineates collateral formation, and lateral or oblique projections, which best illustrate the degree of vessel obstruction. The stenotic lesions are usually seen at or near the vessel origins.

Unusual causes of visceral artery stenosis are fibromuscular dysplasia and median arcuate ligament compression of the coeliac axis and occasionally includes the SMA. Cases of compression of these vessels by the coeliac ganglionic nerve fibres have been reported. These cases are often atypical and are the subject of continuing surgical controversy.

During the past 25 years numerous methods for visceral artery revascularization have been evaluated including retrograde synthetic or autogenous grafts, transvisceral artery thromboendarterectomy and reimplantation. Two basic procedures are now preferred: transaortic thromboendarterectomy and antegrade synthetic graft bypass grafting.

Operative indications and preoperative preparations

Revascularization is indicated in patients with characteristic symptoms and significant stenosis of one or more visceral branches as seen by arteriography. The objectives are to relieve pain and prevent bowel infarction. Prophylactic visceral revascularization may also be indicated in coexisting aortoiliac and aortorenal vascular procedures (Stoney, Ehrenfeld and Wylie, 1977). Intra-abdominal disease of nonvascular origin must be thoroughly excluded before operation. Intravenous hyperalimentation may be required in the catabolic patient with profound weight loss to restore an anabolic state. When prosthetic grafts are used, antibiotics are given intraoperatively and during the next 48 h.

Antegrade prosthetic grafting

Atherosclerotic visceral artery lesions, in conjunction with lesions in the renal arteries, may be part of an unusually extensive atherosclerotic process of the abdominal aortic wall, which can make grafting at this level technically difficult. Antegrade prosthetic visceral bypass reconstructions may be desirable as the grafts will originate from the usually undiseased distal thoracic aorta. Antegrade graft placement is haemodynamically superior to retrograde placement which may predispose to early graft thrombosis. The antegrade route is shorter and usually requires shorter grafts. Retrograde bypass is particularly awkward for revascularization of the SMA since this artery arises from the aorta at an acute angle and is quite mobile, predisposing to kink and occlusion. Arterial autografts are ideal for revascularization procedures involving the renal arteries (Ehrenfeld, Stoney and Wylie, 1982). However, in visceral artery revascularization, synthetic grafts are preferred since the most common autografts, the hypogastric (internal iliac) arteries, constitute part of the visceral collateral system. The hypogastric artery autograft is generally too short for antegrade revascularization of the SMA. Venous autografts are not used, since it is thought that they frequently cause dilatation, stenosis and late occlusion (Stanley, Ernst and Fry, 1973). Flanged knitted Dacron prostheses (5 or 6 mm) are preferred for single vessel bypass, and bifurcated grafts (10 × 5 mm or 12 × 6 mm) are used when both the coeliac axis and the SMA are revascularized. Visceral erosion by these grafts has not occurred in our series. Revascularization of both the coeliac axis and the superior mesenteric artery is preferred when indicated and feasible, since they supply 90% of splanchnic blood flow. This procedure is commonly used in patients with operative risk factors that preclude thoracoabdominal exposure. Despite temporary aortic occlusion of 20–30 min, the results with this procedure are excellent, with a long-term graft patency and durable relief of abdominal angina in over 90% of patients.

Operative technique

An upper midline incision extending from the xiphoid to the umbilicus is used. The coeliac artery and the supracoeliac aorta are reached by first dividing the gastrohepatic ligament. After division of the triangular ligament, the left lobe of the liver is retracted to the right and the oesophagus and the stomach to the left in order to expose the posterior fibres of the diaphragm.

1a–d

Illustration 1(a) shows the anterior approach to the coeliac artery and supracoeliac aorta. The inset depicts a typical coeliac atherosclerotic lesion with contiguous aortic involvement. Isolated coeliac disease is a more common cause of symptoms than isolated SMA disease. The arcuate ligament and diaphragmatic crura are divided in the midline to expose the distal thoracic aorta (*b*). The coeliac ganglionic fibres are dissected and resected from around the artery. The aorta is temporarily occluded at a level 5 cm proximal to the coeliac axis origin and also distal to the origin of the coeliac axis, after intravenous administration of 2000–4000 i.u. of heparin. An elliptical disc of the aortic wall is cut out from the anterior surface of the aorta (*c*). A 6-mm flanged Dacron graft (made from 12 × 6 mm bifurcation graft) is anastomosed to the aortotomy site with a running 4/0 synthetic suture. Thereafter, the aortic clamps are released and a vascular clamp is applied on the proximal portion of the graft. The graft is then anastomosed end-to-end to the undiseased distal artery (*d*).

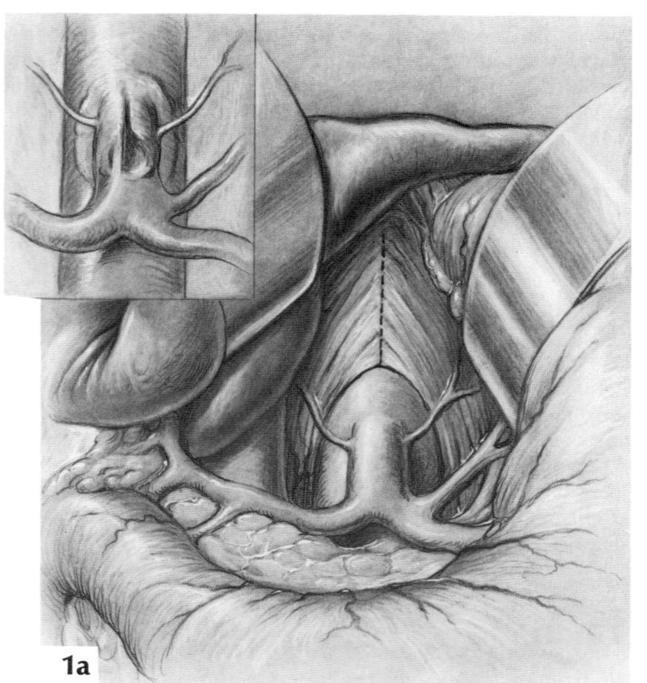
1a

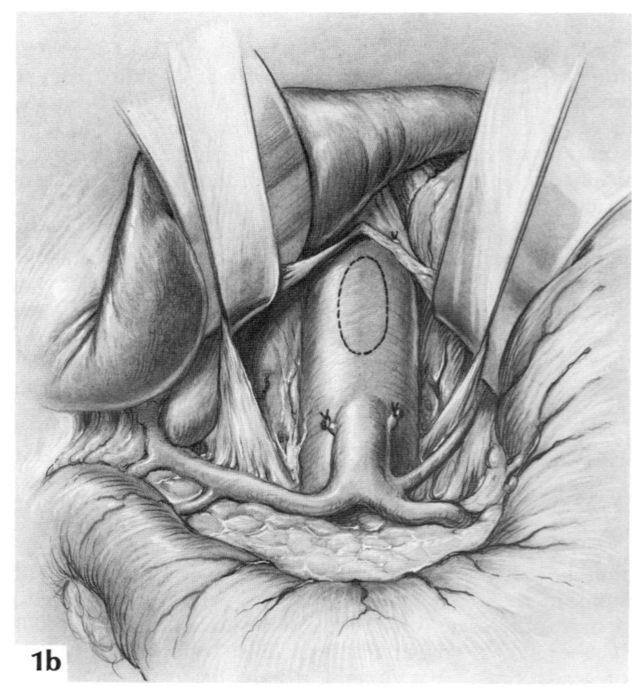
1b

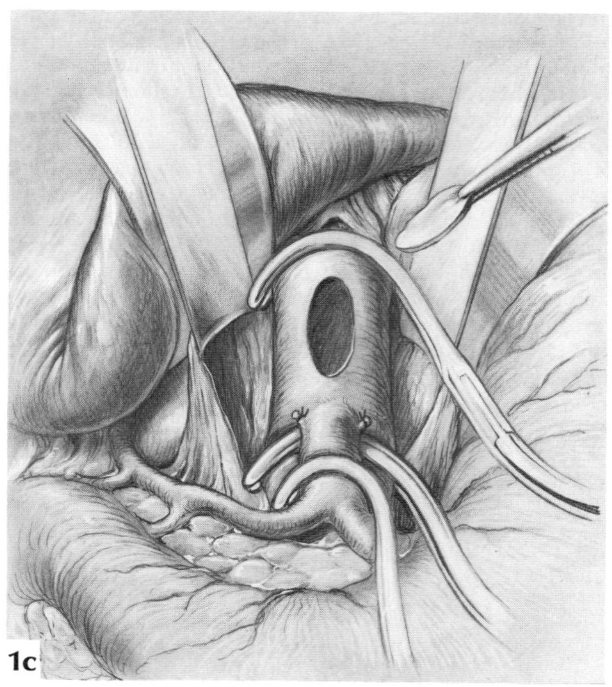
1c

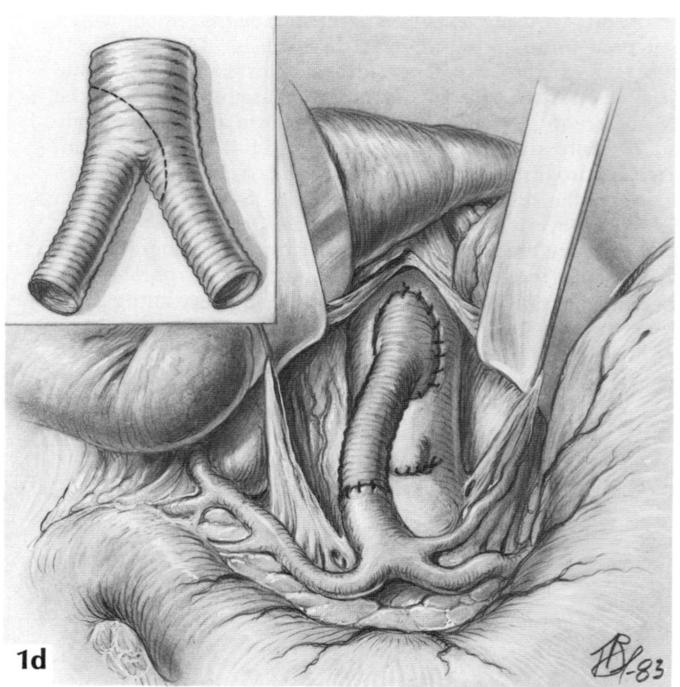
1d

2a–c

If bypass to both the coeliac and the SMA is planned, the SMA is also exposed by further dissection and resection of the coeliac nerve fibres overlying the aorta. This manoeuvre frees the body of the pancreas which can then be elevated from the aorta with ease and retracted caudally, thus exposing the first 4–5 cm of the SMA. An elliptical aortotomy is made on the right anterolateral aspect of the aorta (*a*). With this technique, the two graft limbs will line up parallel to the coeliac axis and the SMA, respectively, without kinking and buckling of the graft. A flanged tubular bifurcation graft (12 × 6 mm) is anastomosed between aortic clamps to the aorta using a 4/0 suture. The body of the graft is then clamped and aortic flow is restored. Thereafter the coeliac axis is clamped, transected and the proximal end is oversewn. An end-to-end anastomosis is performed between the graft limb and the distal, nondiseased coeliac artery using either interrupted or running 5/0 sutures. The clamp is then shifted to the right SMA limb and the same procedure is used for the SMA (*b*). The right (SMA) limb of the bifurcated graft lies behind the pancreas to parallel the course of the SMA (*c*). The full length of the retropancreatic course of the SMA limb is visualized in (*c*) by the artist's cutaway of a section of pancreas. The adequacy of the reconstruction may be assessed by electromagnetic flow probe measurement. Alternatively, intraoperative ultrasound B-mode imaging with Doppler flow velocity measurement can be used. Postoperative arteriography is also performed to verify the operative result.

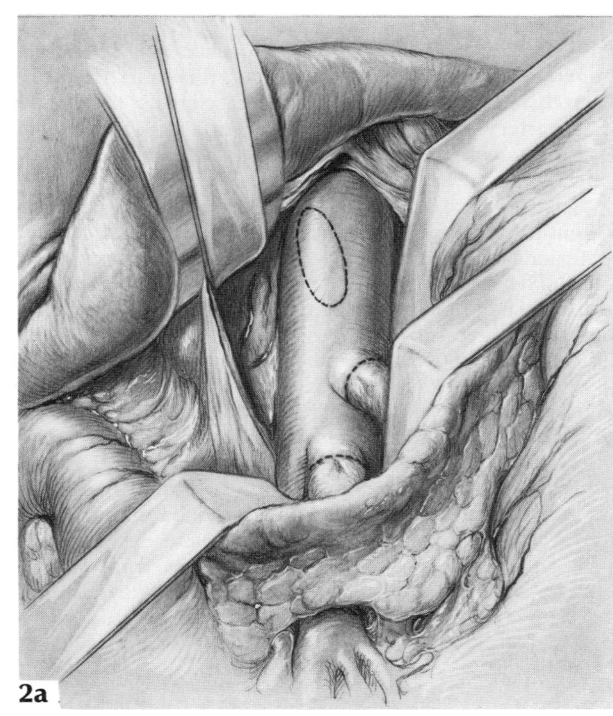
2a

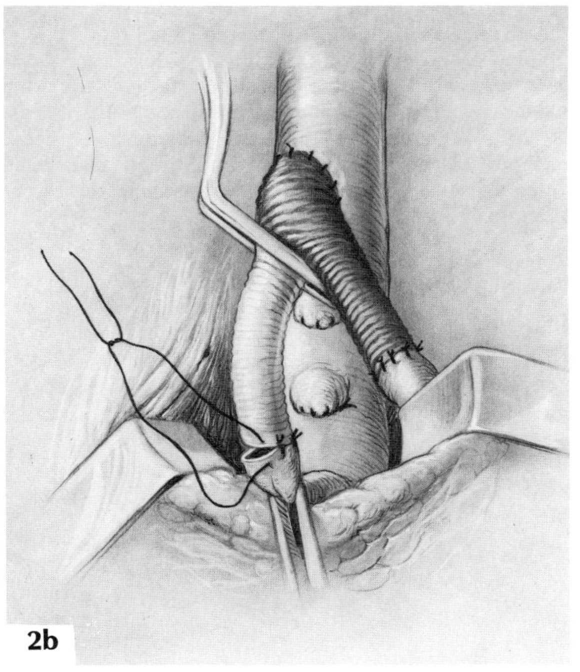
2b

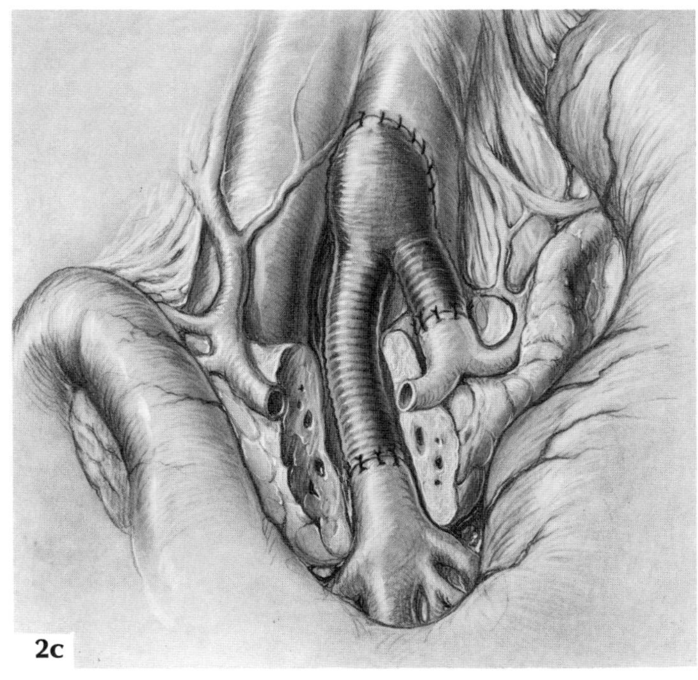
2c

Transaortic endarterectomy

The atherosclerotic lesion in the coeliac axis is invariably limited to the very proximal portion of this short artery. Even when this vessel is occluded by atherosclerosis, the distal half of the artery maintains its patency as a result of collateral flow through its three terminal branches. SMA occlusion is generally more extended. When the orifice is occluded the clot usually progresses to the first major distal branch, 5–8 cm from the origin. The short lesion in coeliac stenosis or occlusion is easily removed by a simple transaortic endarterectomy. The longer lesion in SMA occlusion may require an additional angioplasty. Transarterial endarterectomy through the diseased vessel only is no longer used because of the difficulty in removing the aortic intimal lesion surrounding the visceral artery orifice. The ventral course of the visceral arteries and the position of the SMA under the pancreas make access for endarterectomy of these arteries extremely difficult with the conventional transperitoneal approach. It is technically feasible, but exposure is not optimal. This problem has been solved by the use of the thoracoabdominal retroperitoneal approach which provides complete exposure of the aorta and its visceral and renal branches from the distal thoracic aorta to the aortic bifurcation (Stoney, Ehrenfeld and Wylie, 1977). This approach is particularly advantageous in the presence of coexistent distal aortic or aortorenal atherosclerotic disease requiring additional surgical repair. Recently, we have used a new exposure that eliminates the need for thoracotomy by performing left median visceral rotation.

Operative technique

With the patient in the supine position, a midline incision is made extending from above the xiphoid to the pubis. Using a self-retaining retractor (Omni-Tract, Minnesota Scientific Co., Minnesota) to obtain 'handless exposure', the small intestine is placed in a 'bowel bag' to the right. Mobilization of the descending colon is begun laterally and the plane is developed cephalad with incision of the splenorenal ligament. Combined blunt and sharp dissection are then employed to rotate the spleen, pancreas and left colon to the right. The left kidney, adrenal gland, ureter and gonadal vein are left in place. The left renal vein is fully mobilized to the inferior vena cava allowing for retraction or, if necessary, division. Following division and reflection of the dense autonomic ganglia on the left anterior surface of the aorta, the left diaphragmatic crura is incised longitudinally. The aorta is then circumferentially mobilized together with the superior mesenteric artery, coeliac axis and renal arteries when necessary (Sauer and Stoney, 1989).

3a, b & c

After application of proximal and distal aortic clamps as well as individual clamps on the visceral and renal arteries, excellent exposure of the coeliac and the SMA orifices is provided by a 'trap door' aortotomy in the anterolateral aortic wall. The dissected renal vein is retracted caudally.

If the aortic atheroma is confined to the anterior aorta, the endarterectomy is limited to the undersurface of the 'trap door' as shown here. When advanced atheromatous disease involves the whole circumference of the aorta, a sleeve endarterectomy is performed. The aortic intima is transected to the cleavage plane in the outer media and the aortic endarterectomy is carried out.

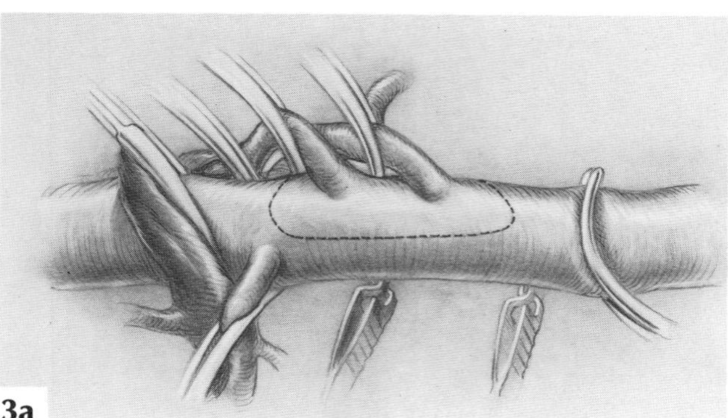

3a

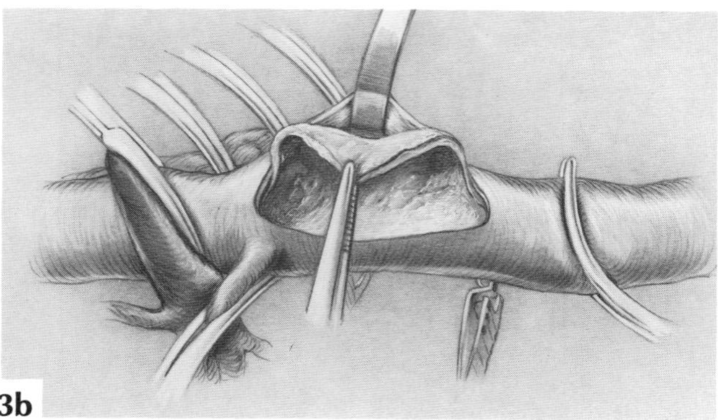

3b

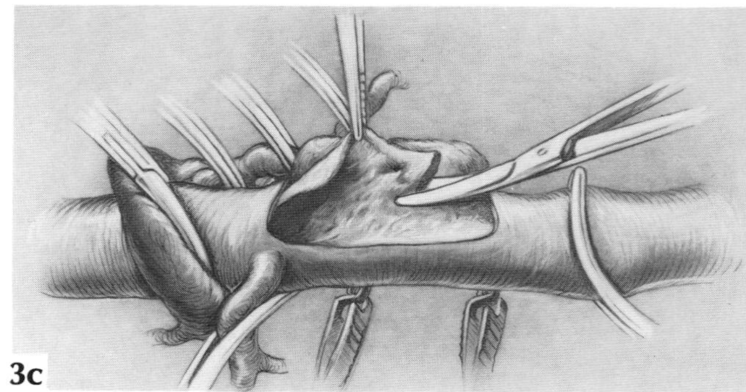

3c

3d, e & f

Removal of the intimal lesions of the visceral artery orifices are then performed individually. Gentle traction is applied to the freed aortic intimal core while the media of the visceral artery is pushed away by a blunt dissection instrument (*d*). In the coeliac axis, the short intimal core separates easily at the end-point under direct vision. Similarly, when the SMA orifice is not occluded, the atheroma is separated and the end-point is visualized using the extraction endarterectomy technique. If the lesion occludes the SMA, organized thrombus propagates to the first re-entry collateral (usually the left colic branch). The separation or end-point may not be visible from the aortic orifice. The aortotomy is closed and aortic blood flow is restored prior to clamping the SMA at its origin. A longitudinal SMA arteriotomy is made to a point beyond the occlusion. The specimen is removed, visualizing the smooth transition to normal intima (*e*), and the arteriotomy is closed with a vein patch to prevent narrowing (*f*). When indications for concomitant renal artery revascularization are present, the longitudinal aortotomy is extended to the infrarenal level to facilitate a contiguous transaortic bilateral renal endarterectomy.

As with the bypass grafting procedures, the adequacy of the endarterectomy is checked by electromagnetic flow probe measurement or ultrasound B-mode imaging with Doppler flow measurement. Intraoperative arteriography is rarely performed.

Transaortic visceral endarterectomy is suitable for most patients and can be extended for simultaneous correction of coexisting renal artery lesions or aortic atherosclerotic ('coral reef') lesions. Left medial visceral rotation allows excellent exposure of the entire abdominal aorta and its four major branches for the employment of this technique. Further, the transabdominal approach allows treatment of occlusive lesions causing acute visceral ischaemia and bowel infarction which require thrombectomy, visceral reconstruction and appropriate bowel resection. Synthetic grafts are usually avoided when gross contamination is present.

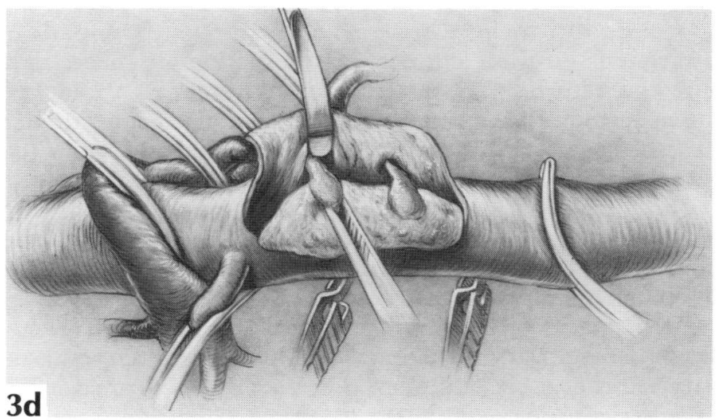

3d

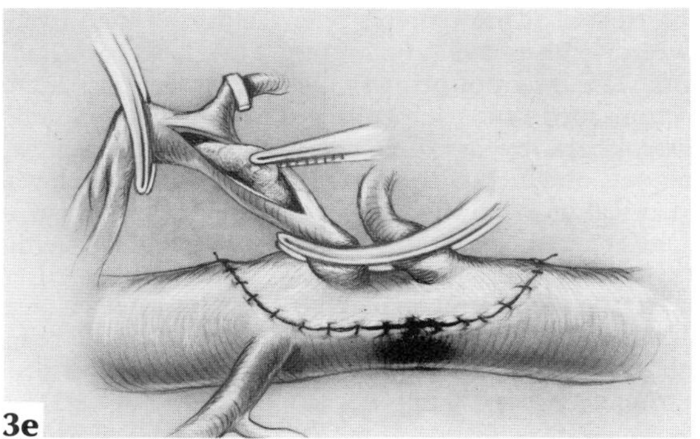

3e

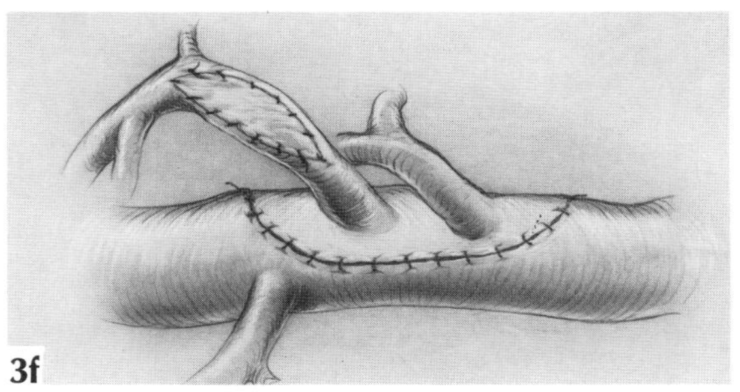

3f

Postoperative care, complications and results

Intravenous infusion and nasogastric suction are maintained until the return of normal bowel movements. Prolonged supracoeliac occlusion of the aorta may cause acute tubular necrosis (rare), and urinary output should therefore be monitored and kept at a high level. Traumatic pancreatitis may occur from excessive manipulation of the pancreas during its dissection and retraction (rare). In over 250 cases requiring supracoeliac clamping other than for pararenal or thoraco-abdominal aneurysmal disease, there have been no instances of paraplegia. Bowel infarction may occur due to graft occlusion or damage of pre-existing collaterals during the revascularization procedure, although this has not been experienced in this series.

Eighty-eight cases of primary chronic visceral ischaemia have been treated at the University of California, San Franciso between 1959 and 1993. Follow-up is available for 97.3% of patients. Treatment of primary chronic visceral ischaemia included transaortic endarterectomy in 51 patients and antegrade aortovisceral bypass in 26 patients. A durable relief of symptoms was obtained with both procedures and which was nearly identical at 1- and 5-year follow-up (Cunningham *et al.*, 1991). Recurrent symptoms of chronic visceral ischaemia developed in eight patients (10%). Five patients were cured after successful repeated revascularization. Antegrade visceral bypass and transaortic endarterectomy provide durable relief of chronic visceral ischaemia and protect patients from progression to acute visceral gangrene.

References

Cunningham, C. G., Rapp, J., Reilly, L. M. Schneider, P. A. and Stoney, R. J. (1991). Chronic intestinal ischemia: Three decades of surgical progress. *Annals of Surgery* **214**, 276.

Dunphy, J. E. (1936). Abdominal pain of vascular origin. *American Journal of Medical Science* **192**, 102.

Ehrenfeld, W. K., Stoney, R. J. and Wylie, E. J. (1982). Autogenous arterial grafts. In *Biologic and Synthetic Vascular Prostheses*. Stanley, J. C., ed. New York: Grune and Stratton.

Mikkelson, W. P. (1957). Intestinal angina: Its surgical significance. *American Journal of Surgery* **94**, 262.

Rapp, J. H., Reilly, L. M., Qvarfordt, P. G., Goldstone, J., Ehrenfeld, W. K. and Stoney, R. J. (1985). Durability of endarterectomy and antegrade grafts in the treatment of chronic visceral ischemia. *Journal of Vascular Surgery* **3**, 799.

Sauer, L. and Stoney, R. J. (1989). Transabdominal exposure of the pararenal and suprarenal aorta by medial visceral rotation. *Seminars in Vascular Surgery* **2**, 209.

Stanley, J. C., Ernst, C. B. and Fry, W. J. (1973). Fate of 100 aortorenal vein grafts: Characteristics of late graft expansion, aneurysmal dilatation, and stenosis. *Surgery* **74**, 931.

Stoney, R. J. and Wylie, E. J. (1976). Surgery of the celiac and mesenteric arteries. In *Vascular Surgery: Principles and Techniques*, 2nd ed. Haimovici, H., ed. New York: McGraw-Hill.

Stoney, R. J., Ehrenfeld, W. K. and Wylie, E. J. (1977). Revascularization methods in chronic visceral ischemia caused by atherosclerosis. Annals of Surgery. **186**, 468.

Stoney, R. J., Ehrenfeld, W. K. and Wylie, E. J. (1977). Revascularization methods in chronic visceral ischemia caused by atherosclerosis. *Annals of Surgery* **186**, 468.
Hobson, R. W. and Williams, R. A. (eds.) New York: McGraw-Hill.

Wylie, E. J., Stoney, R. J. and Ehrenfeld, W. K. (1980). *Manual of Vascular Surgery*, Vol. 1. New York: Springer-Verlag.

Surgical techniques for renal artery revascularization

DOUGLAS L. JICHA MD, *Vascular Fellow*
WILLIAM K. EHRENFELD MD, *Professor of Surgery*
RONALD J. STONEY MD, *Professor of Surgery*
University of California, San Francisco, California, USA

Introduction

Since Goldblatt *et al.* (1934) discovered the impact of renal artery stenosis on hypertension, extensive surgical experience with renal artery lesions has been acquired. Currently, renovascular hypertension is the most common indication for renal artery surgery, although prevention of renal failure and restoration of renal function have become increasingly important goals in recent years. This has been possible due to improved surgical and anaesthetic techniques, as well as precise intraoperative haemodynamic monitoring and perioperative critical care.

Occlusive lesions of the renal artery are predominantly due to atherosclerosis and fibromuscular dysplasia. A variety of historic operative techniques have been used for atherosclerotic lesions with varying results including nephrectomy, arterial reimplantation and transrenal artery thromboendarterectomy with and without patching. We have evaluated and subsequently abandoned these methods because of disappointing early and late failure rates, and currently employ transaortic endarterectomy and aortorenal bypass exclusively to treat hypertension and renal dysfunction due to renovascular disease. Fibromuscular dysplastic renal artery disease involves the middle and distal thirds of the renal artery and causes renovascular hypertension most commonly in young female patients. The use of *in situ* and *ex vivo* aortorenal bypass, depending on the extent of distal involvement, has proven effective and durable. This chapter will describe the common lesions and our preferred methods of revascularization.

1a, b, c, d & e

Following administration of intravenous heparin and mannitol which ensure anticoagulation and a diuresis, the aorta is occluded proximal to the superior mesenteric artery and distal to the renal arteries. Proximal clamping below the superior mesenteric artery is possible in cases where the inferior border of the superior mesenteric artery is greater than 2 cm cephalad to the renal ostia. Individual clamps are used to control back bleeding from the renal arteries, the superior mesenteric artery and the pararenal lumbar arteries. A longitudinal aortotomy of approximately 6–8 cm in length is created on the anterior surface of the aorta and extended proximally, between the renal arteries, and then is curved to the left of the superior mesenteric artery (*1a*).

The endarterectomy is fashioned to remove a sleeve of the pararenal aorta with bilateral opposed or multiple orificial lesions extending into the proximal renal arteries. The endarterectomy is begun in the aortic component of the plaque and follows a plane in the outer portion of the media of the diseased artery. After the aortic atherosclerotic core is freed, the distal end is transected at a point of minimal intimal thickening. When the cylinder of the entire aortic intima is separated just below the superior mesenteric artery, the proximal intimal sleeve is transected. The entire aortic plaque has been dissected before the renal orifice lesions are separated (*1b*).

Removal of the renal artery orifice disease is performed individually. Gentle traction is applied to the freed aortic intimal core while the media of the renal artery is pushed away with a Halle dissector (*1c*). This manoeuvre facilitates prolapse of the renal artery into the aortic lumen. The intimal core separates at the well-defined atherosclerotic end-point under direct vision (*1d*). The battery powered Auto Sector (Omni-Tract Surgical) (*1e*) facilitates these manoeuvres and is preferred since it shortens the endarterectomy and the renal ischaemia. After removal of any residual intimal fragments, the renal arteries are back bled, irrigated with 4°C Ringer's lactate and the aortotomy is closed with a continuous 4-0 suture.

Failure to complete the removal of atheroma by transaortic endarterectomy occurs in less than 1% of patients. If an end-point problem is suspected, following restoration of aortic flow, the renal artery is clamped proximally and distally. The residual atheroma is removed through a transverse arteriotomy under direct vision and a stable end-point is verified. The arteriotomy is closed with interrupted sutures to prevent narrowing.

With experience, renal ischaemia time rarely exceeds 20–30 min. In kidneys with renal dysfunction (creatinine 2.0 or greater), warm ischaemia tolerance is reduced when compared with normally functioning kidneys. To minimize ischaemic damage, we instill 4°C Ringer's lactate solution periodically into the renal arteries during the ischaemic period to produce renal cooling.

Intraoperative evaluation of the results of transaortic endarterectomy is best performed with Doppler ultrasound (B-mode imaging with Doppler flow velocity measurements). This allows visual and haemodynamic confirmation of a satisfactory technical result prior to wound closure.

Pararenal atherosclerotic disease

Transaortic renal endarterectomy

Atherosclerotic renal artery stenosis or occlusion typically involves the pararenal aorta and renal ostia, producing variable degrees of aortic and renal artery narrowing. Typically, disease extends 1–2 cm into the renal artery and has a well-demarcated, palpable end-point. The typical location of the pararenal atherosclerotic lesions makes aortorenal bypass potentially a less suitable option because:

1. A calcified atherosclerotic aorta poses technical problems at the proximal graft anastomosis.
2. Progressive aortic atherosclerosis predisposes the proximal graft anastomosis to late stenosis or occlusion.
3. Approximately 60% of patients require a second graft to relieve bilateral renal ischaemia.

Transaortic endarterectomy is particularly suitable for repair of pararenal atherosclerosis since the aortic component is completely removed with the orificial extension through the open aorta (Wylie, 1975).

Operative technique

A midline incision is made from the xyphoid to the pubis and the pararenal aorta is exposed using an infracolic posterior peritoneal approach. Using a self-retaining retractor (Omni-Tact, Minnesota Scientific Co., Minnesota) to obtain 'hand-less exposure', the pararenal aorta and renal arteries are exposed and circumferentially mobilized.

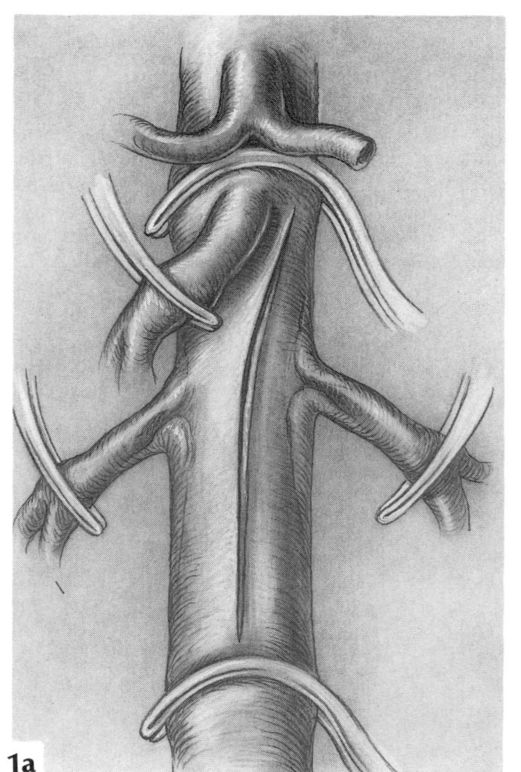
1a

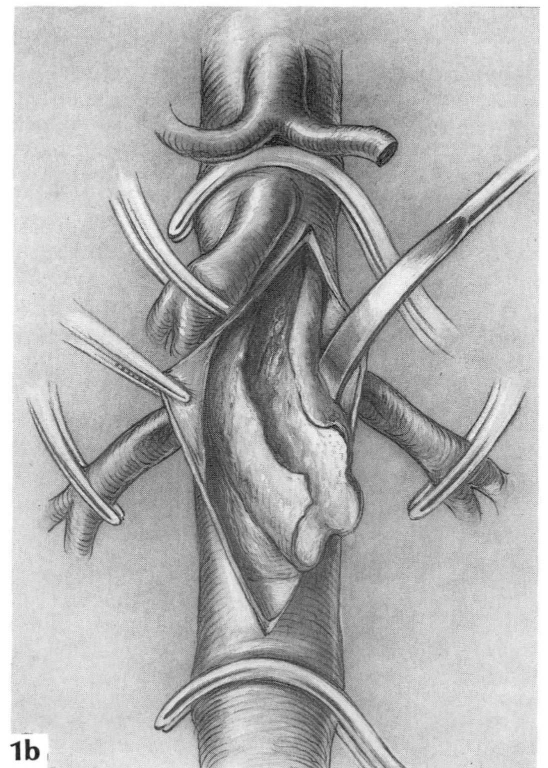
1b

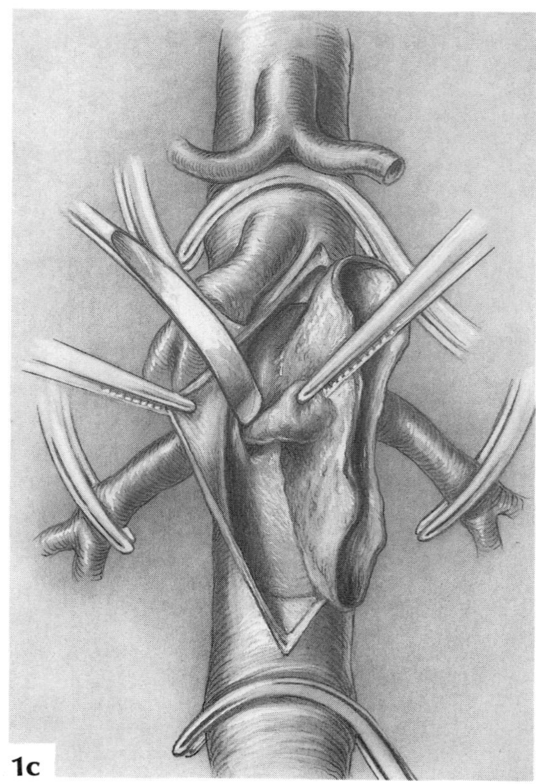
1c

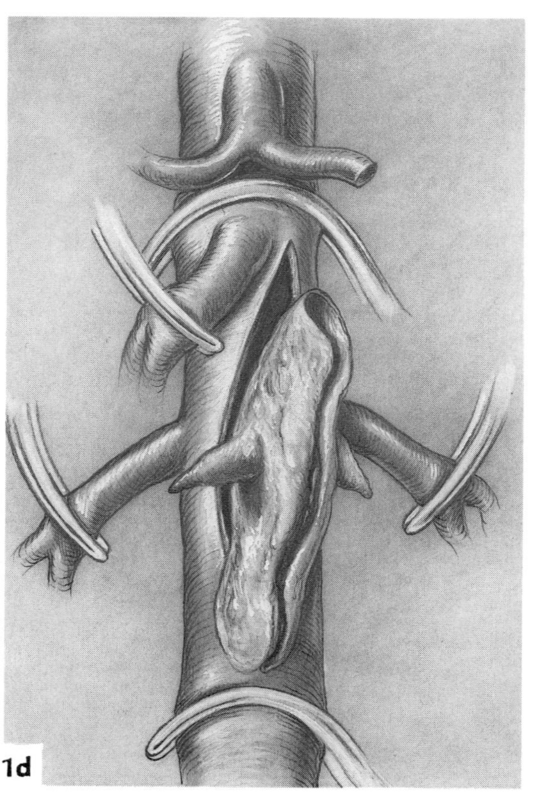
1d

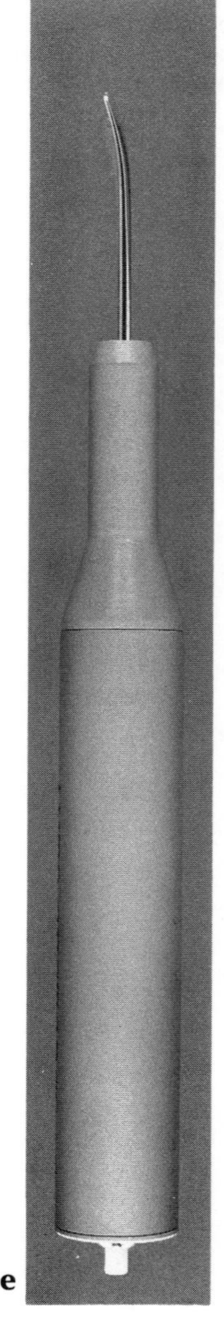
1e

Combined aortorenal atherosclerosis

When transaortic endarterectomy is combined with aortic grafting, as described above, we use the transected aorta for endarterectomy to avoid intersection of suture lines of a longitudinal aortotomy and the end-to-end graft anastomosis. This allows complete revascularization of bilateral single or multiple renal arteries, and aortic continuity is established with prosthetic graft anastomosed to the infrarenal aortic cuff. It can be performed with renal ischaemic times that are comparable with the longitudinal aortotomy approach (Stoney *et al.*, 1989).

Operative technique

Exposure of the pararenal aorta is obtained via a midline incision in the same manner as described with transaortic renal endarterectomy. After identical mobilization of the pararenal aorta, the renal arteries and the superior mesenteric artery, all branches are controlled to allow concurrent disease to be repaired. A self-retaining retractor (Omni-Tract) facilitates this exposure.

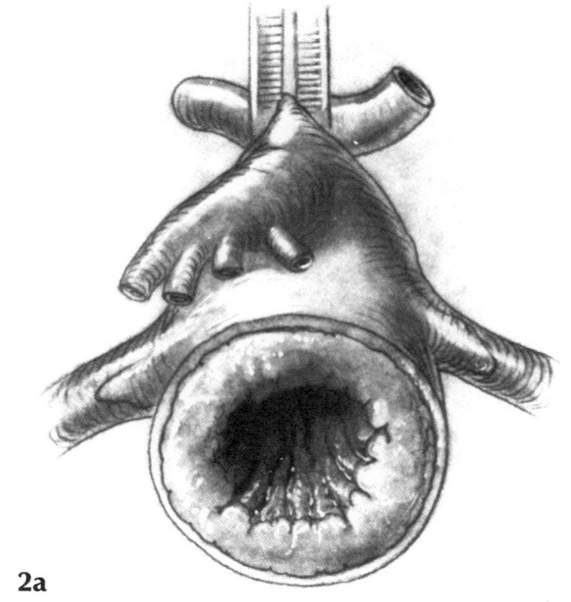

2a

2a, b & c

After complete mobilization, heparin is administered and the aorta and its branches are controlled as described. Transaortic endarterectomy is facilitated by elevating the pararenal aorta to allow inspection of the lumen directly (*2a*). The dissection plane is established between the aortic atheroma and the outer media (*2b*). This plane is developed circumferentially (*2c*). Longitudinal division of the plaque is sometimes helpful. This allows each renal endarterectomy to proceed without the contralateral renal atheroma tethering the specimen in the aortic lumen.

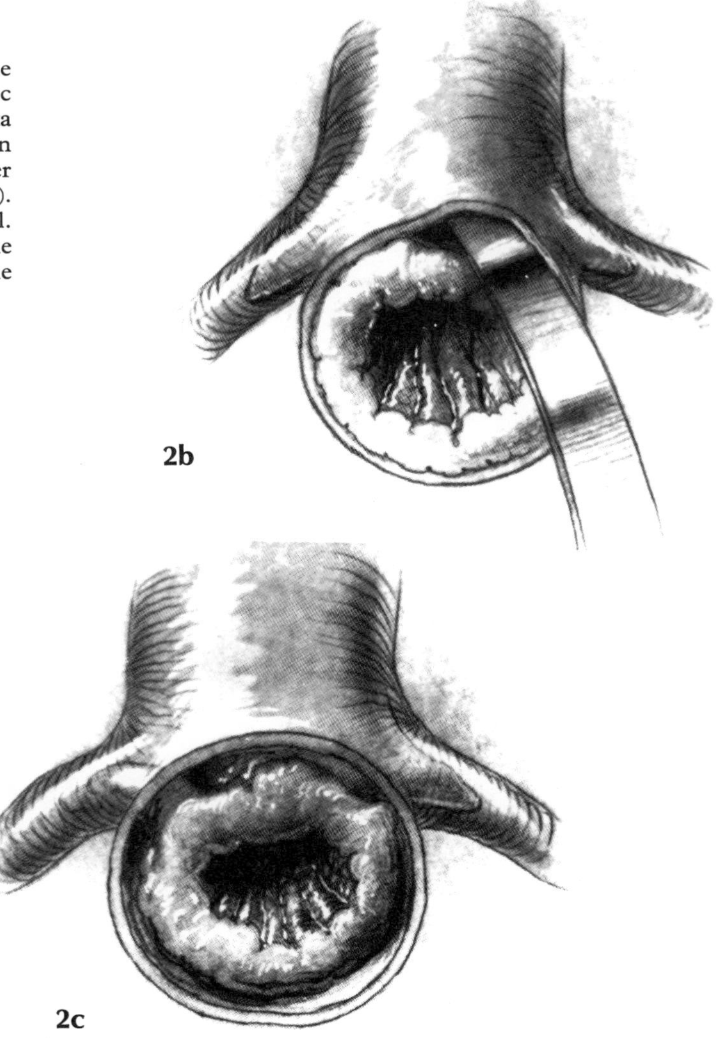

2b

2c

2d & e

The endarterectomy plane is extended cephalad by traction on the mobilized atheromata through the end of the aorta. Further traction on the aortic specimen and the renal artery clamp facilitates prolapse of the renal artery. A well defined end-point is obtained with continued traction and gentle pushing of the residual artery away from the lesion (*2d*). After both renal endarterectomies are completed, the plaque is transected at a level just distal to the superior mesenteric artery orifice and the specimen is removed (*2e*).

The renal arteries are irrigated with heparinized saline and the aortic graft is then attached end-to-end to the aortic stump using continuous braided Dacron suture. Renal perfusion is restored by repositioning the proximal clamp on the graft prior to distal anastomosis to minimize renal ischaemia. Intraoperative duplex scanning is used to assess the technical adequacy of the renal endarterectomy.

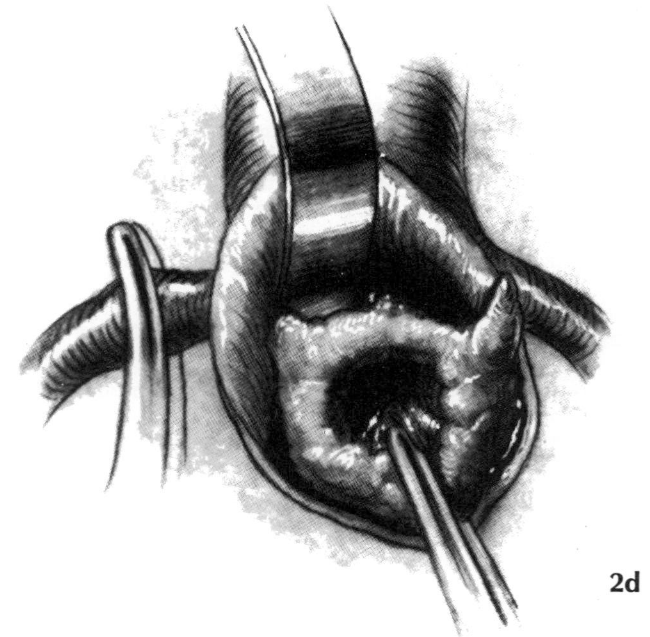

2d

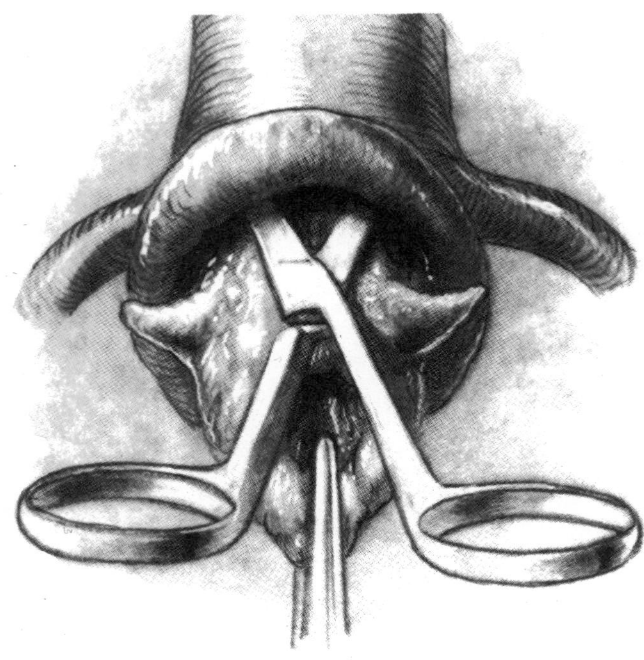

2e

Pararenal aneurysmal disease

Repair of these lesions may be complicated by difficult exposure and associated atherosclerosis that impairs renal blood flow causing hypertension and renal impairment. While simultaneous correction of these coexisting lesions can be formidable, acceptable morbidity and mortality and a durable result can be obtained with careful attention to the pattern of disease requiring operation, the technical details of the revascularization method and the perioperative care of these patients who frequently have serious comorbid disease. The surgical objective of all aortic aneurysm disease is inclusion grafting which relieves the threat of rupture. In addition, renal revascularization is accomplished by bypass or reimplantation of the renal artery to preserve or improve renal perfusion.

Operative technique

A full length midline incision (xyphoid to pubis) is used to expose the aorta. While an infracolic posterior peritoneal approach may suffice, medial visceral rotation is often advantageous and requires mobilization of the descending colon beginning laterally. This plane is developed cephalad with incision of the splenorenal ligament. Combined blunt and sharp dissection are then employed to rotate the spleen, pancreas and left colon to the right. The left kidney, adrenal gland, ureter and gonadal vein are left in place. The left renal vein is mobilized to the inferior vena cava for retraction or, if necessary, division. Following division and reflection of the dense autonomic ganglia on the left anterior surface of the aorta, the left diaphragmatic crura is incised longitudinally. The aorta is then circumferentially mobilized. The pararenal aorta and as much of the superior mesenteric artery and coeliac axis are exposed and circumferentially mobilized as necessary (Sauer and Stoney, 1989).

3a & b

Several configurations of pararenal aortic aneurysmal disease exist. When pararenal aneurysmal disease extends cephalad to a level beyond only one orifice (*3a*), a bevelled aortic transection may be performed. A bevelled graft is then attached end-to-end to the pararenal aorta. Reimplantation of the left renal artery, on a Carrel patch, to the side of the graft is easily performed (*3b*). This technique allows access to the right renal artery orifice as well as the superior mesenteric artery for transaortic visceral endarterectomy if indicated.

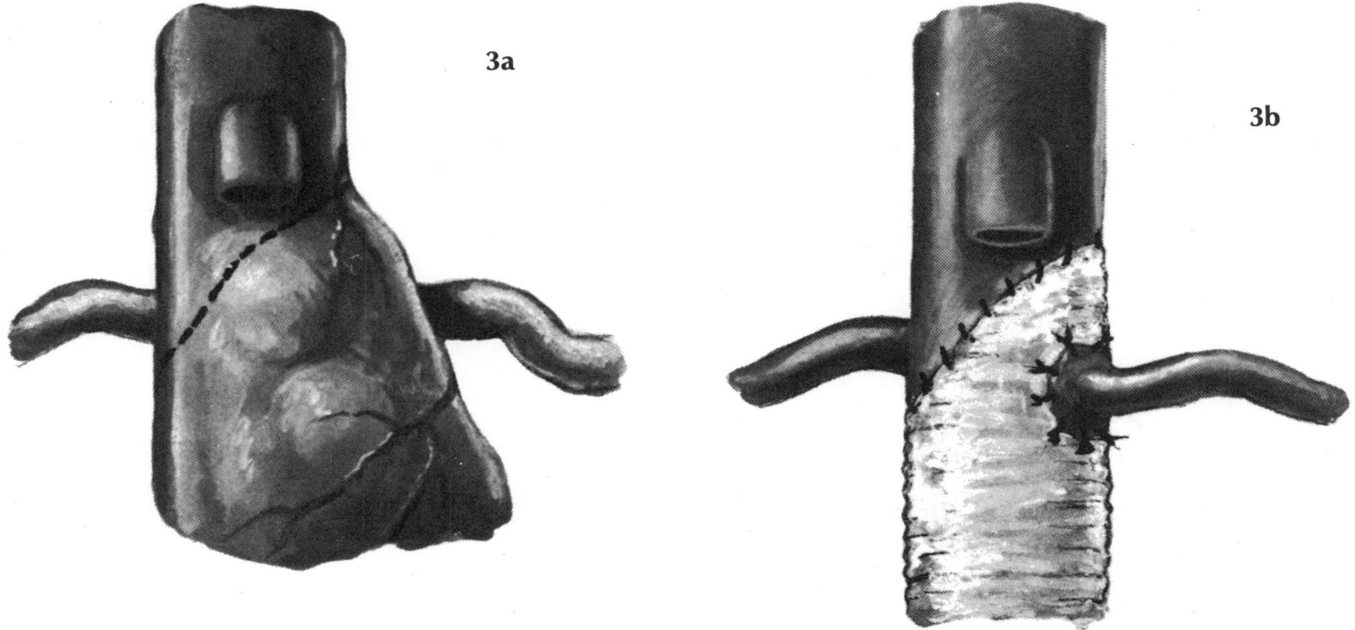

3c & d

Pararenal aortic aneurysmal disease extending above both renal artery orifices can be further complicated by extension of aneurysmal disease into the orifice of the renal arteries (*3c*). In these cases, replacement with a 5 or 6 mm Dacron graft from the aortic graft to the renal artery beyond the diseased segment is preferable. End-to-end anastomosis between the renal artery and the prosthetic graft is preferred. Careful sizing of the graft is necessary to assure a gradual curve to the graft and avoid kinking (*3d*). Intraoperative duplex is used to ensure the accuracy of the procedure.

With more complex reconstructions, special concerns must be addressed in order to minimize renal ischaemia to reduce subsequent deterioration of renal function. In patients with impaired renal function or those requiring complex reconstructions necessitating longer ischaemic periods, renal hypothermia is maintained by placing a balloon catheter in the renal artery and infusing 4°C Ringer's lactate solution. Mean renal ischaemia times with pararenal or suprarenal inclusion grafting are approximately 40 min, when two anastomoses are required.

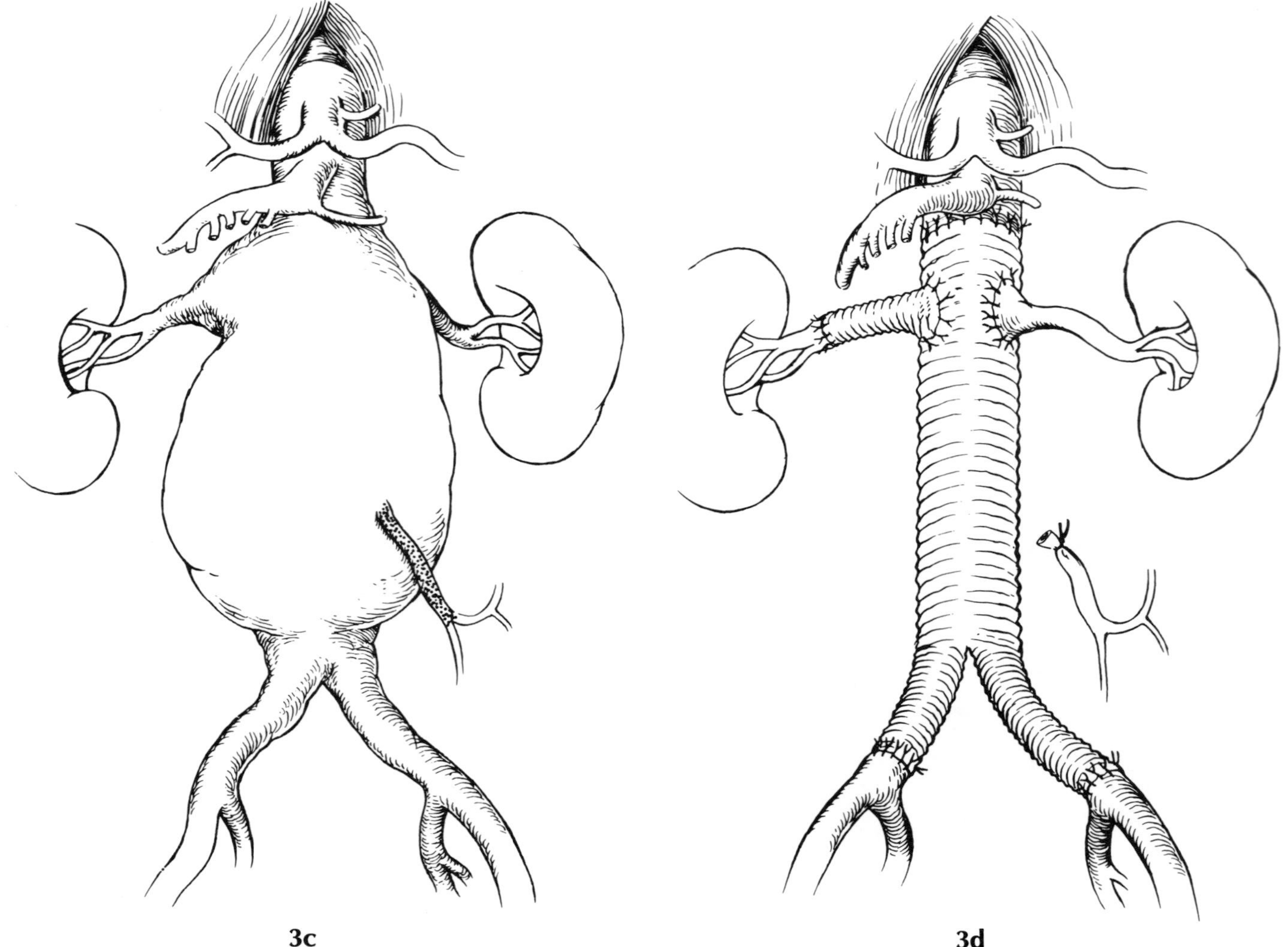

3c **3d**

Non-atherosclerotic renal artery revascularization

Non-atherosclerotic disease of the renal artery encompasses a variety of lesions including fibromuscular dysplasia, congenital bands, strictures, aneurysms and spontaneous or traumatic dissection of the renal artery. Fibromuscular dysplasia, a disease primarily of young women in otherwise good health, predominates. The distribution of these lesions is in the middle and distal third of the renal artery. Restoring normal renal perfusion and relieving or controlling hypertension are achieved using aortorenal grafting. The predominance of young patients demands durable surgical methods that allow patients to live a normal lifespan free of hypertension and the threat of a late failure of the revascularization method. We developed the concept of arterial autograft to replace diseased arterials segments and have used this preferentially for renal fibromuscular dysplasia since 1965 (Wylie, 1965).

All lesions which involve the main renal artery or the proximal renal artery branches can be repaired *in situ* using straight or bifurcated internal iliac autografts. Complex distal renal artery branch lesions or reoperative problems are performed *ex vivo* with hypothermic perfusion preservation and multibranched internal iliac autografts. These strategies achieve durable long-term results with cure of hypertension and renal salvage (Kent *et al.*, 1987). In a recent review of 71 patients at UCSF with 1–19 year follow-up, branched internal iliac autografts allowed salvage of all but two of 78 kidneys with complex renal vascular disease. Further, hypertension was cured or improved in 97% of patients. *In situ* and *ex vivo* repair with iliac artery autograft provides a durable repair of complex distal non-atherosclerotic renal artery lesions.

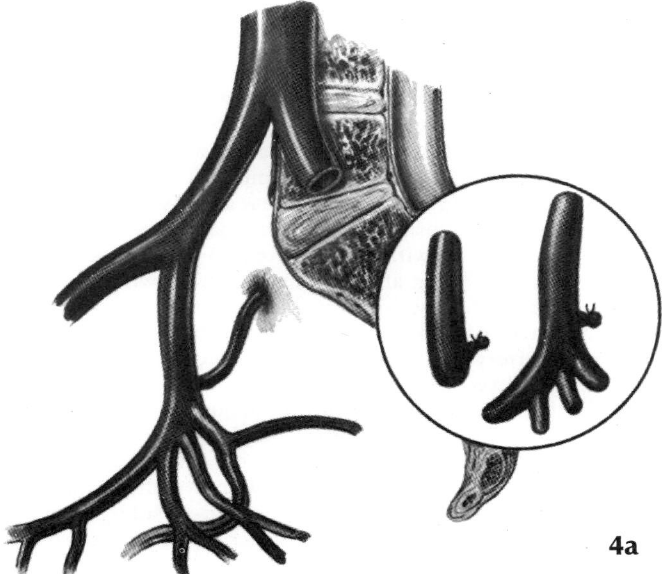

4a

Operative technique

Arterial autograft procurement

Arterial autografts are procured during the transabdominal exposure of the renal artery disease. *In situ* or *ex vivo* techniques are used depending on whether the repair is limited to the primary bifurcation branches (*in situ*) or is necessary in the more distal renal artery complex (*ex vivo*). The internal iliac artery is particularly suitable because its size closely approximates that of the renal artery in adults and children and its branches allow for branched reconstructions. Further, arterial autografts placed in children will grow with the patient. Finally, removal of the internal iliac artery does not require donor site repair because of abundant pelvic collateral circulation.

4a

The donor artery is exposed by an incision of the posterior peritoneum overlying the common iliac bifurcation. The entire internal iliac artery with the requisite number of branches is circumferentially mobilized, excised and stored temporarily in heparinized saline solution (*4a*). A larger diameter arterial autograft may be obtained from the common iliac and its two bifurcation branches. Dacron reconstruction of the donor site is required to preserve blood flow to the extremity.

4b, c, d & e

In situ *repair*

A full length midline or transverse incision allows the initial harvest of the autograft vessel from the pelvis. A self-retaining retractor (Omni-Tract) assists in exposure of the juxtarenal aorta and the renal artery with its hilar branching via the posterior infracolic approach. Mobilization of the inferior vena cava with lumbar vein ligation facilitates retrocaval autograft tunnelling for right side graft placement (*4b*). After heparin anticoagulation, the infrarenal aorta is segmentally occluded.

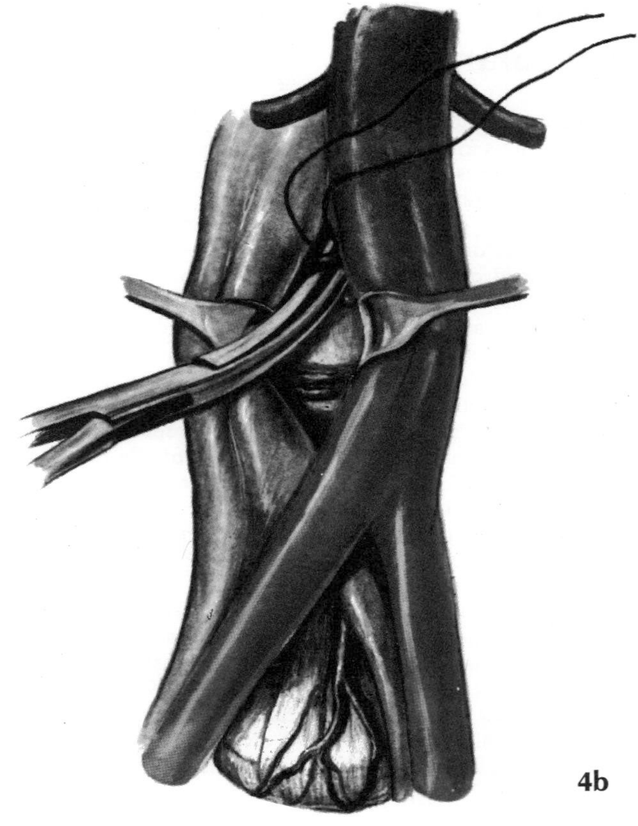

4b

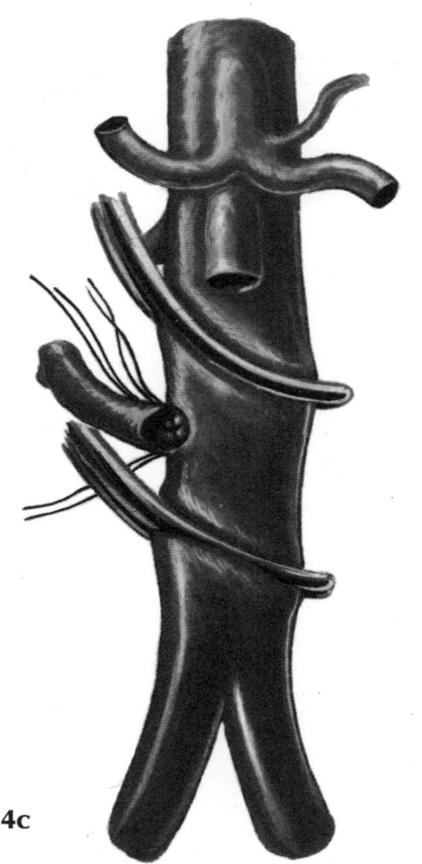

4c

With rotation of the clamps to further expose the lateral aorta, a disc of aorta is excised with an ostial punch on the posterolateral aorta and an end-to-side anastomosis is created using interrupted 5-0 sutures (*4c*). Clamps are then removed from the aorta and the autograft is clamped. The native renal artery is then clamped beyond the disease and divided. Primary end-to-end anastomosis of the native renal artery to the autograft is performed with interrupted 6-0 sutures (*4d*). An unbranched autograft reconstruction is shown but, *in situ* procedures using the bifurcated iliac autograft are used when indicated. After perfusion is reestablished, the diseased native renal artery is excised for pathologic examination and the proximal renal artery is oversewn. Duplex scanning is used routinely to assess the technical adequacy of the repair.

Bilateral renal artery repair employing *in situ* techniques is also technically feasible either with single autograft or one bifurcated autograft as shown with common, internal and external iliac artery in *4e*. The end-to-side common iliac artery to aortic anastomosis is generally positioned so that the longer external iliac artery is used to repair the right renal artery.

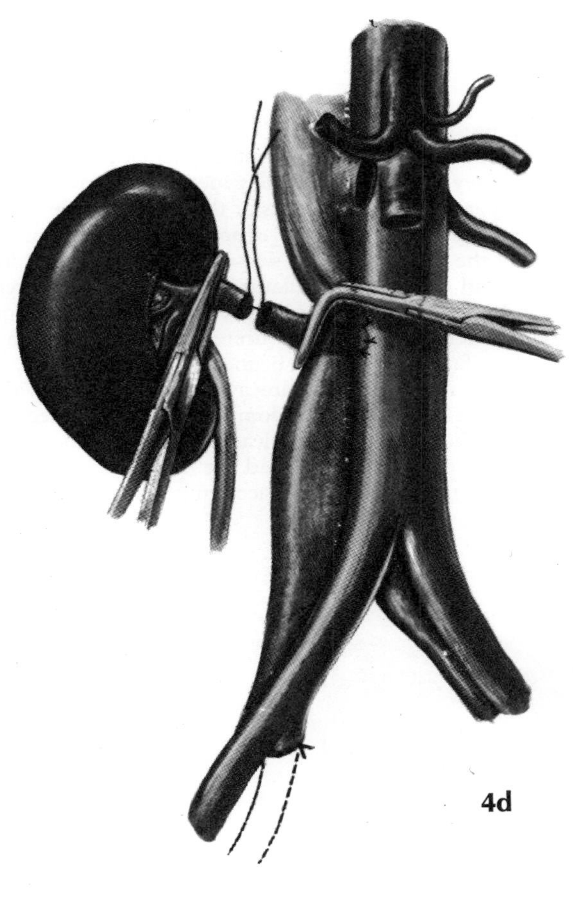

4d

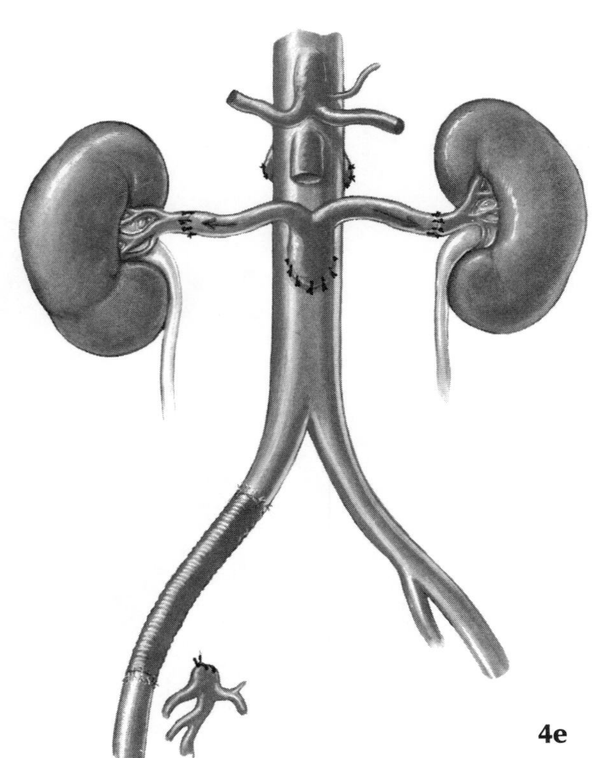

4e

Ex vivo *repair*

Ex vivo repair is employed when renal artery disease is considered unreconstructable by *in situ* techniques. *Ex vivo* repair allows precise dissection because of improved exposure with continuous hypothermic perfusion providing optimal renal preservation. Technical problems or anastomotic leaks during the autograft reconstruction can easily be identified and repaired during perfusion rather than after reimplantation.

5a

A long midline or transverse abdominal incision is made and a self-retaining retractor (Omni-Tract) set up is used to approach the iliac donor site, the renal vasculature, the ureter and the kidney. Using right or left medial visceral rotation, the lateral peritoneal attachments of the colon, on the side of anticipated repair, are freed to expose the retroperitoneum and retract the viscera. Gerota's fascia is incised, the kidney mobilized and the renal vasculature is identified. The renal artery and vein are circumferentially mobilized to the aorta and the inferior vena cava. The ureter is mobilized, with its surrounding fat, to the pelvic brim. After mobilization, the proximal renal artery and the paracaval renal vein are divided. The kidney is elevated to the abdominal wall and flushed with 4°C Ringer's lactate solution to clear the venous effluent. The renal artery is cannulated (*5a*) and the kidney is perfused at 60–75 mmHg to maintain a surface temperature of approximately 10°C.

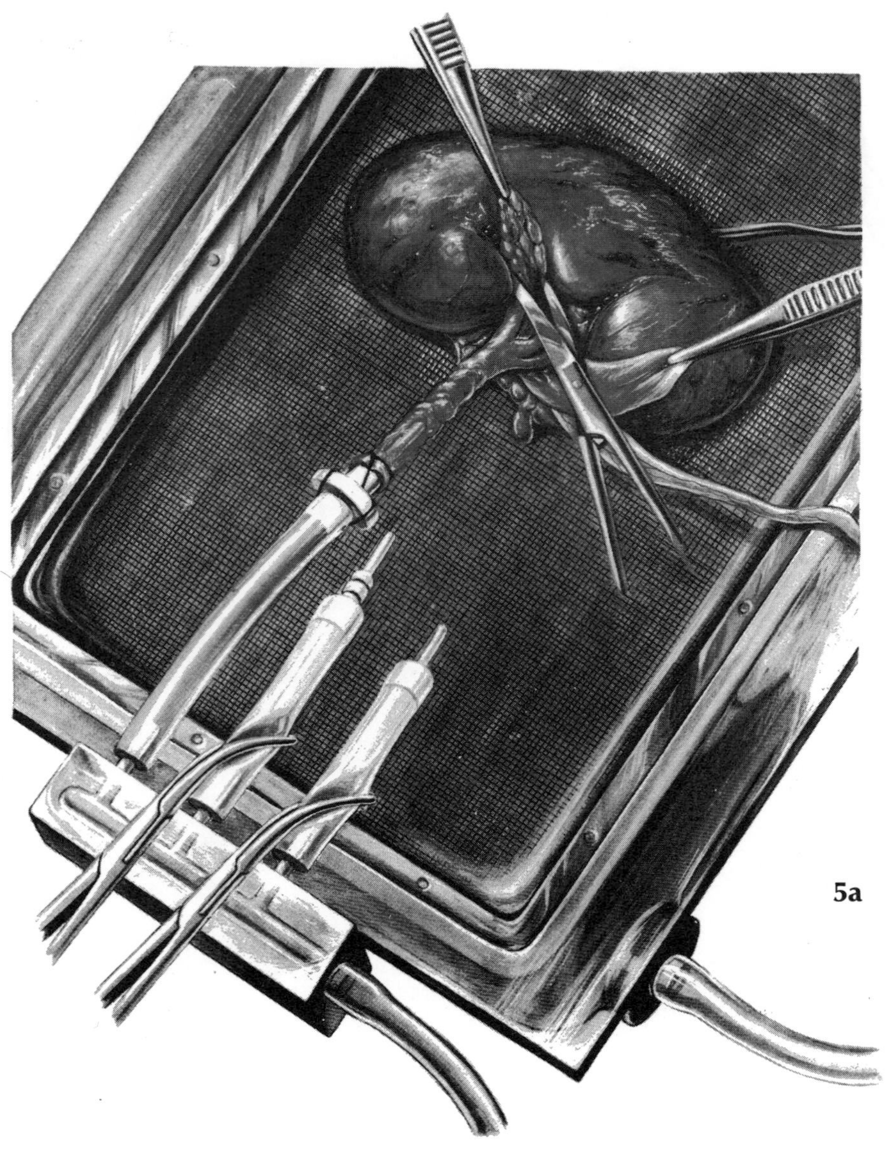

5a

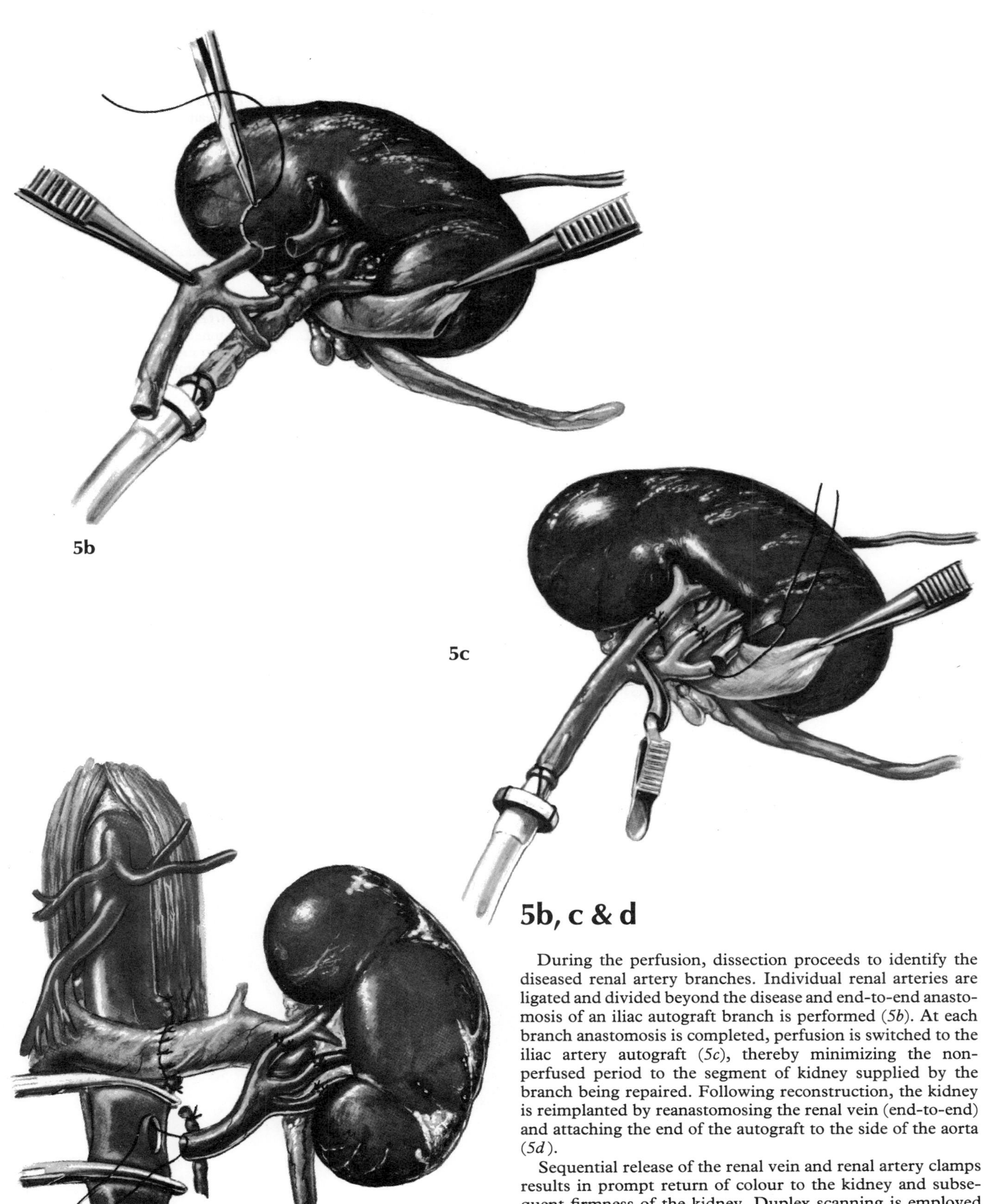

5b

5c

5d

5b, c & d

During the perfusion, dissection proceeds to identify the diseased renal artery branches. Individual renal arteries are ligated and divided beyond the disease and end-to-end anastomosis of an iliac autograft branch is performed (*5b*). At each branch anastomosis is completed, perfusion is switched to the iliac artery autograft (*5c*), thereby minimizing the non-perfused period to the segment of kidney supplied by the branch being repaired. Following reconstruction, the kidney is reimplanted by reanastomosing the renal vein (end-to-end) and attaching the end of the autograft to the side of the aorta (*5d*).

Sequential release of the renal vein and renal artery clamps results in prompt return of colour to the kidney and subsequent firmness of the kidney. Duplex scanning is employed intraoperatively to assess the repair prior to retroperitoneal and wound closure.

Conclusion

The principal diseases of the renal vasculature are atherosclerosis and fibromuscular dysplasia. Their different patterns of distribution necessitate a variety of revascularization techniques to solve problems which they create in renal blood flow. This chapter has attempted to describe those pioneered and used at the University of California, San Francisco during the last four decades.

References

Goldblatt, H., Lynch, J., Hanzel, R. F. *et al.* (1934). Studies on experimental hypertension. I. The production of persistent elevation of systolic blood pressure by means of renal ischemis. *Journal of Experimental Medicine* **59**, 347.

Kent, K. C., Salvatierra, O., Reilly, L. M. *et al.* (1987). Evolving strategies for the repair of complex renovascular lesions. *Annals of Surgery* **206**, 272.

Qvarfordt, P. G., Stoney, R. J., Reilly, L. M. *et al.*. (1986). Management of pararenal aneurysms of the abdominal aorta. *Journal of Vascular Surgery* **3**, 84.

Sauer, L. and Stoney, R. J. (1989). Transabdominal exposure of the pararenal and suprarenal aorta by medial visceral rotation. *Seminars in Vascular Surgery* **2**, 209.

Stoney, R. J. and Effeney, D. J. (1992). *Wylie's Atlas of Vascular Surgery. Thoracoabdominal Aorta and Its Branches*. J. B. Lippincott Co.

Stoney, R. J., Messina, L. M., Goldstone, J. and Reilly, L. M. (1989). Renal endarterectomy through the transected aorta: A new technique for combined aortorenal atherosclerosis. A preliminary report. *Journal of Vascular Surgery* **9**, 224.

Wylie, E. J. (1965). Vascular replacement with arterial autografts. *Surgery* **57**, 14.

Wylie, E. J. (1975). Endarterectomy and autogenous arterial grafts in the surgical treatment of stenosing lesions of the renal artery. *Urology Clinics of North America* **2**, 351.

Juxtarenal aortic occlusion

R. COURBIER MD
Emeritus Professeur Agrégé à la Faculté de Medicine, Hôpital Saint Joseph, Marseille, France

J. M. JAUSSERAN MD
Chef du Service de Chirurgie Cardio-Vasculaire, Hôpital Saint Joseph, Marseille, France

Introduction

In the Leriche syndrome, progressive atherosclerotic disease involves the origin of the inferior mesenteric artery. When this artery becomes completely occluded the clot proceeds up to the level of the renal arteries; this is known as a juxtarenal aortic occlusion. Many reports have pointed to the technical problems involved in treating this (Courbier *et al.*, 1974; 1979; Liddicoat *et al.*, 1975; Starrett and Stoney, 1974; Traverso *et al.*, 1978). A classic thromoendarterectomy (Vollmar, Gruss and Lauback, 1970) necessitates extensive exposure of the aorta and renal branches, which all have to be clamped.

A limited thromboendarterectomy is simpler and avoids extensive dissection, so that the aorta can be clamped at a lower level. Since 1963 we have used this technique in 102 cases (5.4% of cases of aortic reconstruction). Only in a few cases, when there is a high risk to the patient because of renal or respiratory insufficiency or when extensive disease of the visceral arteries cannot be treated, an extra-anatomical bypass is used.

Lower limb revascularization from coeliac or thoracic aorta can be indicated when subrenal aorta or abdominal wall condition prevents direct access (Barral *et al.*, 1991).

Operative technique

The patient is placed in a supine position with the left arm raised, so that a left thoracotomy can be done in case of technical problems.

1

Incision

A vertical midline incision is made. Additional resection of the xyphoid increases the exposure of the upper part.

If it is not possible to expose the upper part or there is a wound in that area, a thoracoabdominal approach through the 8th intercostal space can be used.

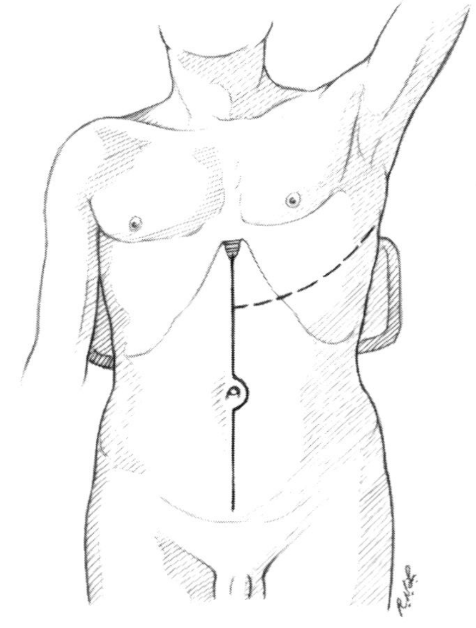

1

2

Dissection of ligament of Treitz

After incision of the posterior peritoneum, the duodenum is retracted to the right and the ligament of Treitz is incised.

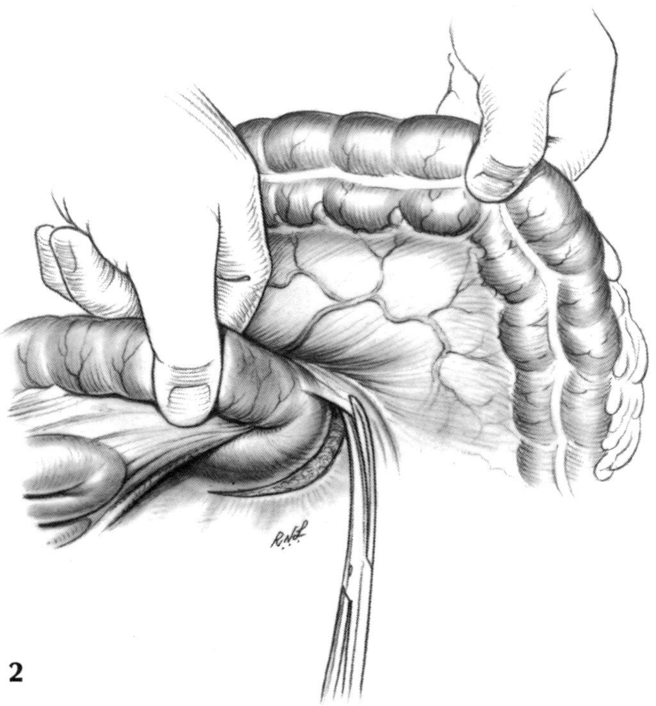

2

3

Limited exposure of the aorta

It is necessary to divide the inferior mesenteric vein, avoiding any arterial anastomotic branch.

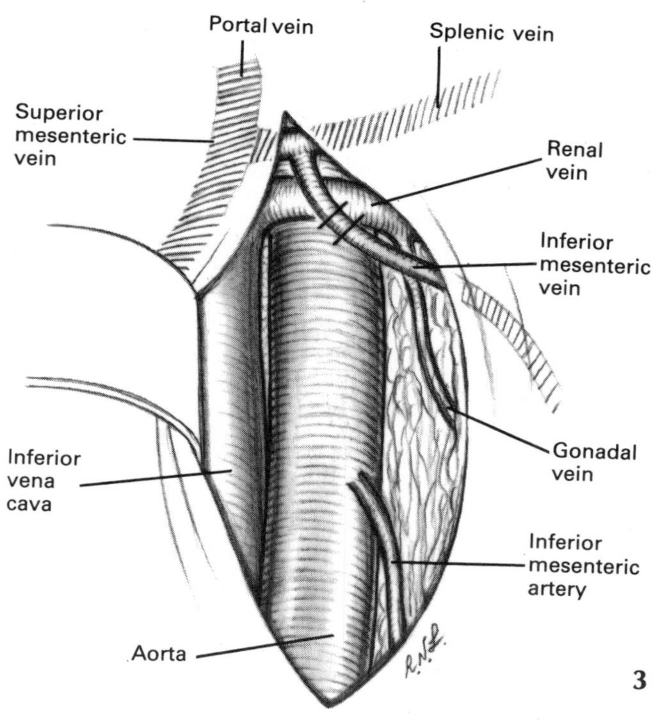

4

The left gonadal vein and capsular vein must also sometimes be divided.

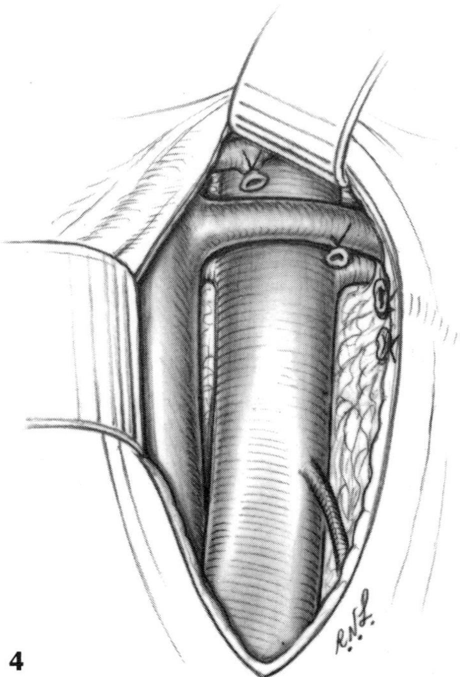

5

Extended exposure of the aorta

This approach is used in case of arterial disease involving the origin of the renal arteries. The left renal vein is retracted and moved up or down so that a tape and a tourniquet can be placed on both renal arteries.

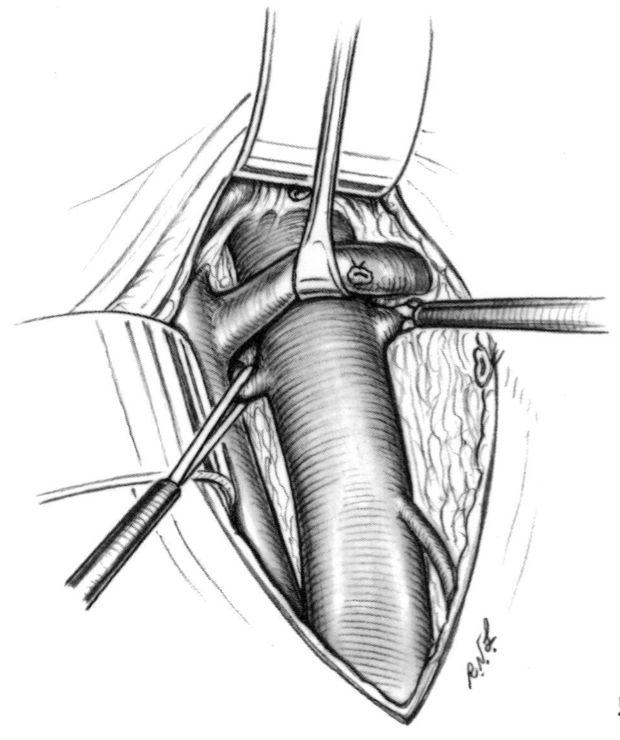

5

6

The left renal vein is divided between two arterial clamps and reconstructed later. The upper limit of the dissection is the origin of the superior mesenteric artery which does not need to be demonstrated. (With this extended dissection it is possible to perform endarterectomy of the aorta, and origins of the renal arteries. The clamp is placed across the aorta above the renal arteries. No clamp is required on the lower end.)

6

7

Illustration 7 shows the usual procedure where it is unnecessary to divide the left renal vein or to control the renal arteries with slings. The aorta is opened transversely, using scissors, 3 cm below the level of the renal arteries, without any posterior dissection. Clamping of the aorta is not necessary.

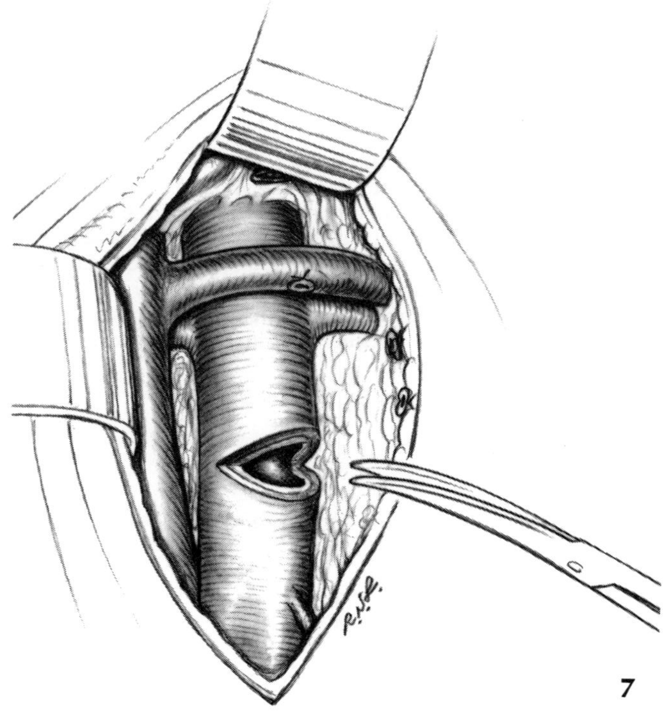

7

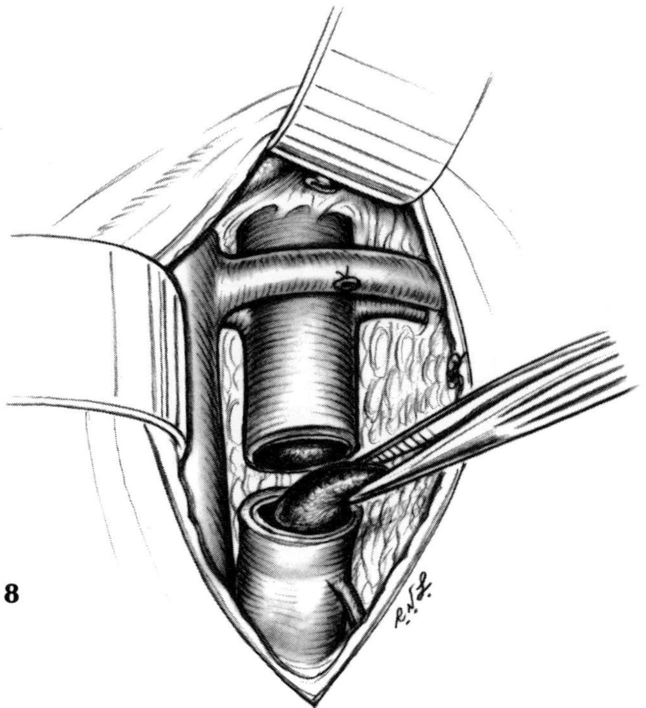

8

8

A small part of the clot is removed from the lower part of the aorta, and the artery is then occluded with a continuous suture.

Thrombectomy

9

This is performed on the upper part of the aorta. The surgeon's 2nd and 3rd left fingers are applied to the pulsating part of the aorta just beyond the upper limit of the thrombus.

Dissection is made with a dissector or with a thin scisccors. It is very important to avoid the plane of thromboendarterectomy, which is too near the exterior of the artery wall, but to use the plane of thrombectomy which leaves enough artery wall behind. Dissection begins anteriorly and posteriorly and continues upward.

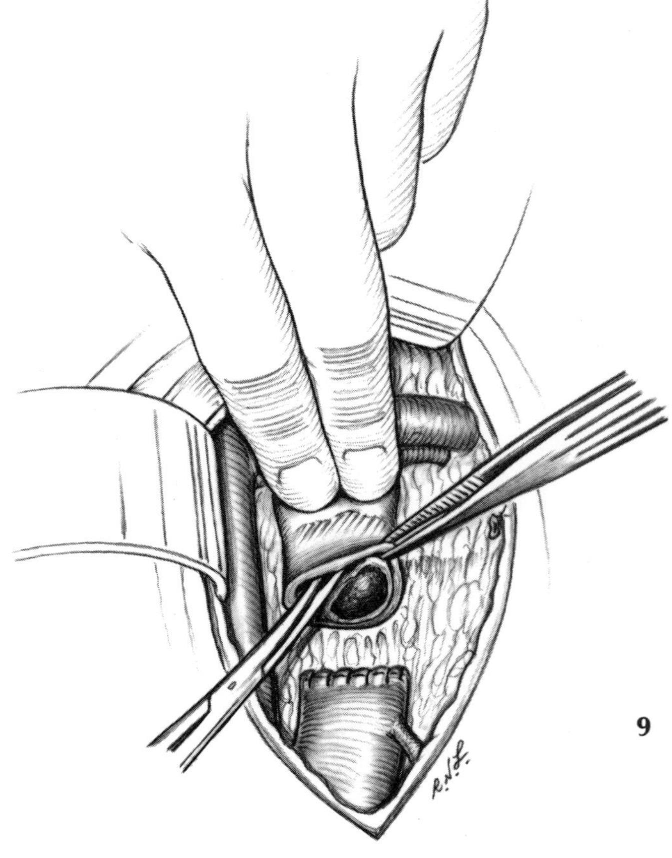

9

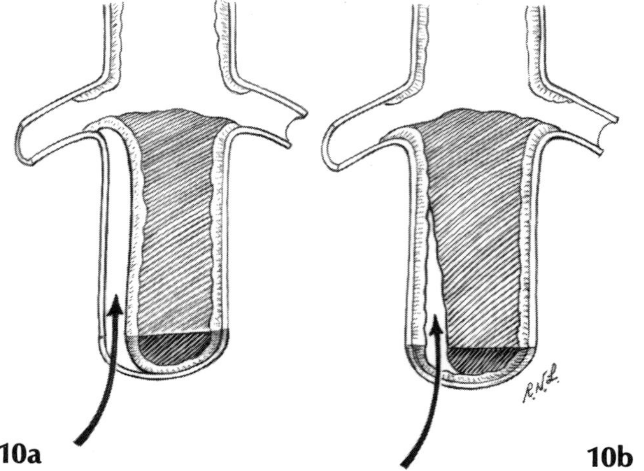

10a 10b

10a & b

The two different dissecting planes

The dissecting plane for thromboendarterectomy cannot be used in a retrograde manner because of the risk of a dissection on the origin of the renal arteries (*a*).

Thrombectomy can be done without any risk. The high flow after reconstruction allows a small part of the aorta to be left without risk of rethrombosis (*b*).

11

When bleeding occurs the two fingers create a temporary haemostasis and feel at the same time the tips of the dissecting scissors.

The total clot is removed *en bloc* with a forceps. The fingers' pressure is released to permit a flush of blood.

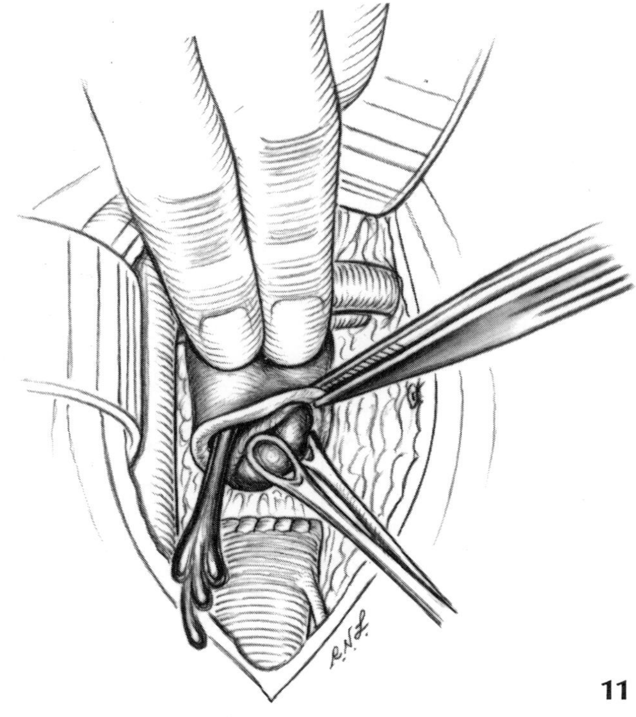

11

12

An aortic clamp is placed between the fingers and the origin of the renal arteries.

The operation can then be continued as for an ordinary aortic occlusion.

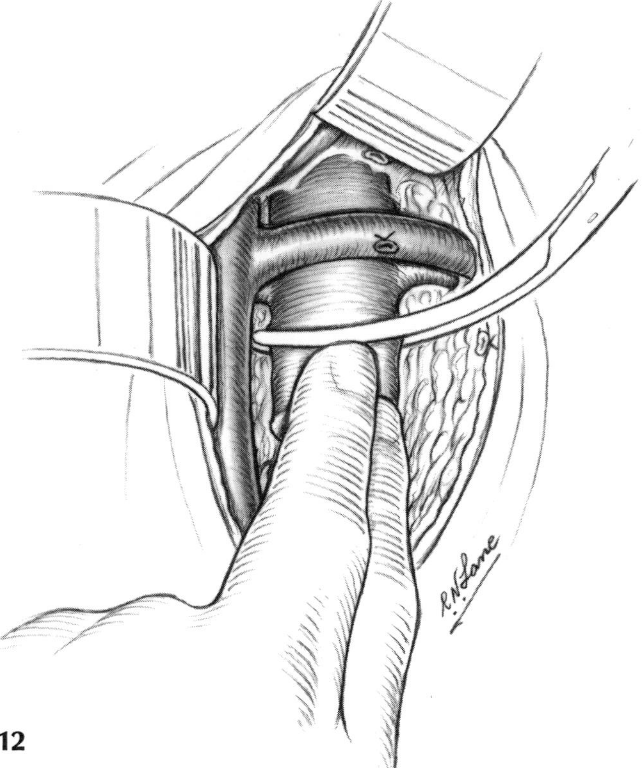

12

13

Supracoeliac aortic access is required for multiple aortic procedures.

A transxiphisternal laparotomy leads to an approach through the lesser sac to the right crus of the diaphragm.

A horizontal clamp of aorta at this level allows the exposure of 4–6 cm above the coeliac axis.

A prosthesis can be passed in front or behind the pancreas.

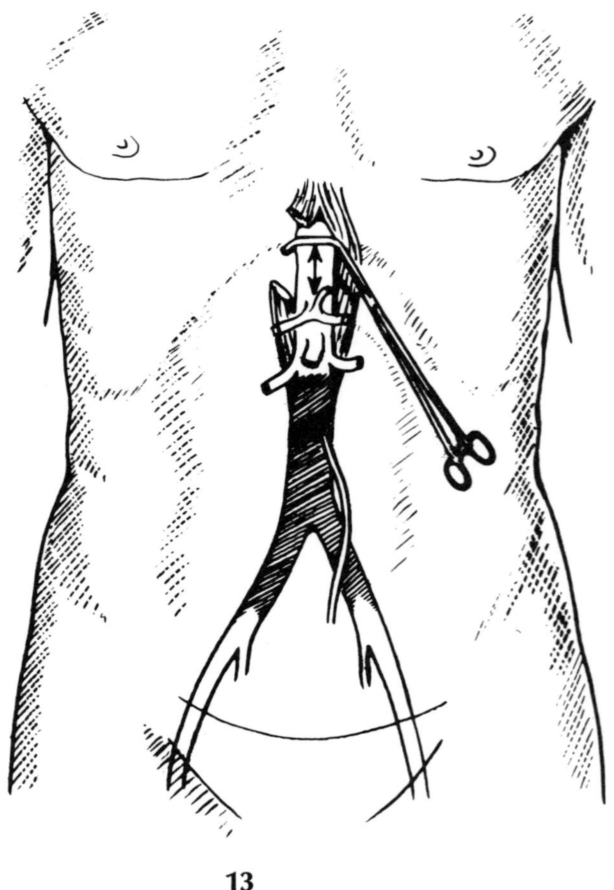

13

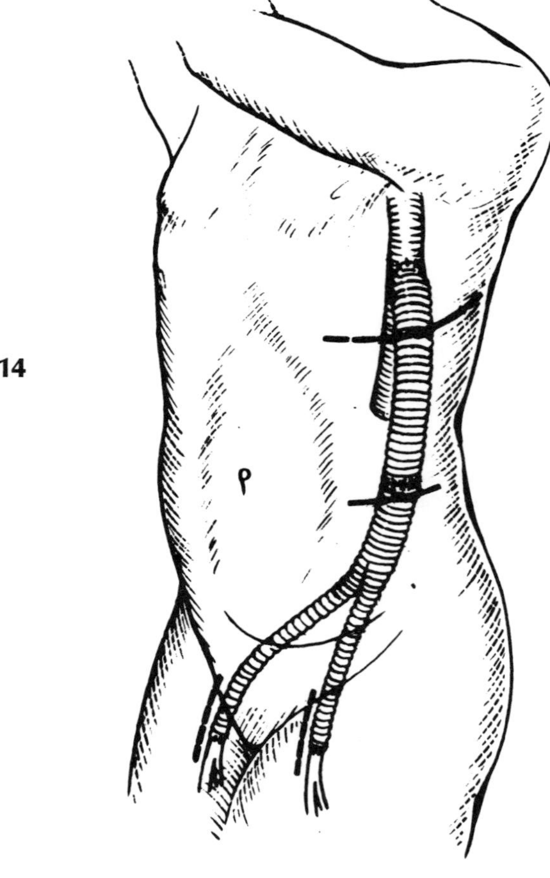

14

14

On occasions it is better to approach the thoracic aorta than to seek the aorta below the diaphragm, e.g. after recent infection or when much scarring is anticipated, the thoracotomy is via the 7th intercostal space. A tunnel can be made behind the diaphragm to pass a prosthesis below in the retroperitoneal space and the right limb can pass in front of the pubis.

References

Barral, X., Gournier, J. P., Favre, J. P. and Rosset, E. (1991). Revascularisation des membres inférieurs à partir de l'aorte thoracique. In *Les lésions occlusives aorto-iliaques chroniques*, Kieffer, E., ed. Paris: A E R C V.

Courbier, R., Jausseran, J. M. and Reggi, M. (1974) Les thromboses aortiques juxta rénales. *Journal de Chirurgie* **107**, 281.

Courbier, R., Jausseran, J. M., Reggi, M., Schlama, G. and Monin, Ph. (1979). Traitement chirurgical des thromboses aortiques juxtarénales – Résultats à long terme. *Journal de Chirurgie* **105**, 545.

Liddicoat, J., Bekassy, S., Dang, M. and De Bakey, M. (1975). Complet occlusion of the infrarenal abdominal aorta: Management and results in 64 patients, *Surgery* **77**, 467.

Starrett, R. and Stoney, R. (1974). Juxta renal aortic occlusion. *Surgery* **76**, 890.

Traverso, L. W., Backer, J. D., Dainko, E. A. and Machleder, H. F. (1978). Infrarenal aortic occlusion. *Annals of Surgery* **187**, 397.

Vollmar, J., Gruss, J. and Lauback, K. (1970). Technique de la thromboendartériectomie. *Journal de Chirurgie* **100**, 67.

Aortic bifurcation grafting for stenosing arterial disease

MICHAEL E. DeBAKEY MD

Olga Keith Wiess Professor of Surgery and Chairman, Cora and Webb Mading Departing of Surgery, and Chancellor, Baylor College of Medicine, Houston, Texas, USA

Introduction

Occlusive disease of the terminal abdominal aorta and common iliac arteries is usually well localized to this segment. The occlusive process may be complete or incomplete (stenosis) with the underlying pathologic lesion being arteriosclerotic or atherosclerotic. Whereas other diagnostic studies may be useful, arteriography is essential in order to obtain precise information regarding the site and extent of the disease, both proximally and distally, and is therefore important in planning the surgical procedure and in indentifying associated occlusive disease of the renal and visceral arteries and unsuspected aneurysmal disease. In our experience, about 30% of patients have secondary segmental occlusion of the distal arterial tree. Preoperative evaluation of the patient's condition should include studies for possible concomitant occlusive vascular disease in the extracranial carotid and coronary arteries. This is emphasized by the fact that about one-third of our patients were found to have significant disease in these arterial segments.

Several methods of surgical treatment or a combination of these methods are available: (1) bypass surgery, (2) thromboendarterectomy, (3) patch-graft angioplasty, and (4) excision with graft replacement. Selection of the appropriate method or combination of methods in an individual case depends upon a number of factors, including the extent and nature of the occlusive process and involvement of the aortic wall. In some occasional patients, for example, usually young women in whom the atheroma is extremely well localized to the abdominal aorta, thromboendarterectomy with patch-graft angioplasty may be employed. In other patients in whom the wall of the abdominal aorta is extensively diseased, as in the presence of periaortic fibrosis, intense inflammatory reaction, or aneurysmal formation, resection of this segment with graft replacement is required.

On the basis of our experience extending over a period of about 40 years, the bypass operation with certain variations according to the extent and nature of the disease, has become our procedure of choice because of its simplicity, avoidance of injury to adjacent structures, and its long-term good results. The technical application of the bypass principle and its modifications or combination with other procedures, depending upon certain factors influencing its use, will be described and illustrated in this presentation.

1a–o

In patients with complete occlusion of the abdominal aorta extending up to the origin of the renal arteries, the following procedure is employed. The peritoneal cavity is opened through a midline incision (*a*). The abdominal aorta is exposed by retraction of the small intestines to the right. A vertical incision is then made in the peritoneum overlying the aorta and separated from the aortic wall on each side, and the renal arteries are exposed. Occluding clamps are then placed on the renal arteries to prevent embolic debris into the renal arteries during the subsequent manoeuvres. The abdominal aorta immediately above the origin of the renal arteries is temporarily occluded manually, and a 4- to 5-cm vertical incision is made through the anterior aortic wall several centimetres below the origin of the arteries (*b*).

The fairly firm thromboatherosclerotic process is recognized, and thromboendarterectomy is performed after the proper cleavage plane in the aortic wall has been identified (*b*). The occlusive lesion is then dissected free proximally and removed. Intermittent release of pressure on the aorta permits flushing of any retained debris (*c*). Careful visualization of the ostia of the renal arteries is important to be certain that no debris is left in the renal arteries and that dissection of the ostia of the renal arteries has not occurred. An aortic clamp is then applied to the abdominal aorta just below the origin of the renal arteries. The clamps on the renal arteries are removed, and the temporary occlusion of the aorta above the renal arteries is released allowing restoration of renal artery perfusion (*d*). This is verified by palpation of good pulses in both renal arteries.

A suitable-sized DeBakey albumin-coated Dacron bifurcation graft is selected, and the aortic end of the graft is anastomosed end-to-side to the opening in the abdominal aorta (*d*). In some cases this may be done as an end-to-end anastomosis to the opening in the abdominal aorta just below the renal arteries. The site for the distal anastomosis is then determined on the basis of the arteriogram and observation and palpation of the distal arteries. If these findings suggest that the external iliac artery is suitable, the anastomosis (end-to-side) is done at this level within the abdominal cavity (*e*). If however, there is significant disease in the external iliac artery, the distal anastomosis must be performed in the common femoral artery in the groin (*o*).

The external iliac artery is exposed through an opening in the peritoneum overlying this artery in the pelvis. The appropriate limb of the previously inserted Dacron graft is passed retroperitoneally to the area of the external iliac artery. Occluding clamps are applied proximally and distally on the external iliac artery, a 1.5- to 2-cm vertical incision is made on the anterior wall of the external iliac artery, and the limb of the bifurcation is then cut at the appropriate length in a bevelled fashion and anastomosed by a continuous suture of 0000 Prolene to the opening in the artery (*e*). After completion of this anastomosis and just before closing to the final suture, the proximal and then the distal occluding clamps are temporarily released to flush the artery from any clot or debris (*f*). The occluding clamps are then reapplied to the external iliac artery, an occluding clamp is applied to the proximal part of this limb of the graft, and the aortic occluding clamp is released for one or two pulses to wash out any clot or debris in the graft (*g*). The end of a suction tube is then inserted into the open limb of the graft to remove any remaining clot or debris (*h*). The occluding clamps on the external iliac artery are then removed, an occluding clamp is applied to the proximal end of the open limb of the graft (*i*), and the occluding clamp in the aorta is removed, a manoeuvre that permits circulation through the anastomosed limb of the graft into that extremity (*j*). The remaining limb of the bifurcation graft is then brought retroperitoneally to the exposed portion of the external iliac artery and is anastomosed to an opening in this artery as previously described (*k*). Just before the suture of this anastomosis is closed, the occluding clamps on the external iliac arteries are temporarily released to flush the graft (*l*), and then the occluding clamp on the graft is temporarily released to flush the graft (*m*), following which the anastomotic suture is tied and all clamps are removed to permit restoration of circulation into this extremity (*n*). In patients in whom the limbs of the graft must be attached to the common femoral artery, this artery is exposed by a vertical incision in the groin, and the graft is tunnelled posterior to the inguinal ligament into the groin (*o*).

In patients in whom the distal limbs of the graft must be attached to the common femoral artery, it is important to determine that there is good outflow through the superficial femoral or profunda femoris or both arteries. This assumes great significance in regard to the profunda femoris when the superficial femoral artery is occluded. In such cases the profunda femoris may require profundaplasty.

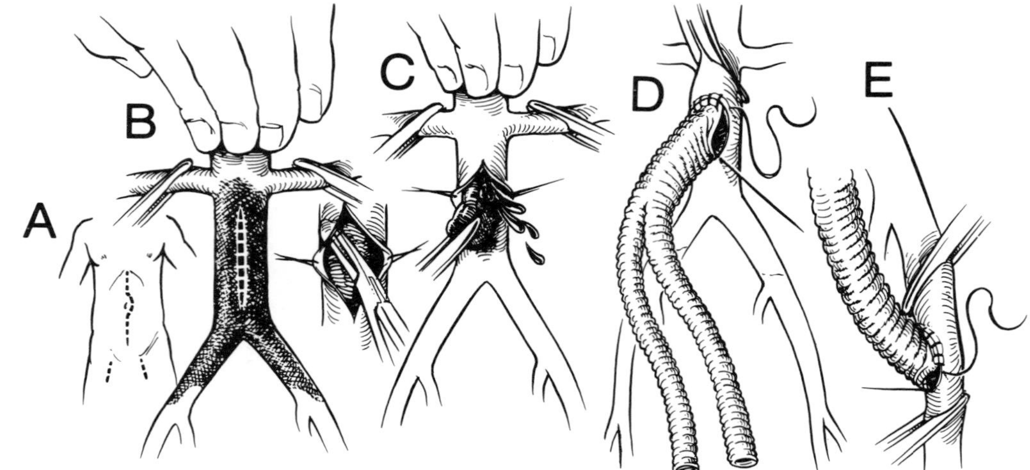

1

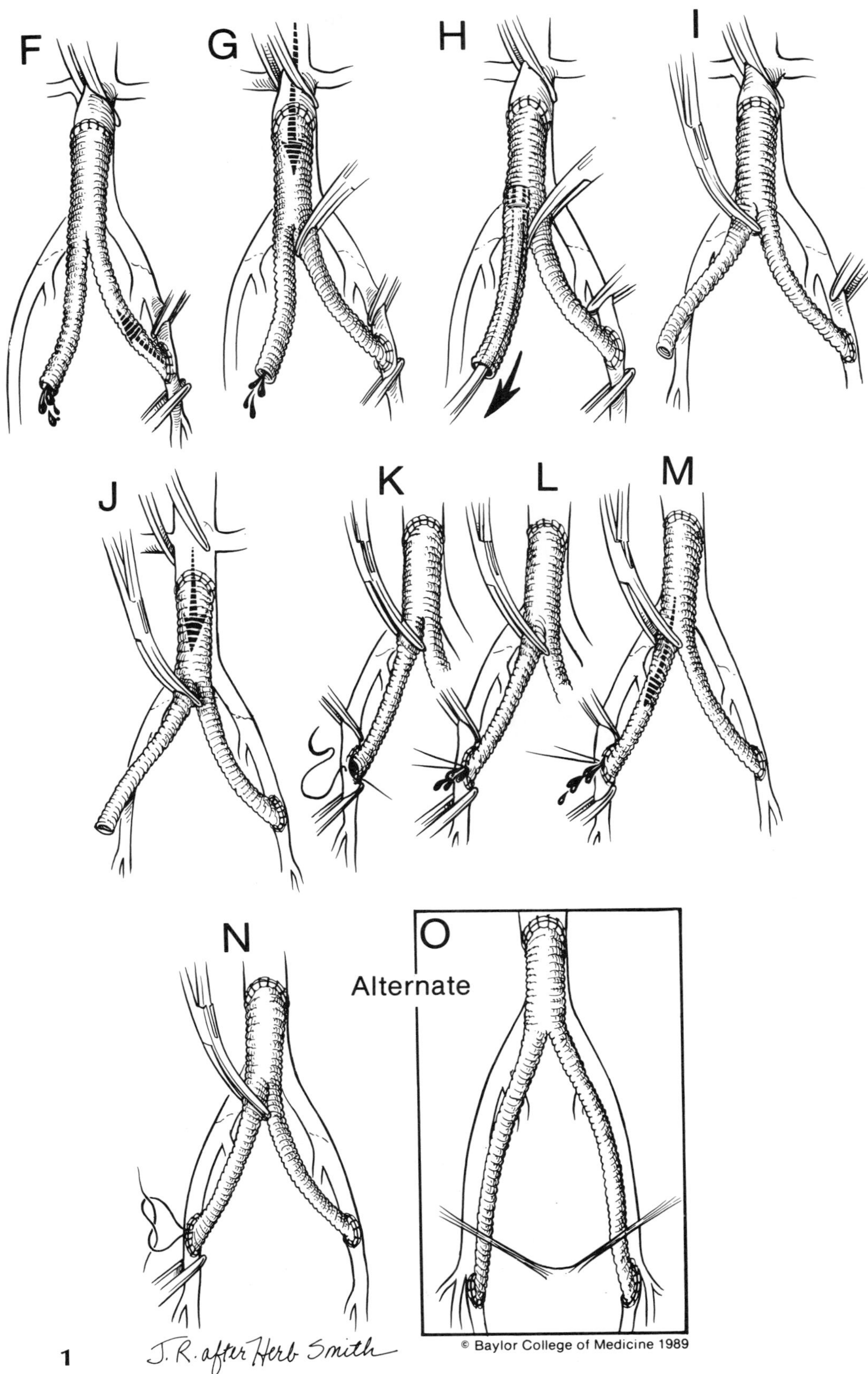
F
G
H
I
J
K
L
M
N
O
Alternate
J.R. after Herb Smith
© Baylor College of Medicine 1989

1

2a–j

In occasional patients in whom the occlusive or associated aneurysmal disease involves the abdominal aorta at or near the origin of the renal arteries, it may be necessary to occlude the aorta above the renal arteries using an aortic occluding clamp (*b*). The abdomen is entered through a midline incision (*a*), and the abdominal aorta is exposed by a vertical incision in the overlying peritoneal layer (*b, c*). In such cases, the renal arteries should be occluded as previously described (*d*). After the endarterectomy is performed and the ostia of the renal arteries are cleared of disease, there many not be a sufficient amount of aorta below the renal arteries to permit the placement of an occluding clamp below the renal arteries. Under these circumstances, after completion of the endarterectomy (*d*), the aorta is cirumferentially incised just below the ostia of the renal arteries, and the opening of the lumbar and inferior mesenteric arteries are oversewn (*e*). In order to prevent retrograde bleeding, occluding clamps are also placed upon the common iliac arteries (*e*).

The aortic limb of the graft is then sutured as an end-to-end anastomosis to the proximal opening in the aorta, care being taken to avoid compression of the ostia of the renal arteries (*f*). This may be assured by placing an appropriate sized dilator into the ostia of the renal arteries during the anastomosis. After completion of this anastomosis, the aortic clamp is temporarily opened to flush the aorta and remove any clots or debris, following which the occluding clamps on the renal arteries are similarly flushed. An occluding clamp is then applied to the Dacron graft just below the anastomosis, and the occluding clamps on the aorta and both renal arteries are removed to permit restoration of circulation to the kidneys (*h*). The attachments of the limbs of the bifurcation to the external iliac or common femoral arteries are then performed as previously described (*i,j*). The distal opening in the abdominal aorta just above the bifurcation is closed by suture (*f*) or the common iliac arteries are closed by suture (*g*) depending upon local circumstances.

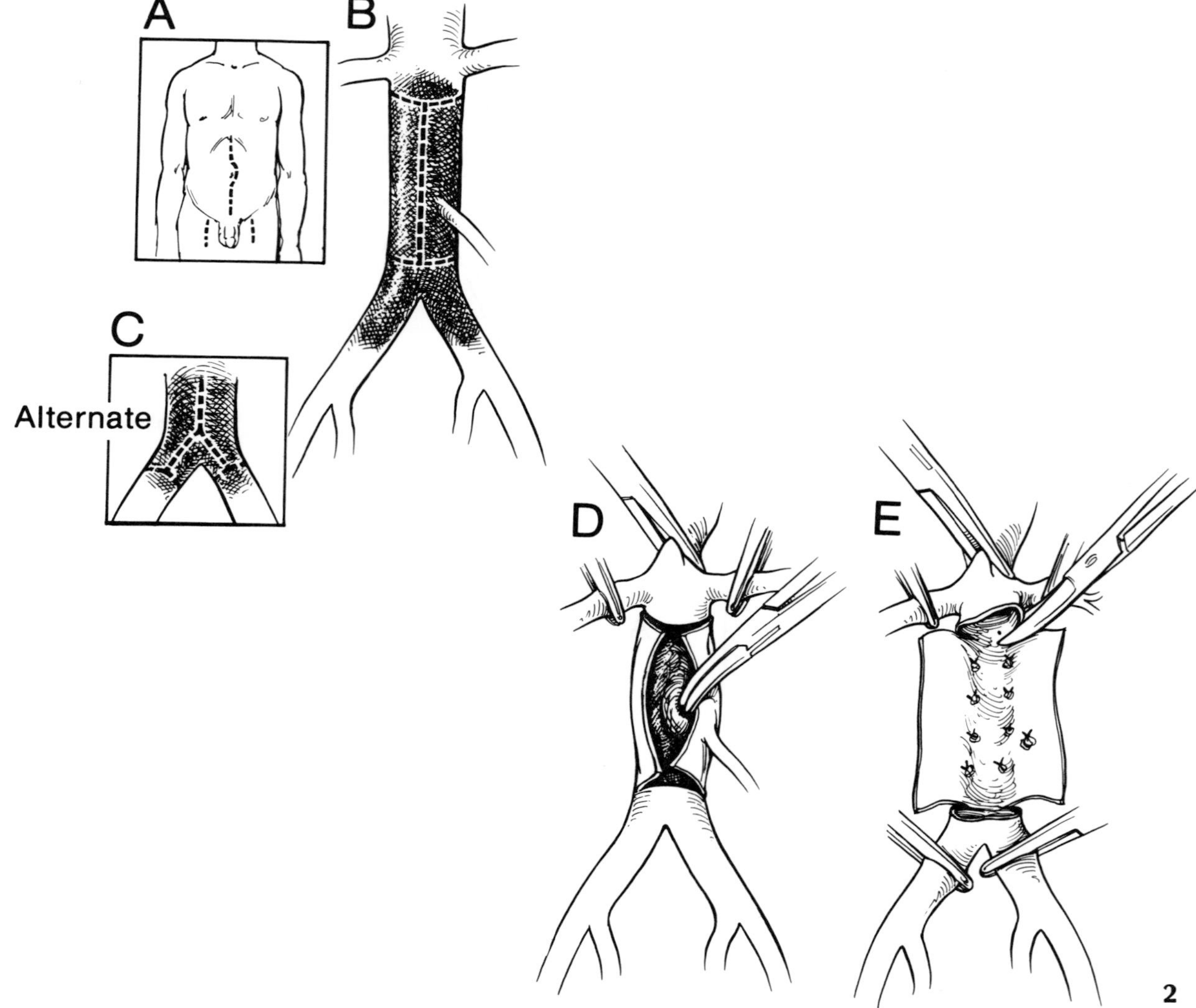

2

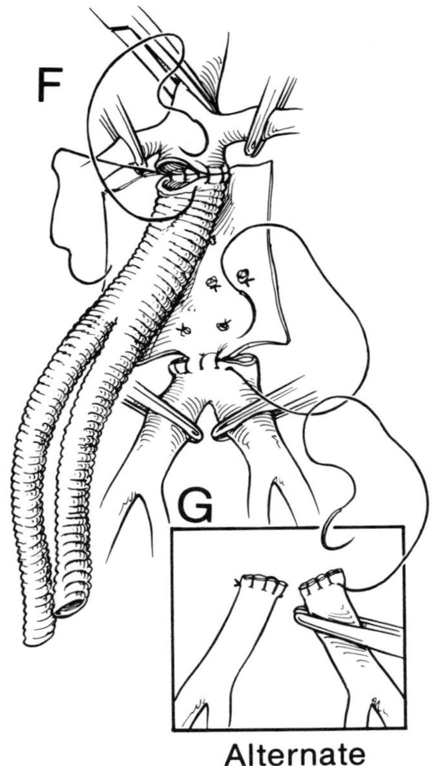
F
G
Alternate

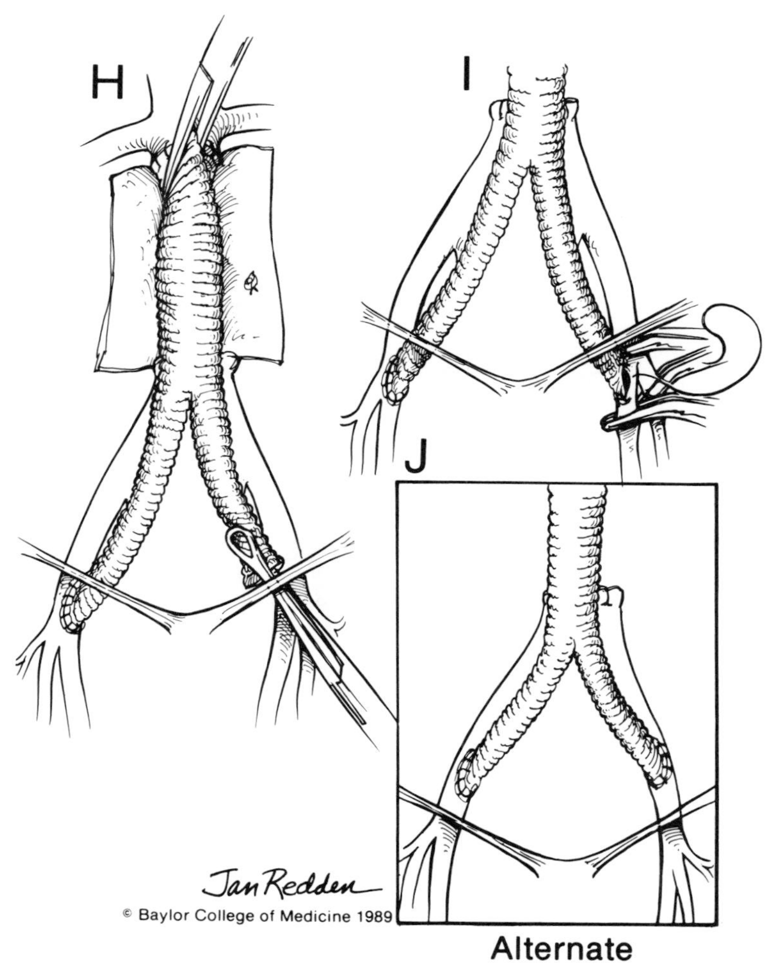
H
I
J
Jan Redden
© Baylor College of Medicine 1989
Alternate

2

3a–b

In still other patients who have incomplete occlusion but significant stenosis, the bypass procedure is usually preferred. In such cases, the abdominal aorta just distal to the renal arteries may be relatively free of disease, and endarterectomy is thus not required. After an occluding clamp is applied to the abdominal aorta just below the origin of the renal arteries and to both common iliac arteries and inferior mesenteric arteries, an aortic occluding clamp is passed under the common iliac arteries to occlude the posterior wall of the abdominal aorta to prevent retrograde bleeding from the lumbar arteries (*a*). A longitudinal incision is then made in the abdominal aorta as close as possible to the proximal aortic occluding clamp (*b*). The aortic limb of the Dacron graft is attached to this opening by end-to-side anastomosis, and the two limbs of the graft are attached to the external iliac or common femoral arteries as previously described.

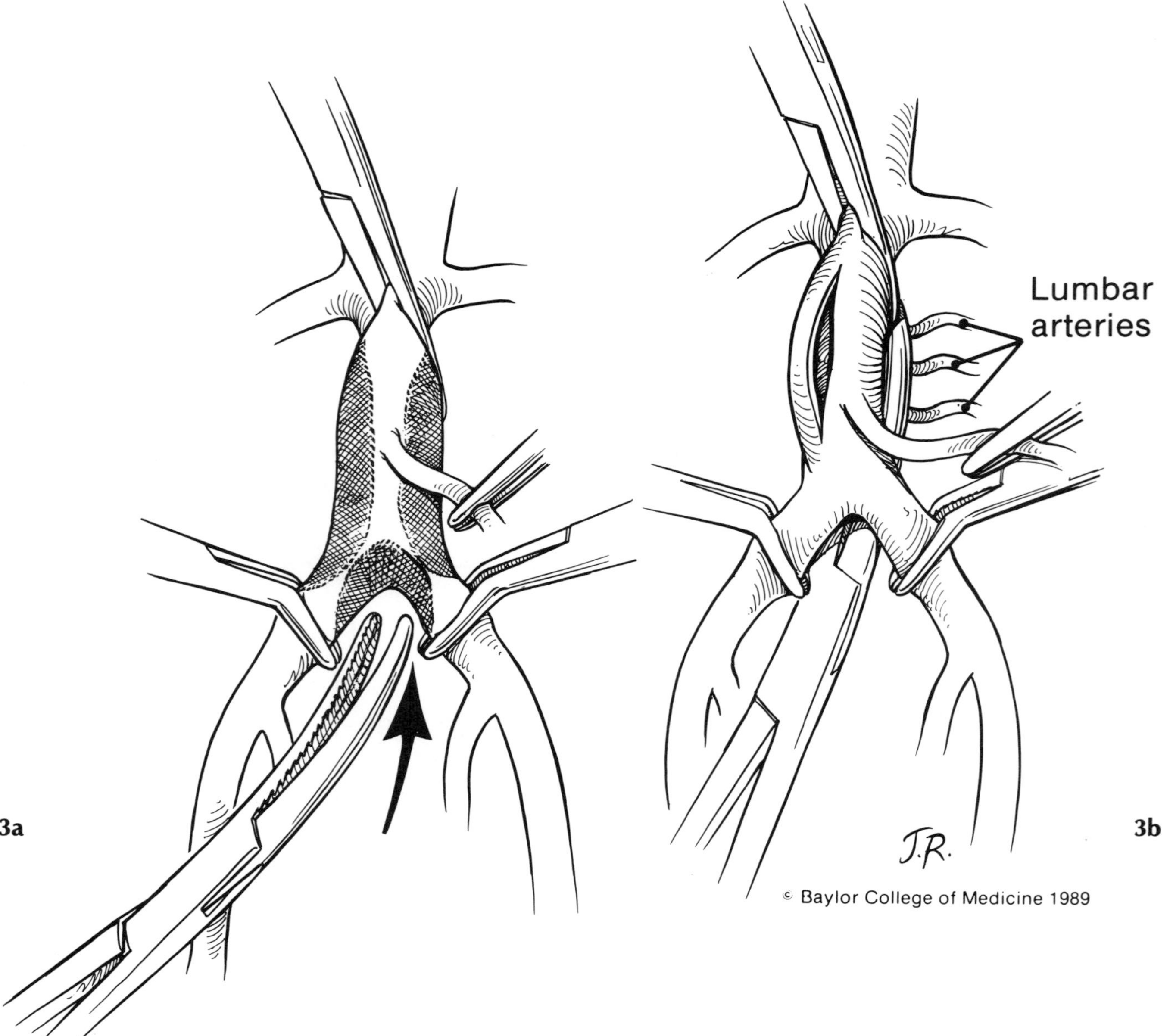

3a 3b

4a–d

There are still other more complicated cases, fortunately encountered only occasionally, that require a different approach. These may be exemplified by patients in whom the infrarenal aorta is densely adherent to surrounding structures owing to previous operation or is associated with intense inflammatory reaction or periaortic fibrosis, thus creating great difficulty or even jeopardy in dissection and exposure of the infrarenal abdominal aorta. In such cases, after the peritoneal cavity is opened through a midline incision (extending up to the xyphoid) (*a*), the abdominal aorta is exposed just below the diaphragm as it passes through the diaphragmatic hiatus by entering the lessor sac and retracting the left lobe of the liver (*b*). A partial occluding clamp is then applied to the aorta just above the celiac axis and a vertical incision is made in the anterior wall of the occluded portion of the aorta (*c*). An appropriate-sized (usually ranging between 10 and 16 mm in diameter) albumin-coated tubular DeBakey Dacron graft is attached to the opening in the aorta by end-to-side anastomosis (*d*).

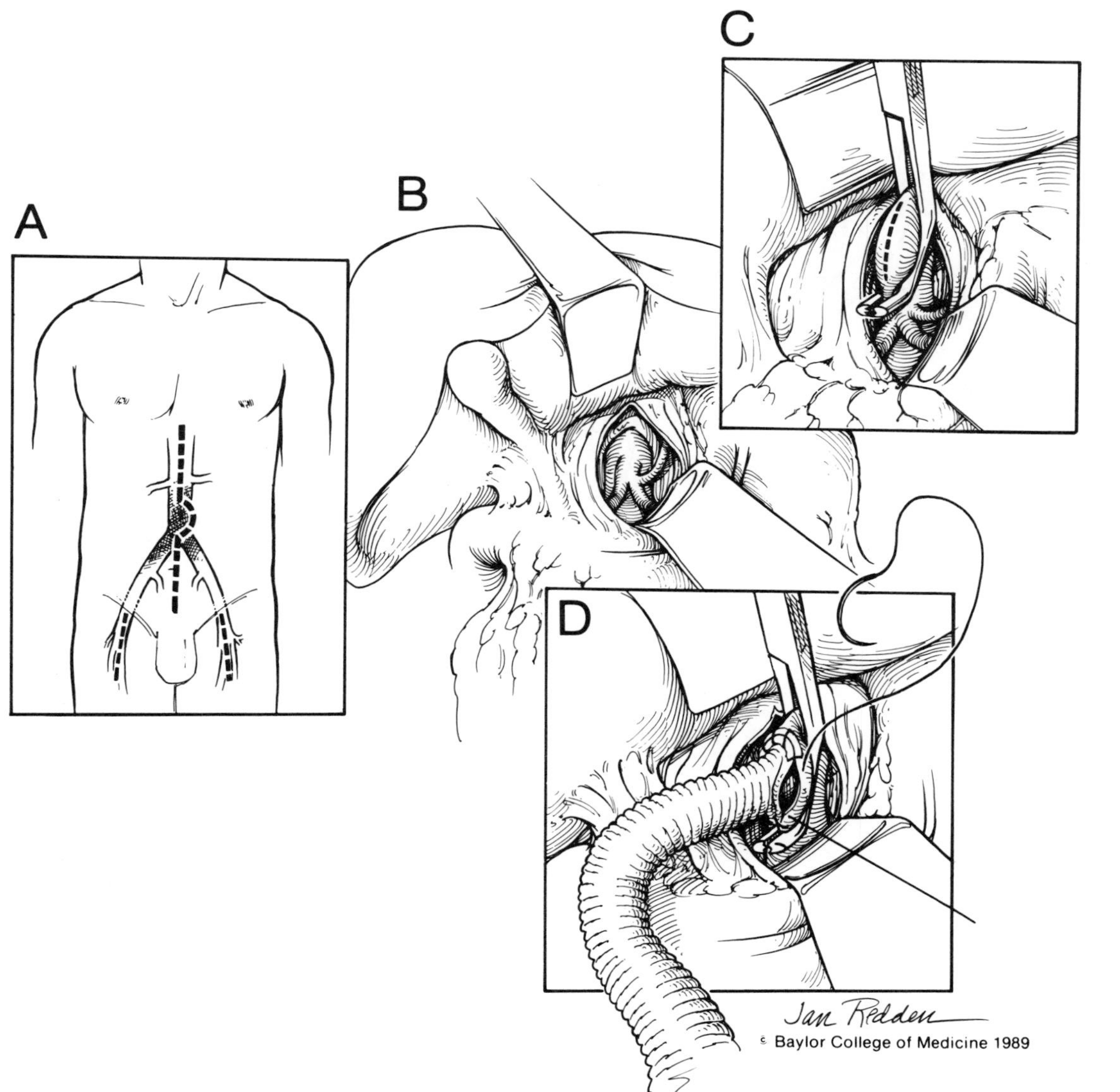

4

4e–h

After completion of this anastomosis, an occluding clamp is applied to the Dacron graft just distal to the anastomosis and the partial occluding clamp on the abdominal aorta is removed. An incision is then made in the peritoneum overlying the iliopsoas muscle to permit entrance into the retroperitoneal space (*e*), and by careful sharp and blunt dissection, a long sponge holder or other comparable clamp is inserted through this retroperitoneal space to the opening in the lessor sac at the site of the graft anastomosis to the aorta, and the distal end of this graft is brought out into the distal retroperitoneal opening (*f*). The left common femoral artery is exposed through a vertical incision, and the Dacron graft is then tunnelled under the inguinal ligament (*g*) and brought into the groin incision (*h*).

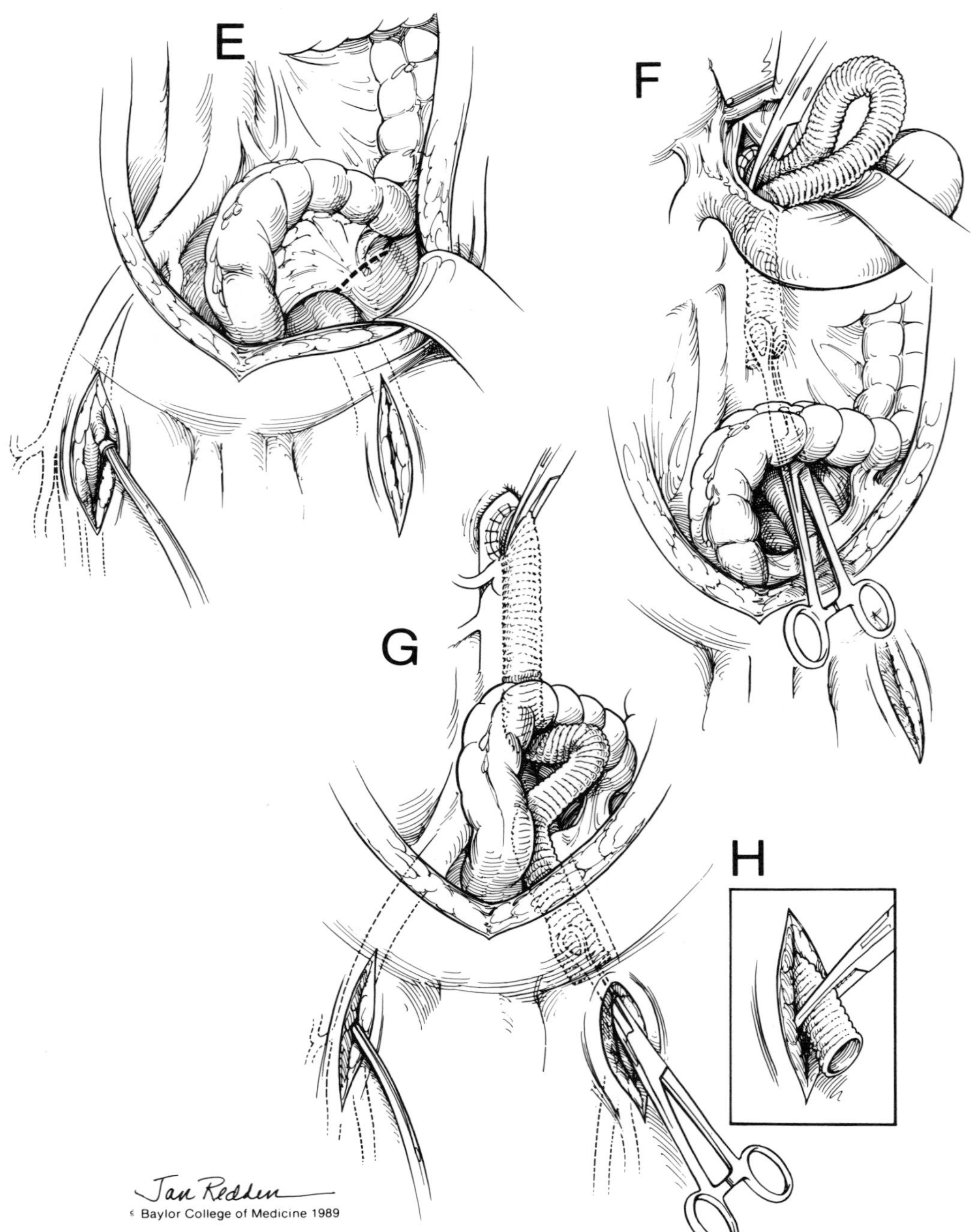

4

4i–l

Here, again, as previously noted, if the distal portion of the external iliac artery is relatively normal, it is preferable to the common femoral artery for anastomosis. Another appropriate-sized (approximately 8 to 10 mm) albumin-coated tubular DeBakey Dacron graft is then attached by end-to-side anastomosis to a vertical opening on the right side of the previously placed aorta to right femoral graft (*i*). This graft is then tunnelled retroperitoneally through an opening exposing the right common femoral artery (*j*). The distal end of the graft that is brought into the left groin incision is then attached to the left common femoral artery by end-to-side anastomosis (*k*). An occluding clamp is then applied to the Dacron graft going to the right groin just distal to its anastomosis to the main graft, and the occluding clamps on this main graft and the common femoral artery are sequentially temporarily released to flush any clots or debris, following which these clamps are removed and circulation is permitted to pass through the main graft into the legs (*k*). The right limb of the graft is then anastomosed to the right common femoral artery as previously described (*l*).

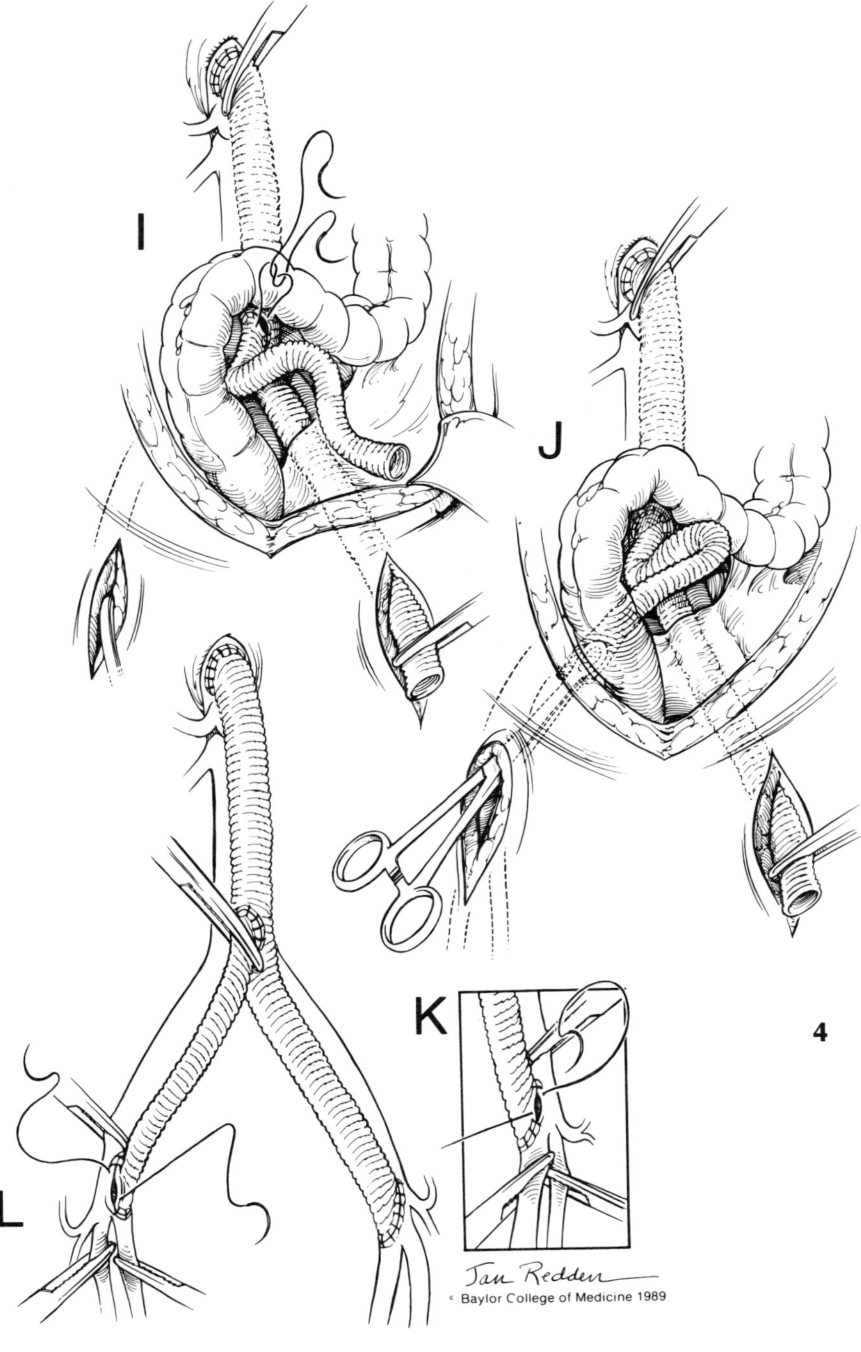

4

5

Occasionally in such cases as just described, it may be necessary to attach the proximal end of the graft to the lower part of the descending thoracic aorta rather than the abdominal aorta just below the diaphragm (*a*). A separate lower left intercostal incision is used to expose the lower descending thoracic aorta. A partial occluding clamp is then placed on the descending thoracic aorta and a vertical incision is made along the left lateral wall of the aorta to which the graft is attached by end-to-side anastomosis. The peritoneal cavity is opened through a separate midline incision, and the graft in the left pleural cavity is tunnelled retroperitoneally through an opening in the diaphragm along the left side of the aorta as it passes through the aortic diaphragmatic hiatus.

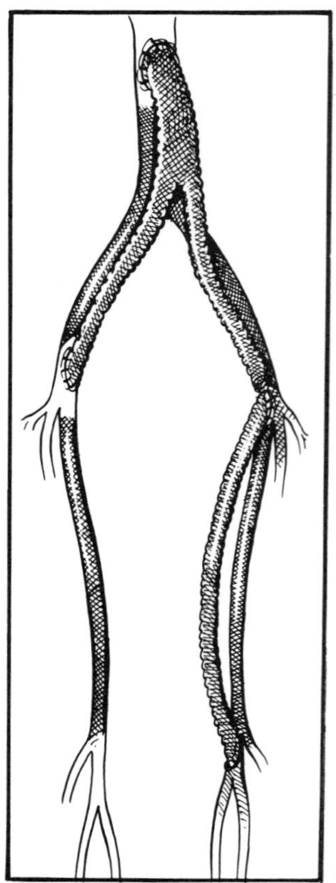

5

Technical modifications in the repair of thoracoabdominal aortic aneurysms

LARRY H. HOLLIER MD, FACS, FACC

Chairman, Department of Surgery and Executive Director of Clinical Affairs, Health Care International, Glasgow, Scotland

Introduction

Thoracoabdominal aortic aneurysms represent extensive deterioration of the aortic wall in patients who generally are elderly and often plagued with other degenerative diseases, especially hypertension and coronary artery disease. Failure to repair these aneurysms results in a 5-year survival rate of less than 20% (Bickerstaff *et al.*, 1982).

The advent of computerized tomography has aided greatly in the detection and delineation of the extent of thoracoabdominal aortic aneurysms. Additionally, simple suprarenal extension of abdominal aortic aneurysms are also being found with increasing frequency. In general, however, these latter aneurysms can be readily repaired by an abdominal approach and are not truly thoracoabdominal aneurysms. For purposes of this chapter, we limit the term thoracoabdominal aneurysm exclusively to mean aneurysms involving the origin of *all* the major visceral arteries. Clearly, these aneurysms require extensive technical reconstruction with revascularization of celiac, superior mesenteric and both renal arteries, as well as the spinal cord and the lower extremities.

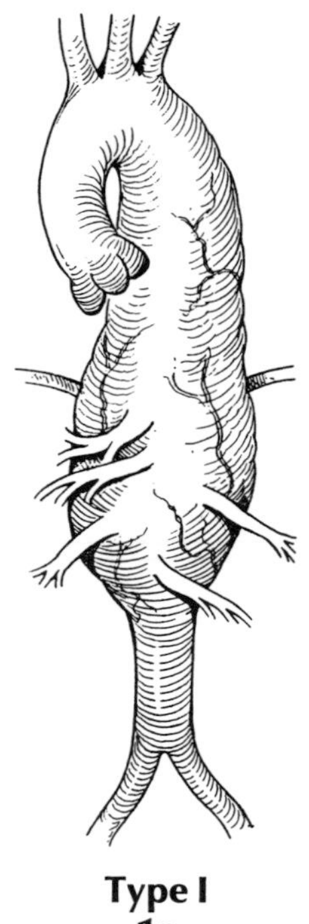

Type I
1a

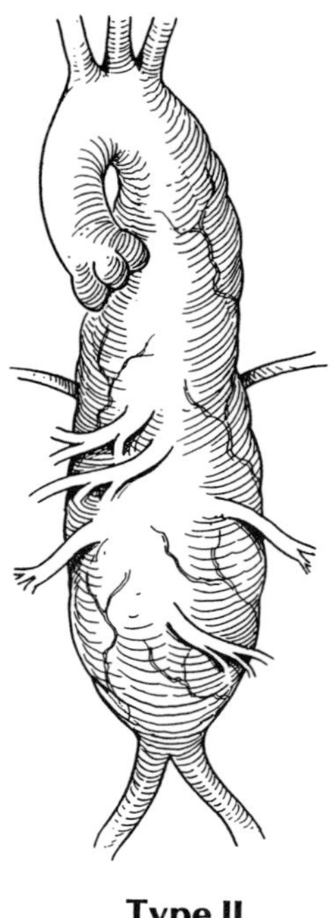

Type II
1b

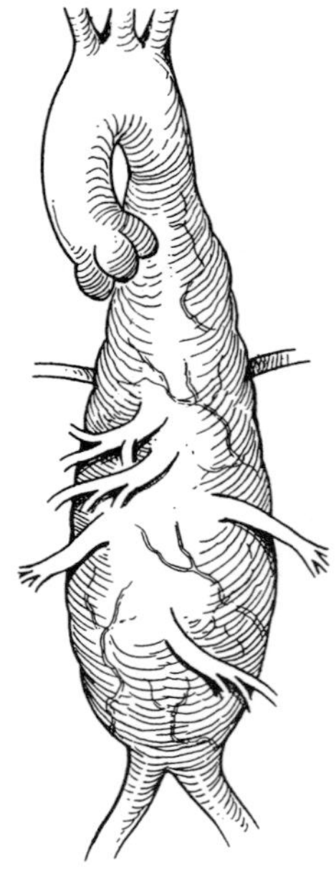

Type III
1c

1a, b, c & d

Using this criterion to delineate thoracoabdominal aneurysms, we find **four** clinical presentations: type I, which is essentially a thoracic aneurysm that extends inferiorly to the extent that it involves the visceral vessels; type II, the classic, diffuse thoracoabdominal aneurysm with extensive involvement of the aorta both above and below the visceral arteries; type III, with aneurysmal changes starting below the middle of the thoracic aorta; type IV, aneurysmal changes that start at the level of the diaphragm and involve the visceral vessels and infrarenal aorta.

The patterns are easily differentiated by computerized tomography, with type III aneurysms being identified most commonly in our experience. Although the type II thoracoabdominal aneurysm is best treated by the classic technique described by Crawford (1974), the other anatomical configurations may allow for modifications in surgical approach so that operative time can be reduced and visceral revascularization can be facilitated. These technical modifications were actually suggested in Crawford's early publications (Crawford, 1974, Crawford *et al.*, 1978), but their utility has not been appreciated by most surgeons.

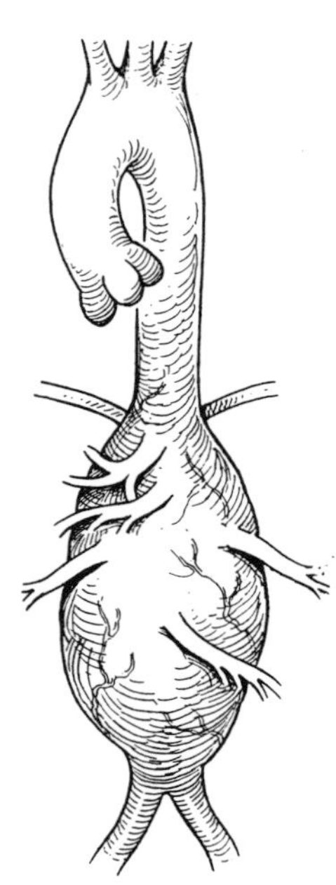

Type IV
1d

Techniques

2a & b

For all cases of thoracoabdominal aneurysm repair, the patient is placed in a semilateral position, with the buttocks resting flat on the operating table, but with the chest and shoulders rotated approximately 45° anteriorly. The left arm is placed on an arm-rest rotated above and anterior to the patient's head.

The chest, abdomen and groins are scrubbed with povidone-iodine solution, then covered with sterile drapes and an adhesive plastic skin barrier. The incision extends upward from the pubis to the umbilicus, then obliquely to the left up across the costal margin and through the appropriate intercostal space. If the aneurysm involves the abdominal aorta and the origin of the visceral vessels but terminates in normal or near-normal aorta near the diaphragm (type IV), the thoracic portion of the incision is usually placed through the 9th or 10th intercostal space. If the mid- or upper thoracic aorta is involved with contiguous aneurysmal change (type I or II), the 4th or 5th intercostal space is incised.

Exposure of the infradiaphragmatic aortic may be accomplished either extraperitoneally or transperitoneally. However, if endarterectomy of the right renal, celiac or superior mesenteric artery is required, the transperitoneal approach allows more thorough inspection of the distal vessel beyond the site of endarterectomy. Except for type I thoracoabdominal aneurysms, it is easier to reflect the left kidney along with spleen, pancreas and left colon, to expose the entire course of the aorta.

To complete exposure of the thoracoabdominal aorta, the diaphragm is divided in a circumferential rather than radial fashion, since this allows function of the left hemi-diaphragm to be preserved. We place alternating green and black marking sutures in the edges of the diaphragm as it is cut so that precise approximation can be achieved at the time of closure.

Prior to manipulation of the renal vessels, mannitol 25 g and lasix 10 mg are given intravenously. This places the kidneys in a diuretic state, thereby lessening the risk of acute tubular necrosis from renal ischaemia. Systemic heparin is not given, but the visceral vessels are irrigated with heparinized saline after opening the aorta later in the operation.

After exposure to the thoracoabdominal aorta, the extent of aneurysmal change in relation to the visceral vessels is assessed. As the greatest risk in thoracoabdominal aneurysm repair is myocardial infarction related to increased left ventricular afterload and subendocardial ischaemia, every effort should be made to minimize clamping time. Some surgeons have suggested the use of femorofemoral bypass or heparin-coated shunts to reduce ventricular strain, but additional complications have been noted as a direct result of these techniques. In our experience, intravenous nitroprusside has been a safe and useful means of pharmacologically off-loading the left ventricle and it avoids the problems of shunts and extracorporeal circulation. Despite vasodilatation techniques, however, prolonged cross-clamping of the thoracic aorta should be avoided, not only because of the cardiac risk, but also to lessen the risk of paraplegia.

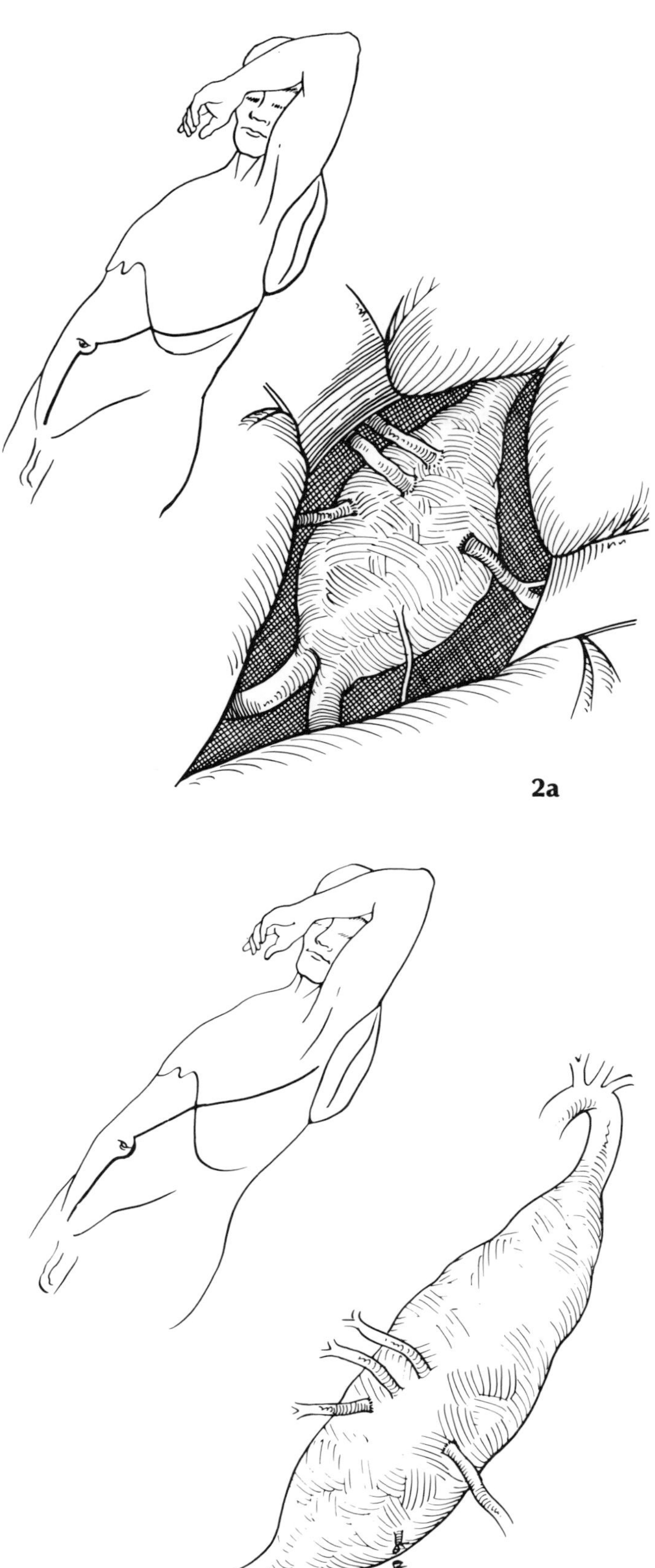

2a

2b

Diffuse thoracoabdominal aneurysm

3

When widespread aneurysmal changes are noted throughout the aorta, we perform graft replacement in the manner popularized by Crawford. The entire aneurysm is exposed, proximal and distal occluding clamps are placed, and a vertical arteriotomy is made through the lateral wall along the entire length of the aneurysm. If the left kidney is left in place, the left renal vein is mobilized so that the graft may be passed beneath it without difficulty. After opening the aneurysm, a catheter is placed in the left renal artery and the kidney is perfused with iced heparinized saline to irrigate and cool it during ischaemia.

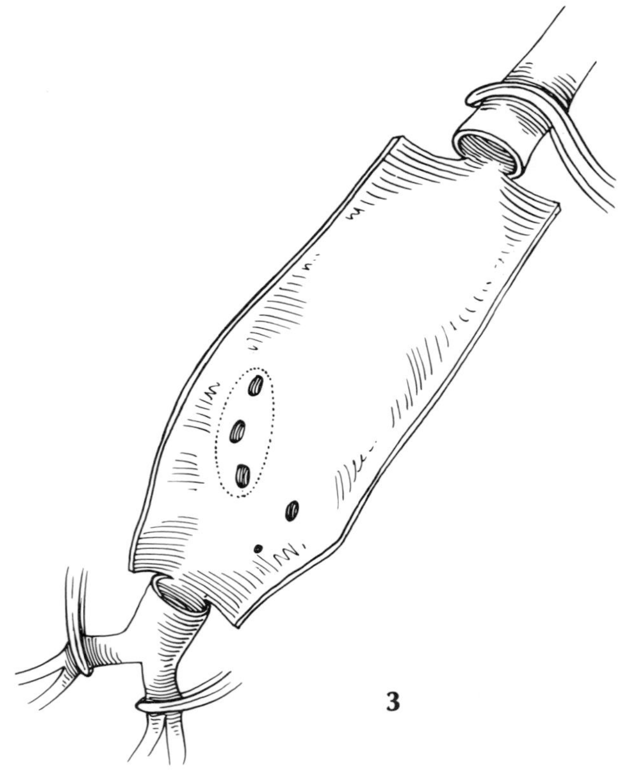

3

4

A low porosity woven graft is then sutured, end-to-end, to the partially transected proximal thoracic aorta using 0-polypropylene suture on a V-7 needle. Felt pledgets are commonly used to reinforce the anastomotic line. After the proximal anastomosis has been completed, any patent intercostal arteries are reimplanted into the graft after excising an elliptical section of the graft posteriorly. It is often possible to re-anastomose two or three pairs of intercostal arteries in one such anastomosis. Occasionally, a proximal intercostal artery can be revascularized by tailoring the proximal anastomosis obliquely to include these vessels. After intercostals have been reimplanted, the clamp is removed distally and flow is restored to the intercostal arteries. A button of graft is then excised opposite the orifices of the celiac, superior mesenteric and right renal arteries. The graft is then sutured side-to-side to the aorta with 0-polypropylene suture, encompassing the origins of all three vessels as a single anastomosis.

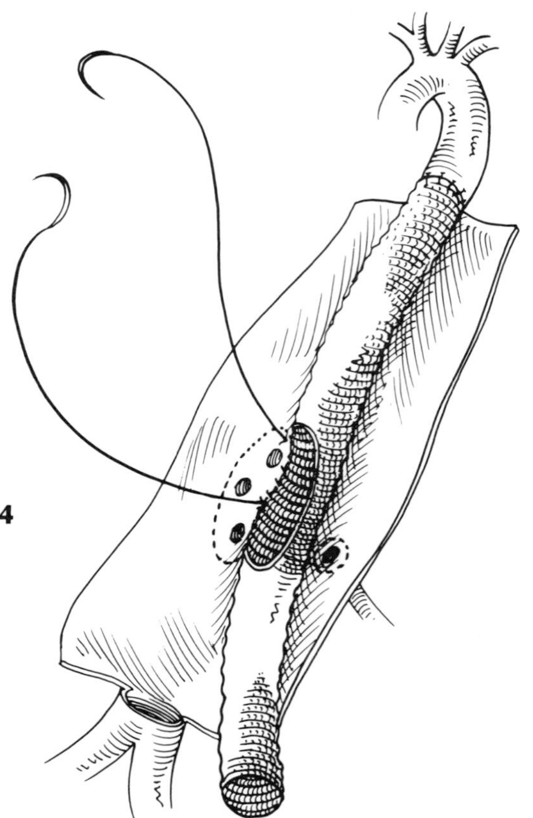

4

5

Flow is then restored to these vessels. The total occlusion time thus far is usually no more than 30 min. Because flow through these vessels is generally more than 2000 ml per min, its early restoration provides excellent off-loading of the left ventricle. The distal anastomosis to the aortic bifurcation is then performed and flow is cautiously restored to the lower extremities. If significant iliac disease is present, a woven bifurcation graft may be used instead of the straight graft.

After lower extremity flow has been restored, the left renal artery may be implanted into the graft directly.

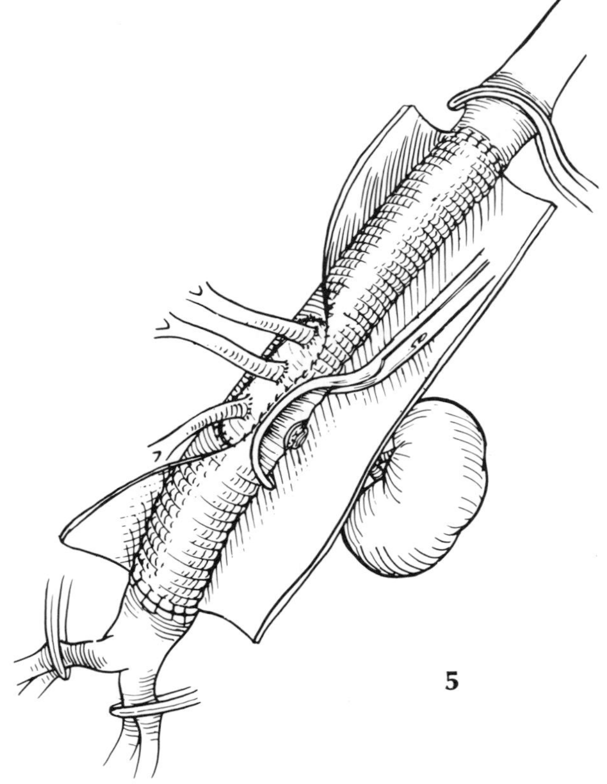

5

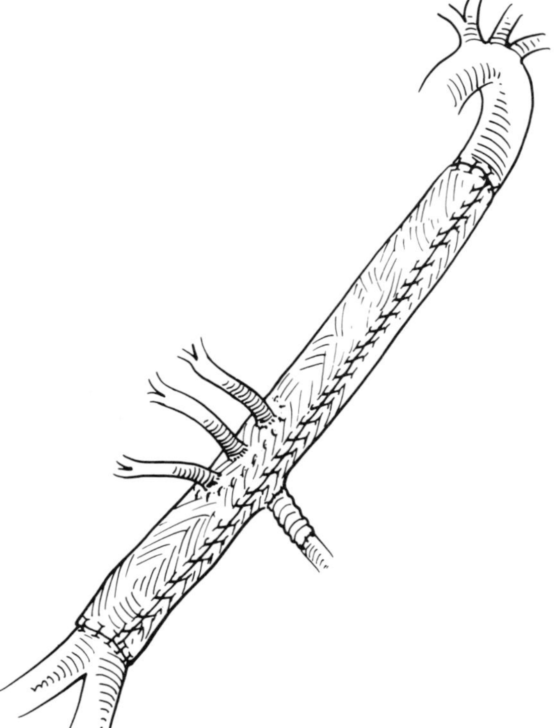

6

6

If stenosis of the left renal artery is noted, we use a short-segment (6 or 8 mm) Dacron graft to revascularize the left kidney. After completion of all anastomoses, the sac of the aneurysm is closed tightly around the graft for added haemostasis.

Vessels are examined for adequacy of pulses, and flows are measured in the revascularized arteries. The abdominal viscera are then restored to their normal anatomical position and the diaphragm is closed with interrupted horizontal mattress sutures of 2/0 braided Dacron. Two chest tubes are placed through separate stab incisions to drain the left chest, and the chest and abdominal incisions are closed in layers in standard fashion.

Low thoracoabdominal aneurysm

With increasing frequency, we see patients who have thoracoabdominal aneurysms which involve the entire abdominal aorta, including the site of origin of the visceral vessels, but in whom the aorta is relatively normal from the diaphragm upwards. In this situation we find that slight technical modifications can significantly reduce the time of increased afterload on the left ventricle.

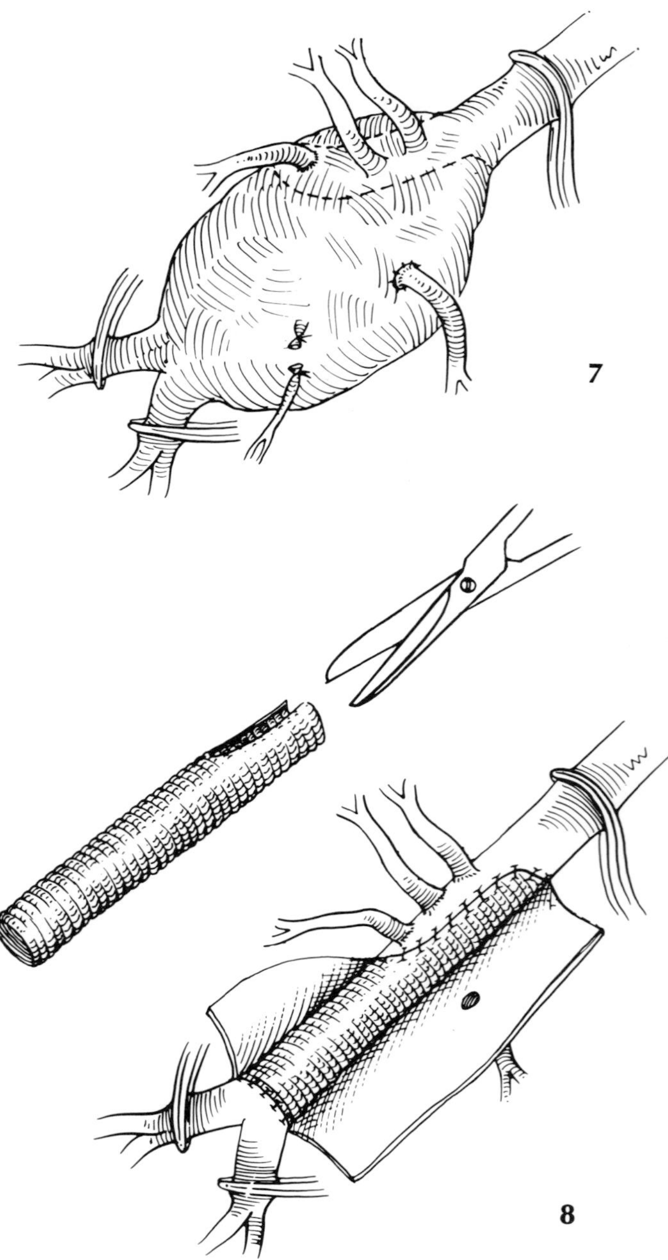

7

8

7

A low thoracoabdominal approach is utilized (see *Illustration 2a*), and the aorta is dissected as previously described, although only the lower third of the thoracic aorta need be exposed in these cases. Because of the proximity of normal aorta to the visceral vessels, clamp time can be minimized by including a tongue of aorta bearing the orifices of these vessels in an oblique proximal anastomosis.

8

The woven low-porosity Dacron graft is trimmed as shown and an anastomosis is fashioned to provide revascularization of the celiac, superior mesenteric and right renal arteries in conjunction with the proximal anastomosis. The proximal clamp can then be repositioned on to the graft below the right renal artery and visceral flow can be restored. Total occlusion time to this stage of the procedure is usually 15 min.

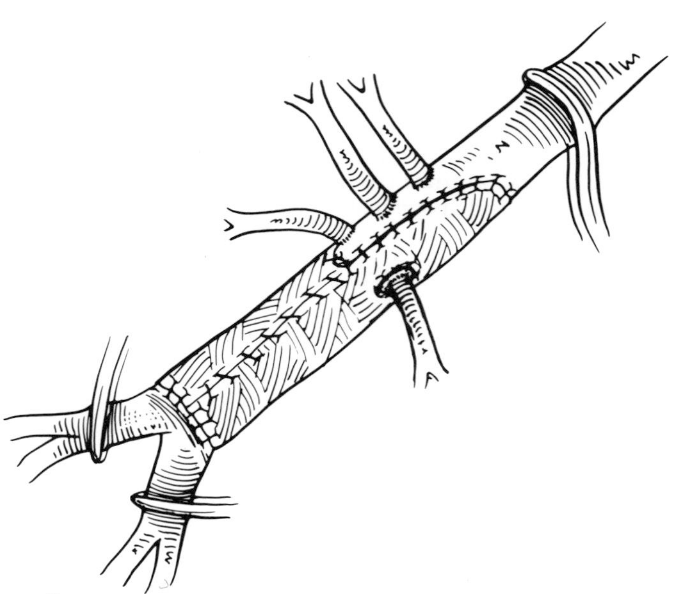

9

9

The distal anastomosis and left renal revascularization are then performed as previously described, and the sac of the aneurysm is closed over the graft with a running suture of 3/0 polypropylene.

10, 11 & 12

Thoracic aneurysm with abdominal extension

Some patients with thoracoabdominal aneurysms that are primarily thoracic aneurysms (type 1), but the aneurysmal changes extend down below the diaphragm and involve the aorta at the site of origin of the visceral vessels. In such cases, operative time may be reduced by incorporating the visceral revascularization with the distal anastomosis. Total aortic occlusion time in these cases is generally no more than 30 min.

In all variations of revascularization procedures described here, the visceral and spinal artery anastomoses are performed in a side-to-side fashion; that is, the aortic wall is not incised in 'button' fashion around the orifices, but the reimplantations are done by suturing into the inside of the intact aortic wall. This is most clearly shown in *Illustration 4*.

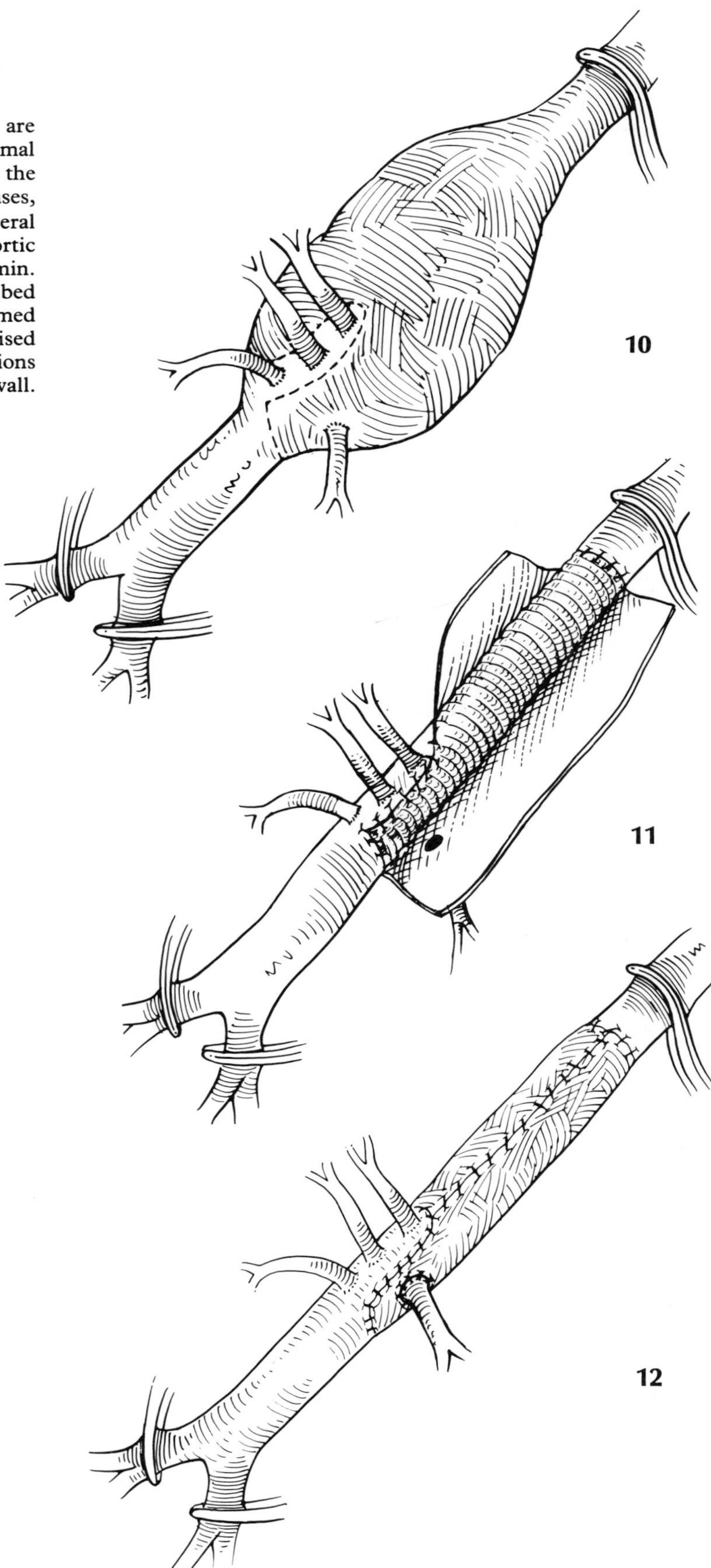

Prevention of paraplegia

Despite the use of evoked potential monitoring, heparin-bonded shunts, femorofemoral or atriofemoral bypass, or routine intercostal reimplantation, paraplegia still occurs. Obviously, when technically feasible, use of shunts or bypass can reduce the risk of paraplegia if clamp time is expected to be prolonged, but they are often ineffective, especially in type II aneurysms.

Recent experimental and clinical experience with spinal fluid drainage has suggested that this technique may improve spinal cord perfusion and may increase the safe clamp time. This may allow a longer safe interval in which to reimplant the intercostal arteries to revascularize the spinal cord.

After endotracheal anaesthesia is instituted, the patient is placed on his right side and an 18 gauge spinal needle is introduced intrathecally between the 4th and 5th lumbar vertebrae and a silastic catheter is introduced. A total of 10–15 dl of spinal fluid is withdrawn and the needle is withdrawn, leaving the intrathecal catheter in place; the catheter is then connected to a pressure transducer for continuous monitoring. If the spinal fluid pressure rises during the case, additional spinal fluid is withdrawn to keep the spinal pressure below 10 mmHg.

It is important to remember that spinal fluid drainage alone does not prevent paraplegia and is not a substitute for intercostal artery reimplantation which is mandatory in some patients. Additionally, it seems unlikely that it will reduce the incidence of paraplegia that sometimes occurs several days after otherwise successful repair of thoracoabdominal aneurysms.

Complications and results

Use of the techniques mentioned above has resulted in expeditious repair of thoracoabdominal aneurysms with acceptable morbidity and mortality. We have now operated on over 200 patients who underwent repair of non-dissecting thoracoabdominal aneurysms. Long-term dialysis was needed in <3% of patients. The most common complicated encounters were pulmonary (20%), particularly the need for prolonged ventilation.

A total of 97% of patients survived sufficiently long to determine neurological function. Overall, paraplegia or paraparesis occurred in 4% of those patients who had type I and type II thoracoabdominal aneurysms. The incidence of spinal cord injury was 6.6%. Spinal drainage was not used in any patient early in the series. Since routine spinal fluid drainage was instituted, we have not yet seen paraplegia occur when intercostal arteries have been reimplanted.

Continuing experience and the relaxation of surgical indications will undoubtedly increase the mortality and morbidity of any series. None the less, careful preoperative evaluation and preparation, careful and expeditious surgical technique, and meticulous attention to postoperative management, will improve salvage in patients with thoracoabdominal aortic aneurysms.

References

Bickerstaff, L. K., Pairolero, P. C., Hollier, L. H., *et al.* (1982). Thoracic aortic aneurysms: A population-based study. *Surgery* **92**(6), 1103

Bower, T. C., Murray, M. J., Gloviczki, P., *et al.* (in press). The effects of thoracic aortic occlusion and cerebrospinal fluid drainage on regional spinal cord blood flow in dogs: Correlation with neurologic outcome. *Journal of Vascular Surgery*.

Crawford, E.S. (1974). Thoracoabdominal and abdominal aortic aneurysms involving renal, superior mesenteric, and celiac arteries. *Annals of Surgery* **179**(5), 763.

Crawford, E. S., Snyder, D. M., Cho, G. C., *et al.* (1978). Progress in treatment of thoracoabdominal and abdominal aortic aneurysms involving celiac, superior mesenteric and renal arteries. *Annals of Surgery* **188**(4), 404.

Hollier, L. H. (1987). Protecting the brain and spinal cord. *Journal of Vascular Surgery* **5**(3), 524.

Hollier, L. H., Symmonds, J. B., Pairolero, P. C., Cherry, K. J., *et al.* (1988). Thoracoabdominal aortic aneurysm repair: Analysis of postoperative morbidity. *Archives of Surgery* **123**, 871.

Hollier, L. H., Money, S. R., Naslund, T. C., *et al.* (1992). Risk of spinal cord dysfunction in patients undergoing thoracoabdominal aortic replacement. *American Journal of Surgery* **164**(3), 210.

McCullogh, J. L., Hollier, L. H. and Nugent, M. (1988). Paraplegia after thoracic aortic occlusion: Influence of cerebrospinal fluid drainage. *Journal of Vascular Surgery* **7**(1), 153.

Abdominal aortic aneurysms

JOHN A. MANNICK MD

Moseley Professor of Surgery, Harvard Medical School;
Surgeon-in-Chief, Brigham and Women's Hospital, Boston, Massachusetts, USA

ANTHONY D. WHITTEMORE MD

Assistant Professor of Surgery, Harvard Medical School;
Surgeon, Brigham and Women's Hospital, Boston, Massachusetts, USA

Introduction

The indication for repair of an abdominal aortic aneurysm is the presence of an aneurysm of significant size in a patient of any age who does not have another non-correctable, life-threatening condition. It is generally conceded that aneurysms which have reached 5 cm in diameter are in danger of rupturing and surgery for such aneurysms is clearly indicated. There is some debate as to whether aneurysms of smaller diameter than 5 cm are likely to rupture. Our own practice has been to operate selectively on aneurysms between 4 and 5 cm in diameter. The decision to operate is based upon evidence of recent expansion in aneurysm size by ultrasound or CT, the ratio of the aneurysm diameter to that of the uninvolved aorta and the age and fitness of the patient. We rarely operate on aneurysms smaller than 4 cm. Patients with tender aneurysms or with symptoms of back pain or abdominal pain suggesting acute expansion of the aneurysm require urgent surgery. Obviously, a patient with the diagnosis of a ruptured abdominal aortic aneurysm should be taken to the operating room immediately.

In addition to standard preoperative preparation, it has been our practice for the past decade to study every patient undergoing elective or urgent aneurysm repair by inserting a Swan-Ganz catheter preoperatively (Whittemore *et al.*, 1980). Several points on the left ventricular performance curve are then determined for each individual so that a pulmonary capillary wedge pressure can be selected which will result in a desirable cardiac index. Volume replacement during surgery can be regulated to maintain this optimal pulmonary capillary wedge pressure and thus ensure adequate tissue perfusion throughout the operation. Declamping hypotension can also be minimized with this technique.

We routinely perform preoperative aortography using the retrograde Seldinger technique in order to define the upper extent of the aneurysm better in relation to the renal arteries and to ensure that there are no anomalous renal arteries arising from the aneurysm itself. We obtain biplane views to ensure patency of the superior mesenteric artery and coeliac axis since aneurysm repair will involve ligation of the origin of the inferior mesenteric artery.

We believe that it is helpful to recover shed blood during the course of aneurysm surgery by the use of a Cell Saver. Since we began using this device 10 years ago, approximately 35% of patients undergoing elective abdominal aneurysm repair have not required banked blood transfusions.

The operation

The technique of aneurysm repair employed by our service is a modification of the graft inclusion technique previously described by Creech (1966) and Javid *et al.* (1982).

1

The abdomen is opened and explored through a midline incision extending from the pubis to the xiphoid. The small bowel is lifted superiorly and to the right, and is packed into the right upper quadrant of the abdomen. Exposure of the operative field is greatly facilitated by a multi-armed mechanical retractor fixed to the operating table. The peritoneum is incised with scissors along the inferior border of the third and fourth portions of the duodenum, and the duodenum is retracted superiorly. The peritoneum and areolar tissue overlying the aorta are opened longitudinally with the scissors or cautery, exposing the anterior surface of the aneurysm.

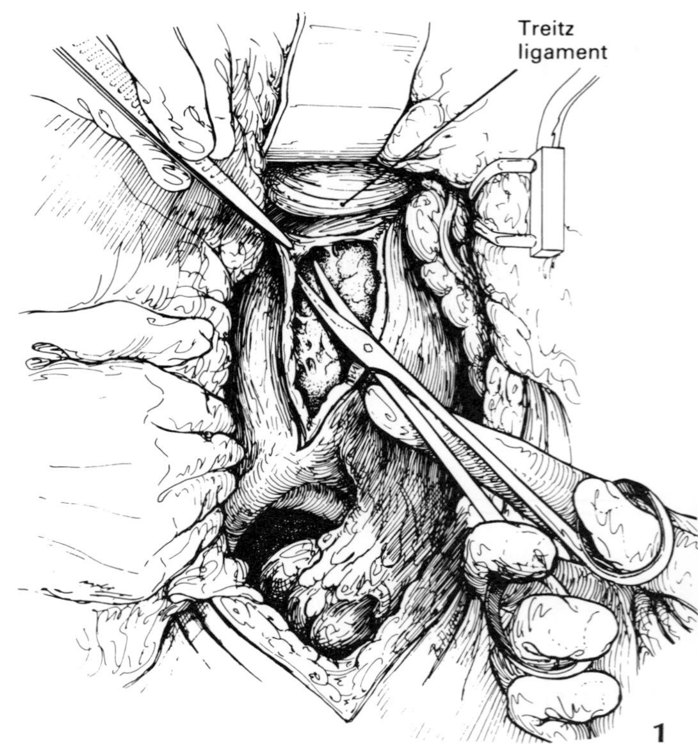

1

2

The incision is carried superiorly to the level of the left renal vein and inferiorly 2.5–5 cm beyond the aortic bifurcation. The aorta just above the aneurysm and below the left renal vein is freed up from its surrounding tissues by sharp dissection anteriorly and laterally. No attempt is made to dissect behind the aorta at this level, nor is the neck of the aneurysm encircled with tape. However, the dissection along each lateral wall of the aorta is continued far enough posteriorly so that the neck of the aneurysm can be compressed easily by an occluding clamp which will be applied at this level.

Inferiorly, the anterior and lateral walls of both common iliac arteries are freed by sharp dissection in a similar fashion without separating these vessels from their attachments to the common iliac veins posteriorly. If it is convenient at this point, the inferior mesenteric artery is temporarily controlled with a bulldog clamp near its origin from the aorta as illustrated. In most instances, the origin of the inferior mesenteric artery is ligated from inside the aneurysm at a later stage. Ligation and division of the inferior mesenteric artery away from its origin is avoided for fear of damage to vital collateral branches which feed the sigmoid colon. Dissection of the lateral walls of the aneurysm is kept to a minimum to eliminate the necessity for ligating multiple small vessels that traverse the surrounding lymphatic and areolar tissue. Dissection of the aneurysm wall from the inferior vena cava is particularly avoided to reduce the risk of injury to that structure.

Heparin is administered to the patient systemically intravenously, 4000–5000 u in an average adult. While it is possible to repair many, if not most, abdominal aortic aneurysms successfully without the use of heparin, it is advisable to heparinize the patient partially when the aorta and iliac arteries are clamped; otherwise, extensive distal thrombosis can occur in patients who have severe distal arterial occlusive disease and in those instances where mural thrombus or arteriosclerotic debris from the aneurysm is inadvertently embolized distally. It has been our experience that retrograde thrombosis is kept to a minimum in such instances before the embolic debris is retrieved if the patient has been prophylactically heparinized.

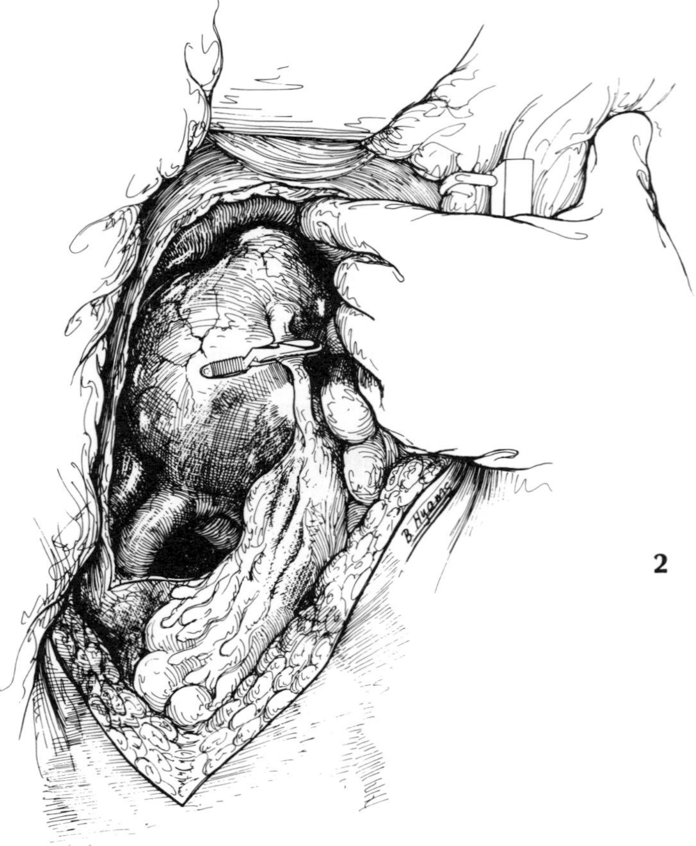

2

3

After heparinization, large straight Fogarty vascular clamps are applied to both common iliac arteries and a deBakey reverse-angle aortic clamp is applied to the aorta above the aneurysm. The aneurysm is then opened longitudinally with a knife or cautery.

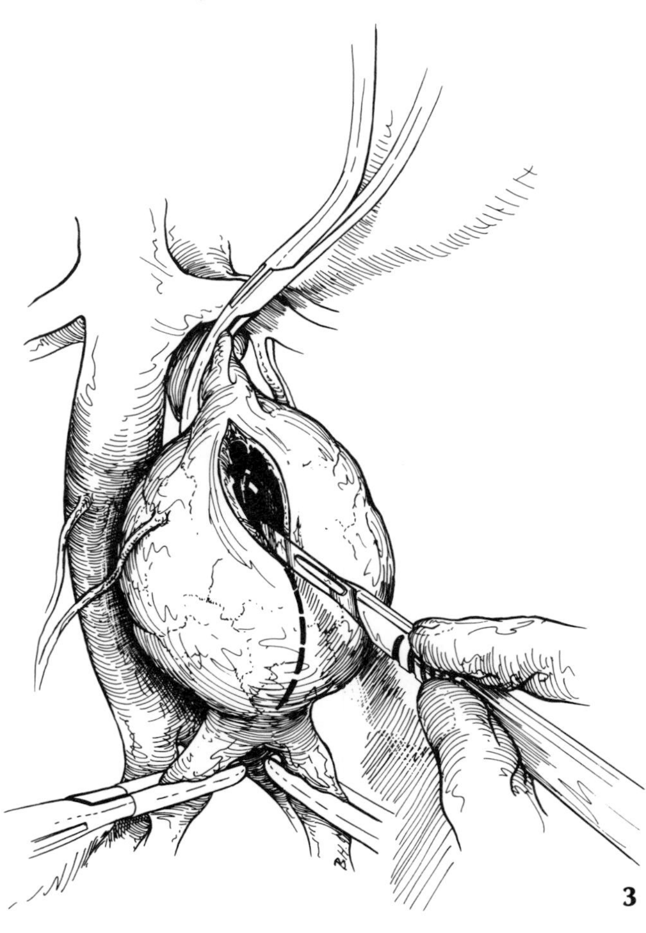
3

4

The incision in the aneurysm is completed with Mayo scissors.

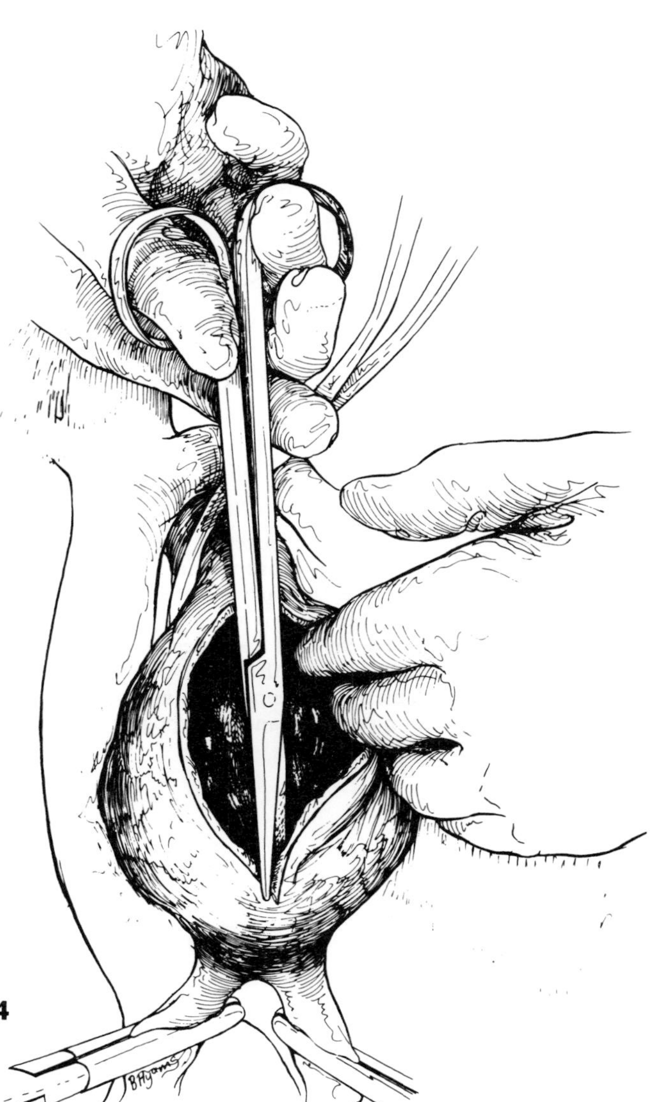
4

5

All mural thrombus and loose arteriosclerotic debris is evacuated from the lumen of the aneurysm.

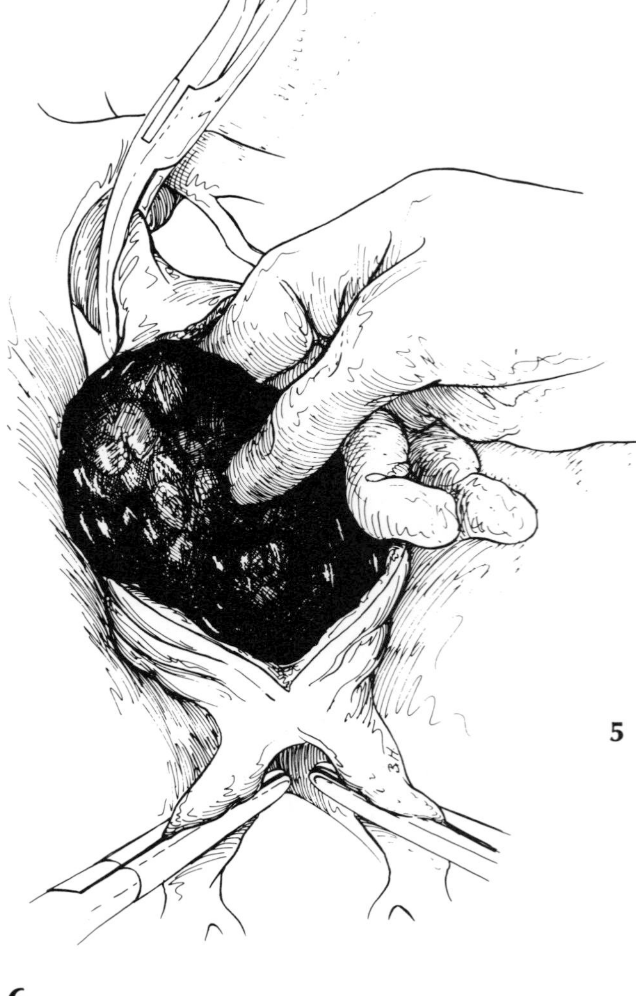

5

6

The origins of bleeding lumbar arteries are oversewn with figure-of-eight sutures of 3/0 polypropylene. The origin of the inferior mesenteric artery is similarly sutured if this vessel is still patent and the backbleeding is vigorous. If the inferior mesenteric is widely patent and backbleeding is sluggish, reimplantation of the artery into the aortic prosthesis should be considered, particularly if preoperative angiograms show disease of the superior mesenteric and/or hypogastric arteries.

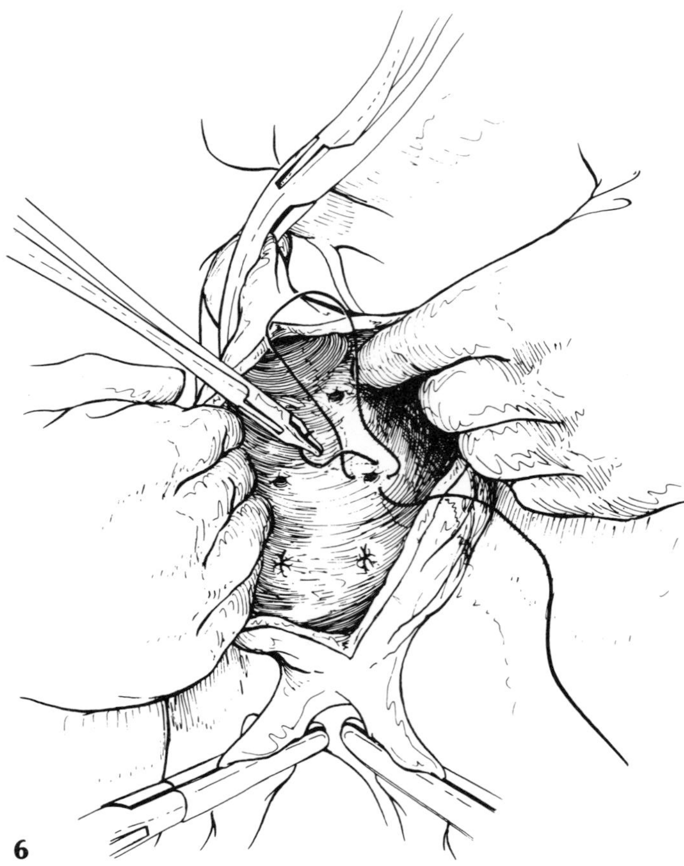

6

7

In patients with no significant iliac aneurysms, a tube graft of woven or collagen-impregnated knitted Dacron is preferred for aneurysm replacement. This graft will be sutured distally to the aortic bifurcation which usually remains of reasonably normal size even when the aneurysm involves the entire infrarenal abdominal aorta. Cuffs may be cut proximally and distally extending partially down each side of the aorta at the neck of the aneurysm above and at the aortic bifurcation below. However, in large aneurysms, we have found it just as convenient to avoid this step and simply to suture the graft to the ring of normal vessel superiorly and inferiorly.

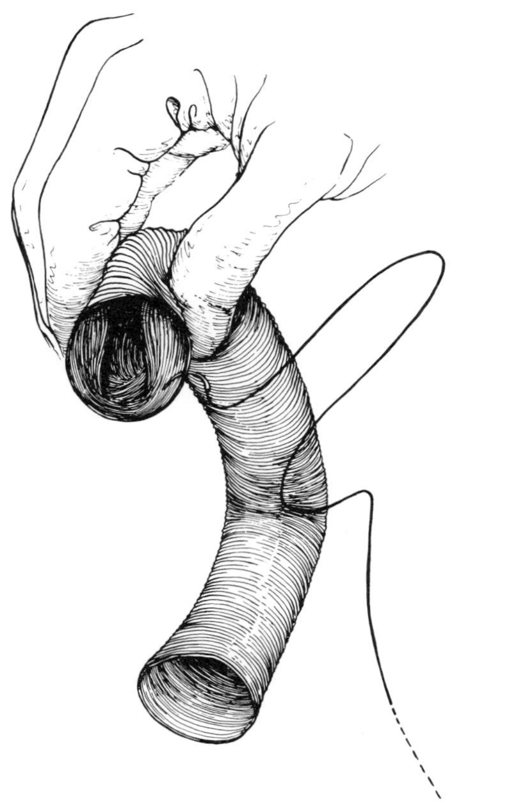

7

8

The posterior wall of the aorta is not divided either proximally or distally. The posterior aortic wall is often a rather tenuous structure and we prefer to add strength to the posterior suture line by including the surrounding fascial tissue in the posterior stitches of the anastomosis. A Dacron tube graft of appropriate size is sewn with a double-armed polypropylene suture to the posterior wall of the aorta at the neck of the aneurysm. A double-thickness of aortic wall is included in each bite posteriorly.

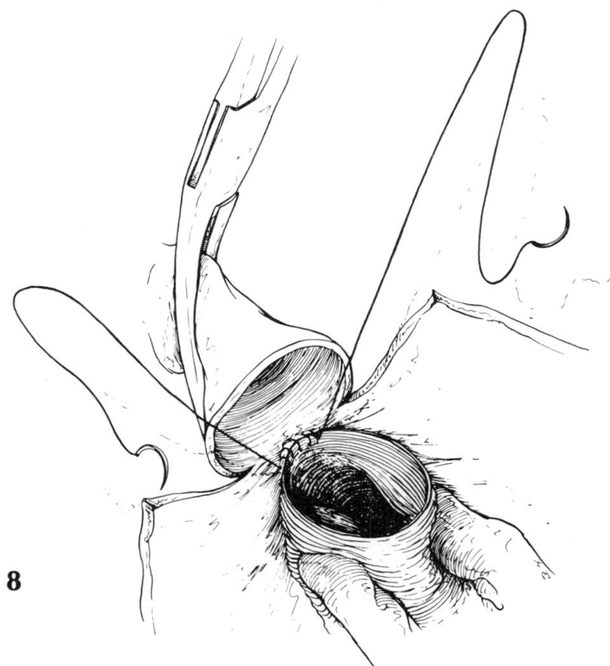

8

9

The suture is carried around each side of the neck of the aneurysm and tied anteriorly.

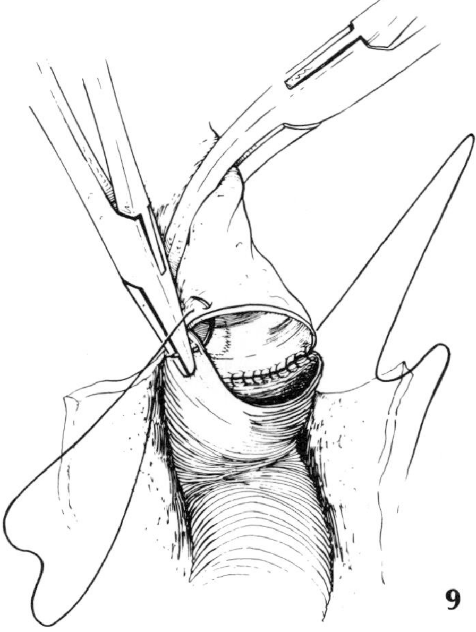

9

10

The proximal anastomosis is then tested for leaks by clamping the tube graft and releasing the aortic clamp briefly. If any leaks are noted in the anastomosis they are repaired with simple or figure-of-eight sutures of 3/0 polypropylene. The aortic clamp may then be reapplied or, if preferred, the graft may be clamped just distal to the proximal anastomosis.

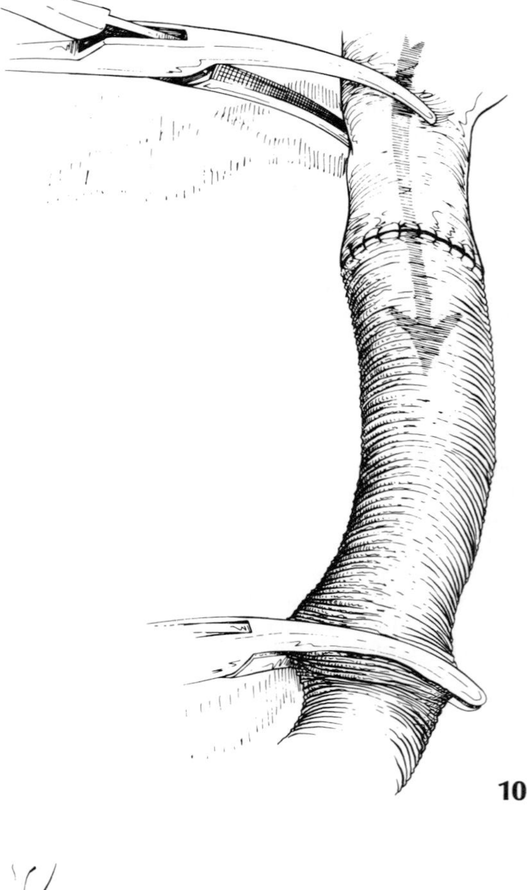

10

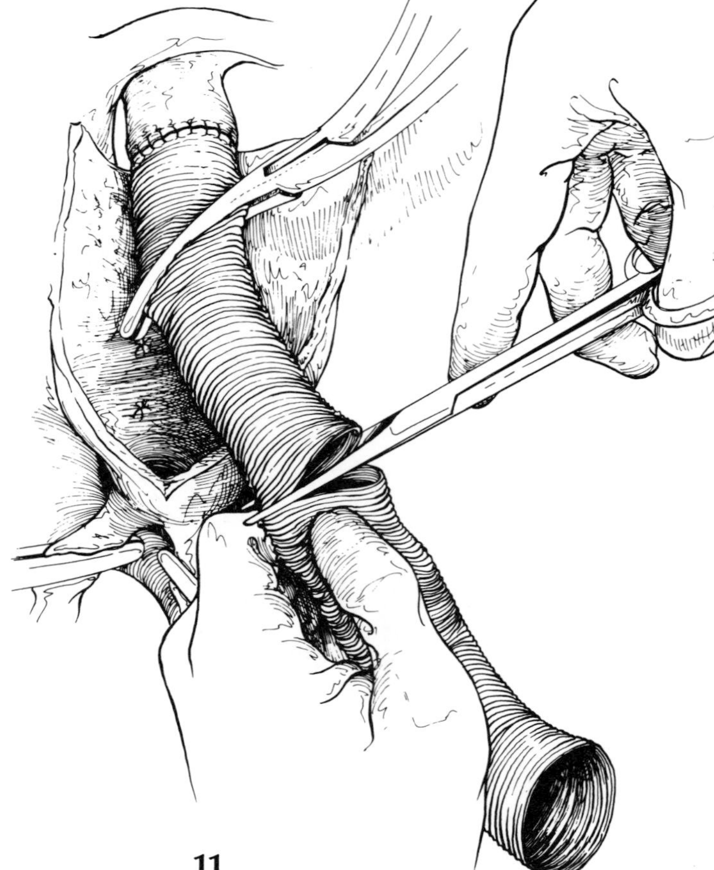

11

11

After being evacuated of all blood with a sucker, the graft is placed under slight tension and cut to the appropriate length for anastomosis with the aortic bifurcation.

12

The lower anastomosis is performed using a double-armed suture of 3/0 polypropylene.

All vessels are flushed before completion of this suture line. If there is adequate backbleeding from both iliac systems no attempt is made to pass Fogarty catheters distally to retrieve possible emboli. The suture line is then completed and tied anteriorly as for the proximal anastomosis. The iliac clamps are released and the lower anastomosis is inspected for leaks which are repaired as for the proximal anastomosis. The proximal aortic clamp is then gradually released while the anaesthetist carefully monitors the patient's blood pressure and infuses extra volume intravenously if needed. If the patient has been maintained with an optimal pulmonary capillary wedge pressure, declamping hypotension is ordinarily not observed. After release of clamps the iliac arteries are inspected for adequate pulsations and the presence of good femoral pulses in the groin is determined by palpation. We seldom find it necessary to neutralize the heparin with protamine.

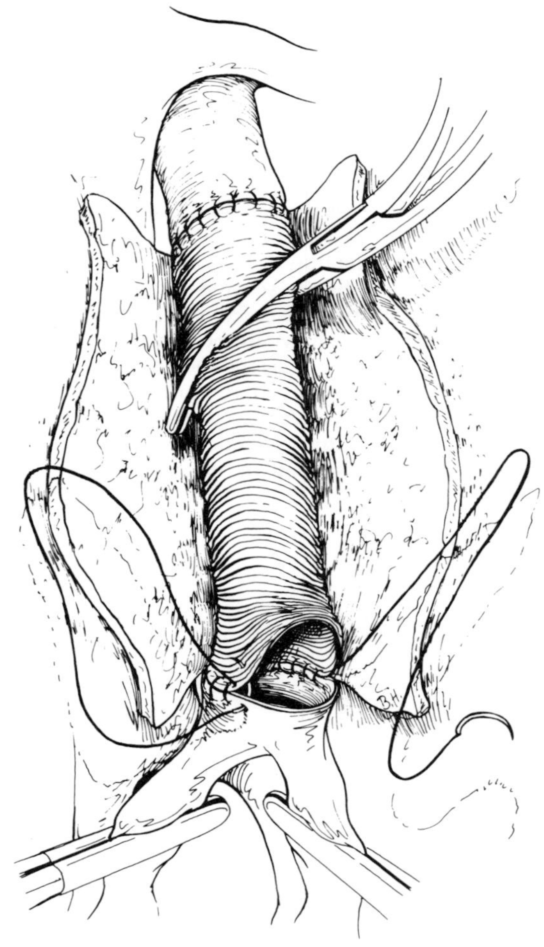

12

13

Any residual bleeding points in the aneurysm wall are sutured, ligated or electrocoagulated and the aneurysm wall is sutured back over the prosthesis with a running stitch of polypropylene. This manoeuvre ordinarily covers both the proximal and distal suture line with residual aneurysm wall.

If the wall is too large to fit snugly around the prosthesis it may be overlapped in vest-over-pants fashion as a double suture line. We have found that this is usually more convenient than trimming the wall, since trimming often produces further bleeding which must then be controlled. The periaortic tissues are then approximated over the aorta, and if possible, over the resutured aneurysm wall by a second running suture of polyglycolate in order to provide further retroperitoneal haemostasis. This also has the advantage of placing yet another layer between the prosthesis and the posterior wall of the duodenum. The posterior peritoneum is then closed over the aorta and resutured aneurysm wall with a running suture of polyglycolate. It is ordinarily possible to interpose the peritoneum as an additional layer between the posterior wall of the duodenum and the aorta. The abdomen is then closed with a continuous suture of #2 polypropylene to the rectus fascia and staples to the skin.

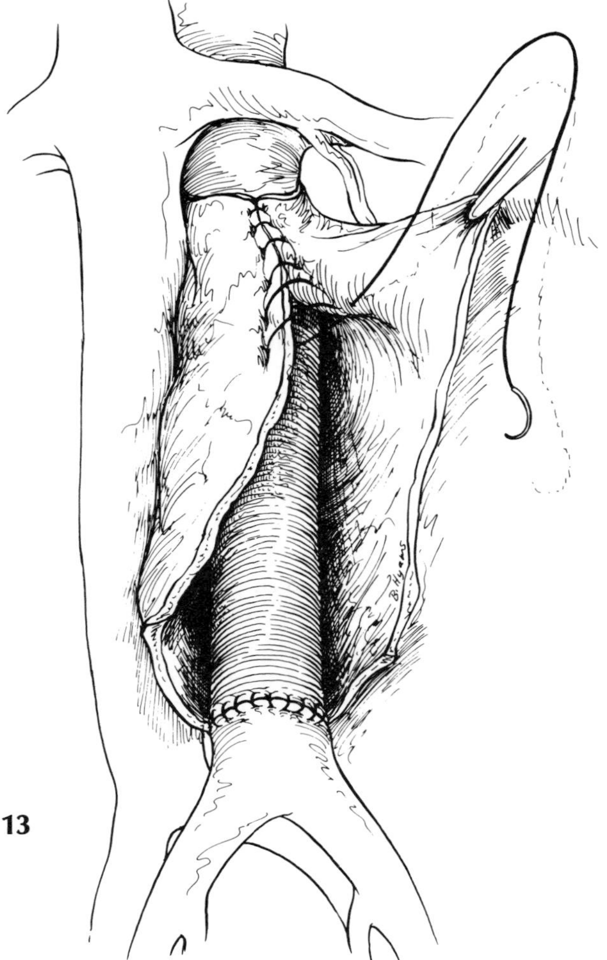

13

14

Iliac aneurysms

If common iliac aneurysms are present, a similar operative procedure is followed. However, the iliac clamps are applied to the iliac bifurcations, taking care to avoid injury to the ureters which usually cross the common iliac arteries distally. Iliac aneurysms are opened longitudinally. A bifurcation graft of Dacron is used and the upper anastomosis is performed as described. The iliac limbs are sutured on either side to the distal common iliac arteries, again from inside the iliac aneurysms. The aneurysm walls may also be sutured back over the graft limbs to provide an extra layer of host tissue between the graft and the abdominal viscera. In the case of a large left iliac aneurysm it may be more convenient to exclude the aneurysm and suture the left limb of the graft end-to-side to the external iliac artery inferior to the sigmoid mesentery.

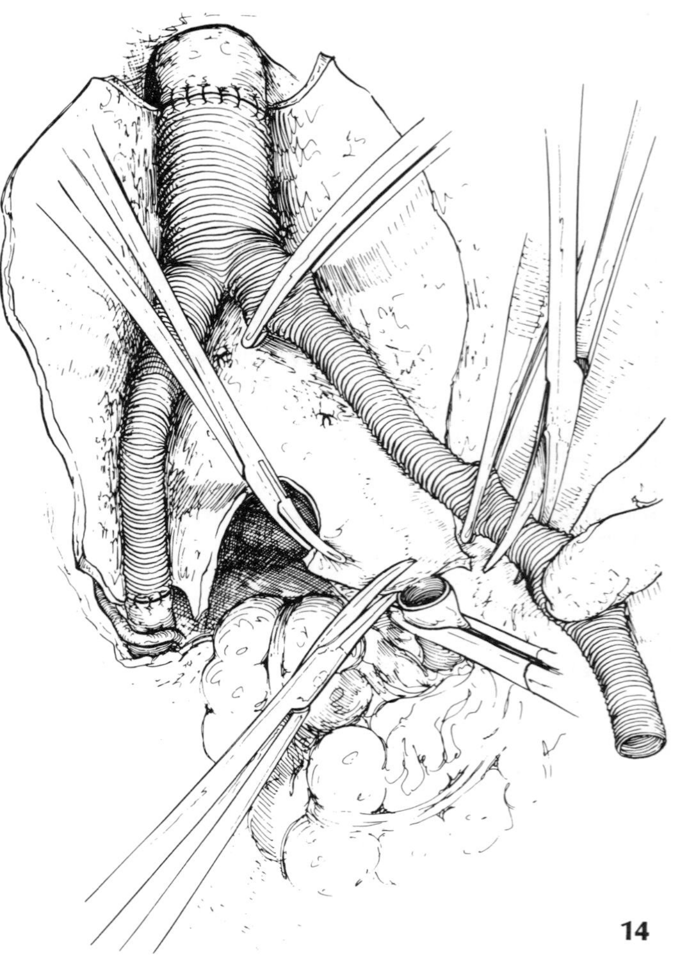

14

Juxtarenal abdominal aortic aneurysms

In cases where the abdominal aortic aneurysm extends more proximally than usual and there is little or no neck of normal aorta between the aneurysm and the renal arteries, it is helpful to place the aortic clamp at the level of the diaphragm while the proximal anastomosis is performed.

15

The aorta at the level of the diaphragm can be exposed by incising the attachments of the left lobe of the liver to the diaphragm and retracting the liver to the right. The lesser sac is entered and the aorta is exposed as it passes underneath the crus of the diaphragm.

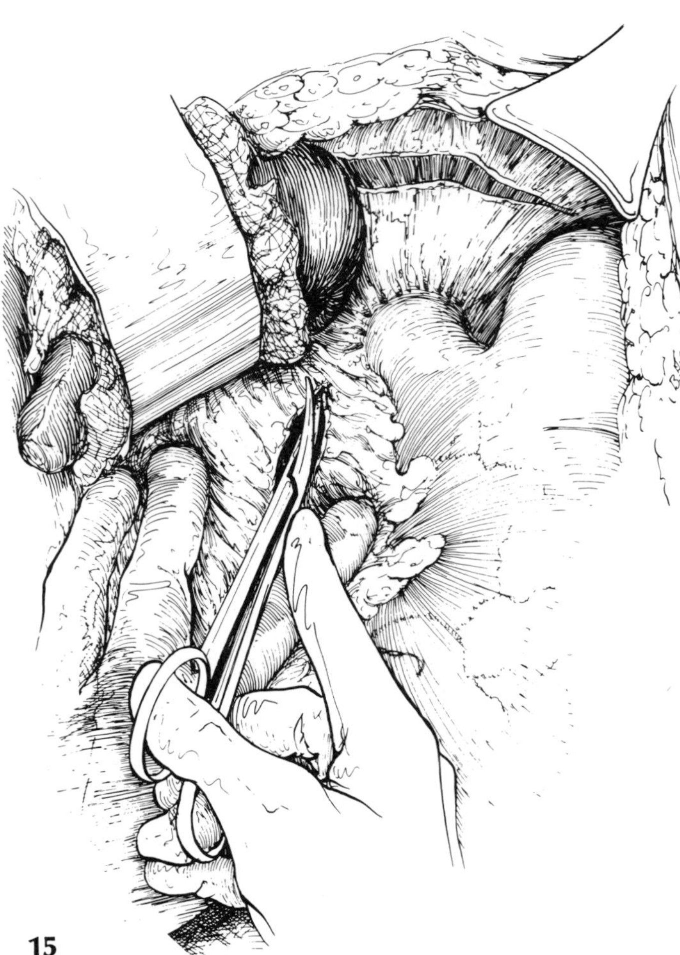

15

16 & 17

With finger dissection, the crus can be stretched and split enough so that a clamp can be applied to the aorta at the hiatus, where this vessel is usually of normal calibre and free of branches.

Backbleeding from the coeliac axis and superior mesenteric artery can be controlled with an intra-aortic balloon catheter inserted from below, and the graft can be anastomosed proximally with excellent visibility from inside the aneurysm into the normal aorta just distal to the renal artery orifices. After completion of the proximal anastomosis, the aortic clamp is released and the prosthesis is clamped, restoring flow to the viscera and to the renal arteries. We believe that this manoeuver is much less hazardous to the kidneys than attempts to clamp the aorta close to the renal artery orifices which may result in arteriosclerotic embolization to one or both kidneys. Some patients with juxtarenal aneurysms have a considerable, 2 cm or more, distance between the renal artery orifices and the origin of the superior mesenteric as indicated by angiography. In such individuals it may be more convenient to free up the aorta just above the renal arteries and left renal vein. The aorta can then be safely clamped below the superior mesenteric thus avoiding even a brief period of visceral ischaemia.

The retroperitoneal approach

In some patients (about 15% of those in our practice) the retroperitoneal approach (Williams *et al.*, 1980) to abdominal aortic aneurysms is preferable. We believe this approach is especially indicated in patients who have had multiple prior abdominal operations in order to avoid the lysis of adhesions which would be necessary in the transabdominal approach. We believe the retroperitoneal approach is also indicated in those rare individuals with a horseshoe kidney and an abdominal aneurysm, and in patients with inflammatory aneurysms since the attachment of the duodenum to the inflammatory aneurysm is not an issue with this approach. We have also found that the thick inflammatory aneurysm wall is usually thinner posteriorly than anteriorly. We now prefer the retroperitoneal approach in many patients with juxtarenal abdominal aneurysms since the crus of the diaphragm is readily visualized by this approach and can be divided with ease for application of a clamp to the supraceliac or suprarenal aorta.

18

For the retroperitoneal approach, the patient is placed in the left lateral thoracotomy position with the hips rotated back toward the supine position. The positioning of the patient is greatly aided through the use of a 'bean bag' moulded by suction. The incision is placed in the left flank beginning at the lateral border of the rectus muscle just below the umbilicus and extending out into the 11th interspace. The abdominal muscles are cut in the line of the incision and the peritoneum and left kidney are retracted medially and to the right. This allows easy visualization of the left posterolateral wall of the aorta, the left common iliac artery, and the origin of the left renal artery.

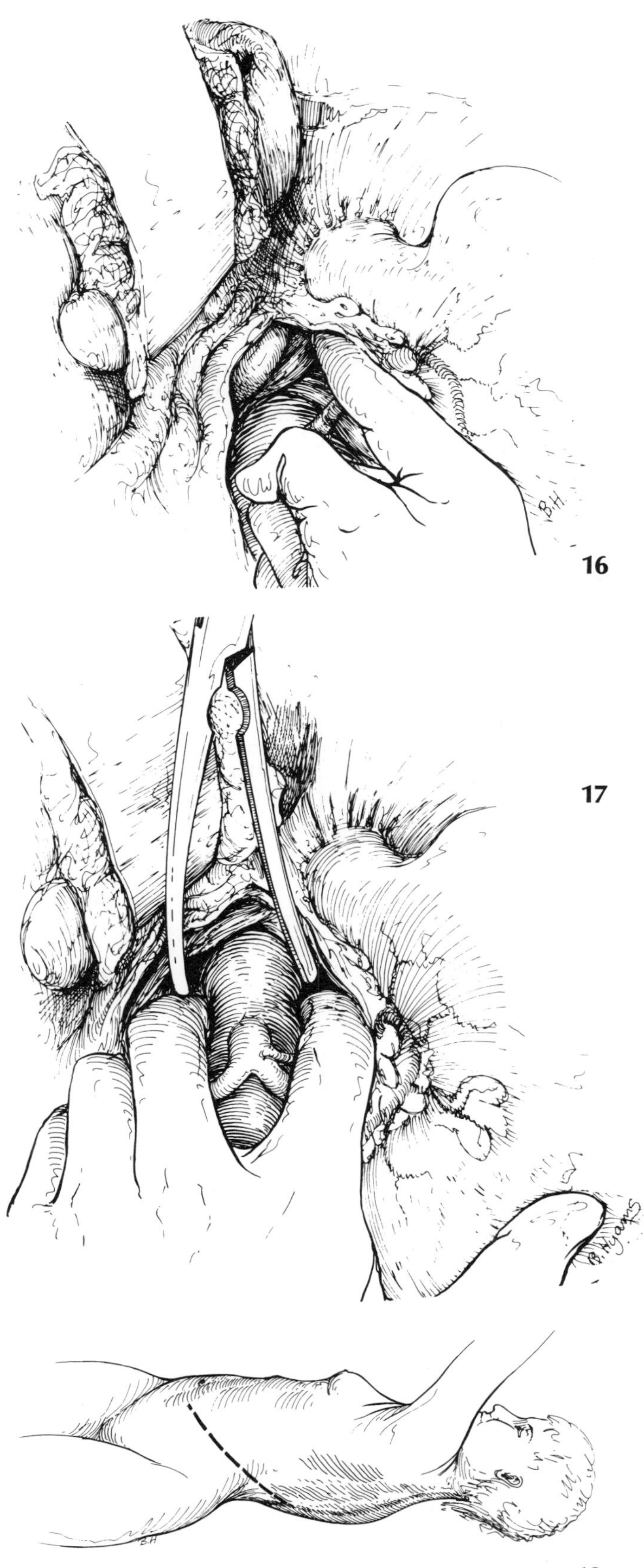

16

17

18

19, 20 & 21

The neck of the aneurysm can be exposed without difficulty below the left renal artery for application of a clamp. In those instances where aneurysmal disease extends to the region of the renal vessels, this approach can be ideal. It enables easy suprarenal control and the Dacron is tailored to enable a single oblique suture line to incorporate the origins of the renal arteries as shown. Exposure of the right common iliac artery is sometimes difficult with this approach and control of the vessel with a balloon catheter after the aneurysm has been opened is sometimes preferable. The operation is otherwise conducted as in the anterior approach. The aneurysm wall is closed back over the prosthesis at the completion of the procedure. Obviously, no closure of the periaortic tissues or the parietal peritoneum is possible or necessary.

We have not found retroperitoneal exposure to reduce operative time, operative blood loss or postoperative hospital stay, as has been claimed by some authors. In fact, postoperative discomfort, in our experience, is greater with this incision than with the midline abdominal incision. However, bowel function does appear to return earlier in the postoperative period with this approach.

We believe the retroperitoneal approach is relatively contraindicated in patients with right iliac aneurysms. These aneurysms would otherwise need to be dealt with through a separate right lower quadrant transperitoneal or retroperitoneal incision. We also believe that adequate exposure with this approach is difficult to achieve in patients with a high narrow costal arch in whom the distance from the incision to the diaphragm is great, mandating that the operation take place almost entirely underneath the shelf of the rib cage.

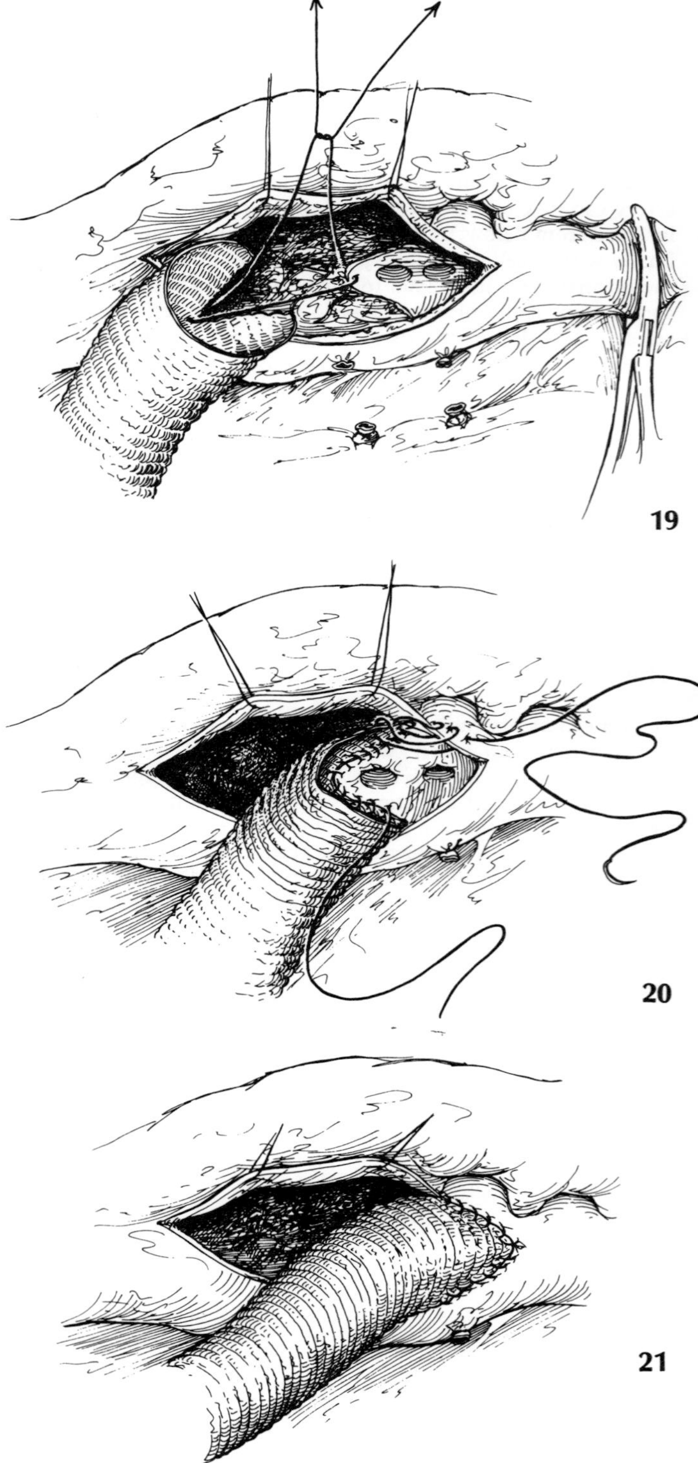
19

20

21

References

Creech, O., Jr (1966). Endo-aneurysmorrhaphy and treatment of aortic aneurysm. *Annals of Surgery* **164**, 935.

Javid, H., Julian, O. C., Dye, W. S., *et al.* (1982). Complications of abdominal aortic grafts. *Archives of Surgery* **85**, 650.

Whittemore, A. D., Clowes, A. W., Hechtman, H. B. and Mannick, J. A. (1980). Aortic aneurysm repair. Reduced operative mortality associated with maintenance of optimal cardiac performance. *Annals of Surgery* **192**, 414.

Williams, G. M., Ricotta, J., Zinner, M. and Burdick, J. (1980). The extended retroperitoneal approach for treatment of extensive atherosclerosis of the aorta and renal vessels. *Surgery* **88**, 846.

Surgery for vasculogenic impotence

RALPH DePALMA MD

Chairman, Department of Surgery, George Washington University Medical Center, Washington, D.C., USA

MICHAEL J. OLDING MD

Department of Surgery, George Washington University Medical Center, Washington, D.C., USA

Introduction

Operations for vasculogenic impotence are performed on large arteries: aortoiliac to distal branching of the internal iliacs, small arteries including the internal pudendal, proper penile arteries, and upon the venous penile drainage. The physiological basis for erection depends on adequate arterial inflow combined with closure of cavernous veins, both mediated by an intact neural mechanism. In selecting candidates for operation, an accurate diagnosis of a physiological defect is essential. Only 5–6% of impotent men are candidates for vascular interventions. Vascular impotence can be purely arteriogenic, purely venogenic, or combined arterial and venogenic. It has recently been shown that arterial inflow mediates cavernosal closure of venous outflow. During normal erection, intracavernosal pressure increases to levels approximating 80 mmHg, with little or no cavernosal venous outflow. Preoperative physiological testing for surgery outlined by De Palma *et al.* (1987) and Michal (1985) is described. Before any microvascular procedure, study of venous dynamics and arteriography are needed (DePalma, 1992).

Preoperative considerations

Penile brachial pressure indices (PBPI)

Reappearance of Doppler signals are detected distal to a pressure cuff placed at the base of the penis. The pressure is noted and expressed as a ratio between pressure in the distal branches of dorsal arteries over systemic pressure. A ratio above 0.75 in the flaccid state suggests that no major obstacle exists to blood flow in the aortoiliac system. PBPI may not detect lesions of the pudendal or penile arteries, which do not become evident until demand is placed on these vessels by the erectile process.

Penile pulse volume recording

Using an air plethysmographic cuff with a transducer contained, penile expansion in response to flow is recorded in the flaccid state. The variables characterizing pulse wave are crest time, waveform and the presence or absence of dicrotic notch. The waveform reflects the pulsatility, i.e. the contribution of all the arterial elements of penile expansion. It more sensitively separates impotent from potent patients in whom borderline PBPIs range from 0.6 to 0.75 (Stauffer and DePalma, 1983). It also detects small vessel disease when PBPIs are normal.

Artificial erection, cavernosal artery closing pressure and cavernosometry

These tests require injection of a pharmacological agent (e.g. papaverine) to produce an artificial erection. Two 19-gauge needles are inserted into the cavernous bodies, one for pressure recording and one for calibrated infusion of warm heparinized saline. Infusion rates to obtain and maintain erection are measured. These rates are compared before and after papaverine injection. A maintenance rate of less than 40–80 ml suggests absence of cavernosal leak or venogenic impotence. During artificial erection, Doppler flow probes placed at the base of the penis and directed toward each cavernosal body respectively can detect disappearance of deep cavernosal flow. The values obtained indicate pressure available for erection through each of the deep cavernosal arteries. The usual pressure obtained on cavernosometry during erection is 80 mmHg; higher pressures are produced during contraction of the muscles of the pelvic floor.

Duplex scanning

Using duplex scanning, both deep cavernosal arteries are examined at intervals before and after papaverine injection. Observation of these arteries and knowledge of the flow diameter and velocity detected by Doppler ultrasound signals provide estimates of total flow. Further experience in duplex scanning is needed to relate abnormalities to sites of vascular obstruction. Failure of cavernosal vessels to dilate can be due to proximal or distal obstruction.

Physiological examinations to provide quantitative data on impaired erectile haemodynamics are essential for proper patient selection. Comprehensive physiological study for surgical candidates cannot be totally non-invasive. Cavernosometry quantitates cavernosal leakage and angiographic studies are needed to display abnormal anatomy.

Preoperative angiographic studies

Cavernosograms obtained during cavernosometry and artificial erection delineate sites of venous leakage. Conventional arteriography demonstrates large vessel occlusive disease and is selected when PBPI is grossly abnormal. Highly selective internal pudendal arteriography using pharmacoangiography is required to display pudendal and penile arterial anatomy.

Neural studies

To ensure intact nervous mechanisms, measurement of bulbocavernous reflex amplitude and time and pudendal-evoked potentials are used. These rule out neurogenic impotence which contraindicates a vascular operation.

Hormonal studies

Abnormalities can be found in serum prolactin and testosterone levels. Most commonly, blood glucose levels are abnormal. Thyroid and renal function tests should be obtained preoperatively.

Operative considerations

This chapter considers procedures for impotence on the internal illiac artery, small arteries (i.e. dorsal penile) and deep dorsal vein arterialization for mixed impotence. Venous ablation for cavernosal leak syndrome use a variety of approaches depending on demonstrated sites of venous leakage. These approaches are still evolutionary and will only be outlined. The candidate for vascular surgical correction of impotence must exhibit an identifiable physiological and anatomic vascular defect in the absence of neurogenic or hormonal causes of impotence.

Operations on large arteries

Operative steps in aortoiliac surgery to prevent sexual dysfunction and restore potency have been described (DePalma, 1985; DePalma *et al.*, 1988). These operations provide flow to the interal ililac arteries and avoid disruption of neural arcs. Operations for impotence *per se* on the large arteries involve mainly those done in isolated internal iliac artery disease.

Internal iliac endarterectomy or bypass

1

With the patient in the supine position, an incision is made just through the fascial layers at the lateral border of the rectus sheath. The peritoneum remains intact and is reflected medially. This method provides a wider exposure than the previously described muscle-splitting incision (DePalma, 1985). The exposure obtained allows proximal control of the origin of the internal iliac and the common and external iliac arteries. The lateral as opposed to a medial approach enhances internal iliac exposure. Distal control of the internal iliac is obtained at its division into anterior and posterior branches as the superior gluteal exits through the greater sciatic foramen.

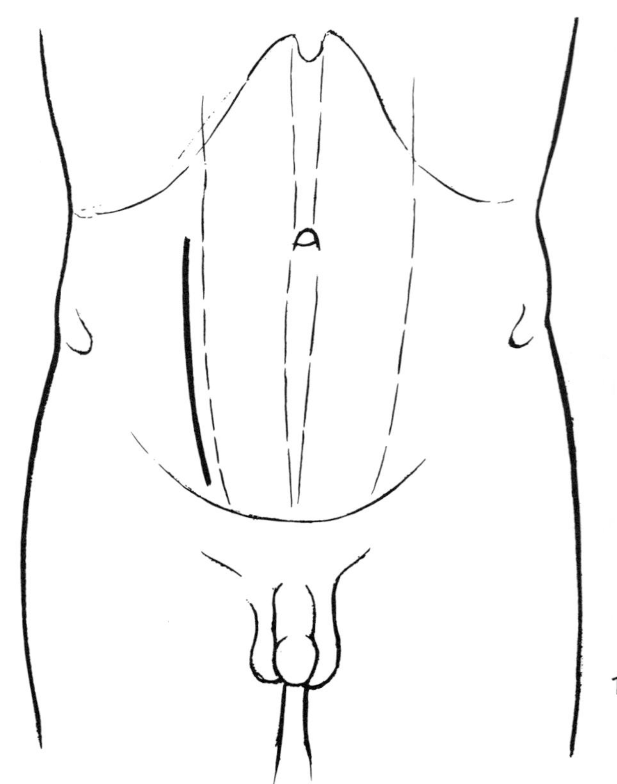

1

2

After systemic heparinization, endarterectomy is carried out and the artery closed with 4/0 or 5/0 prolene.

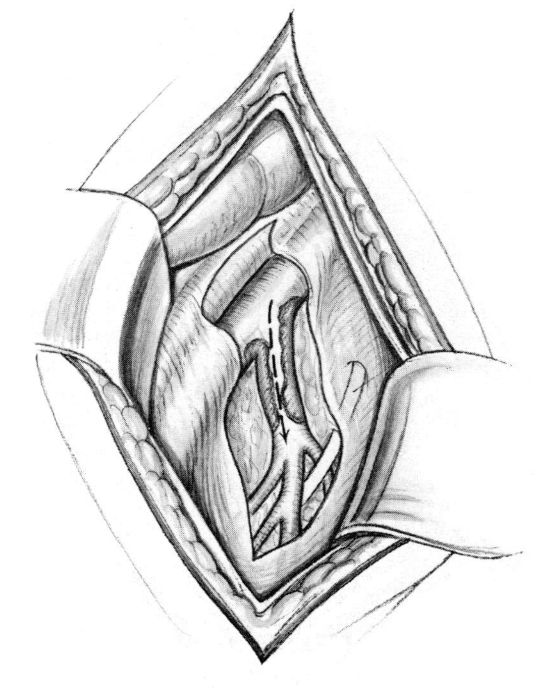

2

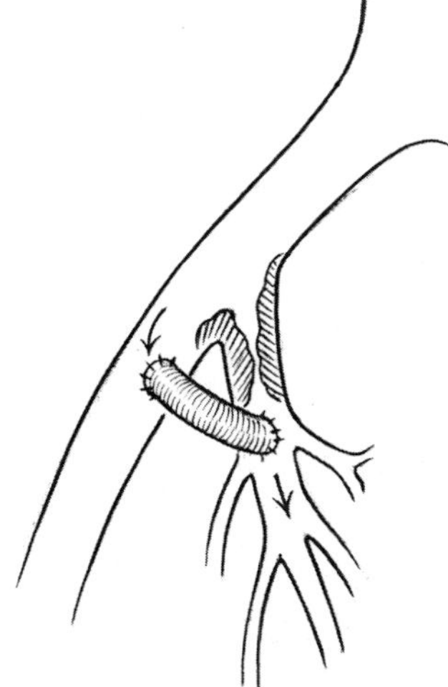

3

3

In cases of diffuse disease, a vein bypass from the external iliac to the branching of the internal iliac can be employed. After bypass heparinization is reversed.

The extraperitoneal incision is closed with 0 polydioxanone (PDS) in the confluence of the layers comprising the edge of the rectus sheath and the combined abdominal layers.

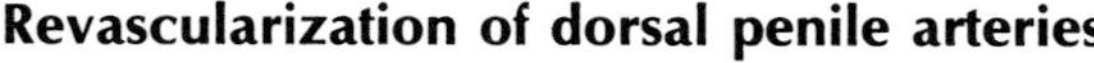

Revascularization of dorsal penile arteries

4 & 5

Revascularization of dorsal penile arteries requires adequate retrograde flow into the deep cavernosal artery or the presence of accessory deep cavernosal branches connecting the dorsal penile and cavernosal systems so that antegrade perfusion occurs. A double end-to-end anastomosis may offer a technical advantage for proximal and distal perfusion when the anatomy permits. The vessel diameter distal to an occlusion site is small, i.e. less than 1.5 mm; however, in most cases it is adequate for anastomosis using standard microvascular techniques. Heparin is not used; the patient is given aspirin 320 mg preoperatively.

Penile arteriographic findings suitable for dorsal bypass must be obtained. These studies are obtained using artificial erection. Intraoperative visual assessment is often quite helpful.

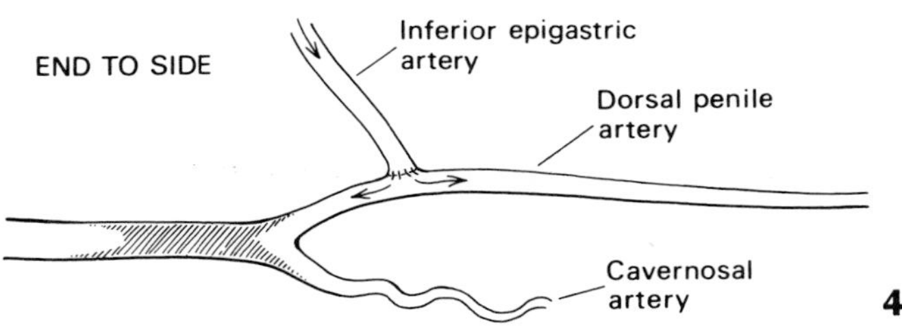

4

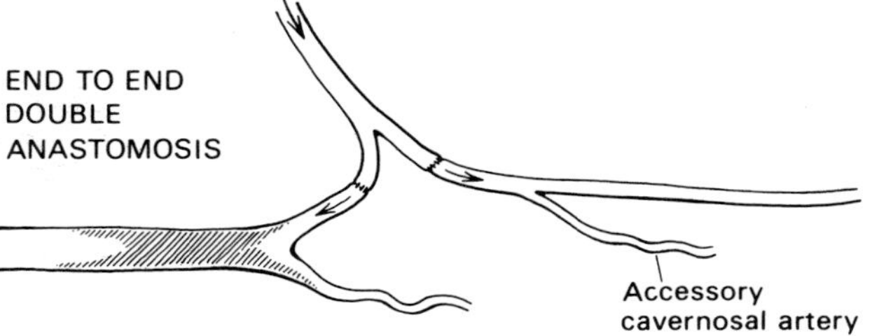

5

6

The inferior epigastric artery is the usual vessel of choice. The length required extends from its origin from the external iliac to 25 mm above the umbilicus. Small vein grafts originating from the common femoral artery or the inferior epigastric artery can be used when this vessel is insufficient. This has not occurred in the senior author's experience. A paramedian incision just medial to the lateral edge of the rectus sheath is used for exposure. The incision extends to at least 25 mm above the umbilicus. A midline incision can also be used to mobilize both inferior epigastric arteries; here exposure is slightly more difficult as more retraction of the recti is needed. Side branches are ligated with fine silk suture and fine vessels closed using bipolar cautery.

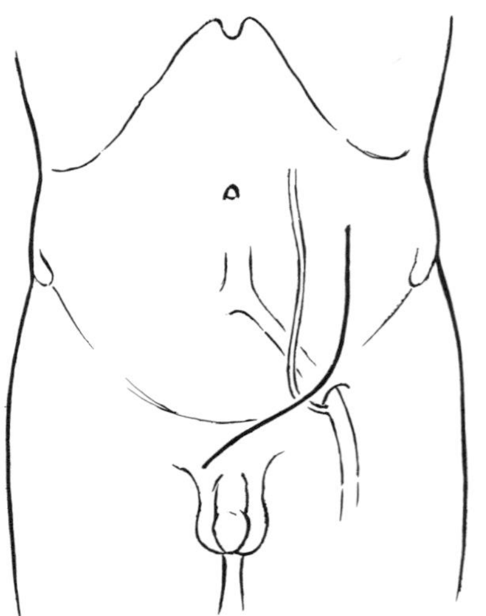

6

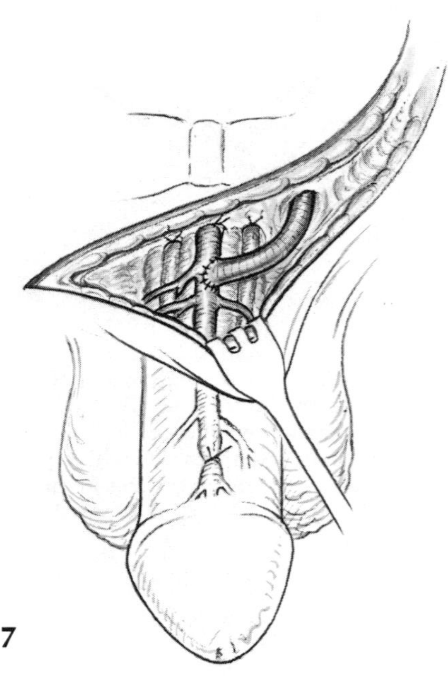

7

7

Bipolar cautery and loupe magnification are essential in penile dissection for precise haemostatic control and to avoid neural damage. Final preparation and anastomosis of the donor and recipient vessel ends are performed with the aid of an operating microscope using standard microsurgical techniques and interrupted 10/0 nylon on a BV 75 μ or BV 50 μ needle. An end-to-side anastomosis is preferred whenever possible, i.e. between, for example, the donor inferior epigastric and one of the laterally placed dorsal penile arteries. This obviates the need to rely on an accessory corpus vessel. Anastomotic patency is assessed using the strip patency test.

The rectus sheath is closed with interrupted 0 PDS. An aperture in the inferior fascial portion is created so that the inferior epigastric graft pedicle passes without fascial impediment to the dorsal penile artery.

Deep dorsal vein arterialization for mixed vasculogenic impotence

8

These operations are used for mixed vasculogenic impotence, i.e. arteriogenic and venous. The usual abnormalities are aplasia or hypoplasia of dorsal penile arteries, distal penile occlusive disease, and venous leakage.

Variations in this technique have been describrd by Virag *et al.* (1983). Their technique is depicted showing the donor artery anastomosed end-to-side to the centrally situated deep dorsal vein of the penis, with distal vein ligation.

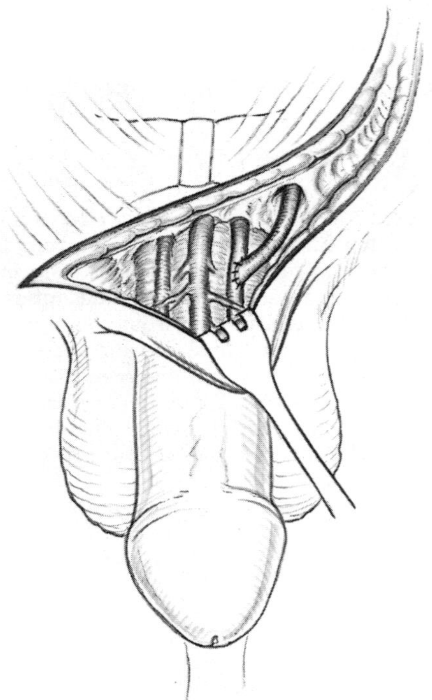

8

9

Other variations include abandoning venocavernostomy. An important pitfall has been found to be the occurrence of glans hyperemia. This now contraindicates valve ablation and suggests wider application of distal vein ligation. The proximal vein is usually ligated.

10

Hauri's (1985) variation is shown, where an arteriovenous fistula is fashioned between a dorsal artery and the dorsal vein for joint anastomosis of these to the end of the donor artery.

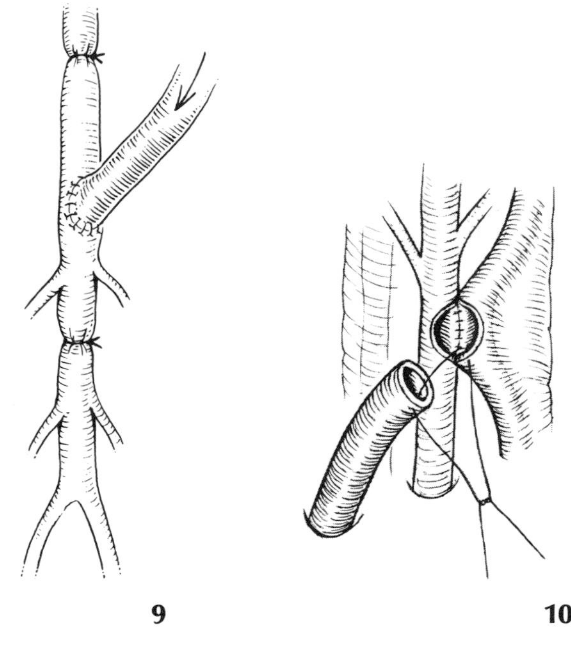

9 10

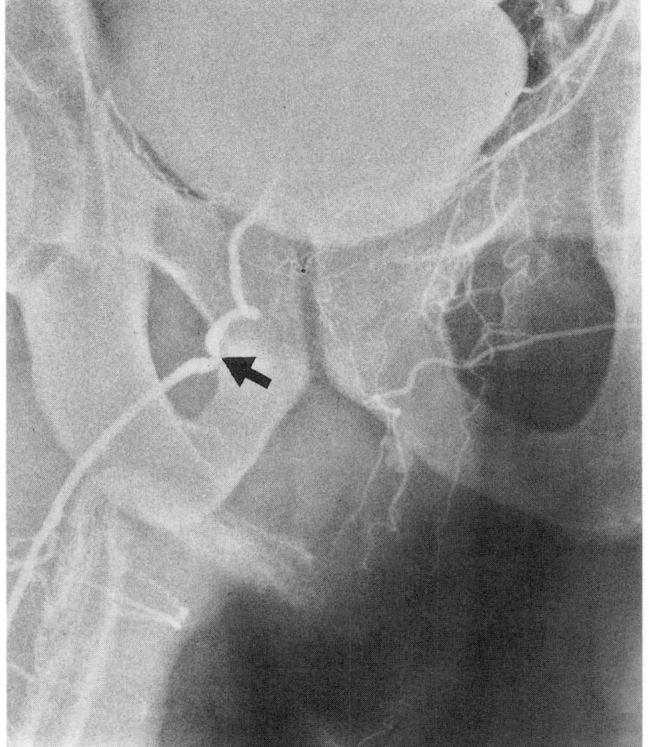

11

11

Postoperative arteriography at 1 year shows a patent epigastric artery to dorsal vein fistula with run-off via the circumflex penile veins into the spongiosum. This patient continued to be potent but later required transluminal angioplasty. Dorsal vein arterialization has been shown to be an effective procedure for mixed arterial and venous impotence (Knoll, Furlow and Benson, 1992; Melman and Riccardi, 1993), as well as for arteriogenic impotence with atretic penile arteries, while large vessel interventions such as internal iliac artery interventions are more securely based.

Venous interruption for cavernosal leak

These operations are useful in increasing response to intracavernous injection. The dorsal penile vein is first resected from the penile hilum to the sulcus behind the glans. Exposure of the deep dorsal vein and its proximal ligation at the hilum of the penis are facilitated by division of the suspensory ligament. For this procedure, either a transverse or a lateral pen-scrotal incision is used. The latter avoids section of lymphatics and produces much less oedema. Ligation of the periprostatic venous plexus in the space of Retzius using an extraperitoneal incision and crural plication using a perineal incision have also been performed. To assess efficacy of venous interruption, postoperative dynamic infusion cavernosometry and cavernosography have been used by our group (Yu *et al.*, 1992). This assures as complete an interruption of abnormal cavernous drainage as possible and documents increased postoperative intracavernous pressure. After the initial response to operation decreases, many of these men now respond to intracavernous injections.

References

De Palma, R. G. (1985). Prevention of sexual dysfunction in aortoiliac surgery. In *Current Operative Surgery – Vascular Surgery*. Jamieson, C. W. ed. London: Baillière Tindall.

DePalma, R. G., Emsellem, H. A., Edwards, C. M., Druy, E. M., Schultz, S. W., Miller, H. C. and Bergsrud, D. (1987). A screening sequence for vasculogenic impotence. *Journal of Vascular Surgery* **5**, 228.

DePalma, R. G., Edwards, C. M., Schwab, F. J. and Steinberg, D. L. (1988). Modern management of impotence associated with aortic surgery. In *Arterial Surgery: New Diagnostic and Operative Techniques*. Bergan, J. J. and Yao, J. S. T., eds. London and San Diego: Grune and Stratton.

DePalma, R. G., Dalton, C. M., Gomez, C. A., *et al.* (1992). Predictive value of a screening sequence for venogenic impotence. *International Journal of Impotence Research* **4**, 143.

Hauri, D. (1985). Operative Moglichkeiten bei der vaskular bedingten Impotenz. *Angio Archiv* **8**, 25.

Knoll, L. D., Furlow, W. L. and Benson, R. C. (1992). Deep dorsal vein arterialization in the management of cavernosal venous leakage. *International Journal of Impotence Research* **4**, Suppl. 2, A133.

Melman, A. and Riccardi, R. Jr (1993). *International Journal of Impotence Research* **5**, 47.

Michal, V. (1985). Arteriogenic impotence. *Angio Archiv* **8**, 4.

Stauffer, D. and DePalma, R. G. (1983). A comparison of penile–brachial index and penile pulse volume recordings. *Bruit* **17**, 29.

Virag, R., Frydman, D., Legman, H., *et al.* (1983). Possibilities chirurgicales dans l'impuissance vasculaire. *Gaz. Med. France* **90**, 2031.

Yu, G. W., Schwab, F. J., Melograna, F. S., DePalma, R. G., Miller, H. C. and Richolt (1992). *Journal of Urology* **147**, 618.

Axillofemoral bypass

SVEN-ERIK BERGENTZ MD

Department of Surgery, Lund University, Malmö General Hospital, Malmö, Sweden

Introduction

Axillofemoral bypass was first performed in 1962 by Blaisdell and Hall (1963) in the USA and by Louw (1963) in South Africa. The former operation was performed for an occluded abdominal aortic aneurysm, the latter for arteriosclerotic occlusive disease.

The technique for this operation should be known by all vascular surgeons, but it should not be used very often. The most important indication is when a standard aortic reconstruction is precluded due to aortic graft infection, an aortoenteric fistula, or intra-abdominal sepsis (Bergqvist *et al.*, 1987). The operation may also be used when there is a colostomy-ileostomy, or other types of enterocutaneous fistula. Another indication is dense abdominal adhesions, following previous surgery or irradiation. Threatening limb loss in high-risk patients due to severe cardiac or pulmonary disease is a rare indication in our institution. A rare and controversial use of axillofemoral bypass is for non-resective treatment of an abdominal aortic aneurysm after induction of acute thrombosis of the aneurysm by bilateral iliac artery ligation (Schwartz, Nichols and Silver, 1986).

Axillofemoral bypass is contraindicated in extensive subclavian or axillary artery occlusive disease. As outflow vessel, a patent deep femoral artery, and/or superficial femoral artery, is mandatory.

Preoperative evaluation

With regard to the inflow vessels, preoperative blood pressure measurements in both arms and auscultation over subclavian and axillary arteries are important. The right axillary artery is usually preferred as inflow vessel since stenotic lesions in the subclavian artery are three to four times more common on the left than on the right side. If, however, the blood pressure is more than about 20 mm Hg higher on the left side, this side should be preferred. If the blood pressure is low bilaterally, or if there are murmurs to be heard over the subclavian and axillary arteries, arteriography of the aortic arch and its branches should be performed.

If an axillofemoral graft is indicated, there is usually a need to vascularize both legs. Originally, this was done by performing one axillofemoral bypass on each side, but now we prefer to use axillofemoral bypass on one side, and add a cross-over graft to the contralateral groin ('axillobifemoral bypass'). This will increase the flow in the long axillofemoral graft, which decreases the risk of occlusion.

The operation

1

Anaesthesia, positioning and draping

Axillofemoral bypass may be performed under local anaesthesia, but light general anaesthesia is preferable. This gives better airway control and ventilation and is usually well tolerated even by debilitated patients.

The patient lies in a supine position with the arm on the ipsilateral side placed on an armboard, at right angles to the body. This arm is draped free and is mobile during the operation. Abduction of the arm moves the clavicle upwards, facilitating access to the first part of the axillary artery. Chest, neck, upper arm, abdomen, both groins, and upper parts of the thighs should be draped. The contralateral arm is used for blood pressure recording, sampling and infusions.

It is sometimes recommended to use two teams to speed up the operation. We prefer using one team, although the dissection of the axillary and femoral vessels may sometimes be carried out simultaneously by two surgeons.

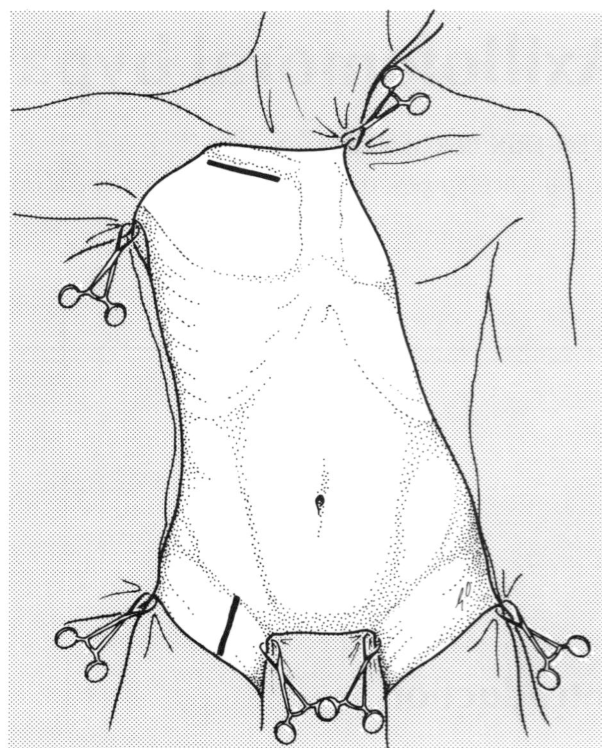

1

2

Axillary artery dissection

The axillary artery lies behind and slightly above the axillary vein. It is divided into three parts, in relation to its relation to the pectoralis minor muscle. The first is located medial to, the second behind and the third lateral to this muscle. The axillary artery is crossed by the lateral and medial anterior thoracic (pectoral) nerves, innervating the pectoralis major muscle. The first part of the axillary artery gives off one branch, the highest thoracic artery. The second part, behind the pectoralis minor, usually gives off two branches. The first and, to some extent, the second part of the artery should be used for the anastomosis, since this is the fulcrum when the arm is abducted. Therefore, traction of the axillary artery by the graft is minimized.

If at least one of the common, deep or superficial femoral arteries are known to be patent, the operation starts by exploring the axillary artery. An incision is made about 2 cm below and parallel to the clavicle. Its length should be about 8 cm. The transversely running fibres of the pectoralis major muscle are split between its clavicular and sternal heads. The pectoralis minor muscle is identified behind the costoclavicular fascia. This muscle might be divided close to the clavicle, but sometimes it is possible to retract at least part of it laterally. The axillary vein is now exposed, lying anterior and inferior to the artery.

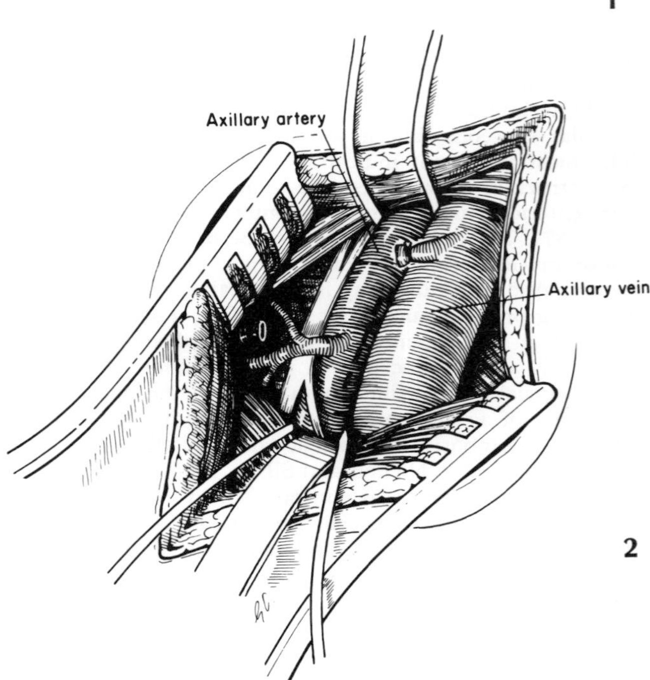

2

Ligation of branches to the vein, particularly those crossing in front of the axillary artery, is necessary for the mobilization. The middle part of the axillary artery now emerges below the clavicle. There are usually two branches from this part, and one from the first part of the artery which should be divided. Polyethylene tubing around the artery facilitates its mobilization. About 5–6 cm of the axillary artery should be mobilized.

3

Femoral artery dissection

The femoral artery is now dissected via a longitudinal incision over the common femoral artery. If it is not known that the common femoral artery or at least one of its branches is patent, the operation should start with a groin dissection. The common, superficial and deep femoral arteries are mobilized. A part of the inguinal ligament may be divided to facilitate a proximal dissection of the common femoral artery if necessary. In the relatively uncommon situation, when it is known from a good angiography that both the superficial and deep femoral arteries are patent and without stenosis in the beginning, the anastomosis may be performed to the common femoral artery. Usually, the superficial femoral artery is occluded and the deep femoral artery is often stenotic at its beginning. In these situations the deep femoral artery must be dissected to, or even beyond, its first muscular branches, thereby also dividing the lateral circumflex vein.

If the groin has been used for previous anastomosis, or is infected, the deep femoral arteries may be approached by incisions a few centimetres lateral and distal to the original groin incision. The sartorius muscle is drawn medially, exposing the deep femoral artery, which can be mobilized to a length of several centimetres.

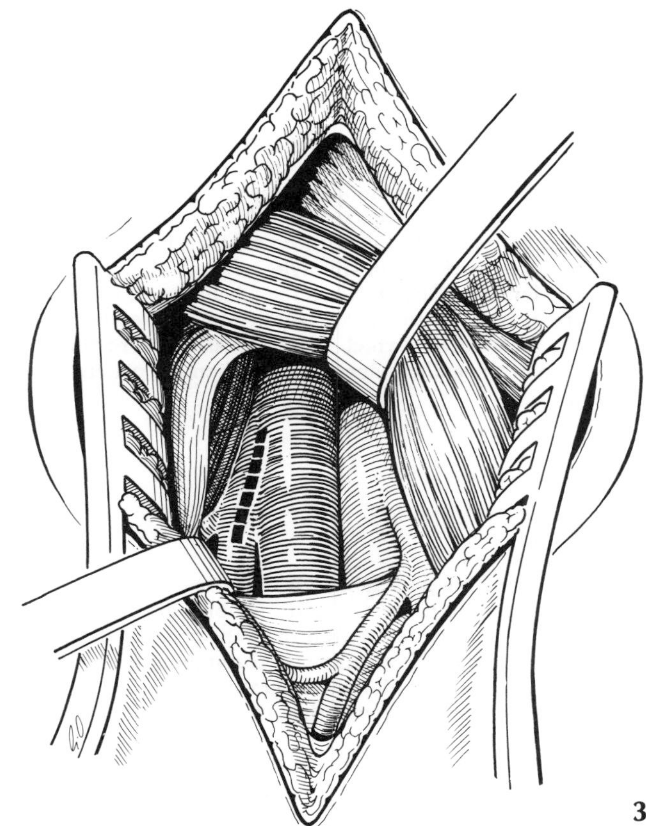

3

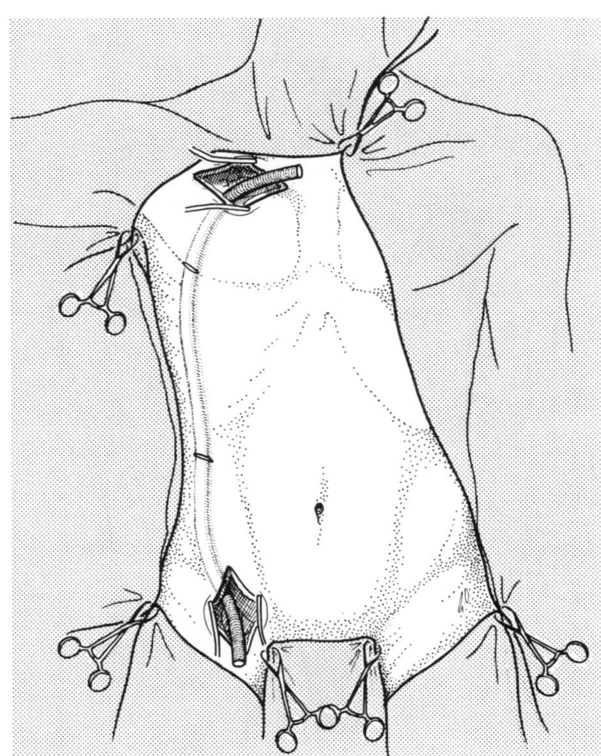

4

4

Axillofemoral tunnel

The tunnel for the graft starts from the axillary incision deep to the pectoralis major muscle. In the beginning it should go in a lateral-caudal direction, the angle to the axillary artery being between 30 and 40°. When the tunnel reaches the midaxillary line (where an incision might be necessary to facilitate the formation of the tunnel), it should be directed caudal to the anterior superior iliac spine, and from there it should continue to the groin. It is important to avoid having the prosthesis anteriorly. This may result in compression of the prosthesis to the costal margin, or kinking when the patient bends.

Selection, preparation and placement of graft

We prefer an 8–10 mm knitted Dacron graft. Careful preclotting is important to avoid haematoma formation in the long tunnel. At least 50 ml of blood is necessary for this long graft. Excellent results have been reported by the use of externally supported grafts but no randomized trial has been performed to prove the superiority of this type of graft. The polytetrafluoroethylene (PTFE) graft has the advantage of precluding preclotting, and it also makes thrombectomy easier. It is, however, non-elastic, which might possibly contribute to disruption of the axillary anastomosis when the patient raises the arm.

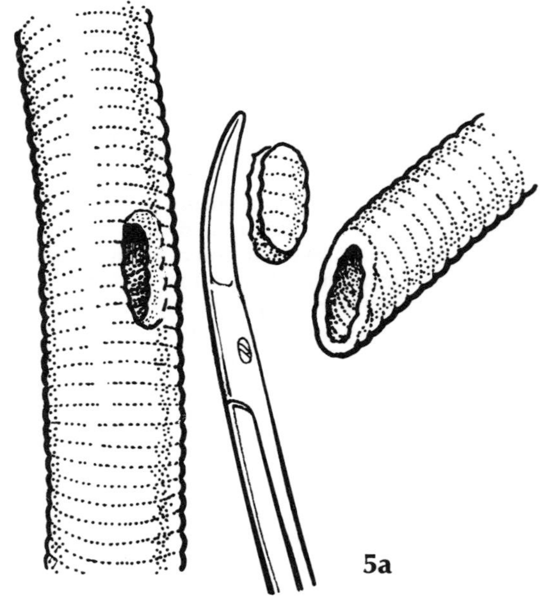

5a

5a & b

Bifemoral grafts are preferable whenever feasible. These can be done with a single graft to the femoral artery with the addition of a femorofemoral graft from the groin of the donor side. This technique allows high flow throughout the length of the main stem of the axillofemoral graft. The femorofemoral graft should be 2 mm narrower than the main graft to obtain a reasonable high flow rate.

There are alternatives to the technique shown in *b*. The femorofemoral branch can be anastomosed to the axillofemoral graft at a right angle or higher up with a more sloping angle. Experimental comparisons between these two techniques have shown that the latter gives a higher flow in the cross-over branch, and also avoids turbulence in the bifurcation. A prospective randomized trial has been performed comparing these techniques. There was no difference regarding the effect on ankle pressure, nor regarding the 2-year patency of the main stem of the axillofemoral graft or the ipsilateral extension of the graft. There was, however, a twofold increase in the occlusion rate of the cross-over branch when the 90° branching was used, compared with the more sloping technique with a higher anastomosis (Wittens, van Houtte and van Urk, 1992). Alternatively a ready made axillobifemoral graft, commercially available, can be selected. This avoids the need for the additional Dacron–Dacron anastomosis shown in *a* and *b*. The ready made axillobifemoral grafts have 90° and also more sloping cross-over angles to meet the surgeon's preference.

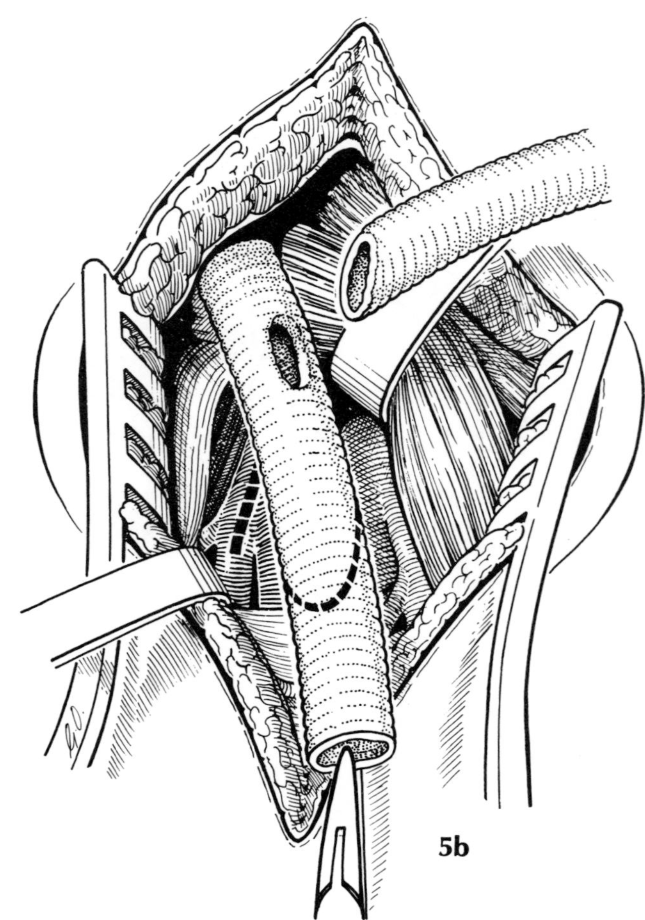

5b

The proximal anastomosis

6

The axillary artery is elevated into the field by traction of the slings encircling the artery. A 2-cm long arteriotomy is made in the anterior and inferior aspect of the axillary artery as far medially as possible. The graft is bevelled at an angle of 30–40°. A 5/0 synthetic double-armed vascular suture is used. The prosthesis is placed anterior to the axillary vein. The sutures are started at the lateral and at the medial ends of the arteriotomy. The back wall of the graft is sutured to the inferior part of the artery from the inside, using one end of the lateral and one end of the medial suture. These two ends are tied together at the midpoint of the back wall.

The other ends of the two sutures, the lateral and the medial, are then used to complete the anterior part of the anastomosis and meet at its midpoint. The clamps on the axillary artery are released. The graft is occluded close to the anastomosis, using a hydrogrip Fogarty clamp before the clamps on the axillary artery are released.

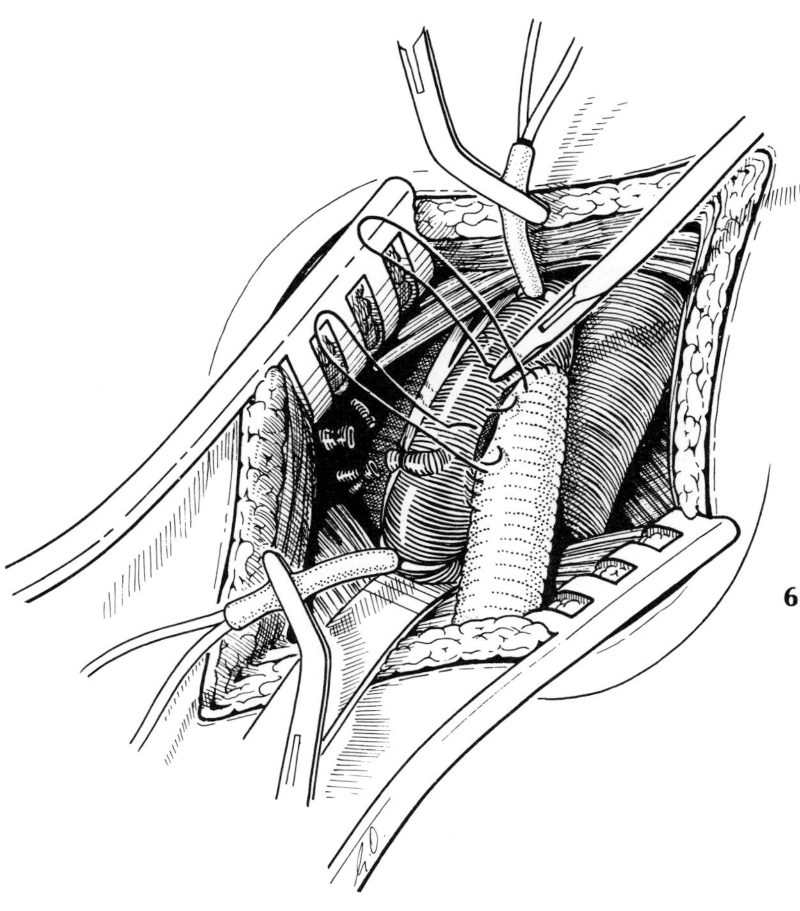

6

7

The distal anastomosis

The prosthesis is drawn from the groin incision, care being taken to avoid any twists and kinks. It is also important to avoid too much tension on the graft, which may draw the axillary artery into a Y configuration. This may result in a thrombosis of the axillary artery, or even disruption of the anastomosis, or a formation of a pseudoaneurysm.

The anastomosis between the graft and the (ipsilateral) femoral artery is made according to the principles described for aortofemoral grafting . If the common femoral artery and the superficial and/or deep femoral arteries are widely patent and without stenosis, the anastomosis is made to the common femoral artery. Very often, however, the superficial femoral artery in these patients is severely diseased or even occluded. The deep femoral artery is often stenotic at its origin. In these cases the arteriotomy of the common femoral artery is carried down 1–2 cm or even further into the deep femoral artery. The graft is formed as an onlay patch in the deep femoral artery. Endarterectomy should be avoided if possible. It it has to be done, it is important to prevent a distal flap development by using several intima-tacking sutures. Several interrupted sutures should be used to prevent purse string constriction when suturing the distal end of the patch on to the rather delicate deep femoral artery.

After completion of the distal anastomosis, the Fogarty clamp on the proximal part of the graft is released. The clamp on the proximal part of the common femoral artery is then removed, forcing the initial blood flow, with any remaining thrombotic material, debris and air bubbles, in the proximal direction. After a few pulses, the superficial and deep femoral artery clamps are removed. If a graft-to-graft anastomosis has been prepared to a femorofemoral graft, this can be used for flushing the axillofemoral graft. After that, a Fogarty clamp is placed on the cross-over graft close to the graft-to-graft anastomosis.

The anastomosis between the cross-over graft and the (contralateral) femoral artery is then performed, following the principles just described.

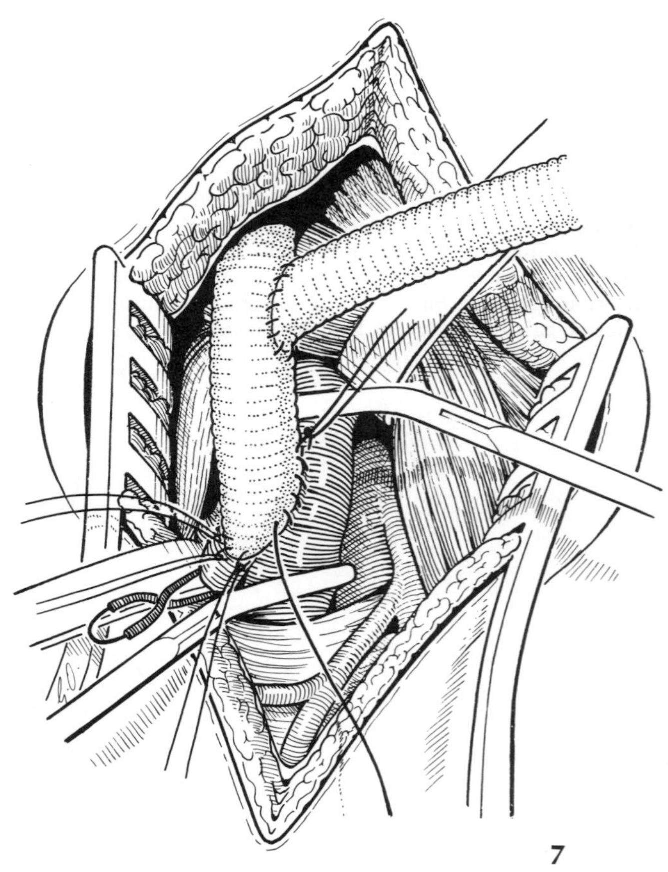

7

Arteriography is considered if there is any question of distal perfusion. A total of 30 ml of contrast medium is injected through a catheter threaded into the prosthesis proximal to the graft-to-graft anastomosis.

The axillary incisions are closed in two deep layers, approximating the fascia of the pectoralis major muscle, and the subcutaneous tissue. We prefer 3/0 synthetic absorbable suture material. The groin wounds are similarly closed in two layers of subcutaneous synthetic absorbable material. The skin is closed with interrupted 3/0 synthetic suture material.

Wound closure

Before closing the wounds, the feet should be inspected. It is usually not possible to feel any ankle pulses, but the colour and the vein-filling in the feet can give some preliminary information about the limb perfusion.

Intra- and postoperative care

Antibiotics

Prophylactic broad spectrum antibiotics, active against staphylococci, is started before surgery and continued for 48 h.

Anticoagulation

We do not use systematic heparinization during these operations. Before occluding a vessel, we irrigate carefully with heparinized saline, and inject 20–40 ml of the solution peripherally. Furthermore, we give dextran 40 in a 10% solution continuously during the operation. The dose is 500 ml during surgery, 500 ml after surgery on the day of surgery, and 500 ml a day for the first 3 postoperative days. We strongly advise the patient to stop smoking. We see no reason to recommend aspirin since it has not been shown to decrease the risk of graft occlusion.

Graft compression

It is not quite clear whether or not compression of the graft plays a role in occlusion. Nevertheless, the patient should be encouraged to avoid constricting clothing and, if possible, lying on the graft. If the patient can cooperate, he may be encouraged to palpate the pulse daily to detect graft occlusion early, which otherwise may be difficult.

Postoperative care and complications

The life-span of an axillofemoral graft can be prolonged by careful monitoring, and early intervention in the case of occlusion. Declotting of an occluded graft is usually a simple procedure, which can be performed under local anaesthesia. An intraoperative angiogram may facilitate complete removal of thrombotic material. Thromboembolic occlusion of the axillobrachial arteries may occur when the graft occludes.

Disruption of the proximal anastomosis, or formation of an anastomotic aneurysm, may occur if this anastomosis is placed too far laterally, and under too much tension.

References

Bergqvist, D., Alm, A., Claes, G., *et al.* (1987). Secondary aortoenteric fistulas – an analysis of 42 cases. *European Journal of Vascular Surgery* **1**, 11.

Blaisdell, F. W. and Hall, A. D. (1963). Axillary-femoral bypass for lower extremity ischemia. *Surgery* **54**, 563.

Louw, J. H. (1963). Splenic-to-femoral and axillary-to-femoral bypass grafts in diffuse atherosclerotic occlusive disease. *Lancet* **1**, 1401.

Schwartz, R. A., Nichols, K. W. and Silver, D. (1986). Is thrombosis of infrarenal abdominal aortic aneurysm an acceptable alternative? *Journal of Vascular Surgery* **3**, 448.

Wittens, C. H. A., van Houtte, H. J. K. P. and van Urk, H. (1992). European prospective randomised multi-centre axillo-bifemoral trial. *European Journal of Vascular Surgery* **6**, 115.

Femorofemoral bypass

P. FIORANI MD

Professor of Surgery, University Hospital of Rome, Rome, Italy

V. FARAGLIA MD
M. TAURINO MD
F. SPEZIALE MD
M. COLONNA MD

Department of Vascular Surgery, University Hospital of Rome, Rome, Italy

Introduction

Cross-over femorofemoral bypass was first proposed in clinical practice by Vetto in 1966 for the treatment of unilateral iliac obstructive lesions. Its indications were subsequently extended to an increasing number of patients with unilateral iliac lesions, obtaining satisfactory immediate and long-term results.

Clinically, there seems to be no doubt about the indications, while special attention should be paid to the haemodynamic assessment of the donor iliofemoral axis due to its involvement with immediate patency and long-term evolution.

Indications

The clinical indications for revascularization by cross-over femorofemoral bypass include unilateral stenotic-obstructive lesions of the iliac axis with claudication of limited autonomy or with rest ischaemia, showing general or local contraindications for conventional revascularization (Eugene, Goldstone and Moore, 1977; Whittemore *et al.*, 1980).

General contraindications are represented by advanced age, severe cardiorespiratory failure, or of other systems, the presence of metabolic imbalance or limited life-expectancy (Vijayanager, Bogudo and Eckstein, 1982). This procedure is extra-abdominal, feasible under local anaesthesia, requires a short operative time and involves only a minor surgical trauma. Local contraindications are represented by the presence, near the aorta, of an infected area or marked sclerosis due to previous surgery, retroperitoneal fibrosis or possible onset of septic foci because of iatrogenic lesions from abdominal surgery as well as from possible peripheral trophic lesions. The presence of extensive lesions of the host femoral axis which may affect the immediate result in terms of patency, can be considered a further local contraindication for major abdominal surgery. Moreover, cross-over femorofemoral bypass is indicated for acute thrombosis of the iliac axis and for occlusion of the branch of a previous aortofemoral bypass (Rutherford, Patt and Pearce, 1987).

Special indications for this procedure include the need to preserve the erectile function by preventing iatrogenic lesions of the pelvic splanchnic nerves of the preaortic plexus, in patients affected by morbid obesity (De Laurentis *et al.*, 1978) or previously treated with radiation therapy at the level of the pelvis or retroperitoneum. Together with clinical indications, problems related to haemodynamic peformance should also be considered. They concern both the host and donor limbs. The host artery frequently shows a femoropopliteal lesion, and thus it should be assessed whether the deep femoral artery is able to ensure adequate perfusion of the limb or not (Nelelsteen *et al.*, 1980; Martinez, Hertzer and Beven, 1980). As for the donor limb, the problem is more complex because obstructive lesions present at this level can be the cause of flow diversion which leads to distal ischaemia (the steal phenomenon).

The steal phenomenon

In 1968, based on observations of patients treated with a cross-over femorofemoral bypass for unilateral iliac obstructive lesions, and who developed ischaemia of the donor limb, explained by a diversion of blood flow between the lower limbs (i.e. the steal phenomenon), and based on other evidence (Harper *et al.*, 1967), Ehrenfeld carried out a canine experiment to try to understand the problem more fully. By modifying the inflow pressure of the donor axis and the peripheral resistance by the creation of an aortovenous fistula, Ehrenfeld was able to demonstrate that lesion-free iliac arteries are able to increase their flow ten fold, allowing them to perfuse proximally as well as contralaterally.

When an iliac artery is significantly stenosed, the flow required by both limbs cannot be satisfied. If distal to the donor axis the peripheral resistance is higher than in the contralateral axis due to femoropopliteal lesions, a femorofemoral revascularization would result in ischaemic symptoms in the donor limb. Therefore, it is important to determine whether a stenotic lesion is present or not. However, even in the presence of a 50% stenosis, this procedure can still be indicated for elderly and non-ambulatory patients. On the other hand, 30% stenosis is considered the limit for young patients with patent infrainguinal arteries who are likely to experience vasodilatation during exercise, and who therefore require an additional blood flow (Hill, Lord and Tracy, 1982).

However, in some cases postoperative ischaemia of the donor limb can be ascribed to a faulty surgical technique (stenosed anastomosis or embolization) or to a progressive distal atherosclerosis.

Preoperative assessment

The integrity of the donor iliac axis is mandatory to ensure perfusion of both limbs. Therefore, clinical, morphological and haemodynamic testing is proposed, both while the patient is at rest and while exercising the lower limbs.

Clinical testing is based on a normal femoral pulse and the absence of bruits both in the iliac artery and iliac fossa, an indication of the integrity of the donor iliac artery, especially when associated with an obstructive lesion of the ipsilateral femoral bifurcation.

The Doppler system is used to detect and assess possible pressure gradients, to examine the iliac vessels and any lesions, and to measure directly the pressure in the iliac and femoral arteries. The criteria proposed are that the Doppler thigh pressure should be equal to but not greater than the brachial pressure, and that the Doppler ankle pressure should be equal to or no more than 15 mmHg below the brachial pressure (McDonald *et al.*, 1978). The iliac axis is considered normal when the pressure in the femoral artery is not more than 10 mmHg below the brachial pressure. A further non-invasive procedure is to study waveform using a Doppler zero-crossing detector.

Nicolaides and Angelides (1981) modified the wave peak of a haemodynamically effective proximal stenosis to determine the pulsatility index. However, in the presence of a diffuse lesion, this procedure is not totally reliable. In the presence of a mildly stenosed lesion which might result in the steal phenomenon after maximal peripheral dilatation, active-passive or intra-arterial papaverine-induced hyperaemia tests have been proposed to stimulate this response (Flanigan *et al.*, 1984).

Angiography is considered the best form of assessment which, when adequately performed, is able to detect with lateral and oblique projections the presence of iliac stenoses not shown up by standard anteroposterior angiography, due to frequent posterior atherosclerotic plaque. Moreover, lesions at this level of the aortic and iliac bifurcation, i.e. where overlapping bone segments can block the view, can also be detected by these projections.

Surgical techniques

1 & 2

The patient is placed in the supine position and general, local or spinal anaesthesia is administered. Most surgeons make an inguinal incision along the projection of the host femoral vessels, preparing and locating with loops the common femoral, superficial and deep femoral arteries, from the orifice to the lateral femoral circumflex vein, which is ligated to expose a portion of healthy artery suitable for the anastomosis or profundaplasty (De Laurentis *et al.*, 1978; Wylie *et al.*, 1980). The donor femoral artery is then prepared using a similar incision, but more limited downwards and more extended upwards to allow the best possible exposure of the common femoral artery.

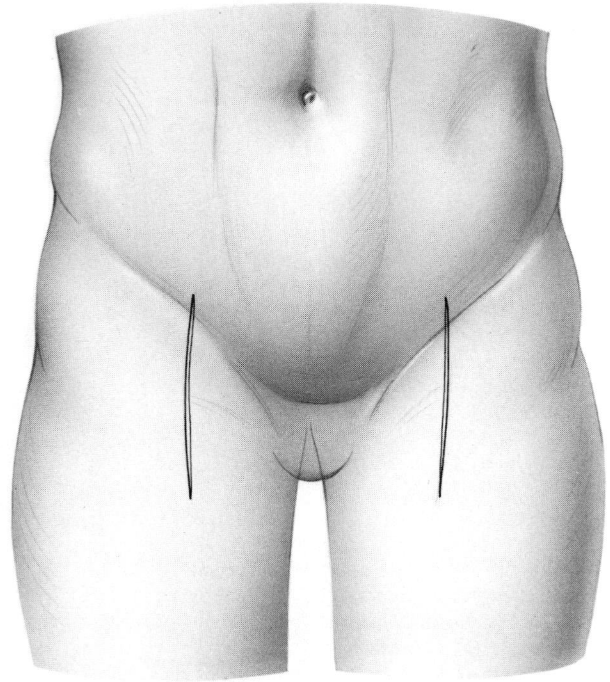

1

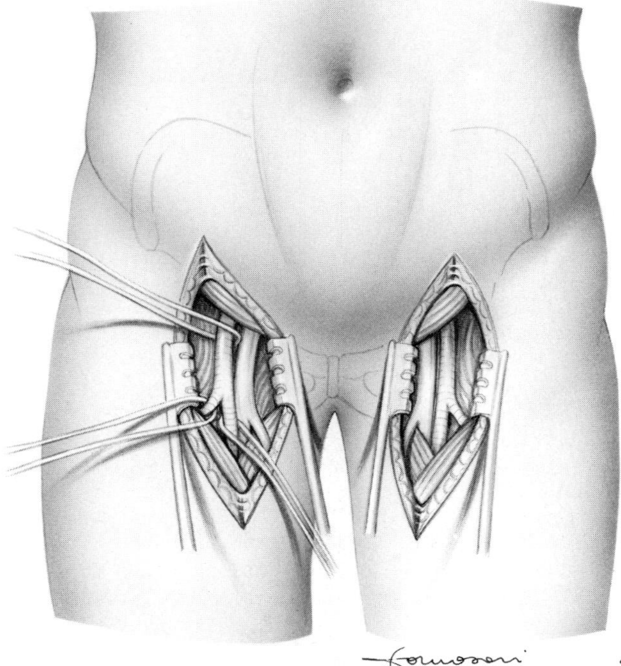

2

3, 4 & 5

The patient is heparinized and preclotted knitted Dacron is used as the prosthesis. PTFE or autologous saphenous vein can also be used, provided that their calibre is not less than 6 mm. In particular instances, it should be possible to use an autologous artery such as an endarterectomized superficial femoral artery (Blaisdell *et al.*, 1970).

Arteriotomies should be performed on the anteromedial aspect of the host vessels to avoid kinking and twisting of the graft. An oblique inflow orifice is also advisable to prevent inflow stenosis (Tyson and Reichle, 1972).

After completion of the donor anastomosis, the prosthesis is canalized bluntly up to the contralateral groin following a subcutaneous course. This is then reversed to form a 'U'-shaped subcutaneous bypass.

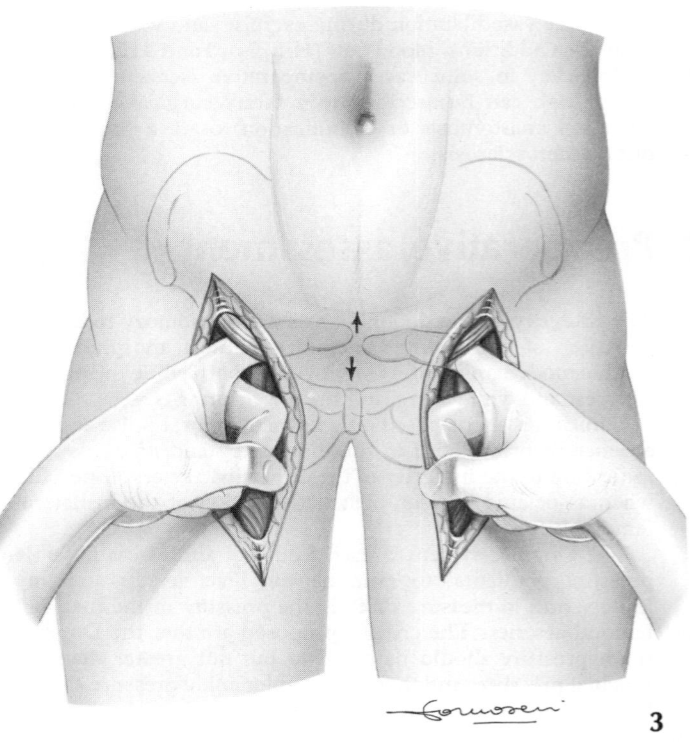

3

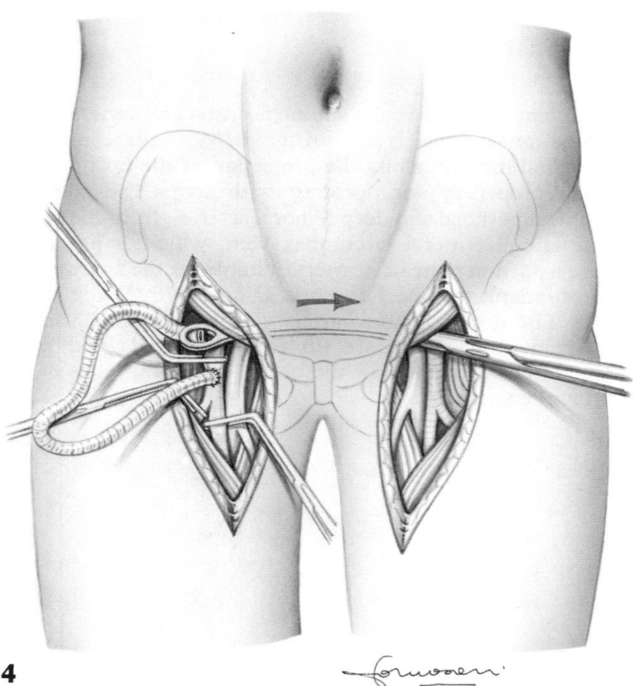

4

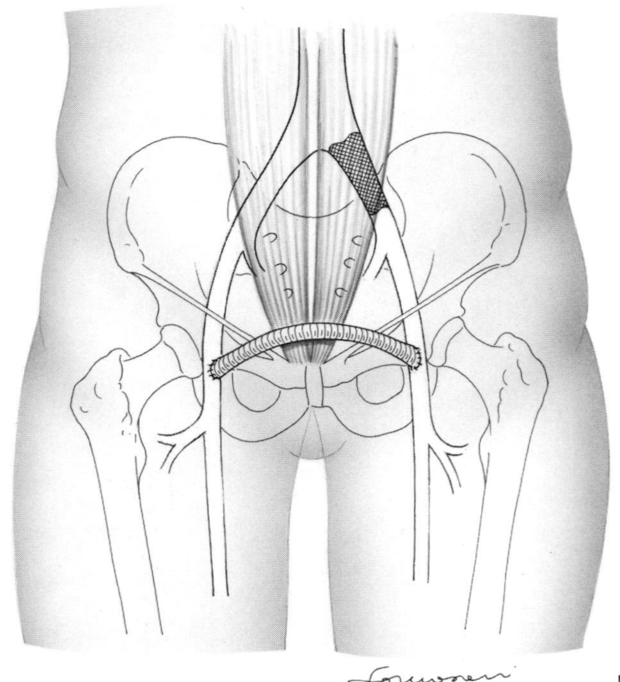

5

6

Other surgeons prefer a deeper positioning of the prosthesis and improved bypass haemodynamics (Courbier *et al.*, 1982). Donor vessels are prepared using an oblique incision parallel to the inguinal ligament, approximately 2–3 cm proximally to permit proximal anastomosis to the external iliac artery. The prosthesis is canalized more deeply behind the rectal muscle in the space of Retzius and below the inguinal ligament, resulting in a 'S'-shaped bypass.

With this procedure, the prosthesis is better protected against external compression, though there is a greater risk of bleeding due to the presence of a rich venous plexus. This cross-over iliofemoral bypass is thus very different from the simple cross-over femorofemoral bypass.

Iliofemoral bypass allows the prosthesis to be positioned outside the donor inguinal region, with its consequent lower risk of bacterial contamination from the the contralateral groin. Canalization in the space of Retzius, which lies at a deeper level than the inguinal ligament, involves the section of the fibrous layer of the ligament. This avoids compression of the prosthesis and traction on the suture line, which is frequently responsible for the formation of anastomotic aneurysms.

In the case of an infected groin, cross-over transperineal bypass can be carried out. This entails a subcutaneous route at the level of the inguino-scrotal folds close to the spongy body, from the common femoral artery to the contralateral superficial or deep femoral artery, far from the site of infection. Autologous saphenous vein is the prosthesis of choice, otherwise PTFE.

Anastomoses are usually performed end-to-side, but with extended lesions of the host deep femoral artery requiring endarterectomy, at this level the anastomosis can be performed end-to-end. The suture material is usually 5/0 or 6/0 monofilament. After completion of the anastomoses with flush to prevent possible distal embolizations, the clamps are released and the pulsatility of the prosthesis and the proximal and contralateral vessels is controlled. Immediate postoperative control is performed by Doppler evaluation of the ankle pressure index (Winsor index) and by intraoperative angiography to evidence possible technical errors, e.g. torsion of the prosthesis or the intimal flap, which can be repaired immediately. After tubular drainage of the area, the groins are sutured by reconstruction of the fascia and section planes. Postoperatively, the antibiotic prophylaxis of infection plays a major role, especially in patients who show trophic lesions.

Contraindications

If adequate haemodynamic testing is carried out, there are no absolute contraindications for cross-over femorofemoral bypass, though particular attention should be paid to the prophylaxis of infection, because the areas involved with the prosthesis are rich in lymphatic vessels and lymph-node stations, and are thus at risk.

In conclusion, femorofemoral bypass should be considered the procedure of choice in the treatment of unilateral iliac occlusion in high-risk patients. An accurate preoperative and haemodynamic assessment provides useful information for obtaining good long-term patency and haemodynamic function.

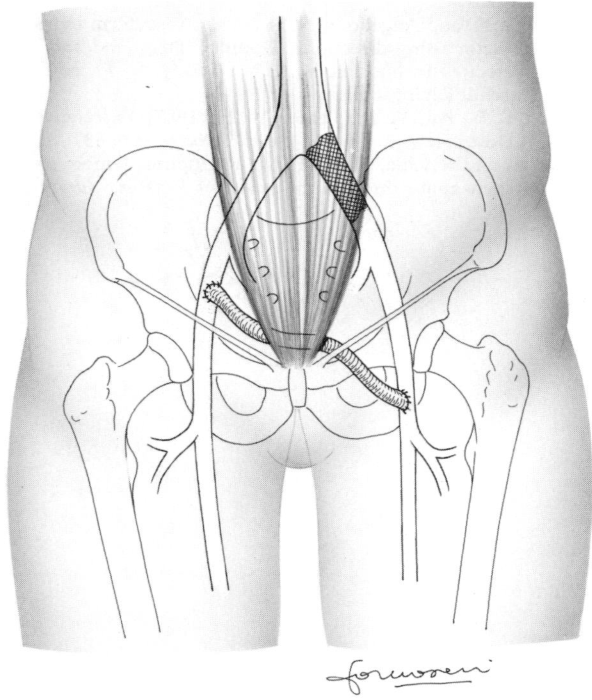

6

References

Blaisdell, R. W., Hall, A. D., Lim, R. C. Jr and Moore, W. C. (1970). Aortoiliac arterial subcutaneous grafts. *Annals of Surgery* **172**, 775.

Courbier, R., Larranaga, J., Ferdani, M., Jausseran, J. M., Reggi, M. and Bergeron, P. (1982). Le faux anévrismes sur prothèse artérielle. *Chirurgie* **108**, 459.

De Laurentis, D. A., Sala, L. E., Russell, E. and McCombs, P. R. (1978). A twelve years experience with axillofemoral and femorofemoral bypass operations. *Surgery, Gynecology, and Obstetrics* **147**, 881.

Eugene, J., Goldstone, J. and Moore, W. S. (1977). Fifteen years experience with subcutaneous bypass grafts for lower extremity ischemia. *Annals of Surgery* **186**, 177.

Flanigan, P. D., Ryan, T. J., Williams, L. R., Schwatrz, J. A., Gray, B. and Shuler, J. J. (1984). Aortofemoral or femoropopliteal revascularization? A prospective evaluation of the papaverine test. *Journal of Vascular Surgery* **1**, 215.

Harper, S. A., Goldin, A. L., Mazzei, E. A. and Cannon, S. A. (1967). An experimental hemodynamic study of the subclavian steal syndrome. *Surgery, Gynecology and Obstetrics* **124**, 1212.

Hill, D. A., Lord, R. S. A. and Tracy, G. D. (1982). Haemodynamic consequences of cross femoral bypass. In *Extra-anatomic and Secondary Arterial Reconstruction*. Greenhalgh, R. M. ed. London: Pitman.

Kalman, P. G., Hosang, M., Johnston, K. W. and Walker, P. M. (1987). The current role for femorofemoral bypass. *Journal of Vascular Surgery* **6**, 71.

McDonald, P. T., Rich, N. M., Collins, J. G., Anderson, A. C. and Kozloff, L. (1978). Femorofemoral grafts: The role of concomitant extended profundaplasty. *American Journal of Surgery* **136**, 622.

Martinez, B. B., Hertzer, N. R. and Bevan, E. G. (1980). Influence of distal arterial occlusive disease on prognosis following aortobifemoral bypass. *Surgery* **88**, 795.

Nelelsteen, A., Suiw, R., Daeneen, W., Boel, A. and Stalpeert, G. (1980). Aortofemoral grafting: Factors influencing late result. *Surgery* **88**, 342.

Nicolaides, A. N. and Angelides, N. S. (1981). Waveform index and resistance factor using directional Doppler ultrasound and zero-crossing detector. In Nicolaides, A. N., Yao, J. S. T., eds. New York: Churchill Livingstone.

Rutherford, R. B., Patt, A. and Pearce, W. H. (1987). Extra-anatomic bypass: A closer view. *Journal of Vascular Surgery*, **6**, 437.

Tyson, R. R. and Reichle, F. A. (1972). Retropubic femorofemoral bypass: A new route through the space of Retzius. *Surgery* **72**, 401.

Vijayanagar, R., Bogudo, D. A. and Eckstein, P. F. (1982). Extra-anatomic bypass operation for aorto-iliac disease in poor risk cardiopulmonary patients. *Angiology* **33**, 69.

Whittemore, K. E., Billig, P. M., Pavlides, C. and Matsumoto, T. (1980). Special considerations in the revascularization for aorto-iliac occlusive disease: Anatomic and extra-anatomic bypass. *Annals of Surgery* **46**, 279.

Wylie, E. J., Stoney, R. J., Ehrenfeld, W. K. and Effeney, D. S. (1980). In *Manual of Vascular Surgery*. Egdahl, R. E. ed.

Subscrotal bypass for the infected groin

ROGER N. BAIRD ChM FRCS
Consultant Surgeon, The Royal Infirmary, Bristol, UK

Introduction

Subscrotal femoro-femoral bypass was described by J. D. Hardy and J. W. Bane in 1975. They reported on the management of a pelvic gunshot injury with massive blood loss by femoral-subscrotal-femoral bypass and 116 units of blood. The bypass was patent 1 year later. The following year, E. Kieffer of Paris reported six subscrotal bypasses, aptly describing their route as 'pontages perineaux'.

Five were for infections following proximal Dacron prostheses implanted to the femoral arteries in the groin; one followed erosion of an external iliac artery by a vesical prosthesis. All were patent during follow-up of up to 8 months. Following this report, Cormier's group, also from Paris, reported 12 subscrotal bypasses for septic complications of Dacron prostheses and endarterectomy. Early graft thromboses occurred in three patients, two required further vascular operations and seven were patent with follow-up of up to 4 years.

In 1982 and 1986, R. S. Taylor and F. Massouh described four cases in which the indication was infection in the groin. Three arose from an infected Dacron prosthesis and one from tuberculous sinuses associated with an ischaemic leg. Two saphenous veins and two polytetrafluoroethylene (PTFE) conduits were used. In three instances the distal anastomosis was to a patent superficial femoral artery; and one to the above-knee popliteal artery. One saphenous vein bypass became stenosed at 2 years and required a patch repair. At the latest report, all four bypasses were patent at 3, 4, 6, and 7 years.

In 1985, P. F. Lawrence and D. Albo published a case report on the use of a subscrotal bypass of an infected groin following an aorto-femoral Dacron graft, which was patent at 6 months follow-up. In 1991, D. P. Newington included a subscrotal bypass in a report of 19 patients with deep groin wound infections.

Indications

With the exception of the first reported case, the indication for subscrotal bypass has been to bypass the infected groin. In many instances, a more conservative approach will succeed, including wound irrigation (Kwaan and Connolly, 1981) and rotational muscle flaps (Perler *et al.*, 1993). However, when the strength of the arterial wall is lost from bacterial arteritis, so that the anastomotic sutures lie slackly causing the discharging sinus to be complicated by haemorrhage, recourse has to be to local removal of the Dacron and ligation of the femoral arteries with revascularization by remote bypass. The subscrotal route is an alternative to oburator bypass, described in the following chapter – Obdurator canal bypass, p. 260. The procedure is unsuitable for women.

The distal attachment of a remote bypass is to the superficial femoral artery above the adductor hiatus, or the popliteal artery below it. The proximal attachment is to the contralateral common femoral artery. An arteriogram may be required to confirm the adequacy of the inflow and outflow arteries.

Operative technique

1

The diagram illustrates a subscrotal bypass from the left common femoral to the right superficial femoral artery. Note the infected right Dacron/femoral artery anastomosis. The patient lies supine with the legs abducted, a urethral catheter in place, the infected groin sealed with op-site, and the scrotum taped to the anterior abdominal wall. Intravenous antibiotics are administered, and the *inflow* common femoral artery, or uninfected limb of an aorto-bifemoral prosthesis, is mobilized, followed by the *outflow* superficial femoral or popliteal artery.

A subcutaneous tunnel is developed retro-scrotally to link the two incisions. Care is taken to avoid the urethra, which is easily identified by the urinary catheter. The bypass conduit, usually saphenous vein or PTFE is placed avoiding kinking and twisting. Excessive tension is avoided. The anastomoses are made end-to-side with 5/0 polypropylene sutures following systemic heparinization and the wounds are closed, and dressings applied.

Attention is then turned to the infected groin. As much as possible of the infected Dacron limb is ligated, excised and sent for culture. The common, superficial and deep femoral arteries are ligated and the wound edges are approximated, with wound drainage if necessary.

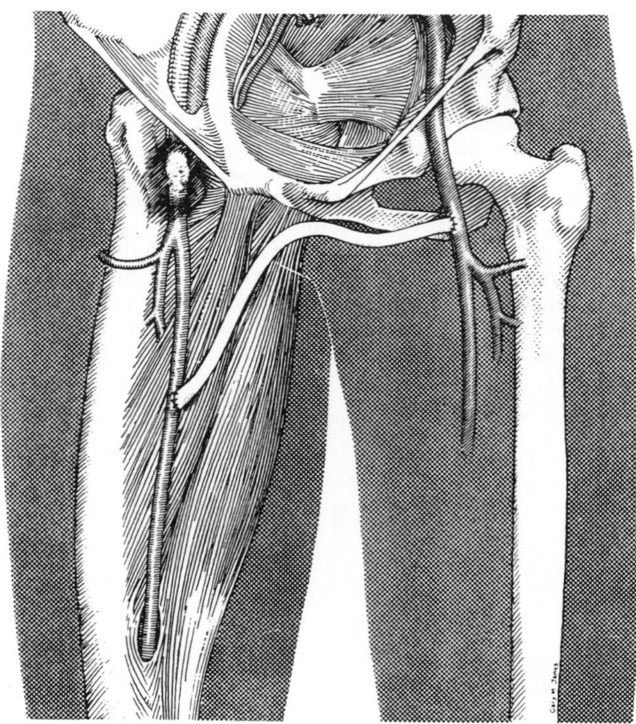

1

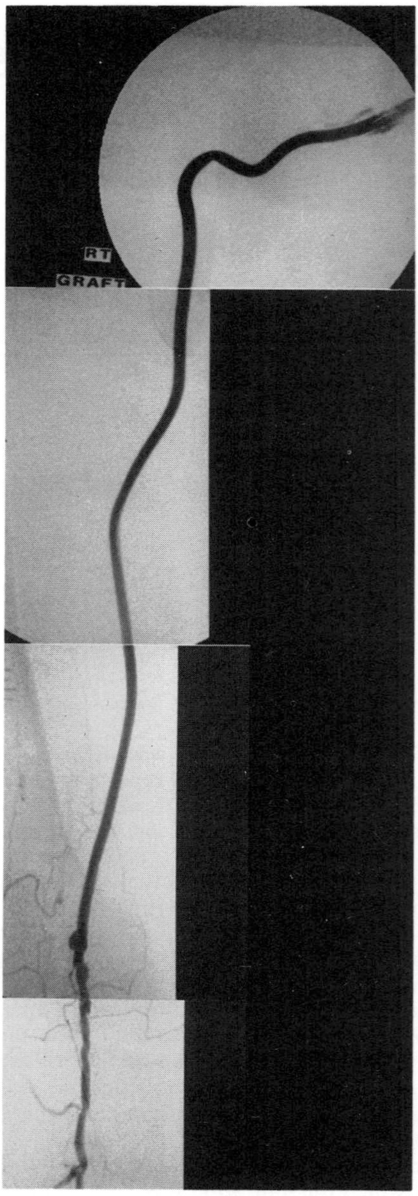

2

Postoperative care

2

Illustration 2 shows postoperative digital subtraction arteriogram of a PTFE subscrotal bypass to the above knee popliteal artery. Note the rounded perineal arch.

Bypass patency is checked by pulse palpation, Doppler ankle pressure measurements and by digital subtraction angiography. The bypass incisions require little attention. However, it may take some time for healthy granulation tissue to appear in the infected groin wound. Routine graft follow-up for infra-inguinal bypasses is undertaken. Cycling is best avoided.

Conclusions

The subscrotal route from the contralateral groin is a useful, and some would say technically easier alternative to the obturator route from the ipsilateral iliac artery, as a remote bypass of an infected groin.

References

Hardy, J. D. and Bane, J. W. (1975). Arterial injury and massive blood loss: a case report of management of pelvic gunshot injury with femoro-subscrotal-femoral bypass and 116 units of blood. *Annals of Surgery* **181**, 245.

Kieffer, E., Laurian, C., Surugue, P. and Natali, J. (1976). Pontage veineux fémoro-fémoral par le perinée. *Chirurgie* **102**, 420.

Kwaan, J. H. M. and Connolly, J. E. (1981). Successful treatment of prosthetic graft infection with continuous povidone-iodine irrigation. *Archives of Surgery* **116**, 716.

Laurian, C., Martino, A. and Courmier, J. M. (1981). *Annals de Chirurgie* **35**, 455.

Lawrence, P. F. and Albo, D. (1985). Femoro-femoral bypass with an infrascrotal perineal approach for the patient with an infected groin wound. *Journal of Vascular Surgery* **2**, 485.

Newington, D. P., Houghton, P. W. J., Baird, R. N. *et al.* (1991). Groin wound infection after arterial surgery. *British Journal of Surgery* **78**, 617.

Perler, B. A., Vander Koek, C. A., Manson, P. M. and Williams, G. M. (1993). Rotational muscle flaps to treat localised prosthetic graft infection: longterm follow-up. *Journal of Vascular Surgery* **18**, 358.

Taylor, R. S. and Massouh, F. (1982). The transperineal graft – an alternative route for femoro-femoral bypass. In *Extra-anatomic and Secondary Arterial Reconstruction*, Greenhalgh, R. M., ed. London: Pitman, pp. 237–243.

Taylor, R. S. and Massouh, F. (1986). Femoro-femoral bypass with an infrascrotal approach for the patient with an infected groin wound. (letter) *Journal of Vascular Surgery* **3**, 555.

Obturator canal bypass

G. KRETSCHMER MD
B. NIEDERLE MD
University Clinics of Surgery, University of Vienna, Vienna, Austria

M. WUNDERLICH MD
Department of Surgery, General Hospital, Hollabrunn, Austria

Introduction

Since obturator canal bypass was introduced by Shaw and Baue in 1963, its indications and techniques have been precisely defined. Today the method is an established standard procedure in vascular surgery, with the results of 250 patients being published. In general, more or less anecdotal reports are available; the largest series comprise 13 and 27 patients, respectively (Van Det and Brands, 1981; Niederle *et al.*, 1988). A survey of the literature concerning long-term results and an evaluation of their own results has been published recently (Sautner *et al.*, 1994). Guidelines and conclusions are drawn from these reports and our own experience (Van Det and Brands, 1981; Prenner and Rendl, 1982; Buchardt-Hansen, Holstein and Krogh-Christoffersen, 1982; Cotton, 1982; Geroulakos, Parvin and Bell, 1988; Niederle *et al.*, 1988; Sautner et al., 1994).

1

Concept

The basic principle is to create an extensive extra-anatomical bypass from the pelvic to the distal femoral or infra-genicular arteries, the site of distal anastomosis depending on the respective morphological conditions.

Graft-conduction through the foramen obturatum, dorsal to hip-joint and adductor muscle group, avoids the femoral triangle so as to prevent any contamination. Accordingly, the procedure allows thorough separation of the graft from the obviously or potentially infected inguinal area through an uncompromised barrier of normal tissue.

Principally, any vascular substitute of adequate dimensions may be acceptable and most have been tested. As would be expected, autologous saphenous vein has been employed in 16% of patients. Although autologous grafts give the most satisfying long-term results, the limited diameter of these conduits often precludes their use. In the remaining patients, the greater distance to be bridged usually requires the use of fabric grafts.

We have found PTFE prostheses (21 out of 27 cases) to have been most satisfactory. Our initial experience with externally reinforced grafts has been promising, due to their greater resistance against kinking and compression.

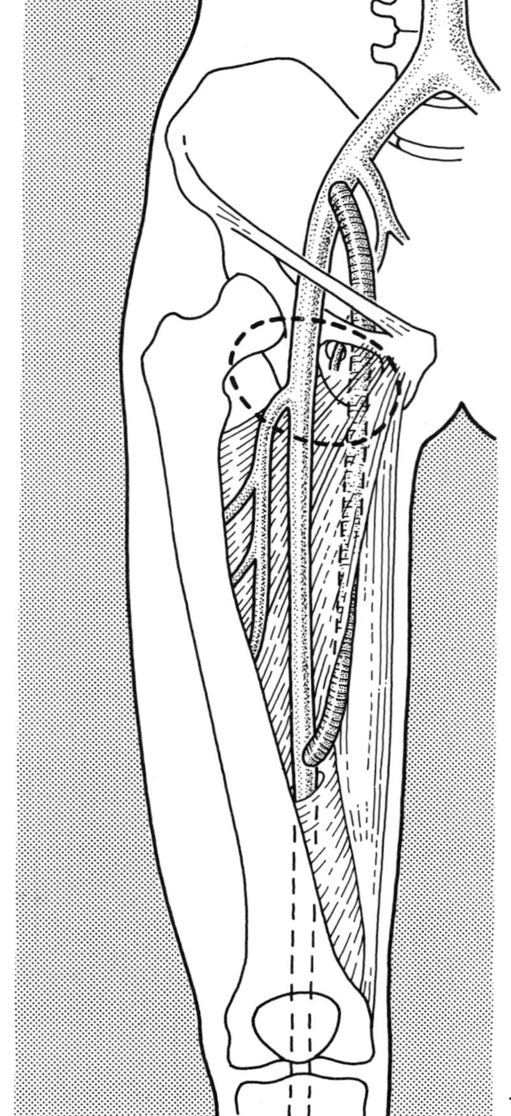

1

Indications

Throughout the literature there is unanimous agreement that the most frequent indication (58%) is unilateral deep infection, strictly confined to the groin (type III according to Szilagyi *et al.*, 1972) as a sequel of vascular surgery of any kind (Brücke and Piza, 1968; Prenner and Rendl, 1982). Less frequent indications are rather evenly distributed between infections subsequent to vascular access surgery (12%; Prenner and Rendl, 1982), inguinal skin and subcutaneous tissue defects after extensive tumour surgery and/or therapeutic irradiation (17%; Niederle *et al.*, 1988) and, finally, complicated (non-arteriosclerotic) aneurysms and severe inguinal scarring (13%; Buchardt-Hansen *et al.*, 1982; Cotton, 1982).

Angiography

The value of preoperative arteriography to identify suitable areas for proximal and distal anastomoses is undisputed. However, in the case of massive bleeding as an emergency indication, valuable time can be wasted waiting for preoperative information. The site of distal anastomosis may then be chosen on grounds of radiology, obtained prior to the primary procedure, or by distal exploration, if necessary with adjunctive on-table angiography during the present bypass procedure.

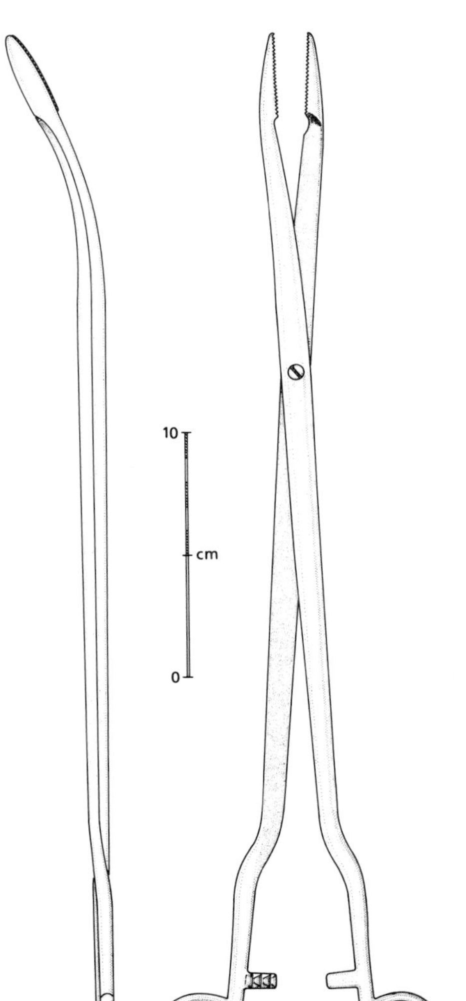

2

2

Instrumentation

In addition to the standard instruments for vascular surgery, we use a slim, long-bladed grasping-forceps, 65cm in length and with a slight bend of 20° for boring the tunnel and guiding the graft into place (i.e. sponge and dressing clamp according to Sims–Meier (Brücke and Piza, 1968)). Of course, any other forceps of adequate length with long blunt jaws will be adequate.

3

Positioning and preparation of the patient

With the patient in the prone position, the spine and hip-joints are slightly over-extended to allow the grasping-forceps to be directed through the obturator canal behind the superior branch of the pubic bone without impediment from the abdominal wall – an obstacle most likely to be met in obese patients.

The entire abdomen and the limb concerned are disinfected and draped in such a way as to permit good access to the abdominal and distal incisions at the medial aspect of thigh and calf. Our practice is to use incisive drapes covering the skin, paying particular regard to the crucial femoral triangle so as to avoid any contamination therefrom.

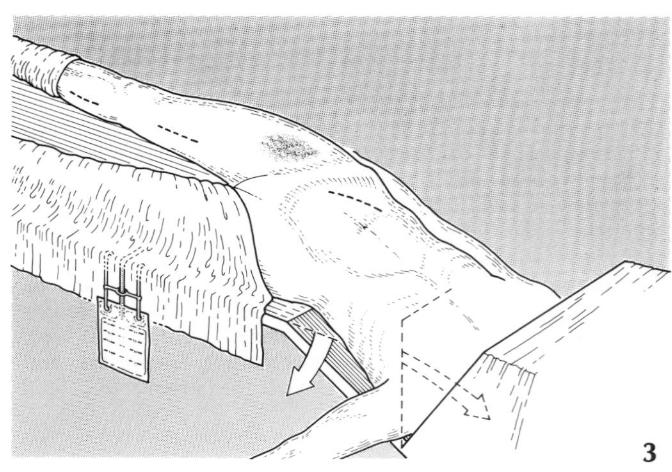

3

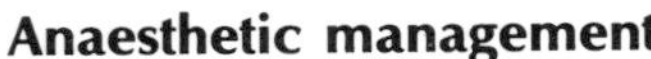

Anaesthetic management

Surgery is performed under general anaesthesia, with the use of at least one or two major i.v. lines, preferably a central venous catheter. A urinary catheter is essential (see *Illustration 3*). The operative strain on the patient can be estimated by using a mean duration of anaesthesia of $3\frac{1}{2}$ h and a mean quantity of blood loss corresponding to 3 units (Kretschmer *et al.*, 1989).

4

Surgical procedure

4

Standard approaches are used for extraperitoneal exposure of the pelvic arteries as well as for medial exposure of the femoral, popliteal or even crural vessles (Leitz, 1981). As a rule, we prefer the extraperitoneal ($n = 17$) to the transperitoneal ($n = 10$) approach, the latter being reserved for redo-surgery.

5 & 6

Gentle sweeping of the peritoneal sac, ureter and bladder to the midline gives access to the foramen obturatum. In male and obese patients in particular, the foramen is often better identified by mere digital palpation of its sharp fascial circumference than by actually viewing it during deep pelvic dissection (Brücke and Piza, 1968). It is our practice to penetrate the membrana obturatoria from the proximal distally, and then bore the tunnel and place the graft, taking care to leave the obturator vessels and the nerve unharmed. In order to avoid blind tunnelling in a heparinized patient, systemic heparin (100 i.u./kg body weight) is administered after graft placement only. Alternative sites for the anastomosis are shown in *Illustration 6*. The proximal anastomosis is constructed by using the side-to-end-technique. Cross-clamping of externally supported grafts is not advisable. The distal end of the graft is cut to shape during full extension of the knee joint. After completion of the distal anastomosis, the vascular clamps are released.

If possible, the external iliac artery should not undergo preliminary ligation from within the pelvis in order to preserve a maximum of collateral circulation to the leg. Suction drains are left in place for 2 days.

Some authors prefer boring the tunnel from the distal proximally (Pearce *et al.*, 1983; Prenner and Rendl, 1982), suggesting that lesions of the obturator artery and vein are better avoided; however, we cannot confirm this.

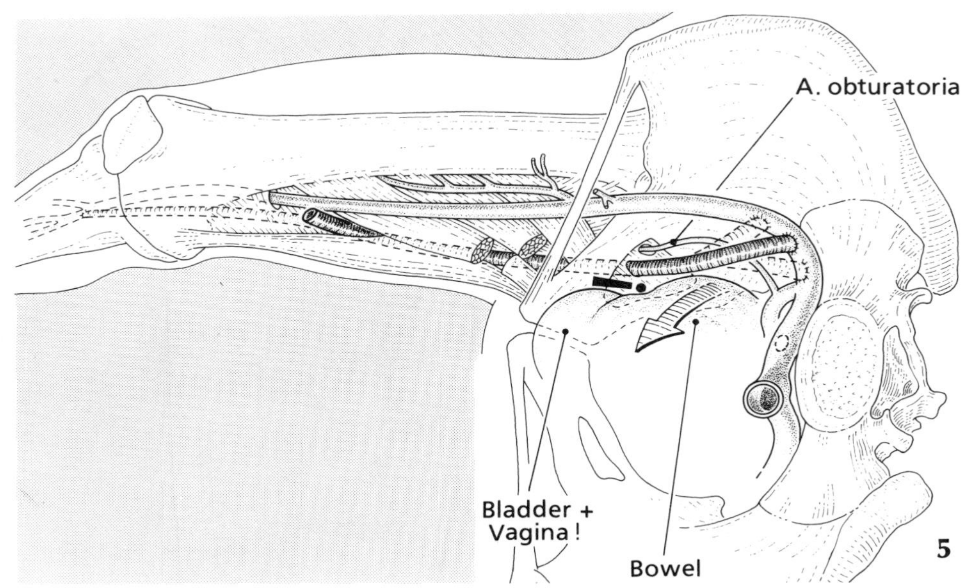

5

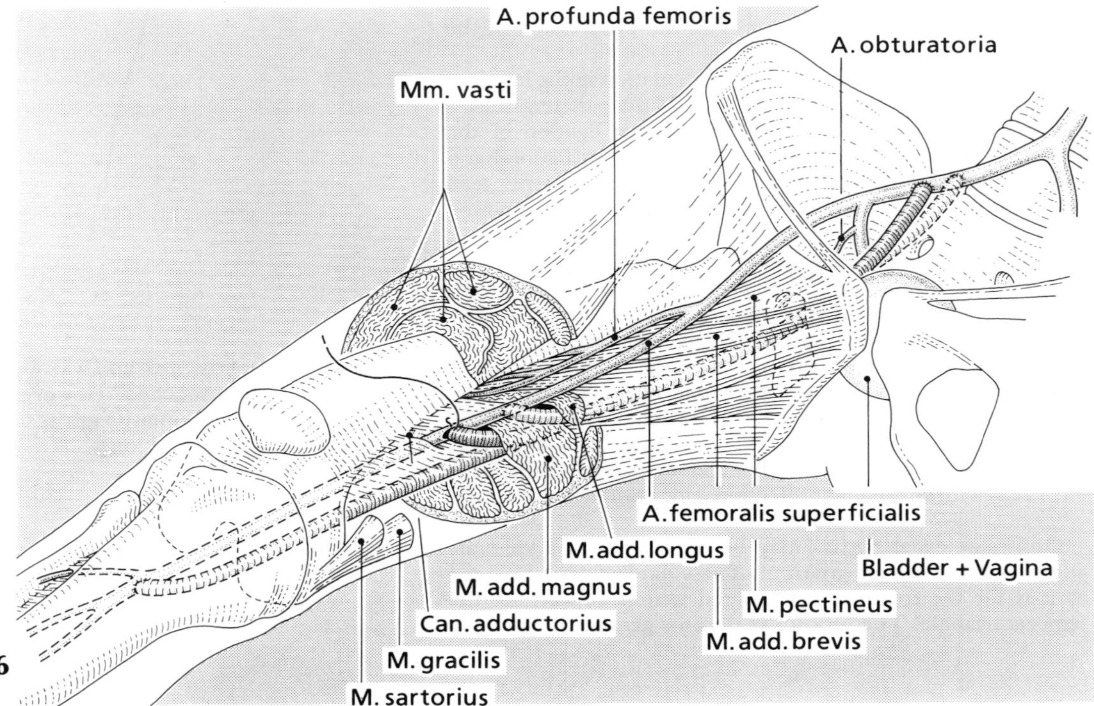

6

7

If it is felt necessary, the bypass procedure is followed by debridement of the inguinal wound by removing the remaining alloplastic material and local suturing of vascular defects, so as to secure haemostasis. At the same time, swabs are taken so as to prescribe antibiotic therapy accordingly.

The operation is rarely indicated; only limited series of patients and/or case reports are available. An evaluation of the operation with the usual techniques of estimating patency, limb salvage and finally patient survival is difficult to obtain. Data from two centres in Austria as well as results derived from the literature were pooled and comparatively assessed (Sautner et al., 1994). The procedure was found to be reliable and durable, but demonstrated the known disadvantages like other operations, in which alloplastic vascular substitutes necessarily bridge long distances thereby crossing a major joint.

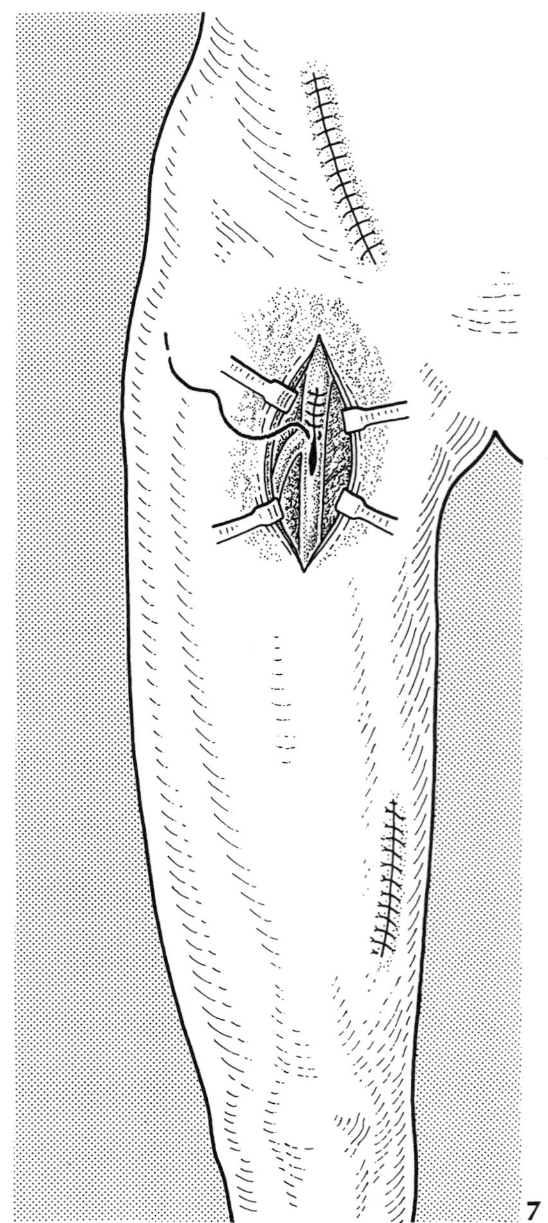
7

Complications

The usual complications following implantation of long-distance fabric grafts are encountered. In the absence of underlying arteriosclerotic disease, long-term graft performance is excellent. However, patency rates cannot be reliably derived from the literature, as most reports do not distinguish if lesions requiring obturator canal bypass have originally been related to chronic occlusive vascular disease or not.

As circulation along the deep femoral artery has to be sacrificed, or is at least severely compromised, graft occlusion will inevitably threaten the entire extremity. Unless prompt surgical correction is feasible, the ischaemic syndrome will necessitate major, it not above-knee, amputation. Therefore, thrombectomy should be attempted without delay, the long-term performance of the graft depending on the availability of the more favourable distal anastomotic site above the knee, the peripheral run-off conditions and the progression of the underlying disease.

The preservation of the collateral circulation in the inguinal area may become of vital importance. If the collateral blood supply is insufficient following preliminary ligation of the external iliac artery, eradication of the common femoral and the superficial and deep femoral at the origin will lead to necrosis of the thigh musculature, the graft remaining obviously patent (Rudich, Gutierrez and Gage, 1979).

If a combination of infection plus haemorrhage demands an extra-anatomical bypass, the procedure will reliably eradicate the danger of exsanguinating haemorrhage while preserving the limb's blood supply (Kretschmer *et al.*, 1989). However, in our series, this combination of events caused two fatalities, the patients with viable limbs having finally succumbed to irreversible sepsis (Kretschmer *et al.*, 1989). Topographical misplacement of the graft was observed, leading to perforation of the bladder or vagina (Szilagyi *et al.*, 1972) with subsequent infection and ultimate loss of limb.

Obturator canal bypass may be considered as a valuable addition to the armamentarium of vascular surgery, designed as it is for the treatment of isolated lesions concerning the femoral triangle. The procedure permits generous bypassing of the inguinal risk area and warrants surgery within operative fields as yet untouched. However, it is not devoid of the disadvantage of alloplastic grafts over long distances, with an increased risk of infection.

Acknowledgement

We would like to thank Mrs Ursula Schattauer for her secretarial assistance.

References

Brücke, P. and Piza, F. (1968). Zur Indikation des Obturator-Bypass. *Zbl. Chir.* **93**, 489.

Buchardt-Hansen, H. J., Holstein, P. and Krogh-Christoffersen, J. (1982). Obturator canal bypass to avoid an infected or scarred groin. In *Extraanatomic and Secondary Arterial Reconstruction*. Greenhalgh, R. M., ed. London: Pitman.

Cotton, L. T. (1982). Obturator canal bypass for aneurysms in the thigh. In *Extraanatomic and Secondary Arterial Reconstruction*. Greenhalgh, R. M. ed. London: Pitman.

Geroulakos, G., Parvin, S. D. and Bell, P. R. F. (1988). Obturator foramen bypass, the alternative route for sepsis in the femoral triangle. *Acta Chir. Scan.* **154,** 111.

Kretschmer, G., Niederle, B., Huk, I., Karner, J., Piza, H., Polterauer, P. and Walzer, L. R. (1989). Groin infections following vascular surgery: Obturator bypass (BYP) versus biologic coverage (TRP) – a comparative evaluation. *European Journal of Vascular Surgery* **3**, 25.

Leitz, K. H. (1981). *Zugangswege in der Gefäßchirurgie*. Heidelberg: Springer.

Niederle, B., Polterauer, P., Kretschmer, G. and Piza, F. (1988). Der Obturatorbypass – Indikation und Ergebnisse bei 27 Patienten. *Angio Arch.* **16,** 90.

Pearce, W. H., Ricco, J. P., Yao, J. S. T., Flinn, W. R. and Bergan, J. J. (1983). Modified technique of obturator bypass in failed or infected grafts. *Annals of Surgery* **197**, 344.

Prenner, K. V. and Rendl, K. H. (1982). Indications and technique of obturator bypass. In *Extraanatomic and Secondary Arterial Reconstruction*. Greenhalgh, R. M., ed. London: Pitman.

Rudich, M., Gutierrez, I. Z. and Gage, A. A. (1979). Obturator foramen bypass in the management of infected vascular prosthesis. *American Journal of Surgery* **137**, 657.

Sautner, Th., Niederle, B., Herbst, F., Kretschmer, G., Polterauer, P., Rendl, K. H. and Prenner, K. (1994). The value of obturator canal bypass; results of 34 consecutive cases and review of the literature. *Archives of Surgery* 128; in press.

Shaw, R. S. and Baue, A. E. (1963). Management of sepsis complicating arterial reconstructive surgery. *Surgery* **53,** 57.

Sheiner, N. M., Sigman, H. and Stilman, A. (1969). An unusual complication of obturator foramen arterial bypass. *Journal of Cardiovascular Surgery* **10,** 324.

Szilagyi, D. E., Smith, R. F., Elliott, J. P. and Vrandecic, M. P. (1972). Infection in arterial reconstruction with synthetic grafts *Annals of Surgery* **176,** 321.

Van Det, R. J. and Brands, L. C. (1981). The obturator foramen bypass: An alternative procedure in iliofemoral artery revascularization. *Surgery* **89,** 543.

Cervical sympathectomy

GIORGIO M. BIASI MD, FACS

Professor of Vascular Surgery, Chief, Division of Vascular Surgery, Bassini Teaching Hospital, University of Milan, Milan, Italy

PAOLO MINGAZZINI MD

Assistant Professor, Bassini Teaching Hospital, University of Milan, Milan, Italy

UGO RUBERTI MD

Professor and Chief, Institute of General and Cardiovascular Surgery, University of Milan, Milan, Italy

Introduction

Although it is a commonly used term, 'cervical' sympathectomy is something of a misnomer, since it has never implied division of the cervical chain. The approach, which is via the neck to the upper thoracic sympathetic chain, has given rise to the term.

Indications

Since the first cervical sympathectomy performed in 1899 by Alexander for epilepsy (White, Smithwick and Simeone, 1952), this procedure has been applied for various indications. Nowadays the surgical ablation of thoracic (dorsal) sympathetic ganglia continues to play an important role in the treatment of a few selected pathologies.

Primary hyperhidrosis refractory to conservative treatment remains one of the main indications for the procedure with good postoperative results (Greenhalgh, Rosengarten and Martin, 1971). Excessive sweating of the hands frequently causes severe psychological and social problems, which can justify the surgical option if all medical measures fail. If abnormal axillary sweating is also present, a resection of the fourth thoracic ganglion, in addition to the second and the third, must be performed in order to obtain a complete sympathetic denervation of the axilla.

True causalgia and other pain syndromes like the post-traumatic sympathetic dystrophies can be relieved by upper thoracic sympathectomy, if diagnosed early and not treated sufficiently by physical therapy and nerve blocks (Witmoser, 1984; Kleinert, Cole and Wayne, 1973).

Ischaemic disorders of the upper extremity were the most common indications in the past; these can be caused by atherosclerotic disease as well as by other less common pathologies, such as Raynaud's syndrome, scleroderma, frostbite, embolism, thrombo-angiitis obliterans (Buerger's disease). The surgeon should always inform the patient that Raynaud's symptoms may recur in 1 or 2 years (Welch and Geary, 1984), a reason to reserve the surgical procedure for digital ulceration.

Raynaud's phenomenon is frequently associated with a collagen disease such as the CREST syndrome and sympathectomy is then of limited value, but sometimes may delay the need for amputation (Harris and May, 1989). An unusual indication for cervical sympathectomy is the Long Q-T syndrome, a congenital disorder accompanied by a high incidence of sudden cardiac death. In this extremely rare disease, when resistant to the use of β-blockers, left cardiac sympathetic denervation obtained by stellectomy resulted in a marked reduction in the incidence of tachyarrhythmic syncope (Schwartz *et al.*, 1991)

Surgical approaches

Access to resect the thoracic sympathetic chain can be gained by several approaches.

The posterior approach described by Smithwick (1940), with excision of part of the third rib and transverse vertebral process, has been almost completely abandoned.

The extrapleural axillary approach through excision of the first rib (Ross, 1980) has low postoperative effects such as postoperative pain, but is technically demanding.

The transaxillary approach through the second or third intercostal space (Atkins, 1954) gives a good view of the sympathetic chain and allows extended resection to the fourth ganglion. (See following chapter – Transthoracic sympathectomy, p. 276.)

The supraclavicular approach is perhaps the classical route. It was proposed by Jonnesco (1923), Bruning (1923), Royle (1924) and later well described by Telford (1935) and Gask and Ross (1937). His approach has less complications for pulmonary function and less postoperative pain and is consequently preferred by many surgeons. The disadvantages are the deep and narrow surgical field which can cause difficulties (e.g. control of deep bleeding), therefore the surgeon must be very familiar with this procedure. Moreover, access to the lower part of the sympathetic chain is difficult, so if the fourth thoracic ganglion must also be resected, the transthoracic route is preferred.

The thorascopic approach is a new surgical technique since the first description dates back to 1943 by Hughes (Adams *et al.*, 1992), but recent improvements in instrumentation and technology have enhanced the possibilities of this minimally invasive approach.

In this chapter we will describe in detail the supraclavicular approach which is the one that we most frequently adopt.

Anatomy

1

The thoracic sympathetic chain passes vertically down the side of the vertebral column deep to the pleura on the rib necks.

The first thoracic ganglion fuses with the inferior cervical ganglion forming the stellate ganglion. Thoracic ganglia receive preganglionic fibres from the thoracic spinal cord via the white rami communicantes from the adjacent spinal nerve. These fibres synapse in the ganglion where postganglionic fibres commence and pass back to the nerve root via grey rami communicantes. The sympathetic outflow to the upper limb is from within the spinal cord at level thoracic 5–9. The fibres either pass up the spinal cord and then cross via rami communicantes at a higher thoracic level or near the original outflow (5–9). To interrupt the sympathetic supply to the upper limb the chain must be transected below the third ganglion and all rami cut including to the second ganglion.

Some consider it necessary to resect the thoracic component of the stellate ganglion (lower one third), for complete sympathetic denervation of the upper limb, but it is not necessary and adds to the risk of Horner's syndrome.

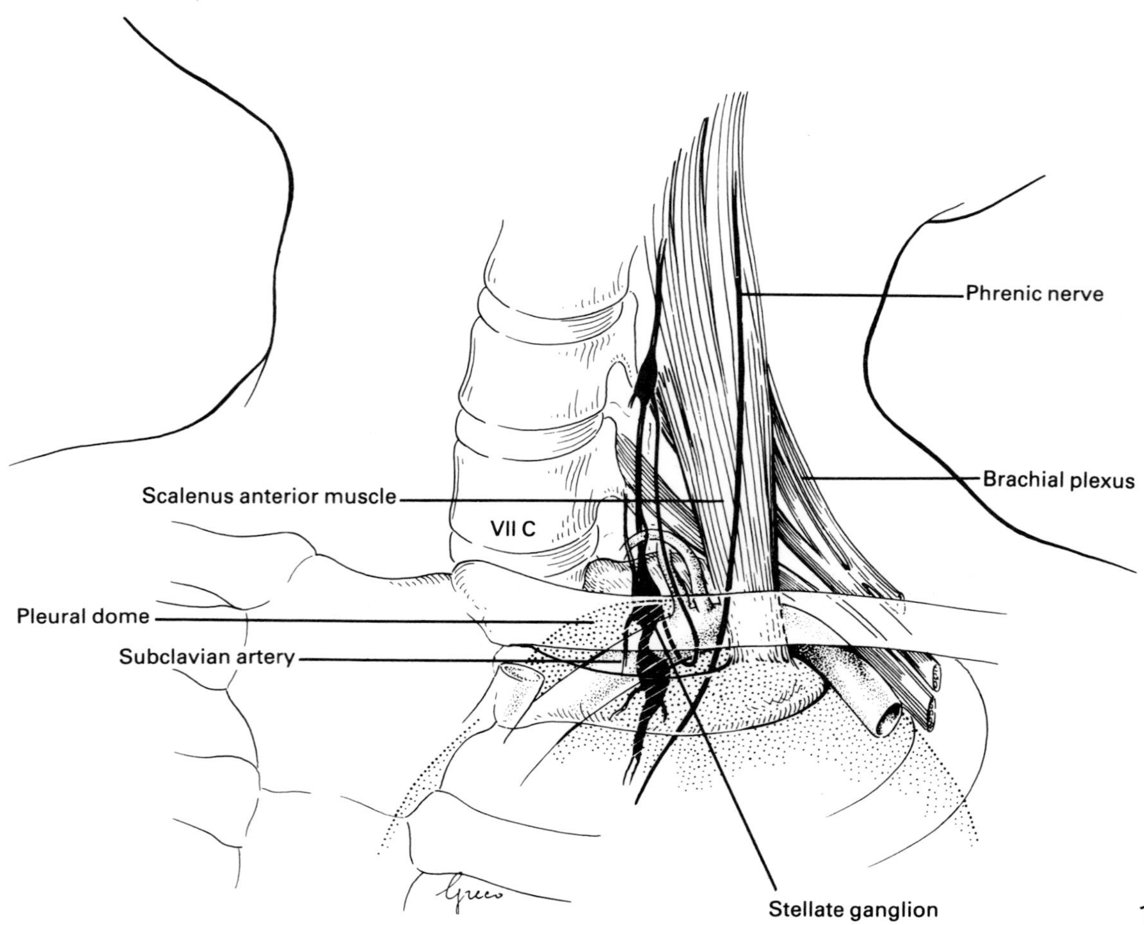

1

The operation

2

The operation is performed under general anaesthesia with tracheal intubation, because accidental opening of the pleural dome can cause a pneumothorax. With the patient's head turned away from the side of the incision and with the neck slightly hyperextended, a horizontal incision is made 1 cm above the superior border of the clavicle, 1–2 cm lateral to the jugular fossa on the anterior face of the clavicular head of the sternocleidomastoid muscle. An incision of 5–6 cm is sufficient to facilitate division of the clavicular head of the sternomastoid. The incision passes through the platysma muscle and the external jugular vein may have to be divided.

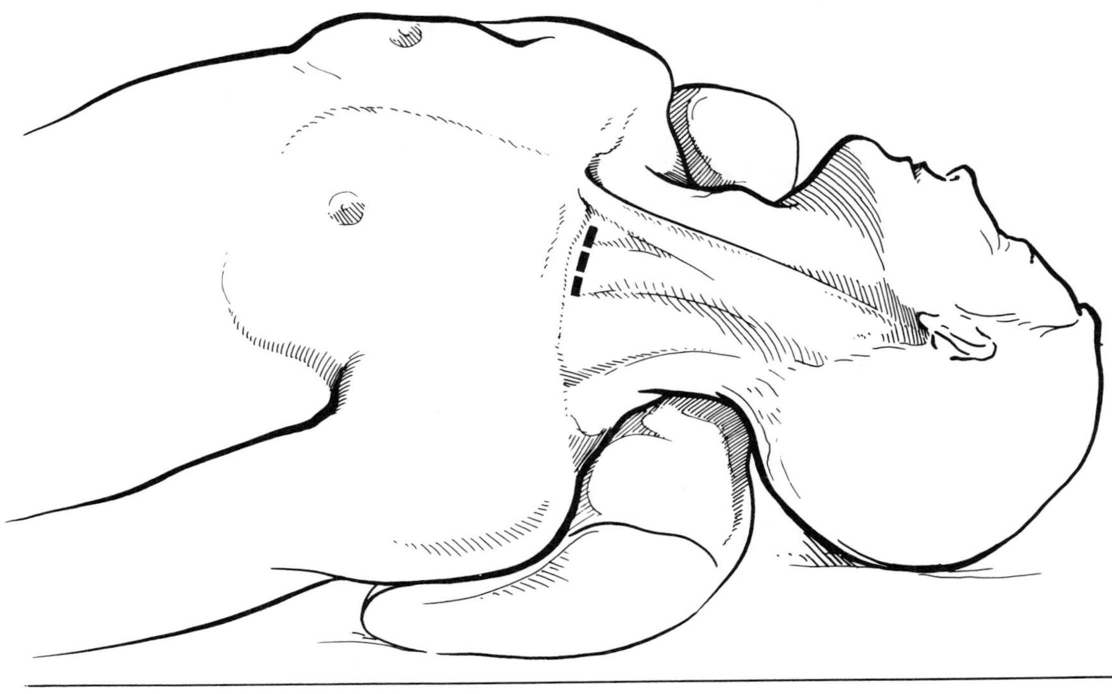

2

3

The clavicular head of the sternocleidomastoid muscle is then divided, leaving sufficient muscle below for the reconstruction. The omohyoid muscle crosses the operative field obliquely and occasionally it may have to be divided.

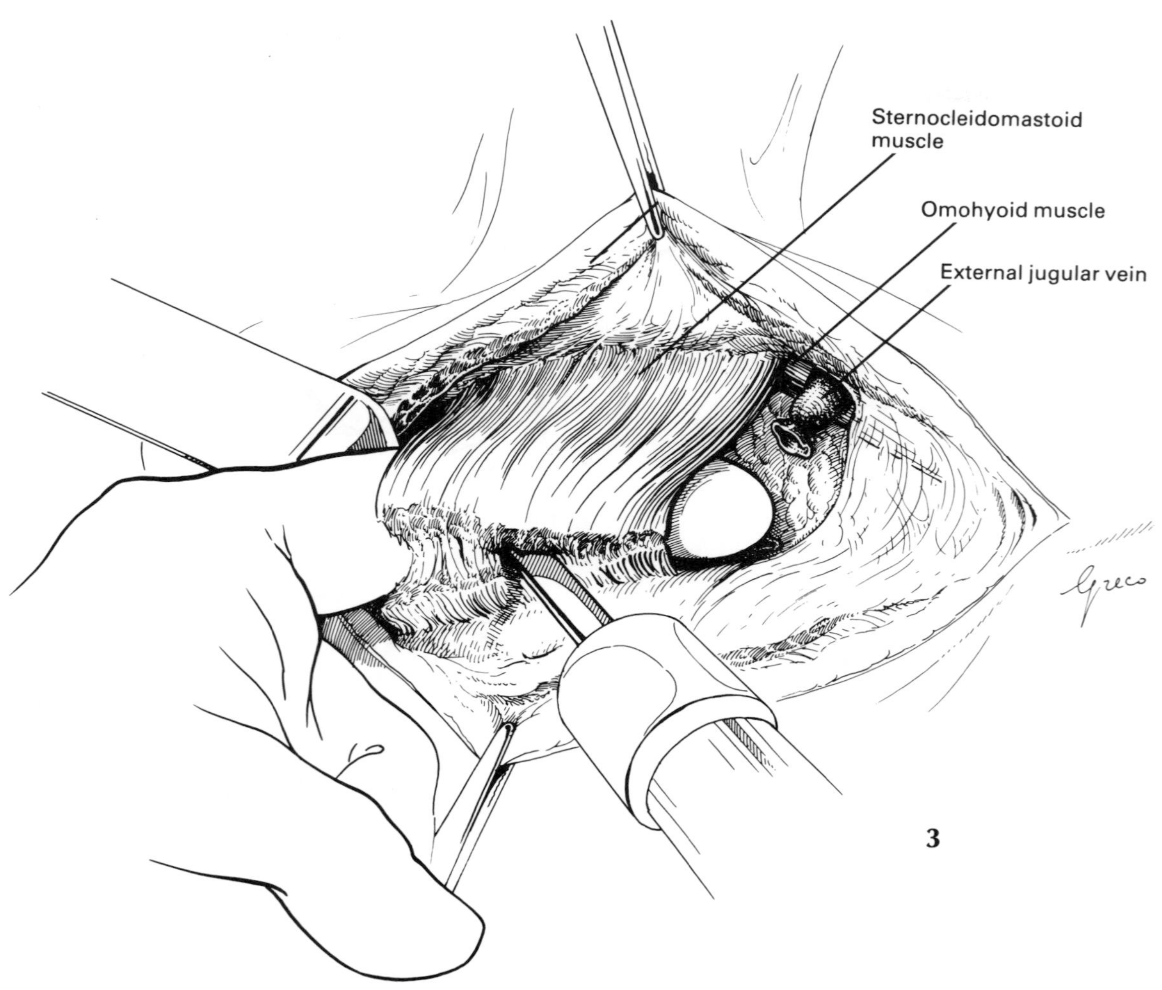

3

4

The internal jugular vein is identified and preserved. The scalene pad of fat with lymph nodes is situated in the centre of the field; this is displaced upwards and must sometimes be divided between clips. The scalenus anterior muscle is now visible. The phrenic nerve, attached to the muscle by fascia, can be seen running from lateral to medial on the muscle from above downwards. The nerve must be dissected free and isolated. Using extreme delicacy it is retracted medially with a small retractor or, preferably, with a Silastic loop. The scalenus anterior muscle is then divided very near its insertion into the first rib. Immediately behind the scalene muscle lies the subclavian artery and from it the vertebral artery branches and runs upward. It is vital, therefore, when dissecting the scalene muscle, to avoid damage to these deep vascular structures. For this reason some surgeons first pass an instrument behind the muscle before dissecting it. However, we prefer not to perform this potentially dangerous manoeuvre, and instead cautiously dissect the muscle with an electroknife, eventually inserting the index finger of the left hand behind the remaining bundles of the muscle. The muscle fibres retract as the dissection proceeds and, when only a few layers remain, the transparent sheath of the subclavian artery can be seen. The last muscle fibres are then cut with dissecting scissors.

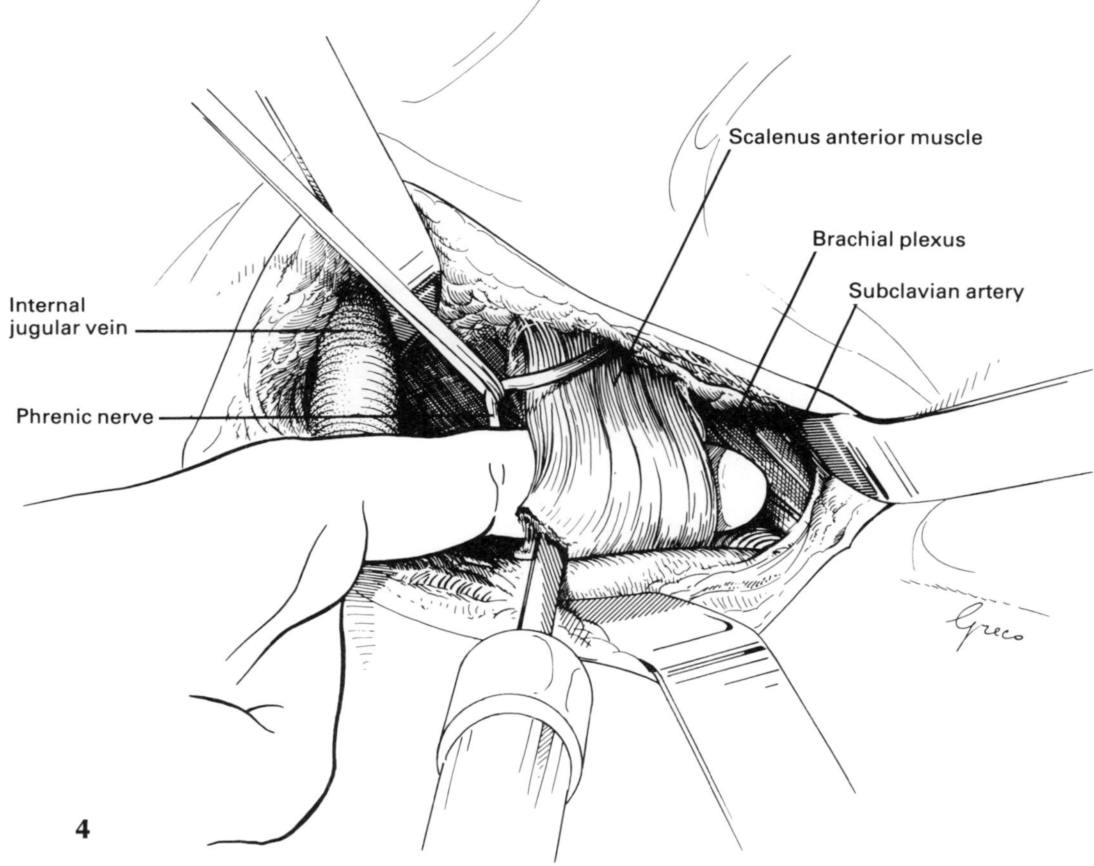

5

The subclavian arch is thus isolated from the internal jugular vein and under it lies the vertebral artery. Distally the thyrocervical trunk, which may be tied, originates from the subclavian artery. Whenever a *left* sympathectomy is performed one should be aware of the presence of the thoracic duct that emerges from the mediastinum and enters the subclavian vein lateral to its confluence with the internal jugular vein. At this point, the subclavian arch is retracted upward to display the apex of the lung, the pleural dome and the suprapleural membrane (Sibson's fascia). Sibson's fascia is bluntly dissected from the rib, thus allowing entry to the retropleural space. It begins to strip more easily below on the medial side. Once the stripping beings a swab is gently pushed into the enlarging space with the index finger until the lung is fully depressed without injury to the pleura.

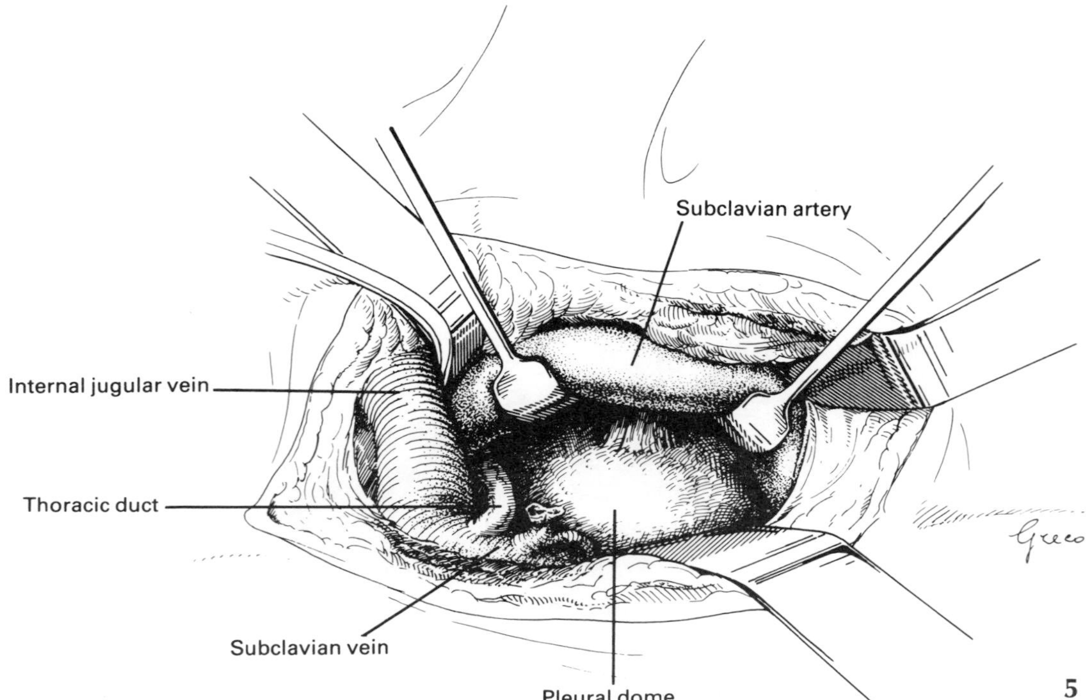

5

6

The sympathetic chain can now be seen but it is more important that the surgeon's hand be guided by a sense of touch in this deep space. The chain is like a thick corded structure that passes across the neck of the first rib. The intercostal artery and vein must be carefully avoided (the first intercostal artery is a branch of the subclavian costocervical trunk). The chain is palpated with the finger and an illuminated lighted retractor is used to view it. A hook is then used to lift the sympathetic chain which is traced as far as possible. Usually, it is easy to reach the third thoracic ganglion and below this the chain is divided and delivered upwards. All of the rami communicantes are divided between neurosurgical metal clips, but the stellate ganglion is not mobilized for fear of producing a Horner's syndrome. Some surgeons divide the chain and take the lower part of the stellate ganglion, but it has been shown that embedding the cut chain into the scalenus anterior muscle with a transfixion stitch is sufficient.

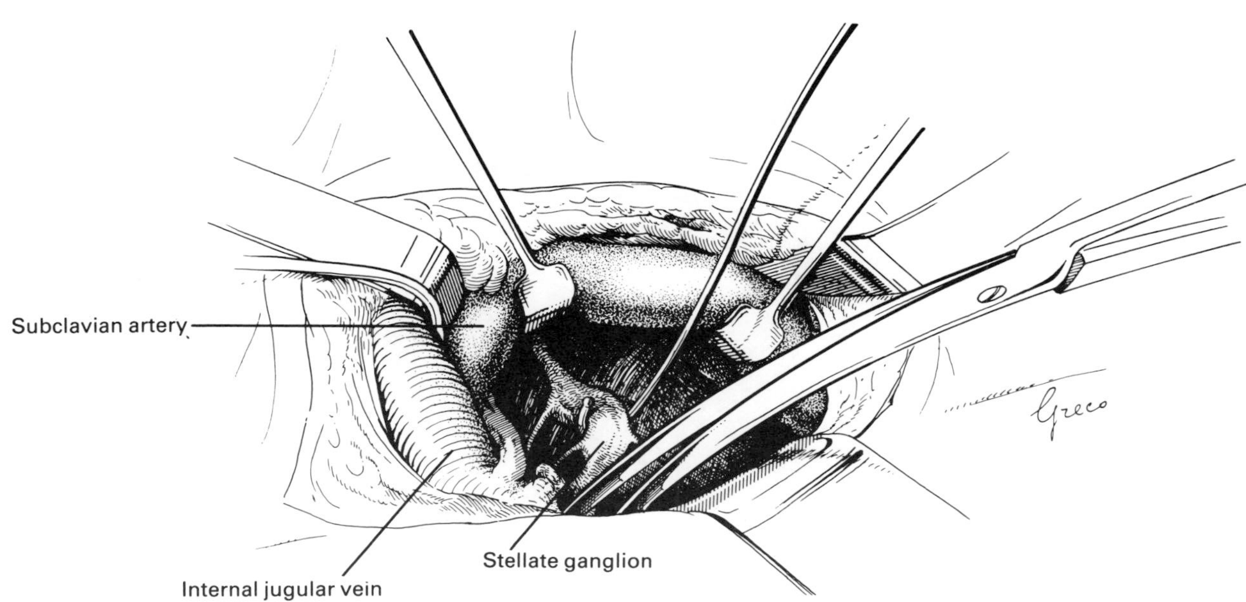

6

7 & 8

Once haemostasis has been secured the incision is closed without drainage. (However, if damage to the pleural dome is suspected, it is advisable to place a slender catheter in the extrapleural space.) The edges of the clavicular head of the sternocleidomastoid muscle are brought together, followed by the platysma muscle, with fine catgut sutures. Finally, the skin is closed, either with Michelle clips or very fine nylon sutures. If a drain is used a Redivac suction drain is usually ideal.

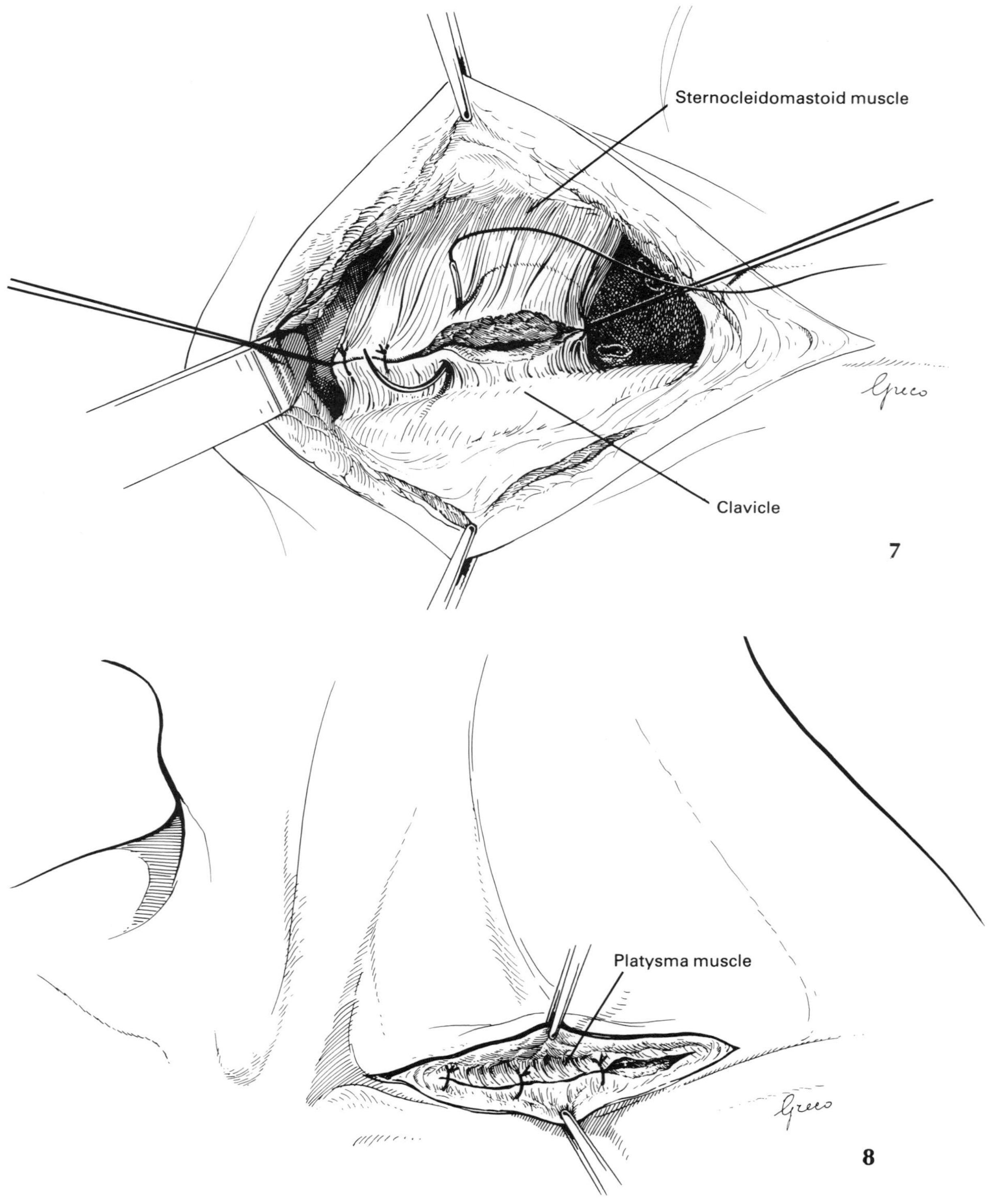

Complications

There are complications of sympathectomy: temporary sweating of the palms in the postoperative period, usually lasts for 1–3 days only; compensatory hyperhidrosis may present on the contralateral side or in other parts of the body after sympathectomy but which reduces in time. Postoperative pain may occur, such as neuralgia of the face, shoulder or chest region; it is more frequent after axillary procedures but seldom lasts more than a few weeks. A postsympathetic neuralgia is fortunately rare, but the severe pain in the upper arm may be really debilitating and may last several months. Horner's syndrome, with ptosis of the lid, endophthalmitis and miosis is more frequent after the supraclavicular procedure, but may affect all approaches. It is mandatory to discuss this possibility with the patient before surgery, as well as other possible complications. Horner's syndrome is associated with nasal congestion and visual disturbance, or with dryness of the nasal mucosa and loss of facial sweating, but is rarely permanent.

Lymph fistula and lymphocoele may occur after the supraclavicular procedure. Chylothorax may also occasionally occur, requiring dissection and ligation of the thoracic duct and chest drainage. Incomplete re-expansion of the lung, or frank pneumothorax are possible but pulmonary complications are more frequent after the transthoracic route.

References

Adams, D. C. R., Wood, S. J., Tulloh, B. R., Baird, R. N. and Poskitt, K. R. (1992). Endoscopic transthoracic sympathectomy. *European Journal of Vascular Surgery* **6**, 558.

Atkins, H. J. B. (1954). Sympathectomy by the axillary approach. *Lancet* **1**, 538.

Bruning, F. (1872). Weitere Erfahrungen uber den Sympathiens. *Klinische Wolkenschrift* **2**.

Gask, G. E. and Ross, J. P. (1937). *The Surgery of the Sympathetic Nervous System.* Baltimore: W. Wood and Co.

Greenhalgh, R. M., Rosengarten, D. S. and Martin, P. (1971). Role of sympathectomy for hyperhidrosis. *British Medical Journal* **1**, 322.

Harris, J. P. and May, J. (1989). Upper extremity sympathectomy. In *Vascular Surgery*, Rutherford, R. B., ed. London: W. B. Saunders.

Jonnesco, T. (1923). *Le Sympatique Cervico-thoracique.* Paris: Masson.

Kleinert, H. E., Cole, N. M. and Wayne, L. (1973). Post-traumatic sympathetic dystrophy. *Orthopaedic Clinics of North America* **4**, 917.

May, J. and Harris, J. P. (1984). Upper extremity sympathectomy: A comparison of the supraclavicular and axillary approaches in evaluation and treatment of upper and lower extremity circulatory disorders. In *Operative Techniques in Vascular Surgery*, Bergan, J. J. and Yao, J. S. T., eds. New York: Grune and Stratton.

Ross, D. B. (1980). Transaxillary extrapleural thoracic sympathectomy. In *Operative Techniques in Vascular Surgery*, Bergan, J. J. and Yao, J. S. T., eds. New York: Grune and Stratton.

Royle, N. D. (1924). The treatment of spastic paralysis by sympathetic ramisection. *Surgery, Gynecology, Obstetrics* **39**, 701.

Schwartz, P. J., Locati, E. H., Moss, E. J., Crampton, R. S., Trazzi, R. and Ruberti, U. (1991). Left cardiac sympathetic denervation in the therapy of congenital long QT syndrome (world-wide report). *Circulation* **84**(2), 503.

Smithwick, R. H. (1940). The rationale of sympathectomy for the relief of vascular spasm of the extremities. *New England Journal of Medicine* **222**, 699.

Telford, E. D. (1935). The technique of sympathectomy. *British Journal of Surgery* **23**, 448.

Welch, E. and Geary, J. (1984). Current status of thoracic dorsal sympathectomy. *Journal of Vascular Surgery* **1**, 202.

White, J. C., Smithwick, R. H. and Simeone, F. A. (1952). *The Autonomic Nervous System: Anatomy, Physiology and Surgical Application.* New York: Macmillan.

Witmoser, R. (1984). Possibilities of using sympathectomy for treatment of pain syndromes. *Applied Neurophysiology* **47**, 203.

Transthoracic sympathectomy

HAROLD ELLIS CBE, DM, MCh, FRCS

Professor of Surgery, Division of Anatomy and Cell Biology, Guy's Hospital, London, UK

Preoperative

Indications

Excision of the upper portion of the thoracic part of the sympathetic chain has, as its main indication, the treatment of severe idiopathic hyperhidrosis of the hands. This has an equal sex distribution, although women with this condition are more likely to complain of the excessive associated axillary sweating. Symptoms usually commence at the time of puberty but may be seen in childhood (Law and Ellis, 1989). All four limbs may be affected but individual patients may complain that the sweating of the axillae, the hands or the feet is the principal nuisance. There is often little difference during summer or winter and the sweating is not usually aggravated by exercise. It is precipitated by emotional or mental stress and ceases during sleep. There is often an associated Raynaud's phenomenon, with the hands and feet being cold and blue as well as sweating.

The cause of this condition is unknown. The sweat glands in the involved areas are normal, both histologically and numerically. Histochemical and electron microscopic changes cannot be detected. The clinical effects of severe hyperhidrosis are most distressing; slippery objects drop out of wet hands, it may be impossible to use a pen and the patient avoids social contact.

Upper thoracic sympathectomy is also indicated in severe examples of Raynaud's phenomenon which do not respond to conservative measures. However, unlike the permanent results of sympathectomy for hyperhidrosis, there is a tendency to progressive relapse following the operation so that only some 50% of patients show persistent improvement when assessed several years postoperatively.

Advantages and disadvantages of the transthoracic approach

The advantages of the transthoracic approach are the almost invisible scar, which lies hidden in the axilla, the avoidance of Horner's syndrome in the great majority of cases, provided that the stellate ganglion is carefully preserved, and the simplicity of the anatomical approach to the chain compared with the transcervical technique.

The disadvantages of the operation are that most surgeons, including the author, consider that it is only safe to perform one side at a time. I usually leave at least a month between the two operations in bilateral cases. Some surgeons, however, have practised synchronous bilateral thoracotomy successfully. The operation is also contraindicated if there has been previous intrathoracic infection, e.g. quiescent pulmonary tuberculosis, with resultant pleural adhesions. In such cases (and I have only encountered one example of this) the transcervical approach becomes mandatory.

Where the expertise and facilities are available, transthoracoscopic diathermy coagulation of the chain is now the operation of choice. The scar is minimal, both sides can be dealt with at the same sitting and, in trained hands, the morbidity is negligible.

This is described in the following chapter – Sympathectomy by thoracoscopy, p. 281. It should be remembered, however, that occasionally adhesions at the lung apex make the endoscopic method virtually impossible – it is important to be familiar with the classical approach.

Surgical anatomy

1

In planning excision of the upper thoracic sympathetic chain for sympathetic denervation of the upper limb and axilla, the surgeon needs to know how much of the chain to remove in order to effect satisfactory denervation and how to prevent a Horner's syndrome. The thoracic portion of the chain continues downwards from the cervical sympathetic chain and lies anterior to the heads of the ribs. It lies immediately external to the parietal pleura, almost invariably immediately anterior to the intercostal vessels. However, the chain lies uncomfortably close to the intercostal veins, which may occasionally cross in front of it. Each ganglion is situated fairly consistently in front of the corresponding rib head. The first thoracic ganglion may be independent or, more usually, is fused to the inferior cervical ganglion to constitute the stellate ganglion. Occasionally, the second thoracic ganglion may be fused into this ganglionic conglomeration. Each ganglion lies below the level of the corresponding intercostal nerve to which it is connected by the white ramus communicans of preganglionic fibres and the grey (postganglionic) ramus. The grey ramus usually lies medially to the white ramus but occasionally these are combined into a single trunk and at times there may be more than two rami.

The fibres in the white ramus communicans of the first thoracic nerve ascend in the chain to the superior cervical ganglion in order to supply sympathetic fibres to the face. Interruption of the sympathetic chain at or above this first thoracic ganglion level will thus result in Horner's syndrome, comprising ptosis, pupillary constriction, flushing of the face and facial anhidrosis on the affected side.

The second thoracic nerve is the highest one to contain preganglionic fibres to the upper limb. There is much more variability to the lower limit and fibres as low as the seventh thoracic nerve may contribute fibres to the upper limb. Although there is this widespread origin of preganglionic fibres to the upper limb, division of the thoracic sympathetic chain immediately below the first ganglion will usually interrupt all fibres that traverse the sympathetic chain to reach the upper limb by distribution through the brachial plexus. In practice, removal of the thoracic sympathetic chain to include the second, third and fourth ganglia, which means removing the chain from the head of the second to the head of the fourth rib, is found to produce effective sympathetic denervation of the upper limb and axilla.

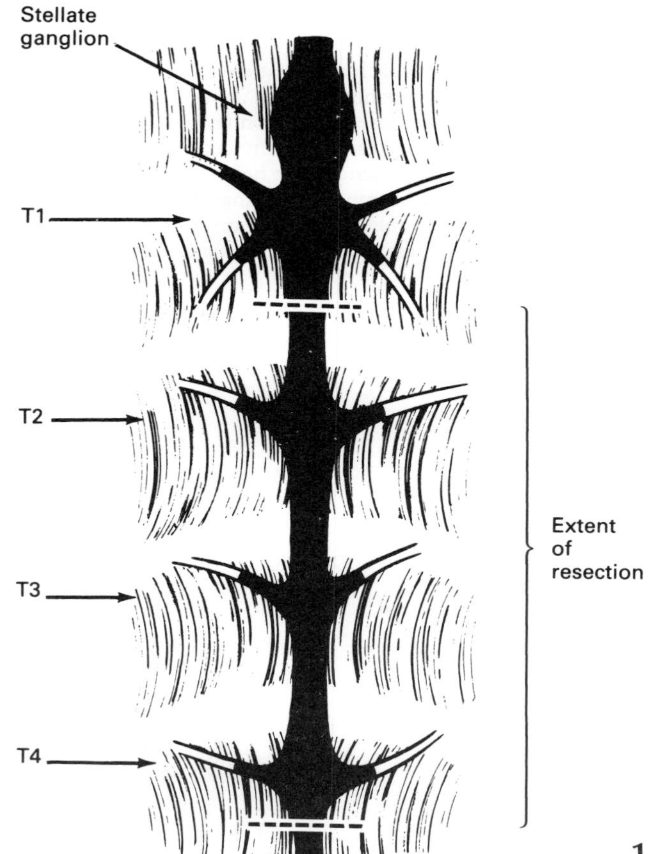

1

Surgical technique

2

The transaxillary approach was first described by Sir Hedley Atkins in 1949. Endotracheal general anaesthesia is used. The patient is placed in the lateral position with the arm abducted to 90°. A suitable right-angled arm support is used. It is convenient to tilt the patient in the head-up position at about 20° to allow adequate illumination of the depths of the wound. It is useful to have a malleable light on a probe to improve illumination if necessary, particularly in an obese patient.

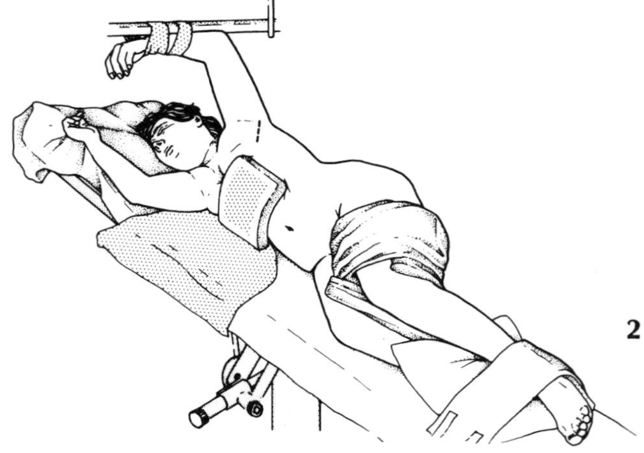

2

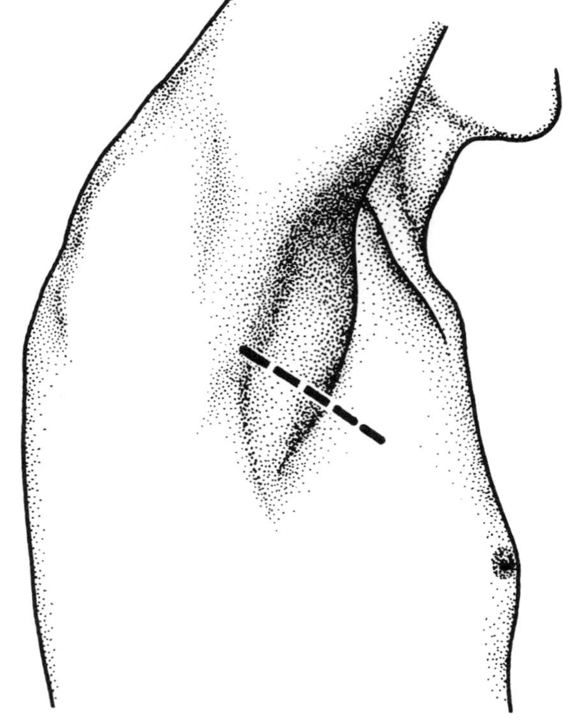

3

3

The incision is made along the line of the second intercostal space from pectoralis major in front to latissimus dorsi posteriorly. The obliquity of this incision varies quite considerably from one subject to another. Because the area is quite vascular, bleeding is controlled by preliminary infiltration of the subcutaneous tissues with a 1:200 000 solution of adrenaline in normal saline and by the use of the diathermy cutting needle. The incision is made through the axillary fat down to the serratus anterior. The nerve to this muscle (the long thoracic nerve of Bell) is identified at the posterior limit of the incision and is carefully preserved. Injury to this nerve will produce winging of the scapula.

The second intercostal space is now palpated and the serratus divided with diathermy over the space. The dissection is then continued through the intercostal muscles down to the pleura. By staying immediately superior to the second rib, damage to the intercostal bundle can be avoided. The pleura is opened, the lung collapses and the intercostal space is opened for the full length of the wound. The ribs are then retracted by means of a Price-Thomas self-retaining retractor which is slowly opened to its full extent. A wet pack is placed over the collapsed lung, which is retracted downwards by means of a suitably bent malleable copper retractor.

4

The sympathetic chain can now be easily identified as it lies beneath the parietal pleura on the heads of the upper ribs. On the right side, the azygos vein is seen lying medially to the chain, whereas on the left side, the aorta and left subclavian artery can be seen.

It is important to identify the sympathetic chain quite precisely before the parietal pleura is opened, otherwise oozing of blood may obscure the anatomy. The line of the chain is indicated on the pleura by two or three scalpel nicks and 2 or 3 ml of the dilute adrenaline solution is then injected via a fine needle beneath the pleura to free it from the underlying ribs.

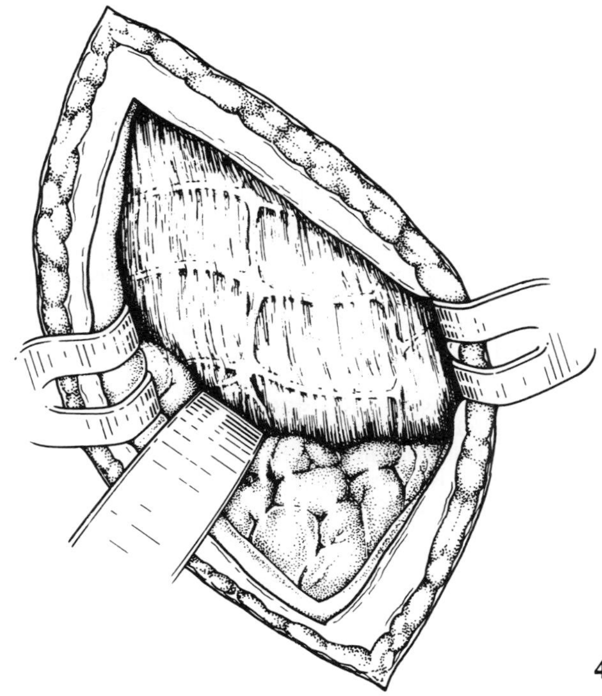

4

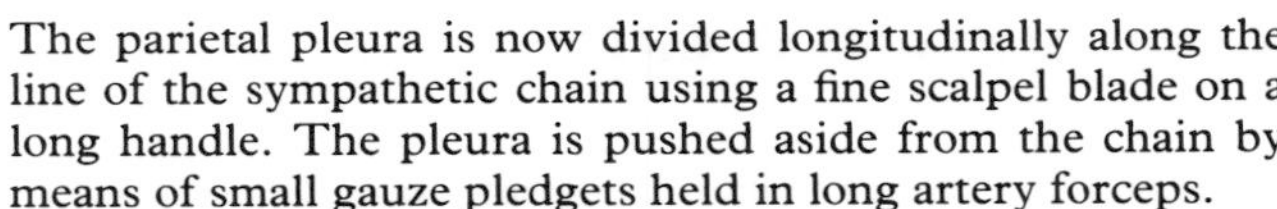

5

The parietal pleura is now divided longitudinally along the line of the sympathetic chain using a fine scalpel blade on a long handle. The pleura is pushed aside from the chain by means of small gauze pledgets held in long artery forceps.

The chain is caught up on a nerve hook and carefully removed from below upwards from the level of the fourth rib to just below the stellate ganglion, thus removing the fourth, third and second ganglia.

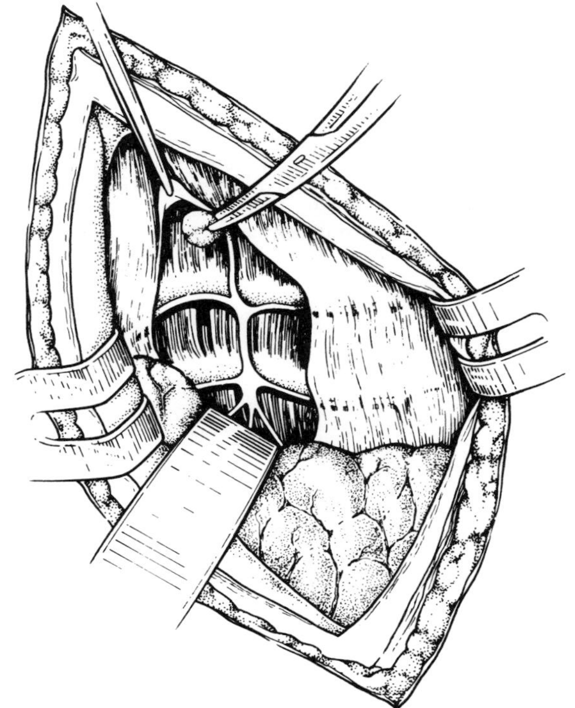

5

6

Bleeding may be encountered from branches of the intercostal vessels, particularly the veins, and haemostasis is effected by means of diathermy coagulation, Cushing's silver clips or a combination of the two.

It is my practice to mark the upper and lower extremities of the chain resection by means of Cushing's clips so that subsequent radiology can confirm the extent of the resection.

A check is made to ensure complete haemostasis before the anaesthetist is asked to inflate the lung.

A plastic intercostal tube is inserted through the second space and brought out through a small stab wound. The wound is closed in layers using catgut, the skin sutured and the intercostal drain connected with an underwater seal. Meanwhile, the anaesthetist continues to ensure that the lung is completely inflated in order to obliterate the pneumothorax.

The patient is transferred to the recovery room and, when conscious, a check X-ray of the chest is carried out. If this confirms that complete expansion of the lung has occurred, the chest tube can be removed in the recovery room before the patient is returned to the ward.

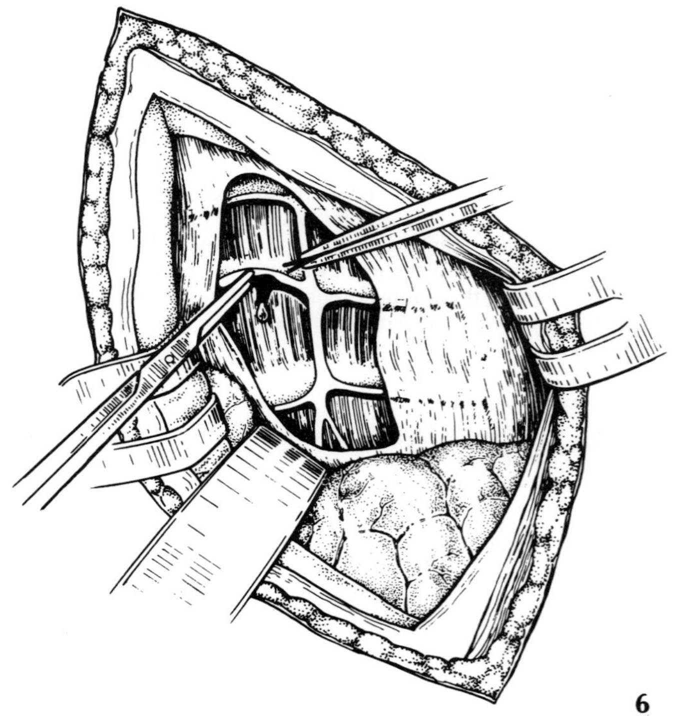

6

Postoperative care

The patient requires vigorous postoperative chest physiotherapy and a repeat chest X-ray the day following operation ensures the absence of a pneumothorax or pleural effusion. The great majority of patients can leave hospital 3 or 4 days postoperatively.

References

Atkins, H. J. B. (1949). Per axillary approach to the stellate and upper thoracic sympathetic ganglia. *Lancet* **2**, 1152.

Ellis, H. (1979). Transaxillary sympathectomy in the treatment of hyperhidrosis of the upper limb. *American Surgeon* **45**, 546.

Law, N. and Ellis, H. (1989). Transthoracic sympathectomy for hyperhidrosis in children under the age of 16. *Annals of the Royal College of Surgeons* **71**, 70.

Sympathectomy by thoracoscopy

WILLIAM P. HEDERMAN MCh, FRCSI

Consultant Surgeon, Mater Misericordiae Hospital, Dublin

Introduction

Ablation of the upper dorsal sympathetic chain has long been accepted as the definitive treatment for troublesome excessive sweating of the palms of the hands. However, the traditional surgical approaches, supra-clavicular, axillary, or posterior, are all major procedures which many surgeons have been slow to undertake for what is a non-lethal, albeit distressing condition.

Endoscopic sympathectomy has been available for some time (Kux, 1978). An excellent view of the upper dorsal sympathetic chain can usually be obtained through a thoracoscope and simple diathermy coagulation of the chain produces excellent results (Malone, Duignan and Hederman, 1982; Byrne, Walsh and Hederman, 1990).

Selection of patients should rule out those with more generalized hyperhidrosis due to any cause and those who are likely to have extensive pleural adhesions. The sweating should be severe enough to interfere significantly with the patient's occupation or enjoyment of life (Blumberg, 1986).

The results of sympathectomy for Raynaud's phenomenon, causalgia and other vascular conditions tend to be disappointing in the long term and should only be undertaken in severe cases when all other methods of treatment have failed.

Preoperative

Chest X-ray, thyroid function tests and general assessment for systemic disease which might cause sweating should be carried out.

The operation

1

The patient lies supine with the head of the table slightly elevated and the arms abducted on arm boards to a right angle.

General anaesthesia, preferably with a double lumen endotracheal tube, is employed. A Verres needle is inserted through a small stab incision in the anterior axilla just behind the pectoralis major muscle in the third intercostal space and about 0.5 litres of carbon dioxide gas insufflated. A telescope is passed through a cannula of appropriate size inserted at the same site and the upper pleural cavity inspected. A second small cannula is introduced under direct vision through the third or fourth intercostal space in the mid-clavicular line and an insulated monopolar diathermy electrode introduced through it. Further amounts of gas are insufflated as required to gain a clear view of the upper mediastinum. The diathermy electrode can be used to depress the apex of the lung if necessary. Pulse rate, blood pressure and blood gases are continuously monitored. Two litres or less of gas are usually sufficient.

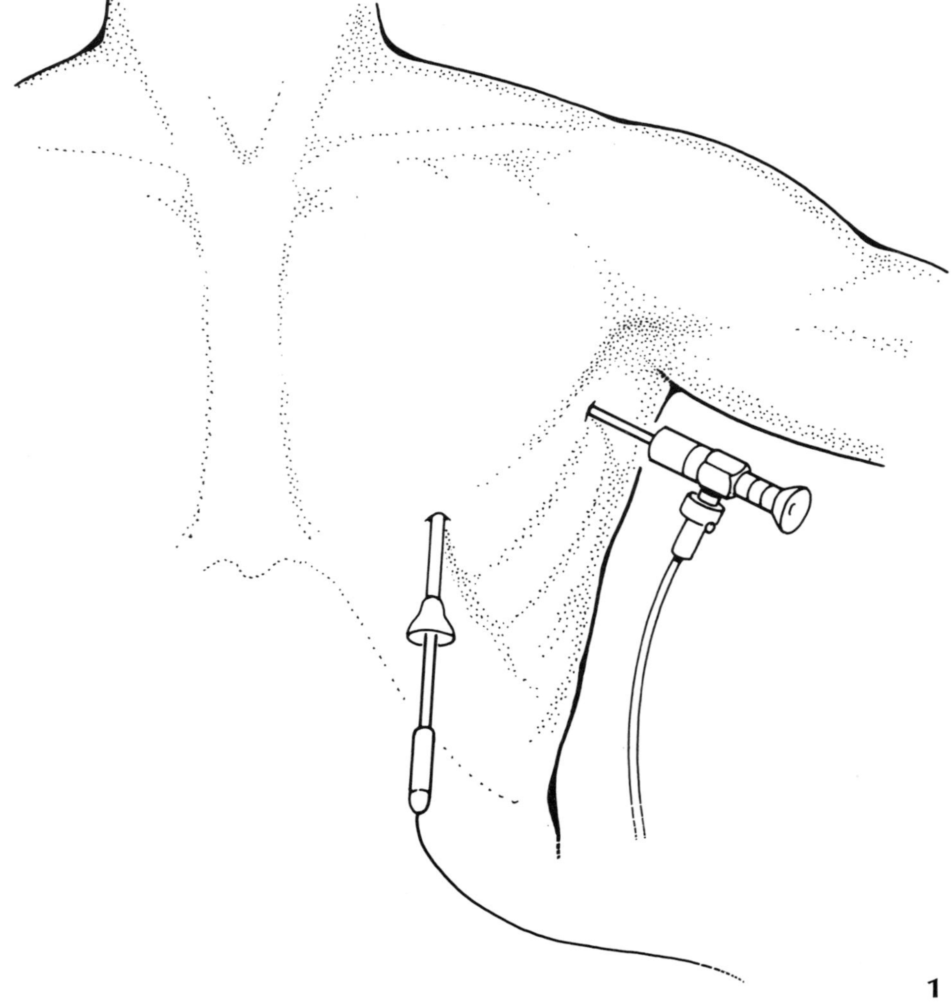

1

2

The neck of the second rib is first identified. It is the highest rib that is visible there, as the first rib and the overlying stellate ganglion are covered by a characteristic yellow pad of fat. The sympathetic chain should be visible beneath the pleura, running over the necks of the second and third ribs. If it is not easily seen, gentle palpation medially along the neck of a rib with the tip of the diathermy electrode will enable it to be identified as it slips out under the tip of the instrument in much the same way as one would palpate for it with the tip of one's index finger in an open operation. A slight bulge is visible on the rib at the site of its articulation with the transverse process and the sympathetic chain lies immediately lateral to this. On the left side the subclavian artery and vagus nerve should be identified medially and on the right side the superior vena cava and the vagus nerve and the azygos vein should be similarly identified.

Fine pleural adhesions can be divided with diathermy scissors but very extensive or dense adhesions can make the operation impossible by this route.

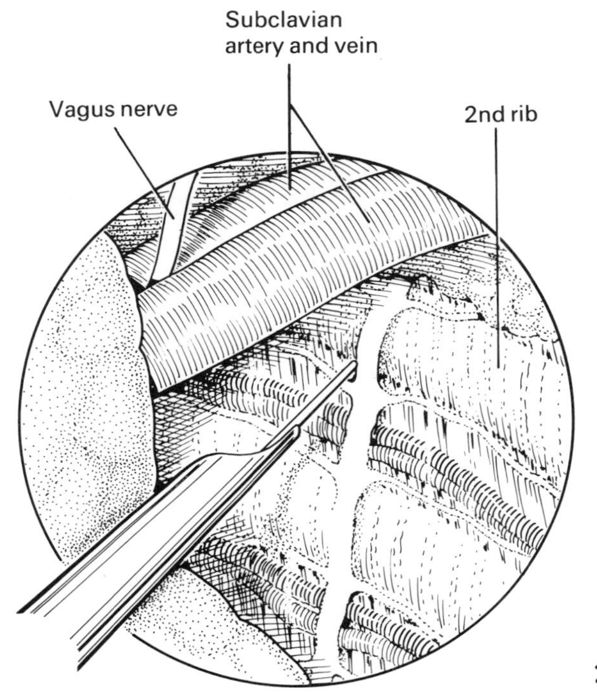

2

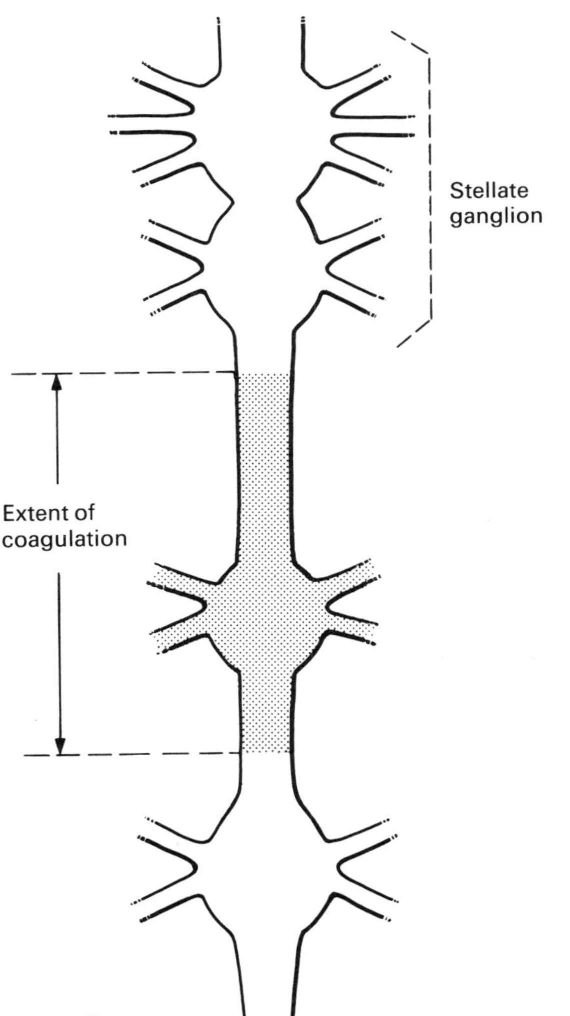

3

3

The pleura is incised with diathermy immediately over the chain and the second ganglion and the chain immediately above and below it is coagulated until it gives a charred appearance. Coagulation should be carried laterally for an inch or so along the neck of the second and third ribs to deal with the possible presence of a nerve of Kuntz (Kuntz, 1927).

The diathermy probe is removed, the gas is disconnected and the lung is reinflated under direct vision by the anaesthetist who reconnects the ipislateral half of the double lumen endotracheal tube which had been disconnected at the outset. No drain is used. The incisions are closed with a single skin suture.

Both sides can be operated on the same occasion provided there is no problem with the first side.

In recent years we have restricted the extent of the sympathectomy to the second dorsal ganglion and the adjoining chain as described above when dealing with cases of palmar hyperhidrosis. This has been found to be fully effective and reduces the amount of compensatory postoperative hyperhidrosis in the trunk and head. Axillary hyperhidrosis has been greatly improved in most cases. (O'Riordan *et al.*, 1993).

Complications

Occasional pneumothorax will be revealed on the postoperative chest X-ray but is usually not significant. Bleeding from an intercostal artery has been reported but should not occur if coagulation is confined to the sympathetic chain and the surface of the ribs. Horner's syndrome is not a problem if one keeps clear of the yellow fat pad, staying well below the stellate ganglion which need not be approached.

References

Blumberg, L, (1986). Endoscopic thoracic sympathectomy in the treatment of upper limb hyperchidrosis. *Annals of the Royal College of Surgeons of England* **68**, 293.

Byrne, J., Walsh, T. N. and Hederman, W. P. (1990). Endoscopic transthoracic electrocautery of the sympathetic chain for palmar and axillary hyperhidrosis. *British Journal of Surgery* **77**, 1046.

Drott, C., Gothberg, G. and Claes, G. (1993). Endoscopic procedures of the upper-thoracic sympathetic chain. *Archives of Surgery* **128**(2), 237.

Kuntz, A. (1927). Distribution of the sympathetic rami to the brachial plexus: its relation to sympathectomy affecting the upper extremity. *Archives of Surgery* **15**, 871.

Kux, M. (1978). Thoracic endoscopic sympathectomy in palmar and axillary hyperhidrosis. *Archives of Surgery* **113**, 264.

Malone, P. S., Cameron, A. E. P. and Remie, J. A. (1986). Endoscopic thoracic sympathectomy in the treatment of upper limb hyperhidrosis. *Annals of the Royal College of Surgeons of England* **68**, 93.

Malone, P. S., Duignan, J. P. and Hederman, W. P. (1982). Transthoracic electrocoagulation: A new and simple approach to upper limb sympathectomy. *Irish Medical Journal* **75**, 20.

O'Riordan, D. S., Maher, M., Waldron, D., O'Donovan, B. and Brady, M. P. (1993). Limiting the anatomical extent of upper thoracic sympathectomy for primary palmar hyperhidrosis. *Surgery, Gynaecology and Obstetrics* **176**, 151.

Embolectomy for acute lower-limb ischaemia

HANS O. MYHRE MD, PhD
Professor and Chairman, Department of Surgery, Trondheim University Clinic, Trondheim, Norway

OLA D. SAETHER MD
Consultant Vascular Surgeon, Department of Surgery, Trondheim University Clinic, Trondheim, Norway

Introduction

In the Scandinavian countries, embolectomies for acute limb ischaemia have increased. Approximately 50% of the procedures are performed by junior staff. The reasons for the increasing incidence of embolism may be due to an increase in the elderly population and the fact that more patients survive major cardiac disease.

In acute limb ischaemia the differential diagnosis between emboli and acute arterial thrombosis is important, because the treatment must be selected accordingly. Thus, an aggressive surgical approach is justified in most cases with emboli, whereas initial conservative treatment may be preferred following acute arterial thrombosis provided the limb is viable (Dale, 1984).

1

The diagnosis of embolism is based on the presence of a potential source and the sudden onset of symptoms. The location of the arterial obstruction may also indicate the source. Thus, an embolus leading to ischaemia of an isolated toe usually arises from atherosclerotic changes in the aorta or the iliac arteries, whereas an embolus in the aortic bifurcation most likely has a cardiac origin. An embolus usually lodges where the artery divides and its calibre reduces.

In arterial thrombosis the onset of symptoms is gradual, often with a previous history of intermittent claudication without signs of cardiac disease. In addition, the pulses may be absent on the contralateral limb.

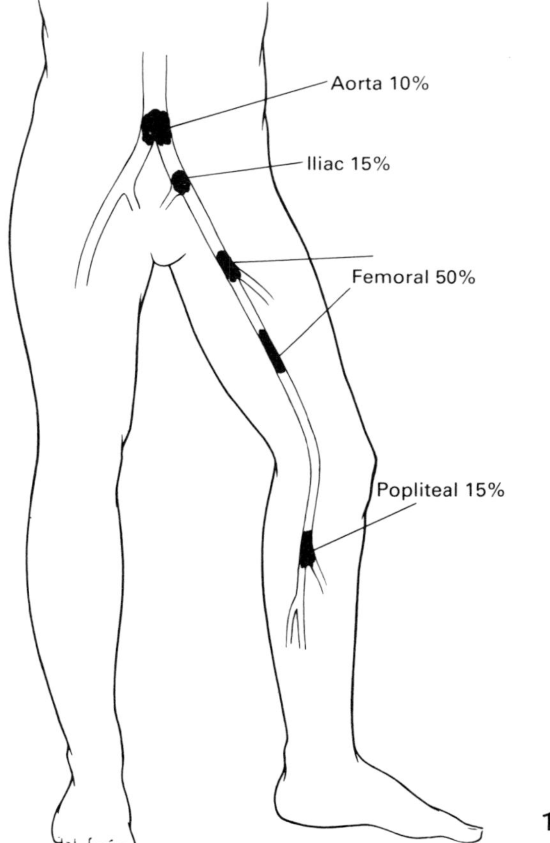

1

Preoperative considerations

Critical ischaemia is indicated by loss of sensitivity, discolouration that blanches with pressure, decreased skin temperature and moderate rigour of the calf muscles. It is generally agreed that embolectomy is indicated even in these patients (Tawes *et al.*, 1985). Although early diagnosis and treatment is important, the time from onset of symptoms to admission is of less importance than the clinical status of the limb. Thus, the time factor does not contraindicate embolectomy by itself.

In irreversible ischaemia there is blotchy cyanotic discolouration which is not influenced by digital pressure. The calf muscle has a firm consistency and, in addition, there is anaesthesia and paralysis of the extremity. The treatment of choice for patients with irreversible ischaemic changes is primary amputation.

Patients with a clear-cut history of emboli are not referred to preoperative angiography. Angiography should, however, always be done when there is doubt about the diagnosis or when acute arterial thrombosis is suspected.

If present, cardiac insufficiency and dehydration should be corrected preoperatively, but the operation should not be delayed by lengthy evaluations.

Heparin is given intravenously as a bolus of 100–150 i.u. per kg bodyweight, taking into consideration that heparin may influence the selection of anaesthesia. Blood is typed and cross-matched and the patient is transferred to the operating room.

In general, the patient is prepared from the nipples to the toes of both feet, keeping in mind that more extensive surgery can become necessary and that multiple emboli often occur. For unilateral femoropopliteal embolectomy when the femoral pulse is palpable, some surgeons prepare the groin and limb only.

Anaesthesia technique and monitoring

Local anaesthesia with lidocaine 0.5–1% is recommended when the embolectomy can be completed via the common femoral artery. Local anaesthetics with adrenaline must be used with care in patients with severe coronary heart disease. Should clinical signs or angiography indicate that additional proximal or distal surgery becomes necessary, local anaesthesia may be a disadvantage. Epidural anaesthesia is contraindicated if the patient is already heparinized, but spinal anaesthesia by a thin needle can be used in these patients without risk of intraspinal bleeding. However, most surgeons prefer general anaesthesia when the operation cannot be completed with local anaesthesia.

Since there is a high incidence of concomitant cardiovascular disease, close monitoring is necessary, especially to detect the systemic effects of revascularization. Monitoring of central venous pressure, systemic arterial pressure and urine output is recommended. In patients with advanced ischaemia, monitoring of central haemodynamics by a Swan-Ganz catheter is justified. Prior to re-establishment of blood flow in such patients, a high urinary output should be obtained by volume therapy and osmotic diuretics. The acid–base status should be closely monitored and sodium bicarbonate added in case of acidosis (Tawes *et al.*, 1985).

The operation

Femoropopliteal embolectomy

2

The advantage of the Fogarty balloon catheter is that emboli can be removed from the aorta as well as the leg arteries via a local arterteriotomy in the common femoral artery. Most femoropopliteal embolectomies can be performed by this approach.

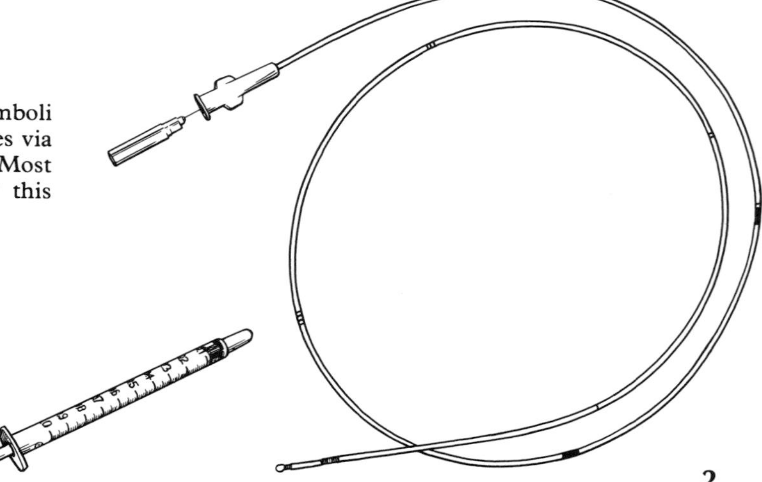

2

3a & b

A vertical incision in the groin is used (*a*), and the common, superficial and the deep femoral arteries are dissected (*b*). Elastic vascular tapes are applied to these arteries for vessel occlusion rather than vascular clamps, so as to minimize blood loss during repeated introductions of the embolectomy catheter. Furthermore, vascular clamps may break the embolic material making it more difficult to remove.

A small incision in the common femoral artery is performed using a No. 11 scalpel blade. A longitudinal arteriotomy of about 1.5 cm is made using fine-angled scissors just proximal to the orifice of the profunda femoris artery. Stay-sutures are applied to the edges of the arteriotomy to facilitate repeated introductions of the Fogarty catheter without damaging the artery, which should not be handled by forceps (*b*).

The stylet of the embolectomy catheter is removed and the patency of the balloon is tested by inflation of saline as recommended for each catheter size. A 1-ml tuberculine syringe is useful for the inflation of a No. 4 embolectomy catheter. Various modifications of the balloon embolectomy catheter have been presented. A channel at the end of the catheter can be used for intraoperative angiography and for irrigation with heparin saline solution. Side-ports central to the balloon may be advantageous for the removal of adherent embolic material and will probably minimize intimal damage. Resterilized catheters should not be used.

The end of a deflated No. 3 or 4 Fogarty catheter is dipped in heparin saline solution or blood and then introduced into the superficial femoral artery (*b*). In patients without atherosclerosis, the catheter can usually be advanced to the foot. The catheter is withdrawn 0.5–1 cm and the balloon is then inflated while moving the catheter to prevent excessive shear forces (Dobrin and Jorgensen, 1985). The grade of inflation must be varied according to the calibre of the artery. Extra caution is necessary during embolectomy of small arteries to avoid overdistention of the balloon. The catheter should be inflated and pulled back by the same surgeon.

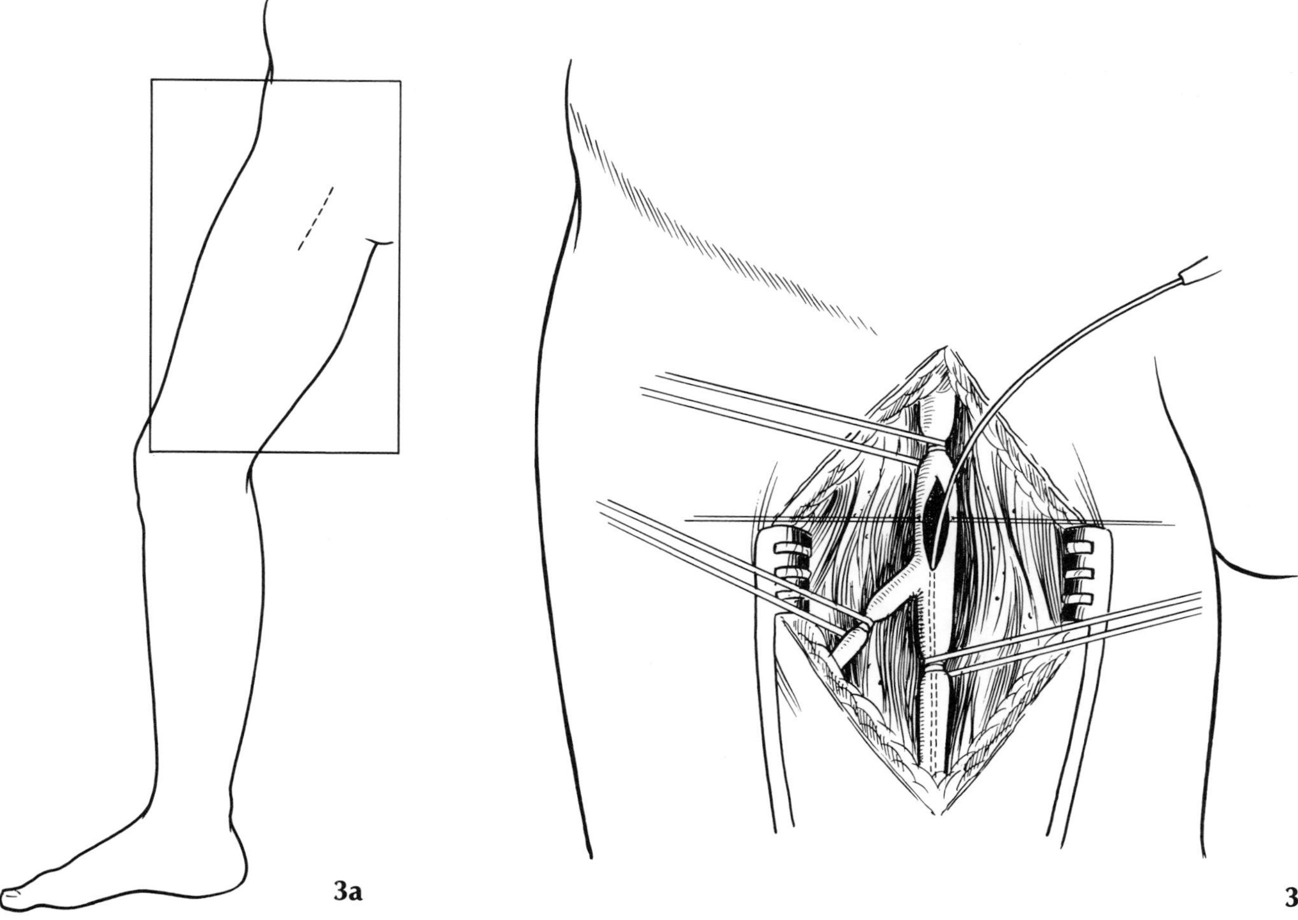

3a

3b

3c, d & e

The embolic material is now removed through the arteriotomy (*c*). The procedure is repeated until no residual embolic material is found, keeping in mind that several withdrawals with a high shear force can induce subsequent intimal hyperplasia (Bowles *et al.*, 1988; Schwarcz *et al.*, 1988). Coagulated blood and debris must be cleaned off the catheter between each introduction. Brisk backbleeding from the distal arterial tree can now be expected, but is not synonymous with a complete embolectomy.

Embolectomy of the profunda femoris artery is now performed. It is extremely important that this artery is free of embolic material. The catheter can usually be advanced about 20 cm from the orifice of the artery. The arteries are flushed with heparine saline solution (1000 i.u. in 100 ml saline) and blood flow from the proximal arteries is tested before the arteriotomy is closed. Provided the artery is unaffected by atherosclerosis and of good calibre, the arteriotomy can be closed by direct suture using 5/0 or 6/0 monofilament suture material (*d*). A patch graft angioplasty is preferred to avoid stenosis during closure of narrow arteries or when there are atherosclerotic changes in the arterial wall (*e*). The saphenous vein is harvested at the ankle and used for patch graft material.

Completion angiography is mandatory following femoropopliteal embolectomy, since incomplete embolectomy has been found in 25–40% of the cases when judged by backbleeding only (Bosma and Jorning, 1990).

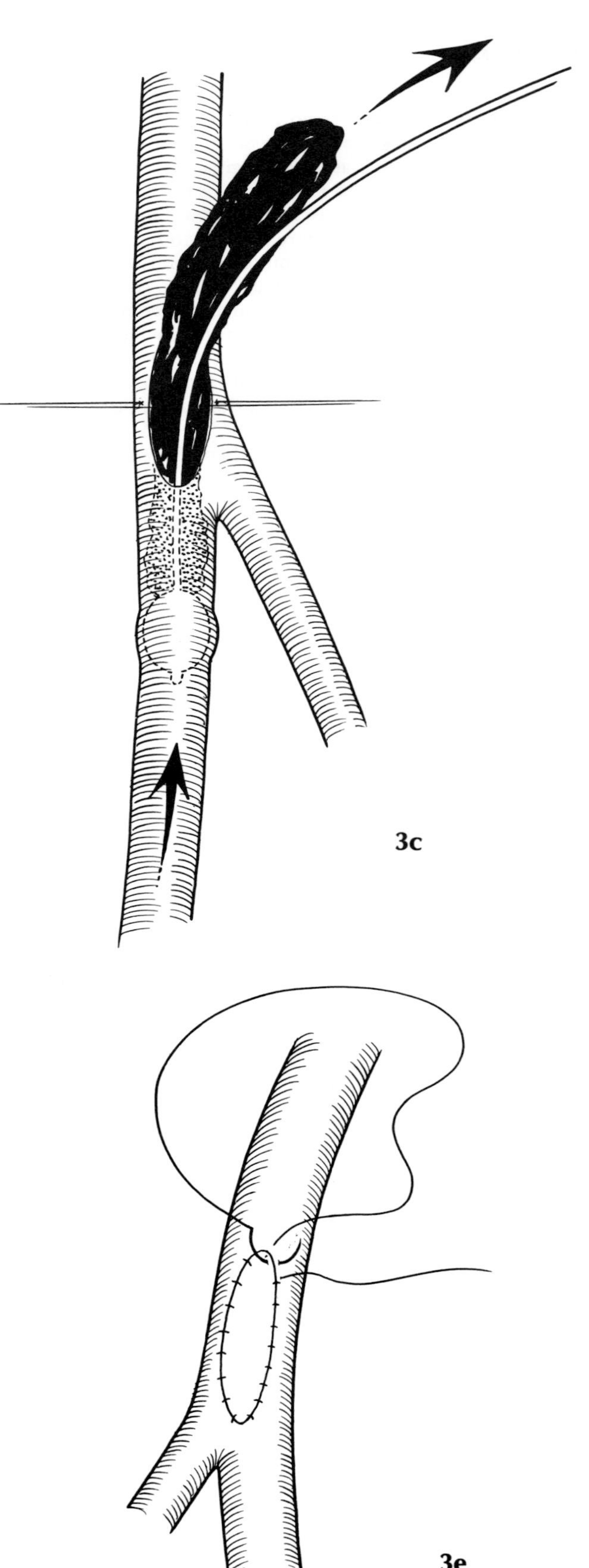

3c

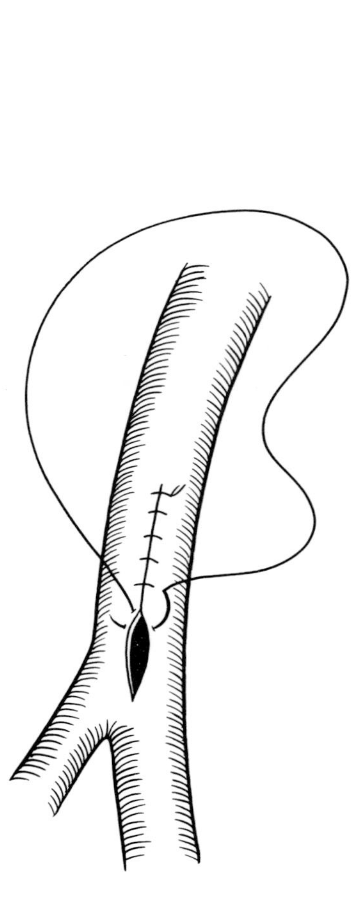

3d

3e

4a, b & c

The peroneal and posterial tibial arteries may be embolectomized through the common femoral artery by bending the tip of the catheter. However, not all types of catheters can be manipulated in this way (Gwynn, Shearman and Simms, 1987). The anterior tibial artery is not readily accessible by this approach. When the popliteal pulse is palpable preoperatively, we explore the popliteal artery below the knee (*a, b*). Following arteriotomy, a No. 3 embolectomy catheter can then be introduced into the different leg arteries. The arteriotomy is closed by patch graft angioplasty (*c*) (Abbott *et al.*, 1984).

In all cases, embolic material should be investigated by microscopy for verification of the aetiology.

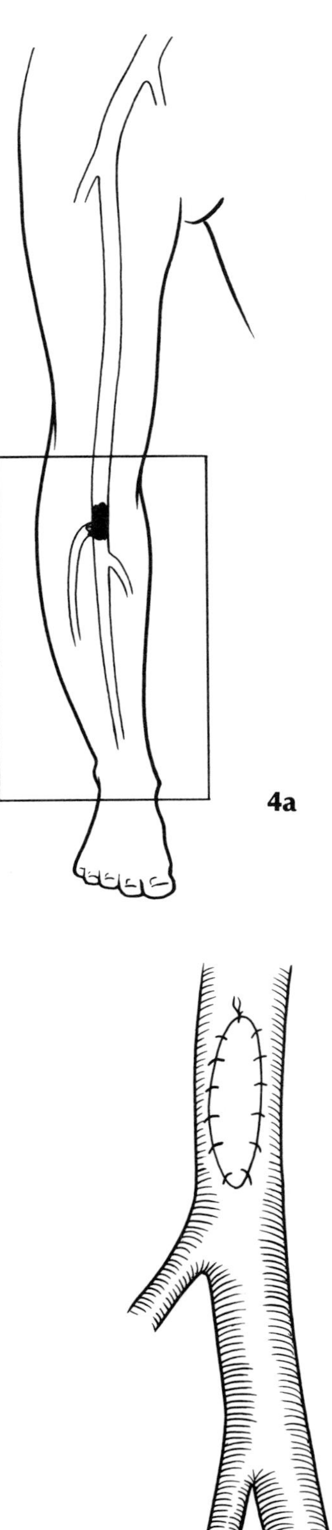

4a

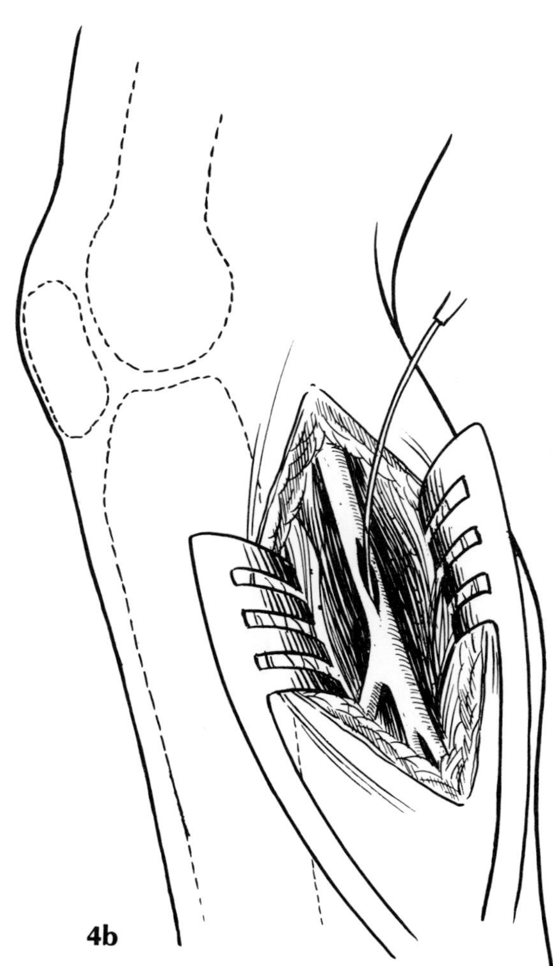

4b

4c

5a & b

Aortoiliac 'saddle' embolectomy

Patients with emboli at the aortic bifurcation or the iliac arteries have a more serious prognosis than patients with femoropopliteal embolism (Busuttil *et al.*, 1983). The abdomen and the lower extremities are prepared as previously described. Vertical incisions are made in both groins and the femoral arteries dissected as described for femoropopliteal embolectomy, preferably by two surgeons working simultaneously (*a*).

A deflated No. 5 or 6 Fogarty catheter is introduced into the aorta through the arteriotomy of the common femoral artery. The balloon is distended and the catheter withdrawn, thereby removing embolic material. The risk of losing embolic material into the contralateral limb can be reduced by compressing the common femoral artery, thereby reducing the blood flow of the contralateral iliac system. When sufficient blood flow from the iliac artery on the embolectomized side is obtained, the embolectomy is repeated on the contralateral side (*b*).

A No. 3 or 4 catheter is then introduced into the superficial femoral and profunda femoris arteries on both sides to remove possible embolic material. The arteriotomies are closed as previously described. A suction drain is routinely left close to each arteriotomy and can usually be removed on the following day.

A similar approach as described for the removal of saddle embolus is used for iliac embolectomy. It is usually sufficient to expose the arteries of one groin only, but great care is taken not to push embolic material into the opposite leg.

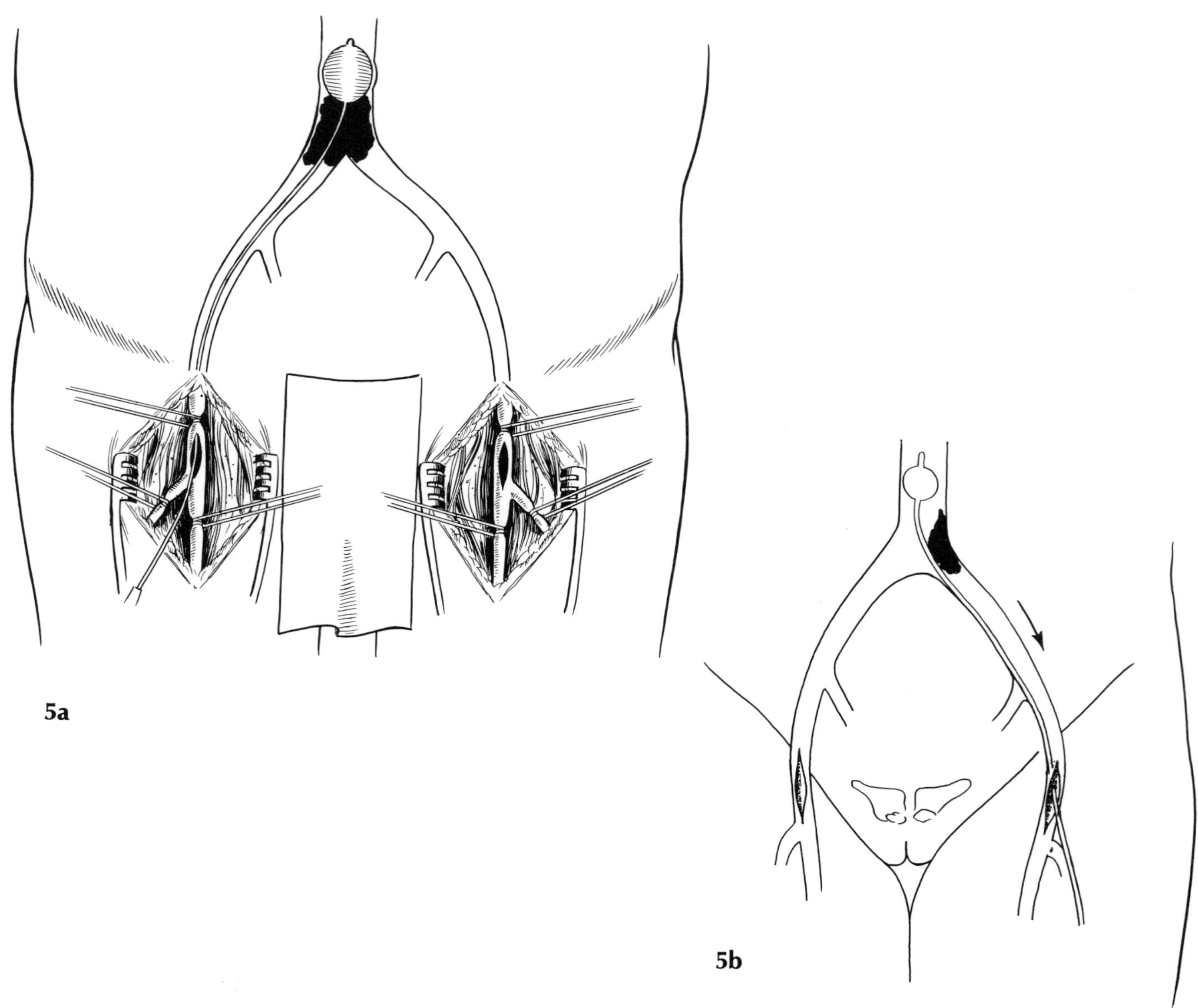

5a

5b

Percutaneous aspiration thromboembolectomy (PAT)

PAT is performed through a specially designed catheter–sheath system for clot extraction. The advantage is that it can be used at the time of diagnostic angiography. It is not within the scope of this presentation to describe the technical details of PAT, which is preferably used for removal of smaller emboli from the distal arterial tree (Wagner and Starck, 1992).

Handling of special problems

Intraoperative thrombolysis appears to be a safe and effective way of removing a residual embolus (Beard *et al.*, 1993).

During delayed embolectomy a cleavage plane between the embolus and the arterial wall may be difficult to identify. A ringstripper can then be used as a supplement to the balloon catheter, or a bypass graft is applied for revascularization.

Sometimes, the embolus may consist of atherosclerotic material from the proximal arterial tree. Removal of the source of embolus is indicated in most of these patients on an elective basis. If the limb ischaemia is caused by aortic dissection, revascularization of the extremity is performed, the anticoagulation therapy must be reversed and further investigation of the aortic dissection is carried out. When acute arterial thrombosis is found to be the cause of critical ischaemia during operation, the surgeon should be prepared to proceed with arterial reconstruction following angiographic investigation. Thrombosis of a popliteal aneurysm may also be the cause of ischaemia. The aneurysm is excluded from the circulation and arterial reconstruction is performed.

Complications

Complications following use of the balloon catheter include rupture of the balloon, intimal injury, arteriovenous fistula, fragmentation of the clot with distal embolization and inadequate removal of the material. Furthermore, dissection of arterosclerotic plaques may occur. Perforation is indicated by difficulties during withdrawal of the catheter. The balloon should be deflated immediately and the catheter removed.

Fasciotomy is performed in cases with preoperative severe ischaemia when repeated postoperative examinations indicate a closed compartment syndrome.

The post-perfusion syndrome can be suspected in the same group of patients. This syndrome is indicated by a urine specimen with Guajac positive pigments, but without red blood cells on microscopy. Prophylaxis by isolation of the femoral vein followed by withdrawal of 300–500 ml of blood during the first pass of arterial blood has been recommended and may be indicated in selected cases (Tawes *et al.*, 1985).

Postoperative considerations

The patient should be observed in the intensive care unit during the first 24 h following the operation. In addition to general monitoring, the circulation of the first toe should be recorded continuously by a non-invasive technique. The patient can be mobilized on the first postoperative day. Heparin is given postoperatively by continuous infusion according to body weight, sex and age. Warfarin-sodium is started immediately following the operation. When a protrombine time of 5–10% of normal value is obtained heparin therapy is discontinued. In most patients, including those with cardiac disease, we find lifelong treatment with warfarin-sodium indicates prevention of recurrent emboli.

References

Abbott, W. M., McCabe, C., Maloney, R. D., Wirthlin, L. S. (1984). Embolism of the popliteal artery. *Surgery, Gynecology and Obstetrics* **159**, 533.

Beard, J. D., Nyamekye, I., Earnshaw, J. S., Scoth, D. J. and Thompson, J. F. (1993). Intraoperative streptokinase: a useful adjunct to balloon-catheter embolectomy. *British Journal of Surgery* **80**, 21.

Bosma, H. W. and Jorning, P. J. (1990). Intra-operative arteriography in arterial embolectomy. *European Journal of Vascular Surgery* **4**, 469.

Bowles, C. R., Olcott, C., Pakter, R. L., Lombard, C., Mehigan,, J. T. and Walter, J. F. (1988). Diffuse arterial narrowing as a result of intimal proliferation: A delayed complication of embolectomy with the Fogarty balloon catheter. *Journal of Vascular Surgery* **7**, 487.

Busuttil, R. W., Keehn, G., Milliken, J. *et al.* (1983). Aortic saddle embolus. A twenty-year experience. *Annals of Surgery* **197**, 698.

Dale, W. A. (1984). Differential management of acute peripheral arterial ischemia. *Journal of Vascular Surgery* **1**, 269.

Dobrin, P. B. and Jorgenson, R. A. (1985). Balloon embolectomy catheters in small arteries: A technique to prevent excessive shear forces. *Journal of Vascular Surgery* **2**, 692.

Fogarty, T. J., Cranley, J. J., Krause, R. J., Strasser, E. S. and Hafner, C. D. (1963). A method for extraction of arterial emboli and thrombi. *Surgery, Gynecology and Obstetrics* **116**, 241.

Gwynn, B. R., Shearman, C. P. and Simms, M. H. (1987). The anatomical basis for the route taken by Fogarty catheters in the lower leg. *European Journal of Vascular Surgery* **1**, 129.

Schwarcz, T. H., Dobrin, P. B., Mrkvicka, R., Skowron, L. and Cole, M. B., Jr (1988). Early myointimal hyperplasia after balloon catheter embolectomy: Effect of shear forces and multiple withdrawals. *Journal of Vascular Surgery* **7**, 495.

Tawes, R. L., Harris, E. J., Brown, W. H. *et al.* (1985). Arterial thromboembolism. A 20-year experience. *Archives of Surgery* **120**, 595.

Wagner, H. J. and Starck, E. E. (1992). Acute embolic occlusions of the infrainguinal arteries: percutaneous aspiration embolectomy in 102 patients. *Radiology* **182**, 403.

Initial lysis and catheter clot removal for occlusive disease in critical ischaemia

B. NACHBUR

Department of Thoracic and Cardiovascular Surgery, University of Berne, Berne, Switzerland

F. MAHLER
DO-DAI-DO

Medical Department of the University of Berne, Berne, Switzerland

E. SCHNEIDER

Division of Angiology, Medical Department of the University of Zürich, Zürich, Switzerland

Introduction

Catheter clot lysis (CTL) is gaining increasing acceptance as it becomes evident that not all cases of critical ischaemia are best treated surgically. Our own experience in Berne comprises well over 250 cases with streptokinase, urokinase and tissue plasminogen activator (rt-PA) being used in that order. Although success rates, i.e. patency rates, have risen from 73 to 85%, the differences are statistically not significant, there being no proof that any one fibrinolytic agent is superior to the other as far as efficacy is concerned. If the results with streptokinase are somewhat less favourable it should be borne in mind that this is most likely attributable to a period during which experience with this new form of treatment had to be gained. In the light of this we look back upon our results with streptokinase with satisfaction and are actually using either this drug or urokinase again.

No doubt streptokinase is no less potent than urokinase, but the latter is generally preferred over streptokinase because it is associated with fewer side-effects (slightly less bleeding complications) and because streptokinase cannot be used repeatedly if anaphylactic reactions to antibodies are to be avoided.

Although Hess and others (Hess, Mietaschk and Ingrisch, 1982; Hess *et al.*, 1982; Schneider and Largiadèr, 1987) have advocated local clot lysis in the treatment of arterial occlusions with symptoms of complete ischaemia, we feel that it is best indicated for treatment of viable limbs presenting with acute thrombotic occlusion associated with localized or widespread atherosclerotic lesions.

It is agreed that acute thromboembolic occlusion of the iliofemoral segment is best treated by the Fogarty balloon extraction catheter, local thrombolysis is especially suitable for acute thrombotic lesions involving the femoral and/or popliteal arteries including the popliteal trifurcation. Furthermore, CTL is indicated in the treatment of early re-occlusions after percutaneous transluminal angioplasty (PTA) and recanalization of acute occlusions of femoropopliteal grafts.

As the clot is gradually being dissolved, underlying stenotic lesions are uncovered and thus become amenable to PTA, which on its own merit must be considered an integral part of catheter clot lysis therapy because it deals with the causative mechanism of thrombotic occlusion. The rate of local thrombolysis can be considerably hastened by aspiration or extraction of loosened clots (CTE) whereby clearance of the vessel is more actively promoted. As a consequence short-term CTL has become the rule, long-term lytic therapy on the other hand the exception.

Method of CTL and CTE

Following preliminary studies by Demski and Zeitler in 1978 the concept of local intrathrombus catheter lysis was developed by Hess and co-workers in 1980. By placing the catheter directly into the thrombus activated plasmin remains where it is needed in high concentration for a lengthy period. Thus smaller doses of fibrolytic agents are needed and the effect greatly enhanced when compared with the regional fibrinolysis applied by Dotter earlier in 1974. If systemic or regional lysis is compared with digestion without chewing, then the combined procedure of CTL and CTE would correspond to digestion *with* chewing (Mahler, 1990).

Methodology

The technical requirements and therapeutic steps are listed as follows:

1. Fluoroscopy.
2. Seldinger technique for introduction of a percutaneous catheter.
3. Percutaneous catheter introducer (PCI kit), for use with a 0.035–0.038 inch diameter guidewire, manufactured by Argon, containing:
   6–9 (=2.8 mm) French radiopaque sheath;
   removable haemostasis valve with side-port extension for injection of heparin or dye and removable stopcock;
   vessel dilator (*Illustrations 1* and *2*).
4. Introduction of a French 5 or 6 polyethylene catheter under fluoroscopy.
5. Gradual infusion of fibrinolytic agent.
6. Stepwise advancement of catheter tip.
7. Suction of fresh, loosened thrombi.
8. Percutaneous dilatation of atherosclerotic plaque.

1 & 2

For introduction of a percutaneous catheter the Seldinger technique is used with anterograde puncture of the common femoral artery. This can pose problems in obese patients because the puncture site should be below the inguinal ligament in order to avoid retroperitoneal haematoma.

The superficial femoral artery (or graft) is catheterized selectively in local anaesthesia. Primary introduction of a radiopaque sheath (6–9 French) is performed to avoid excessive trauma of the vessel wall during repetitive catheter manipulations. Any bleeding tendency is increased in any case because of the drugs in use (heparin and lytic agents). CTL is usually performed by introducing an angiography catheter (5 or 6 French) in the vessel dilator shown in *Illustrations 1* and *2*.

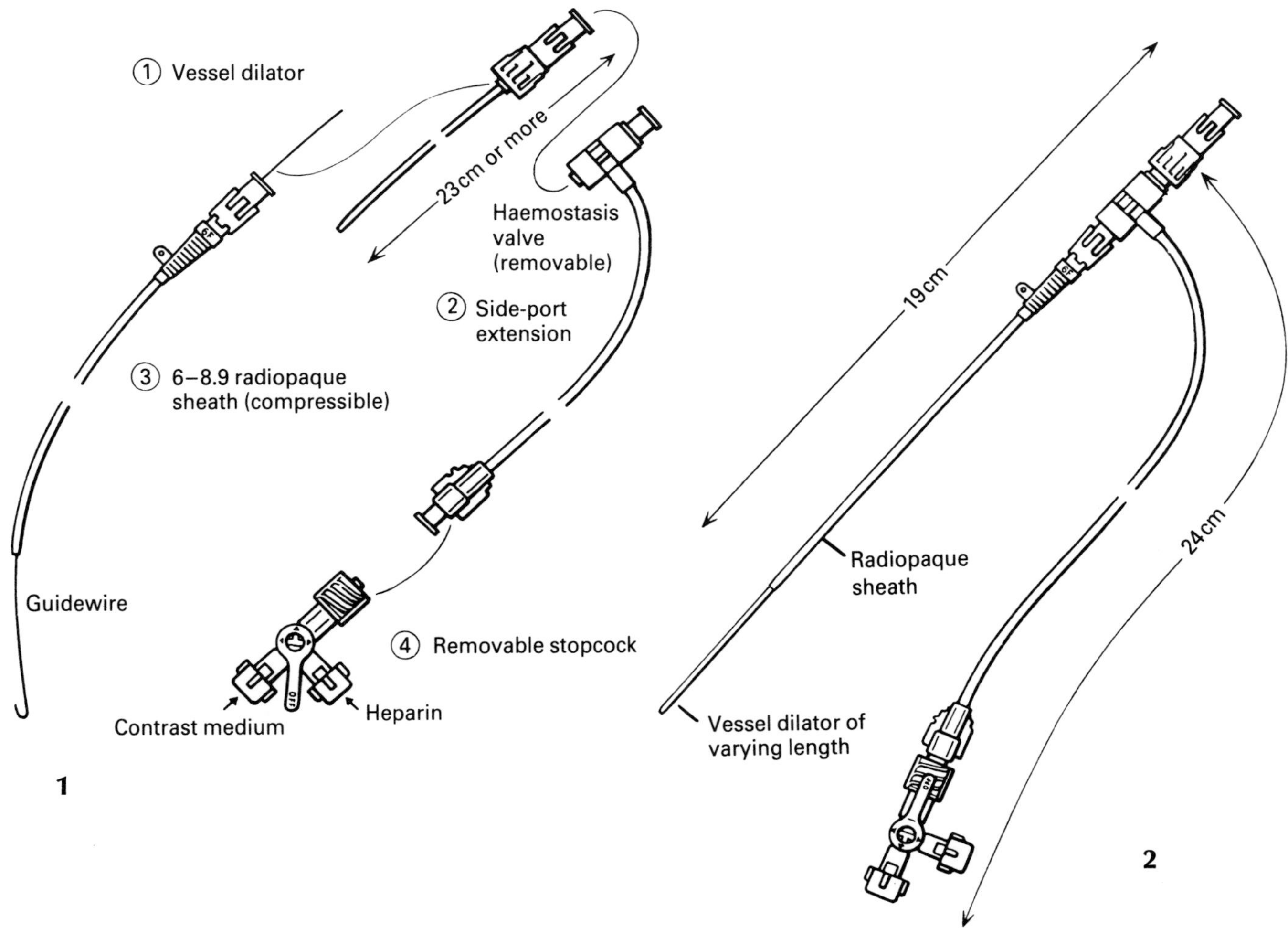

1

2

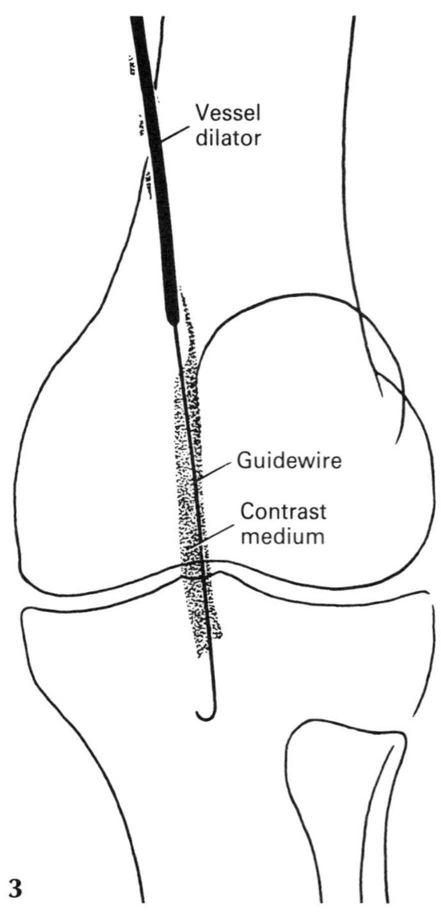

3

3

The tip of the catheter is placed 3–4 cm into the thrombus without piercing through it. The infusion of a fibrinolytic agent is begun, preferably by using an infusion pump providing a volume of 20 ml/h. The catheter is advanced stepwise cm by cm every 2–5 min under fluoroscopic control. The result is checked radiologically with diluted contrast medium at least once an hour. As soon as the distal end of the occluding thrombolic mass is reached the lytic agent flows into the distal vasculature. For increased efficacy of lysis a catheter tip with side holes enabling sprinkling is advantageous.

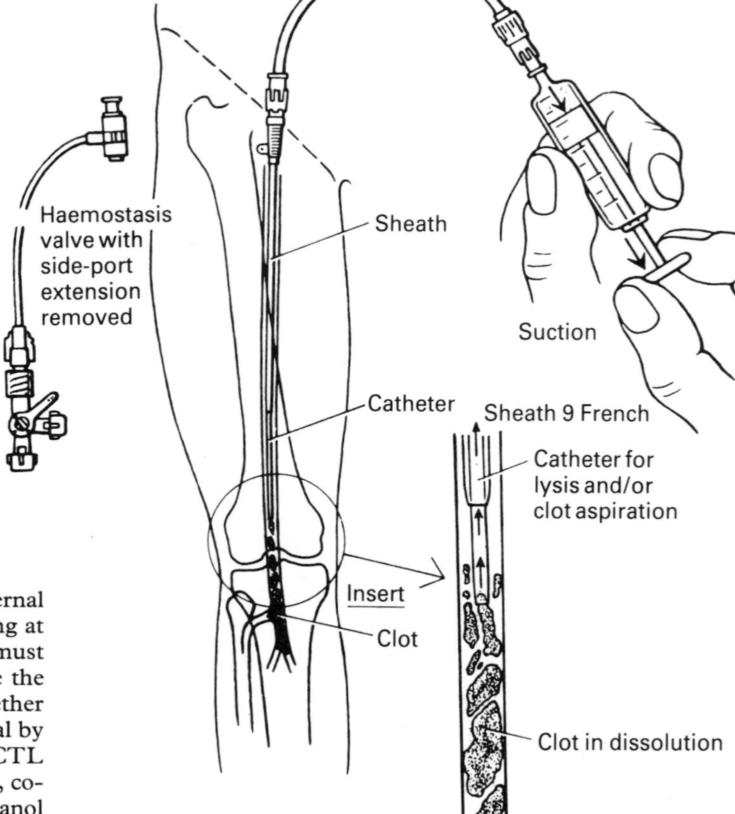

4

4

For aspiration of loosened thrombi a catheter with an internal diameter of 2 mm is used. It should have a single opening at the end and no side holes—as used for sprinkling—and must be attached to a 20 ml or even 50 ml syringe to achieve the necessary suction force. The thrombus is withdrawn together with the catheter. The mechanism of catheter clot removal by suction is depicted. Laboratory examinations during CTL include the analysis of prothrombin time, thrombin time, coagulation factors II, V, VII and X, reptilase time, an ethanol test and fibrinogen levels. During long-term lysis the thrombin time values are kept from exceeding twice the normal by adjusting the doses of heparin given.

Dosage

Streptokinase

In our hands we have used between 2000 and 4000 international units per cm length of clot keeping the catheter in one place for at least 5 minutes. Thus we apply between 40 000 and 100 000 units of streptokinase in one 90-min session. When patency is achieved the procedure is terminated, and 5000 units of heparin are given.

If, after 90 min, the flow through the initially occluded segment is unsatisfactory, the procedure is continued on the ward as a long-term regional thrombolysis after insertion of a 3 French catheter via the introducer sheath. The dose of streptokinase is 4000 units per hour for 8–72 h. Heparin is infused through the side branch of the introducer sheath to prevent pericatheter thrombolysis. Clinical assessment is confirmed by contrast injection through the indwelling catheter at intervals of at least 24 h.

Clinical success is defined by either a return of pedal pulses or a reduction in the arterial ankle pressure deficit of at least 50 mmHg.

Urokinase

If lytic therapy has already been performed once before then thrombolysis will have to be performed using urokinase which is—as opposed to streptokinase—a physiological lytic substance. It is 2–5 times less active than streptokinase per unit. Therefore we use per cm length of clot 5000–10 000 units. For long-term lysis we apply 10 000 units per hour. The total dose should not exceed 500 000 units per day.

Tissue plasminogen activator (rt-PA)

In our own series we have used 10 mg rt-PA per hour successfully. We noted with the doses used by us, with an average of 15 mg rt-PA for an average of 15 cm occlusion, a drop of fibrinonogen levels from 2.7 ± 0.8 g/l to 2.3 ± 1.0 g/l which serves to prove that systemic activity is relatively low. Hess (1988) has decreased his dosage recently to 2.5 mg rt PA/h.

Table 1 Fibrinogen levels before and after CTL with three fibrinolytic agents; bleeding complications

	Streptokinase	*Urokinase*	*rt-Pa*
Fibrinogen (g/l)			
before CTL	2.7 ± 0.7	2.6 ± 0.7	2.7 ± 0.8
after CTL	2.0 ± 0.5	2.5 ± 1.2	2.3 ± 1.0
Bleeding complications	8%	4%	4%

5

Illustration 5 shows clot material retrieved by catheter extraction (suction) after initial intrathrombus lysis in a patient successfully treated by combined CTL and CTE.

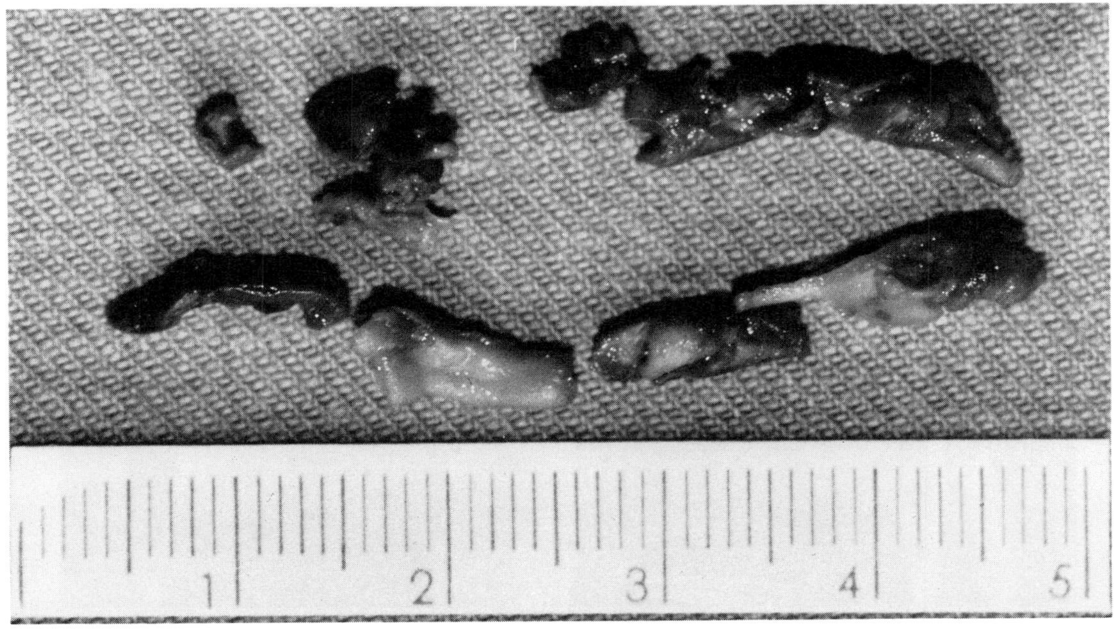

5

6a, b & c

Illustration 6a shows an anteriogram of a long popliteal occlusion of thrombotic origin in a 74-year-old male patient. Clinically, the patient presented in a state of critical ischaemia. The percutaneous catheter shown in *Illustrations 1* and *2* is introduced via the common femoral artery into the superficial femoral artery. A vessel dilator, 40–60 cm in length, can be introduced directly into the superficial femoral artery or with the help of a bent guidewire, which in PTA is advanced through the occluded segment down to the patent vessel lumen beyond the occlusion to ensure avoidance of subintimal catheterization. A guidewire is used in this case for better orientation.

In *6b* the guidewire can be seen approximately 3 cm below the knee joint in the same patient as shown schematically in *Illustration 3*. The tip of the catheter is recognizable at the level of the upper border of the knee cap. By comparison with *Illustration 6a*, one can see that the catheter has been unmistakably advanced into the proximal part of the clot. This manoeuvre is performed very slowly and without undue force. Thrombolysis is induced by gradual infusion of streptokinase in doses of 2000–4000 units for each advancement of the catheter tip, allowing about 2–5 min/cm. If urokinase is used, the average dose necessary for each advancement is between 5000 and 10 000 units. For rt-PA, 1 mg is required. From time to time a little contrast medium is injected via the stopcock (see *Illustrations 1* and *2*) to ascertain the progress of clot lysis. It is possible to identify some contrast medium within the formerly totally occluded popliteal artery. The important aspects of this are shown.

The completion angiogram for the same patient as in *6a, b* shows the lower level of a formerly occluded popliteal artery 24 h after initiation of CTL. The popliteal trifurcation can now be seen clearly.

Note the well-defined circumscribed atheromatous plaque near the origin of the anterior tibial artery. This lesion might have been the reason for thrombotic occlusion. Once it is uncovered by thrombolysis, it can be dealt with by PTA, which is an integral part of the treatment modality.

6a 6b 6c

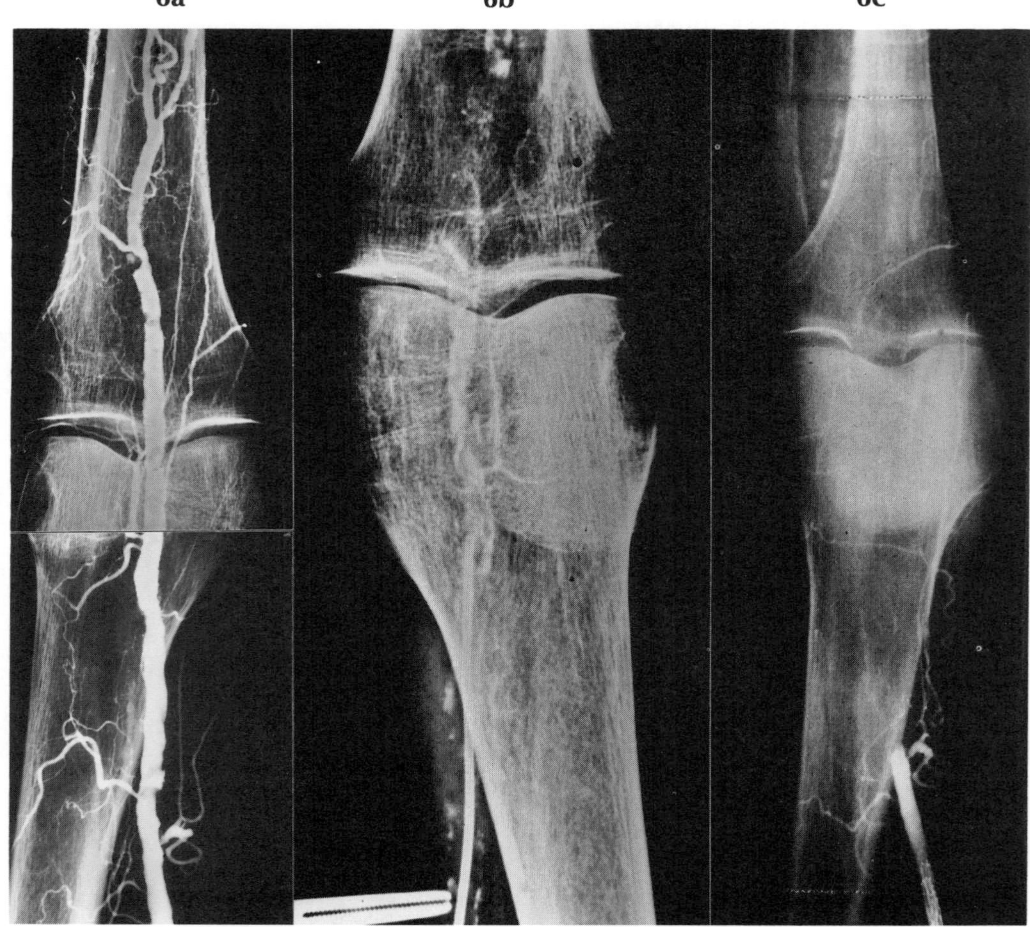

Further examples of initial lysis and catheter clot removal for occlusive disease in critical ischaemia

7

Example 1

Illustration 7 shows a sequence of angiograms performed before, during and after thrombolysis and catheter clot removal in a female patient (64 years old) presenting with acute arterial occlusion with subtotal ischaemia. Radiologically there is clear evidence of thrombotic occlusion attending extensive atherosclerotic disease. Initial local CTL with streptokinase was followed by CTE and completed with percutaneous PTA. Repeat angiogram and clinical evaluation 1 year later confirmed patency.

This example illustrates how even long thrombotic occlusions can successfully undergo percutaneous catheter lysis with the added advantage that the underlying cause for thrombotic occlusion (a plaque) can thereafter be localized and flattened by PTA.

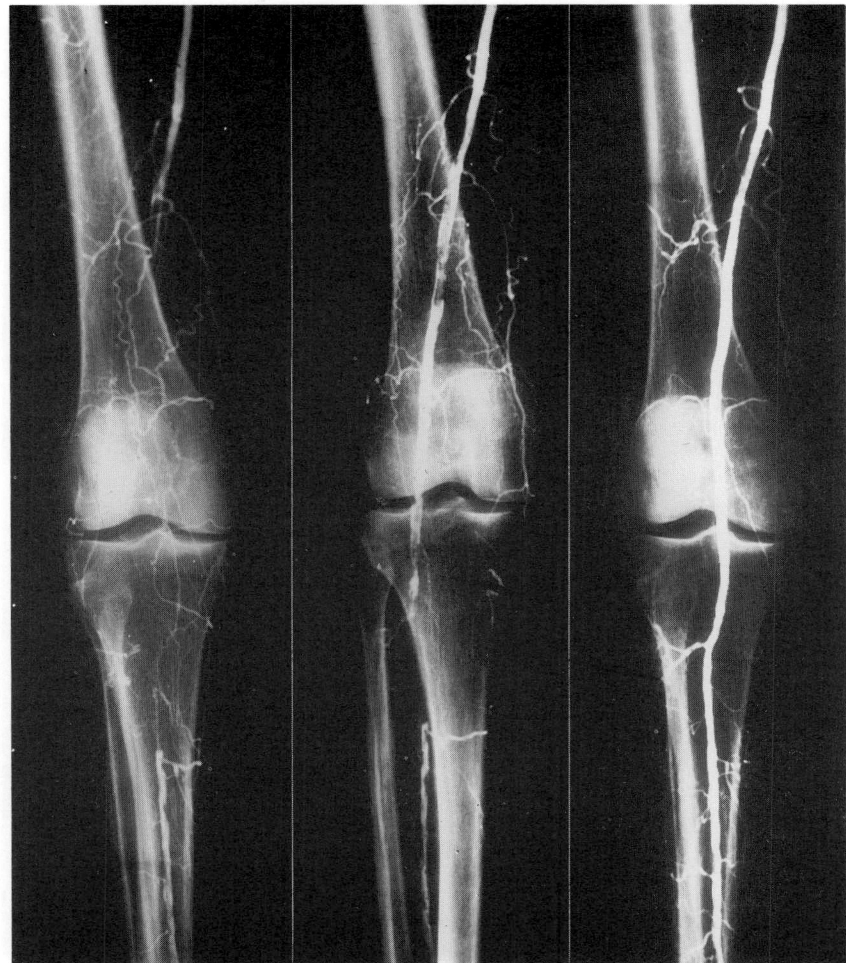

7

8a, b & c

Example 2

This case involved a 76-year-old female patient with sudden onset of arterial occlusion. Angiograms show (*left*) before, (*centre*) during and (*right*) after local thrombolysis and PTA.

Catheter clot lysis was started immediately after performing the initial angiogram on this 76-year-old female patient. Thrombolysis was accelerated by extracting considerable amounts of clot. In this case, an open distal run-off segment can be identified at the upper level of the femur condyles. As soon as complete thrombolysis is achieved, there is suddenly considerable reflux when the haemostasis valve is removed (see *Illustrations 1* and *2*). Loosened clots can then only be suctioned or extracted if the haemostasis valve is regularly removed and replaced afterwards for further manipulation. In the example presented here, there is residual subtotal occlusion of the proximal popliteal artery and a protruding plaque in the distal part of the superficial femoral artery. Both lesions underwent successful PTA. One year later, a control angiogram showed clear evidence of sustained patency of the femoropopliteal axis.

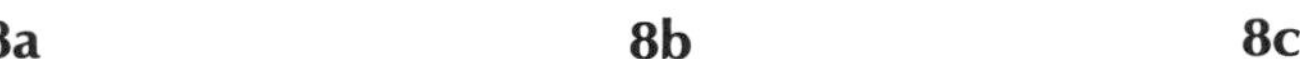

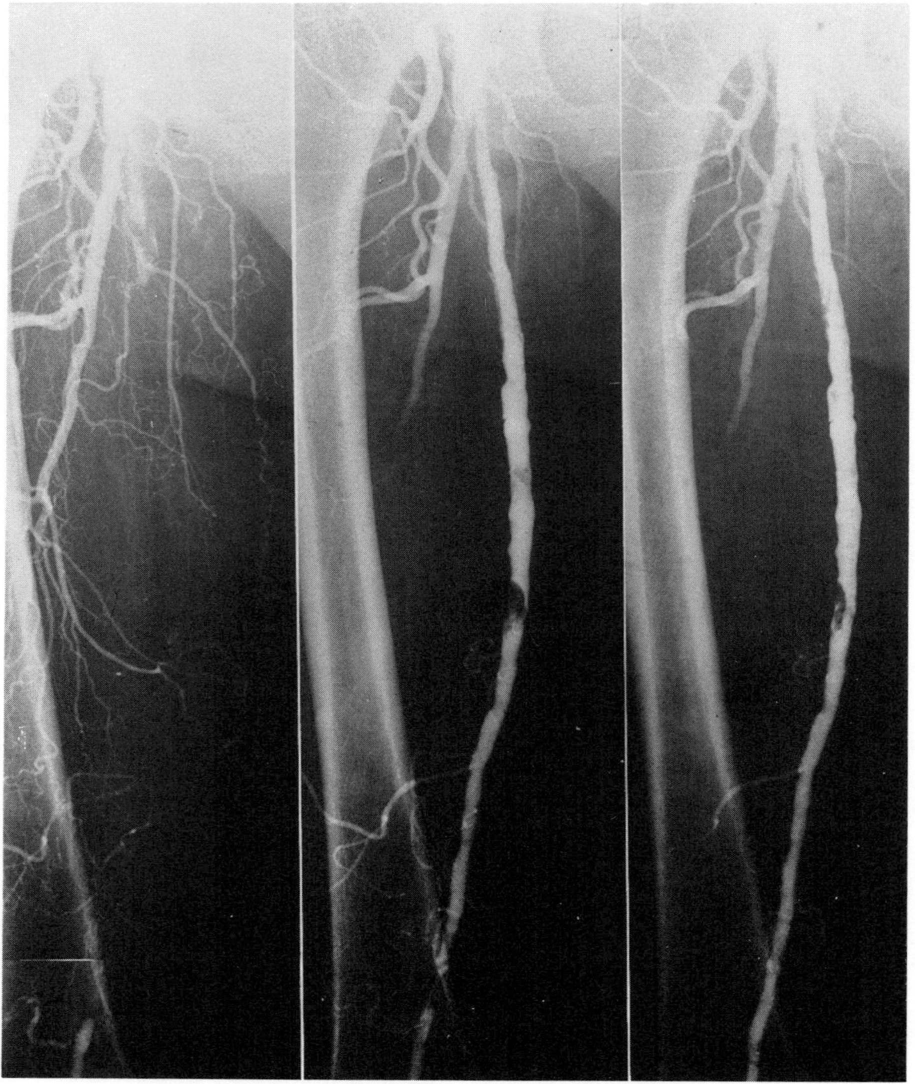

9a, b & c

Example 3

Illustrations 9a, b and *c* show how rapidly embolic occlusions of the popliteal trifurcation can be lysed successfully within 1 hour (in this case with 200 000 units of urokinase and without the accessory help of clot suction or extraction). The vascular wall is smooth, slight traces of small atherosclerotic plaques can nevertheless be observed.

9a **9b** **9c**

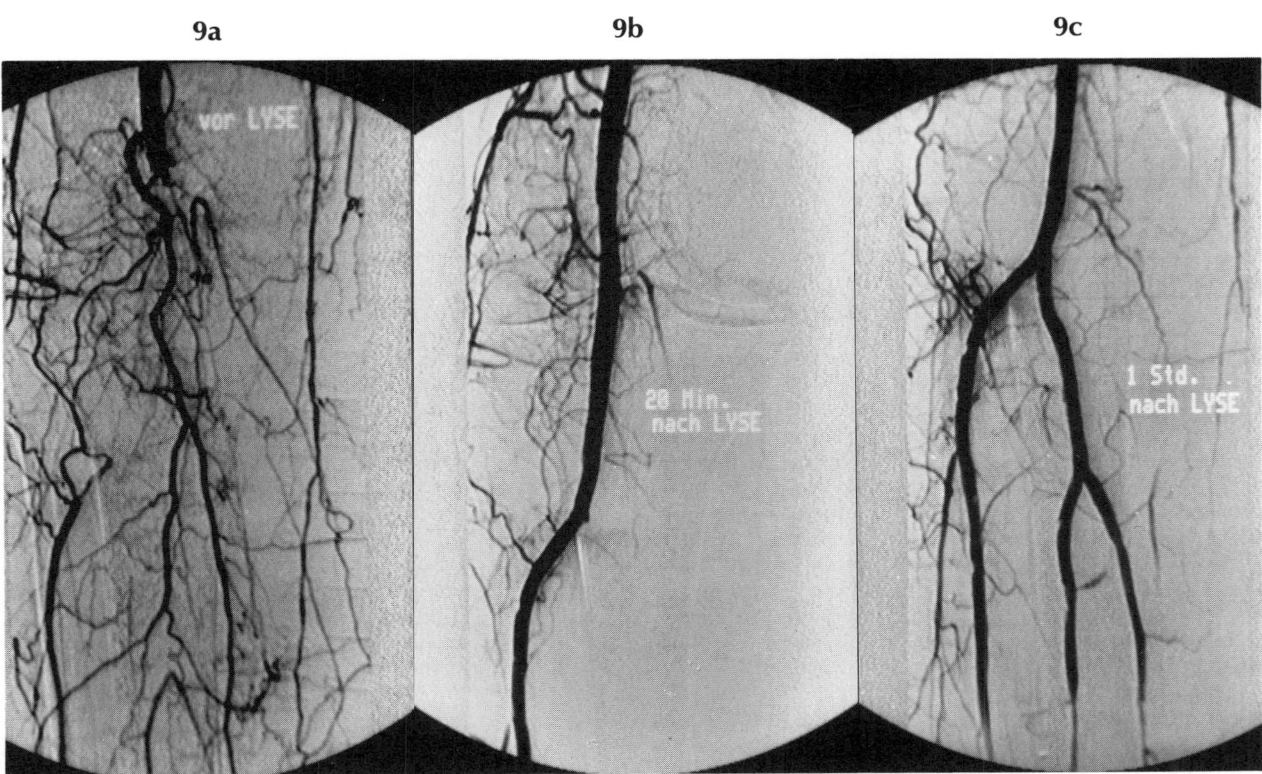

References

Do, D. D., Mahler, F. and Triller, J. (1989). Catheter thrombolysis with streptokinase, urokinase and recombinant tissue plasminogen activator for peripheral arterial occlusion. In *Pros and Cons in PTA and Auxiliary Methods*, Zeitler, E. eds. Berlin: Springer pp. 157–159.

Do, D. D., Mahler, F., Probst, P. and Nachbur, B. (1981). Combination of short and long-term catheter thrombolysis for peripheral arterial occlusion. *European Journal of Radiology* **1**, 235.

Demski, J. C. and Zeitler, E. (1978). Selective aterial clot lysis with angiography catheter. In *Percutaneous Vascular Recanalization*, Zeitler, E., Grüntzig, A., Schoop, W. eds. Berlin: Springer pp. 157–159.

Dotter, C. T., Rösch, J. and Seaman, A. J. (1974). Selective clot lysis with low-dose streptokinase. *Radiology* **111**, 31.

Hess, H., Mietaschk, A. and Ingrisch, H. (1982). Niedrig dosierte thrombolytische Therapie zur Wiederherstellung der Strombahn bei arteriellen Verschlüssen. *Dtsch Med Wschr* **105**, 787.

Hess, H., Ingrisch, H., Mietaschk, A. and Roth, H. (1982). Local low-dose thrombolytc therapy of peripheral arterial occlusions. *New England Journal of Medicine* **307**, 1627.

Mahler, F. (1990). *Katheterinterventionen in der Angiologie*. Stuttgart: New York: Georg Thieme Verlag pp. 113–131.

Schneider, E, and Largiadèr, J. (1987). Therapiekonzept beim akuten Verschluss von Extremitätenarterien. *Therapeutische Umschau* **44**, 653.

Improving profunda femoris flow

CRAWFORD JAMIESON MS, FRCS

Consultant Surgeon, St Thomas' Hospital, London, UK;
Honorary Consultant Surgeon, Hammersmith Hospital and Royal Postgraduate Medical School, London, UK

Introduction

The surgical importance of the profunda femoris artery, has long been recognized (Morris *et al.*, 1961). Early experience of direct reconstruction of stenosis of the origin of this artery was recorded by Natali in Paris, and direct endarterectomy was popularized by Martin and Cotton. Martin published a large series of patients treated by 'profundaplasty' but 80% of them had a simultaneous proximal endarterectomy, or bypass of an iliac arterial stenosis or occlusion (Martin, Renwick and Stephenson, 1968). Cotton favoured an extended approach to the operation, patching the artery well down into the thigh, and claimed that the results were better the longer the reconstruction (Berguer, Cotton and Sabri, 1973). Martin, however, had preached the opposite, feeling that when disease extended beyond the first perforating artery, reconstruction tended to be unsuccessful owing to the prevalence of disease in distal branches. This dichotomy of opinion has never been resolved but, in the course of time, the operation of extended profundaplasty has fallen from favour and most surgeons now confine their attentions to stenoses localized to the proximal few centimetres of the artery.

This is an operation which is relatively safe and easy to perform, is capable of producing a new limited increase in the circulation of the limb but has excellent long-term patency (Hopkins *et al.*, 1983).

Indications

Profundaplasty is indicated only in the presence of a significant stenosis of the profunda femoris artery. This statement may appear obvious but it has been claimed that limb flow may be improved by widening a totally normal profunda femoris origin in the presence of a superficial femoral arterial occlusion (Berguer, Higgins and Cotton, 1975). The logic upon which this decision is made remains, however, rather dubious. It appears from the authors' interpretation of their haemodynamic model that a stenosis exists in the arterial tree which consists of the normal profunda femoris origin but, the branching arterial tree maintains, by an increase of area at each branch, a standard and even linear resistance. The decrease in resistance of the arterial tree from the heart to the foot achieved by a local profundaplasty of 2–3 cm is only an alteration in resistance, compared with the 1.3 m of artery from heart to foot, and cannot therefore be expected to be significant, and the operation of profundaplasty of an unstenosed vessel has generally been abandoned.

The operation is not indicated in patients with a patent superficial femoral artery, although theoretically they might suffer from intermittent claudication of the thigh with severe disease of the profunda femoris. This does not, however, seem to occur, and another cause must be sought for the aetiology of pain in the thigh if the superficial femoral artery is widely patent, even if disease exists in the profunda femoris. The operation is therefore indicated in patients with a stenosis of the origin of the profunda femoris artery and a co-existent superficial femoral arterial occlusion with or without proximal iliac or aortic disease. In the former circumstances, proximal reconstruction plus profundaplasty is indicated, whereas in the latter and less common situation, profundaplasty alone is indicated.

The most important and difficult decision lies in whether a patient with a profunda femoris stenosis and a superficial femoral arterial occlusion should be treated by profundaplasty, femoral popliteal bypass or a combination of both.

Successful femoral popliteal bypass restores flow in the foot to normal levels which profundaplasty in the presence of an untreated superficial femoral artery occlusion will never do (Jamieson, 1983). Bypass is therefore peferable to profundaplasty where circumstances are favourable and where a major increase in flow is necessary, either to relieve crippling intermittent claudication or to heal extensive ischaemic lesions of the foot. Profundaplasty is indicated in the relatively uncommon but well-defined alternative circumstances, particularly where there is critical ischaemia and where a rise of ankle blood pressure by 20 or 30 mmHg can be expected to relieve rest pain or allow healing of mild trophic lesions (Hill and Jamieson, 1977). Carefully selected profundaplasty in exactly this group of patients can produce excellent results and the general disenchantment with the procedure has, to a great extent, been due to unrealistic hopes for an increase in circulation by relief of such a local stenosis. Bernhard (1979) has pointed out that patients with a significant drop in pressure in the thigh, as opposed to across the knee on segmental thigh pressure, may be predicted to obtain a better result from profundaplasty than the latter group. Published results of the operation uncombined with a proximal reconstruction indicate that the mean increase in ankle pressure lies around 20% of the rise in the ankle brachial pressure index. The long-term patency of profundaplasty is excellent, late occlusion being rare within the life-span of the patient.

The major indication for a profundaplasty is as an adjunct to aortofemoral grafting or associated with reconstruction of a unilateral iliac arterial stenosis by direct endarterectomy or angioplasty. Profundaplasty may be vital to maintain an adequate flow and protect long-term patency of a proximal reconstruction, in addition to improving the results of the major proximal operation by increasing flow into the muscles of the thigh.

Simultaneous profundaplasty and femoral popliteal bypass

This is tempting when a superficial femoral block with a good run-off is associated with a severe stenosis of the origin of the profunda femoris artery, but is probably unnecessary, and may even be unwise, because theoretically it reduces the pressure gradient between the common femoral and the popliteal artery and, therefore, the flow rate through the femoral popliteal bypass. Although there is only shaky evidence that patency of femoral popliteal bypass is directly in proportion to the flow, there is no doubt that long-term patency is very poor when flow falls below the critical level of around 150 ml/min (Law and Roberts, 1983). It is probably better to perform the femoral popliteal bypass first, keeping profundaplasty in reserve in case of long-term failure of the bypass.

Preoperative preparation

In addition to the general assessment of the patient for fitness for surgery and the degree of ischaemia of his limb, it is important that angiograms be obtained in two planes, particularly an oblique view, as the profunda femoris origin may be obscured by dye in the origin of the superficial femoral artery in the conventional anteroposterior projection of an angiogram (Beales *et al.*, 1971). Intravenous digital subtraction angiography (DSA) is frequently adequate in this preoperative assessment and direct arterial punture may be avoided, although DSA may not give adequate information on the popliteal run-off and patency of calf vessels when the choice lies between a long bypass and profundaplasty, in which case an intravenous DSA to examine the iliac arterial system followed by a direct femoral puncture and conventional angiogram which gives the best view of the distal vessels of the leg is ideal. Bacteria swabs should be taken of necrotic lesions of the foot and appropriate treatment commenced prior to surgery.

The operation may be performed under local anaesthetic when a proximal reconstruction is not required and is, therefore, highly suitable for the frail patient.

Position of patient

The patient should be positioned supine upon the operating table with the leg slightly abducted. The whole limb should be prepared and exposed and the abdomen prepared to the costal, or even subclavian region, if there is any doubt over the quality of the inflow through the iliac artery. A patch of vein is required and it is inadvisable to remove this vein from the saphenous vein at the ankle, as the wound may not heal well. We prefer to prepare a segment of forearm to harvest a vein patch rather than sacrifice the saphenous vein itself in its more proximal course.

1

Incision

The incision follows a vertical route, slightly convex laterally, over the course of the iliac and femoral vessels to avoid lymphatic damage.

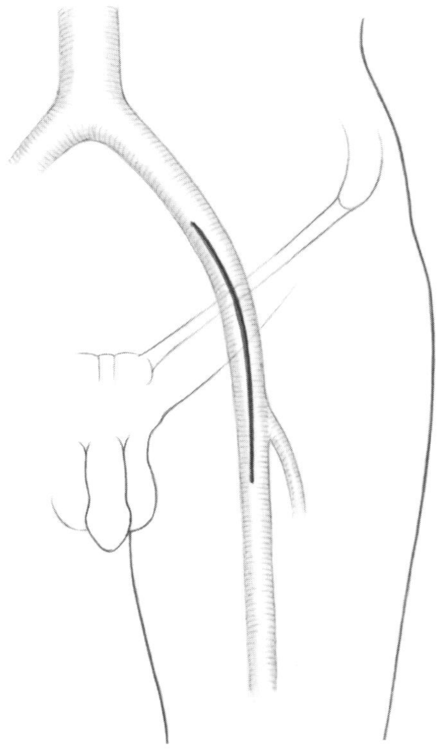

1

2

Exposure

The excision is deepened to the deep fascia and the common femoral artery exposed. The inguinal ligament is defined and the femoral pulse reassessed. If the femoral pulse is weak, it may be advisable to perform direct intrafemoral arterial pressure measurements with an intra-arterial injection of papaverine to assess the adequacy of iliac inflow. This test may be misleading when the superficial femoral artery is occluded and the profunda femoris artery is severely stenosed, because even following injection of papaverine peripheral resistance may be so high that a good femoral pulse may exist in the presence of a severe iliac stenosis. Inadequate flow may then only be detected when the artery is opened.

The superficial femoral artery is exposed and the common femoral artery and superficial femoral artery are snared and elevated. This exposes the origin of the profunda femoris artery which may be multiple and is crossed approximately 1 cm from its origin by a large vein, the circumflex femoral vein, draining into the termination of the profunda femoris vein. This vein may be up to 1 cm in diameter and must be carefully controlled and divided before the distal artery can be exposed. The exposed course of the vein is very short and it is safer to oversew both ends than ligate them. Distal to this vein, the artery tends to run more parallel to the superficial femoral artery, and as it plunges gradually into the muscles of the thigh, it is crossed by further veins at regular intervals which may require division. The branches of the artery, the circumflex femoral artery and the perforating arteries, tend to arise around the level of these veins and should be controlled individually by snares.

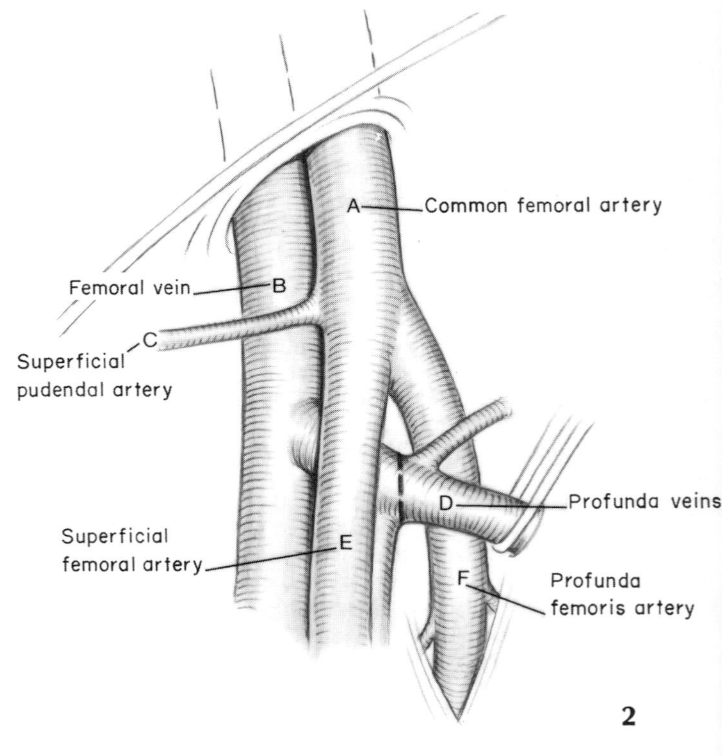

2

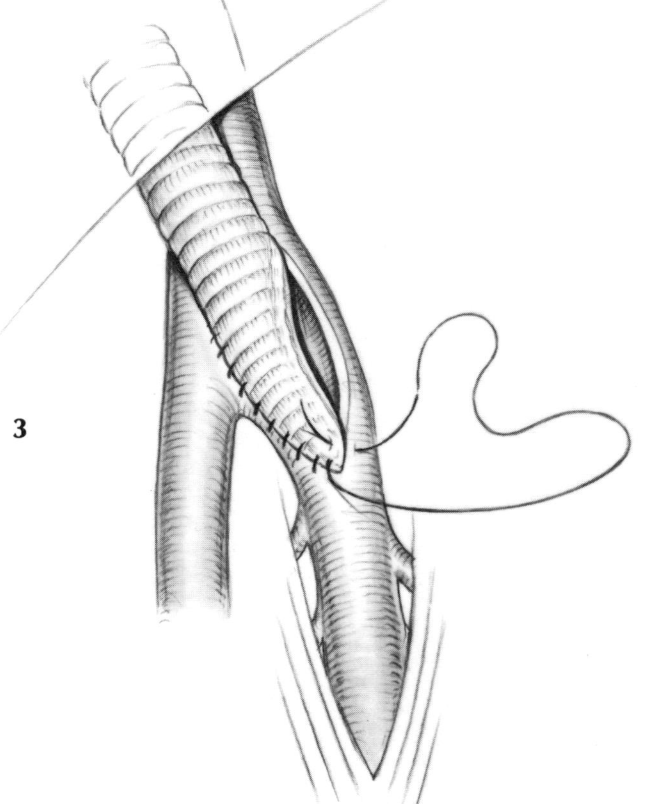
3

3

Reconstruction

The arteries are clamped following intravenous administration of heparin 1.5 mg/kg. The direction and shape of the arteriotomy depends upon which method is selected, but it commences in the distal common femoral artery and is extended down the profunda femoris artery until an adequate lumen is reached. Local endarterectomy may then be performed if necessary, tailing off distally, making quite certain that there is no flap of intima to cause local occlusion. The loose intima should be anchored by a mattress suture inserted in through the endarterectomized segment and out through the unendarterectomized distal intima, to be tied on the exterior surface of the vessel. Avoidance of flaps is best achieved by avoiding endarterectomy where possible as Martin preferred. The adequacy of downflow and backflow are assessed – if downflow is inadequate, proximal reconstruction may be added at this stage, and the profundaplasty is then closed by Dacron end-to-side.

4

If backflow is inadequate, in spite of the gentle passage of Fogarty catheters, it may be necessary to reconsider the decision to perform a femoral distal bypass, but otherwise the arteriotomy is closed with a suitable vein patch. It can be an advantage to cut the vein square-ended as shown. The clamps are removed and anticoagulation is reversed. Operative angiography may be performed to assess the success of the reconstruction. The wound is closed over a suction drain.

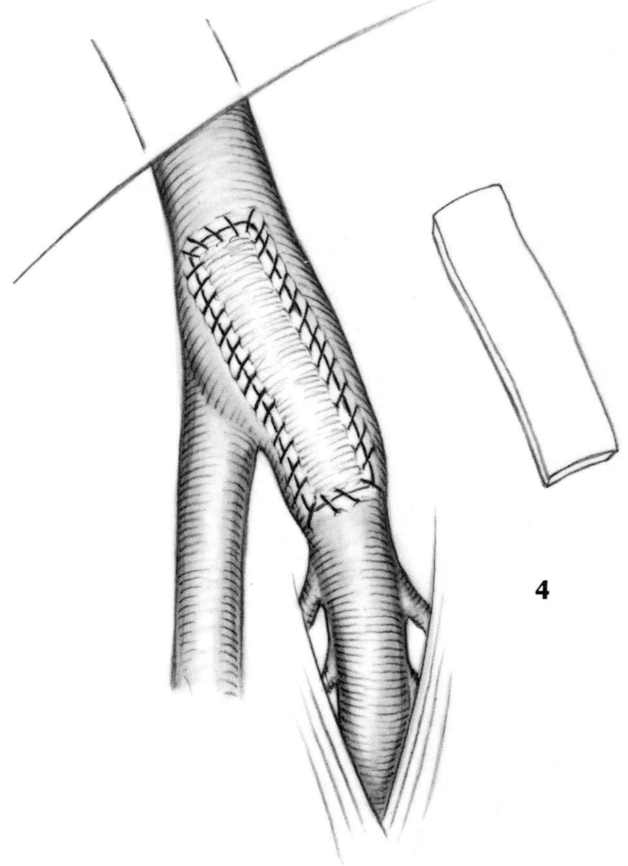

4

5

A variety of permutations exist by which a stenosis of the profunda femoris origin can be relieved. These include use of the segment of endarterectomized occluded superficial femoral artery as a patch, dissected fully free as shown.

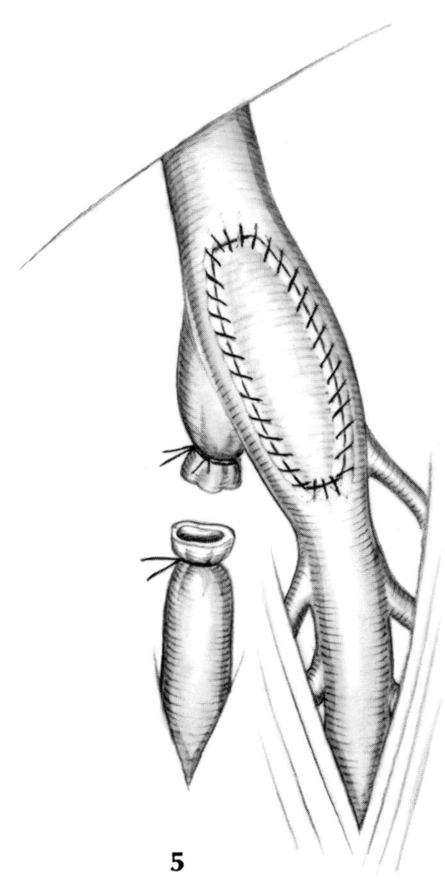

5

6

Alternatively, the endarterectomized superficial femoral artery is left attached and flapped over to widen the profunda origin as a square patch.

7

Widening of the profunda femoris origin can be achieved by suture of a patent or endarterectomized superficial femoral artery to a V-shaped arteriotomy between the superficial femoral artery and the profunda femoris.

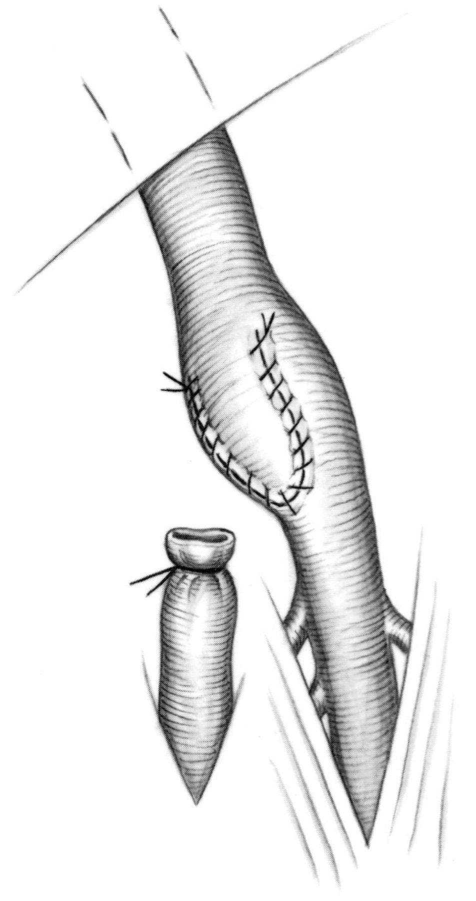

6

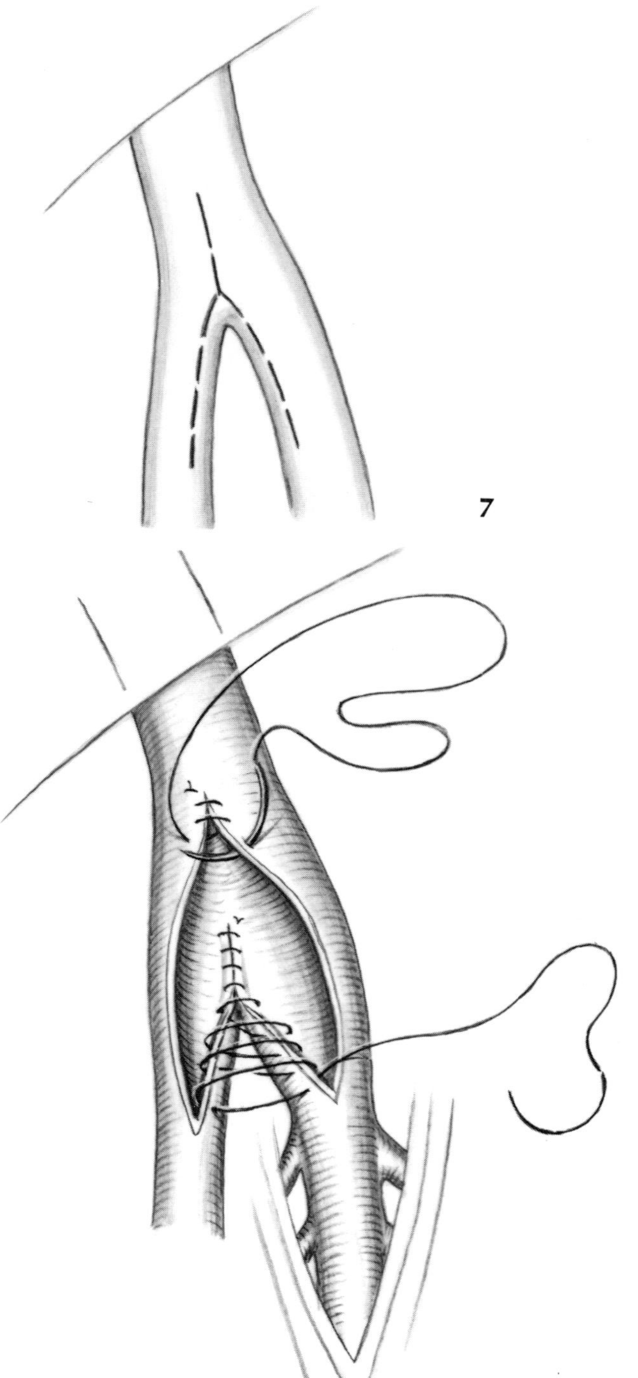

7

Postoperative management

There is little systemic disturbance from this operation and gastrointestinal function is normal. A urinary catheter is not required unless the iliac artery has been exposed, and the patient is allowed up after 24 h, provided there is no excessive lymph leak from the drain. If lymph drainage is considerable it is probably best that the patient be nursed supine until it decreases, as lymph flow is stimulated by exercise of the limb.

Ankle blood pressure is monitored daily for the first few days, though early failure of the reconstruction is most unusual. Antibiotic cover is not necessary as autogenous material alone has been used.

Complications

Apart from the general complications of any anaesthetic in a patient with a diffuse vascular disease and wound infection, the only significant complication is a lymphocoele, which is unusual, and almost always settles with time. It sometimes, however, develops after the suction drain has been removed and if it is large it is best treated by insertion of a further suction drain percutaneously by an oblique route which is left in until the drainage settles. Very rarely, this may take several days.

Profundaplasty combined with proximal reconstruction

The permutations of operation available in profundaplasty plus aortofemoral grafting are covered in elsewhere, but in spite of the popularity of bypass grafting there is still some place for local endarterectomy of iliac occlusions when the contralateral iliac artery is good. This operation may be performed by an extraperitoneal approach. It is safer, quicker and less traumatic than aortofemoral grafting (Martin, Renwick and Stephenson, 1968) and is associated with less systemic disturbance and ileus. Endarterectomy is technically more demanding than bypass, but it is a skill which should be available to every peripheral arterial surgeon and, although its detractors state that it only postpones the inevitable, similar operation on the contralateral side, this is not the case, as most patients treated by unilateral iliac endarterectomy do not survive to require an aortobifemoral graft within their limited life-span.

The preoperative preparation and positioning of the patient are identical to those of pure profundaplasty. The patient lies flat on the operating table.

8

Incision

A thin patient with external iliac occlusion is best treated by an incision carried vertically through the inguinal ligament and muscle layers of the abdominal wall just lateral to the origin of the common femoral artery, and extended proximally along the linear semilunaris. This incision, although apparently traumatic, gives excellent exposure of the external iliac artery and the distal common iliac artery, and is associated with a very low incidence of incisional hernia provided it is sutured carefully with continuous non-absorbable material of adequate strength. The incision is deepened through the external oblique aponeurosis and the conjoint muscles of internal oblique and transversus. A finger is inserted under the inguinal ligament and the peritoneum gently swept medially, taking great care to avoid damage to the deep circumflex iliac vein which crosses anterior to the distal part of the external iliac artery. The peritoneum becomes more adherent superiorly and medially to the posterior aspect of the rectus sheath and must be mobilized with great care to avoid opening the peritoneal cavity. It is, however, easily separated posteriorly from the anterior aspect of the vessels. The ureter is mobilized anteriorly with the peritoneum until the surgeon's fingers detect the normal pulse proximal to the iliac stenosis.

A Goligher retractor is inserted with a short blade against the iliac crest and a long blade protected by a large swab retracting the peritoneum and viscera. It is most important that this retractor should not exert pressure distally upon the femoral nerve which lies hidden under the fasica just lateral to the termination of the external iliac artery. The blades are opened giving excellent exposure of the external and internal iliac arteries and the common iliac artery. The inferior epigastric artery and deep circumflex iliac artery are controlled by snares as they originate from the distal part of the external iliac artery, and the deep circumflex iliac vein is divided. Lymphatic tissue is cleared from the external iliac artery completely exposing the vessel. The internal iliac artery is snared taking great care to avoid damage to the internal iliac vein which lies deep to it. The distal part of the external common iliac artery is mobilized from the common iliac vein and similarly snared. Venous bleeding at this stage presents the only major hazard of the procedure and the common iliac artery may be so closely tethered to the common iliac vein by periarteritis that snaring is inadvisable, though it is difficult to control it adequately with a clamp unless it is mobilized.

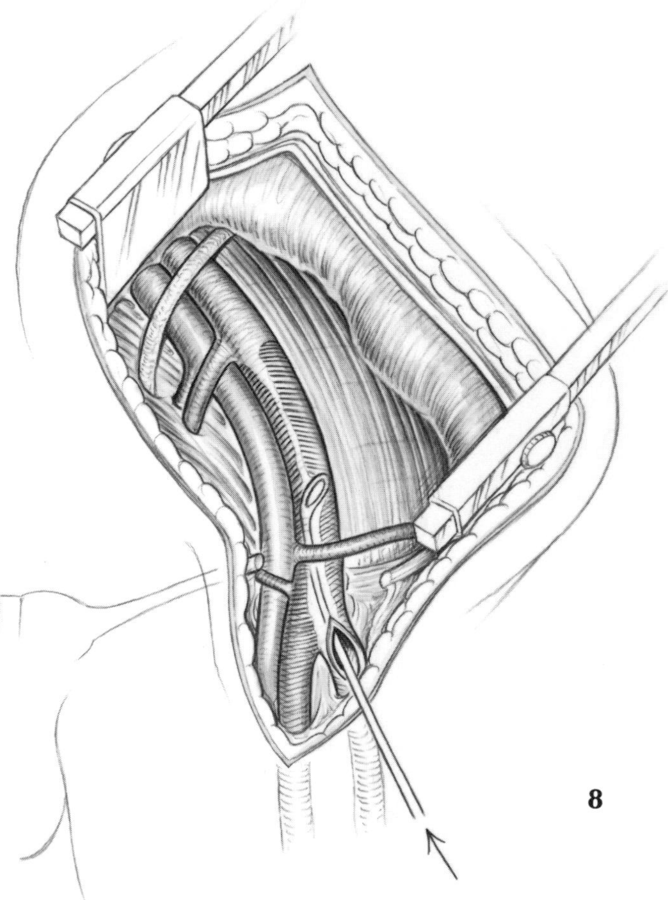

8

Endarterectomy

The patient is anticoagulated with heparin 1.5mg/kg intravenously. The common iliac artery, internal iliac artery and branch of the common femoral artery are clamped and the distal common femoral artery is then opened in the same manner as for profundaplasty, but the arteriotomy is carried proximally to the distal extremity of the external iliac artery. Local endarterectomy is performed upwards from this point using loop or arc strippers to the patent common iliac artery. The arc stripper is extremely valuable for traversing a vessel or varying calibre but has the potential risk of catching in the arterial wall and must not be twisted during its upwards and downwards course in the plane of endarterectomy. It is best located by the surgeon's two fingers on each side of the points of its arc, as it is passed upwards. When the plaque has been loosened by one passage of the ring stripper or four passages of the arc stripper, an arterial clamp is gently closed on the unopened artery at the site of proximal mobilization of the plaque. The gentle closure combined with pressure from the fingers breaks the endarterectomized core, leaving the outer wall intact, and the core may be milked from the endarterectomized vessel.

The manoeuvre is not always successful and excessive force must not be used in attempting to break the plaque as it will result in damage to the external wall. If the plaque does not break open further, arteriotomy must be made at the proximal level of endarterectomy, the plaque divided under direct vision with scissors and the arteriotomy closed with continuous 4/0 polypropylene. Downflow is then assessed and if it is adequate the arteriotomy and the common femoral and profunda femoris arteries are closed with a vein patch as before.

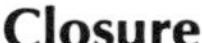

Closure

The abdominal wall is closed with a continuous 2/0 nylon suture in two layers over a suction drain passed along the common femoral artery under the inguinal ligament to lie along the external iliac artery, and the groin wound is closed in layers.

Postoperative course

It is very similar to profundaplasty. Ileus is usually very slight unless the peritoneum has been inadvertently opened.

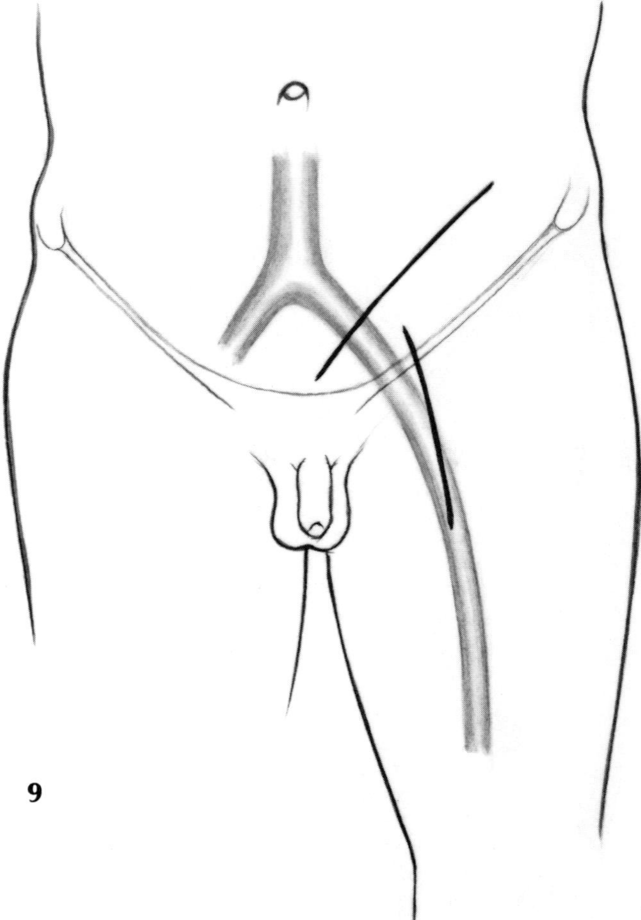

9

Combined common iliac endarterectomy and profundaplasty

9

The patient lies with a sandbag to raise the buttock if preferred. The incision described above does not give good exposure of the origin of the common iliac artery without such proximal extension that it risks weakening the muscles of the abdominal wall, and it gives less good exposure in the obese patient. Extensive unilateral iliac arterial occlusion is better treated by a combination of an incision over the common femoral artery and a separate oblique incision in the abdominal wall. The common femoral arterial exposure is extended proximally by division of the inguinal ligament for approximately 1 cm to allow control of the inferior epigastric and deep circumflex iliac arteries.

The abdominal incision is commenced at a point 3 cm above the pubic tubercle over the conjoint tendon and directed upwards and laterally towards the costal margin. It is deepened through the linear semilunaris in its lower part by a combination of splitting the external oblique and cutting the internal oblique and transversus muscles more proximally. The peritoneum is mobilized medially, as in the previous approach, and retracted by a Goligher rectractor as before. This exposure gives much better access to the common iliac artery and even the aortic bifurcation, and division of the inguinal ligament permits control of all the branches in the segment to be endarterectomized.

10

Common iliac endarterectomy requires a separate arteriotomy situated over the distal part of the common iliac artery. The external iliac endarterectomy is performed from a common femoral arteriotomy to the proximal arteriotomy, and common iliac endarterectomy is carried out using loop or preferably arc strippers. The atheromatous plaque in the common iliac artery is ruptured by gentle compression of the origin of the common iliac artery with an arterial clamp. It is obviously vital that this manoeuvre is performed with care, for rupture of the vessel at this point without adequate aortic control might be fatal. The atheroma in the proximal part of the common iliac artery is, however, in unilateral arterial occlusion, frequently soft and virtually non-existent. Frequently, the vessel occludes because of a development of atheroma in its distal part and, following a distal occlusion, thromboses back to the origin.

In rare circumstances, where external iliac endarterectomy proves to be impossible, it is convenient to insert a Dacron bypass from the common iliac arteriotomy to the common femoral arteriotomy as a unilateral iliofemoral bypass and, in the even rarer circumstance where flow cannot be restored to the common iliac artery, an aortofemoral graft must be used. This last alternative is used to rescue an incorrect clinical decision. These patients are better treated by an aorto-bifemoral graft if there is extensive distal disease.

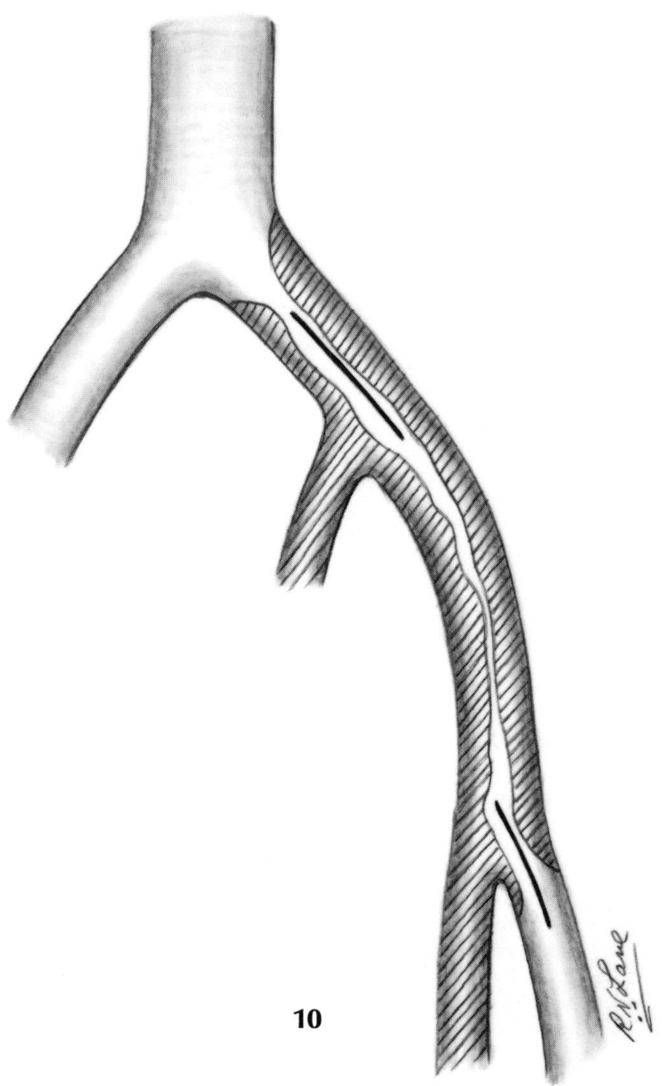

10

The arteriotomy at the lower end of these procedures is always taken into the profunda origin if the superficial femoral artery is occluded and closure is by patch or Dacron graft as for a profundaplasty. Proximal reconstruction of one sort or another is always combined with profundaplasty if the aortoiliac disease significantly limits inflow to the profunda femoris artery.

References

Beales, J. S. M., Adcock, F. A., Frawley, J. S. *et al.* (1971). The radiological assessment of disease of the profunda femoris artery. *British Journal of Radiology* **44**, 854.

Berguer, R., Cotton, L. T. and Sabri, S. (1973). Extended deep femoral angioplasty. *British Medical Journal* **1**, 469.

Berguer, R., Higgins, R. F. and Cotton, L. T. (1975). Geometry blood flow and reconstruction of the deep femoral artery. *American Journal of Surgery* **130**, 68.

Bernhard, V. M. (1979). The role of profundaplasty in revascularisation of the lower extremities. *Surgical Clinics of North America* **59**, 681.

Hill, D. A. and Jamieson, C. W. (1977). The results of arterial reconstruction using the profunda femoris artery in rest pain and pre-gangrene. *British Journal of Surgery* **64**, 359.

Hopkins, N. F. G., Polyrakis, S., Jamieson, C. W. and Vaughan, G. M. M. (1983). Assessment of later patency of profundaplasty. *Surgery* **94**, 814.

Jamieson, C. W. (1983). Profundaplasty: An incomplete alternative to femoro-popliteal bypass. In *Controversies in Surgery* Vol. 2. Delaney, J. P., Varcos, R. L., eds. London and Philadelphia: W. B. Saunders.

Law, Y. F. and Roberts, V. C. (1983). Per-operative haemodynamic assessment of lower limb arterial surgery. *Journal of Biomedical Engineering* **5**, 194.

Martin, P., Renwick, S. and Stephenson, C. (1968). On the surgery of the profunda femoris artery. *British Journal of Surgery* **55**, 539.

Morris, G. C., Edwards, W., Cooley, D. A., Crawford, E. S. and DeBakey, M. E. (1961). Surgical importance of profunda femoris artery. *Archives of Surgery* **82**, 52.

Reversed saphenous vein for femoropopliteal bypass grafting

K. G. BURNAND MS, FRCS
Professor of Vascular Surgery, Department of Surgery, St Thomas' Hospital, London, UK

N. L. BROWSE MD, PRCS
President, Royal College of Surgeons of England

Introduction

Rest pain, pregangrene and frank gangrene of the digits or forefoot in the presence of a good femoral inflow and an adequate run-off via the popliteal artery constitute an absolute indication for the operation. The combination of severe ischaemia and an isolated femoropopliteal occlusion rarely exists. There is almost always some concomitant aorto-iliac, profunda or distal vessel disease in limbs with severe ischaemia. Staged or simultaneous aortic reconstruction may then be required and the distal end of the bypass may have to be taken below the popliteal trifurcation if there is a marked stenosis of the popliteal artery or occlusion of the crural vessels.

Intermittent claudication remains a relative indication for the operation: a good early symptomatic improvement must be weighed against the risks of operation and the uncertainty of long-term benefit. Younger, fit and fully employed patients with a unilateral block, a disease-free popliteal segment and a good-calibre saphenous vein are obvious candidates for surgery, although many would claim that such a combination of circumstances is unusual. Patients should ideally have given up smoking for a reasonable period of time and have stable or deteriorating symptoms of several months' duration, which are interfering with their occupation or hobbies to such an extent, that even after a full explanation of the risks and uncertain long-term benefits of procedure, they continue to request operation. Initial enthusiasm for operating in all patients with claudication has now waned in the UK, and more stringent selection criteria are applied to potential candidates for surgery.

Ischaemic leg ulceration, traumatic damage to the superficial femoral artery, cystic change in the popliteal artery, and popliteal aneurysms are alternative indications for vein bypass surgery.

A good-calibre long saphenous vein remains the conduit of first choice for bypassing atherosclerotic obstruction of the femoropopliteal segment. There appears to be little difference in patency between *in situ* and reversed saphenous vein bypasses to the popliteal artery (Harris *et al.*, 1987) and the decision on which method to use appears therefore to be a matter of personal preference. Reversed grafts often lie better when made to the popliteal segment, whereas *in situ* grafts are almost always preferable below the trifurcation.

Assessment

Patients being considered for femoropopliteal bypass should have the basic screening tests outlined in the chapter Planning the intervention, p. 1, carried out before proceeding to aortography or digital subtraction angiography. If this shows a satisfactory aorto-iliac segment with an isolated femoropopliteal occlusion and satisfactory run-off, we obtain bilateral saphenograms (Senapati, Lea Thomas and Burnand, 1983) to assess the morphology and diameter of both long saphenous veins before surgery is considered. Duplex Doppler scanning is an alternative method of assessing the calibre and branches of the long saphenous vein. Confirmation of a single lumen saphenous vein of adequate length and diameter in either leg makes recommendation of vein bypass surgery much easier in patients with moderate claudication, whereas a multichannelled or narrow vein mitigates against surgery in all but the severely handicapped. In patients with rest pain, demonstration of a poor saphenous vein on saphenography may prevent an extensive dissection through poorly vascularized tissue. A prosthetic graft of human umbilical vein, Dacron or polytetrafluoroethylene can then be selected as an alternative bypass.

Preoperative preparation

The affected limb should be fully shaved together with the genitalia and iliac fossa of the same side. Naseptin drops are administered twice a day to the nasal passages for 48 h before operation and the patients have chlorhexidine added to their bath water for the same period. Flucloxacillin 250 mg four times a day is started 24 h before operation and 2 u of blood are cross-matched.

Anaesthesia

The operation is carried out under normotensive general anaestheisa. Good peripheral intravenous access for fluid and blood replacement is essential and an ECG recording and central venous pressure monitoring may be indicated if severe cardiac disease coexists. A Swan–Ganz catheter, an arterial line and continuous bladder drainage are not routinely required, but may be used on certain occasions.

The operation

1 & 2

Position of patient

The patient lies supine on the operating table with the end flap of the table lowered to remove the opposite leg from the operating field and provide better access to the popliteal space. The affected leg is supported by a rubber-padded steel strip which is held in place between the metal base of the operating table and the weight of the patient on the antistatic rubber cushion. A large sandbag is placed under the thigh to produce slight knee flexion which aids access to the popliteal space, but excessive knee flexion is avoided because this makes tailoring of graft length difficult. Dissection of the popliteal fossa can then be carried out from the opposite side of the table with the surgeon seated on an adjustable stool. The leg is painted with chlorhexidine or iodine from ankle to mid-abdomen. The unprepared foot is wrapped in a sterile plastic bag, which allows its colour to be inspected and the pulses to be palpated when the reconstruction has been completed. The prepared skin is covered with one or two large plastic drapes.

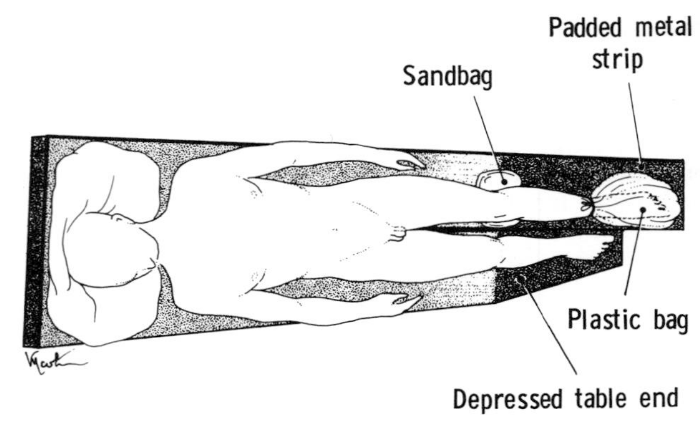

1

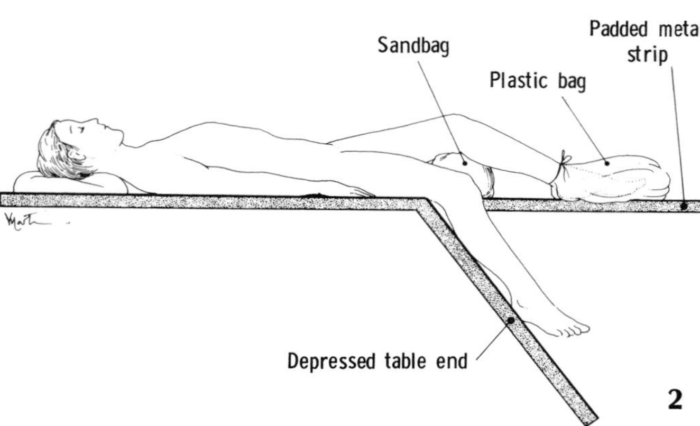

2

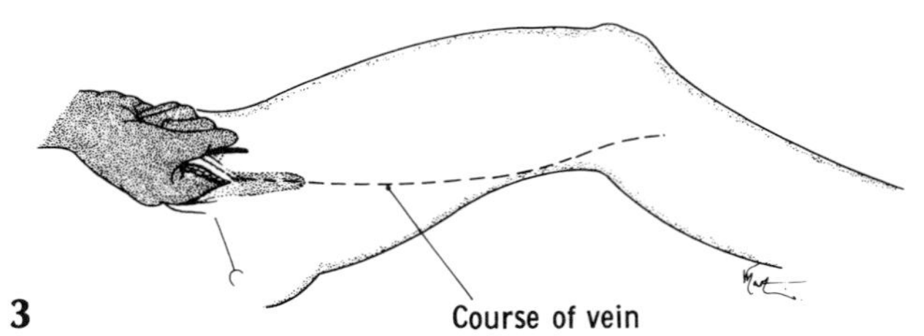

3

3

Exposure of the vein

Confirmation of an adequate saphenous vein and avoidance of vein damage are the first two steps of the operation. Our preference is to find the upper end of the vein by a vertical incision placed over the saphenofemoral junction which is then extended up across the front of the inguinal ligament. This incision also allows adequate access to the common femoral artery. Using a combination of blunt and sharp dissection, the vein should be found in the subcutaneous fat as it dips down through the cribriform fascia. The junction of the saphenous with the common femoral vein must be confirmed. If this step is omitted it is possible to trace a large anteromedial or posterolateral thigh vein instead of the main saphenous trunk. Once the vein has been exposed and dissected to its termination, the initial short incision may be extended along the course of the vein by sliding a finger along the perisaphenous space superficial to the vein and carefully incising the skin overlying the surface of the finger with a scalpel. The subcutaneous fat can then be divided with scissors. The finger prevents inadvertent damage to the vein and identifies the direction of its course, so preventing an inaccurate incision and undercutting of the wound edges which predisposes to skin necrosis.

4 & 5

Dissection of the vein

The skin and subcutaneous tissue over the vein are divided, exposing the appropriate length required for the bypass, using the sliding finger technique already described. It is advisable to over-estimate the length of a vein which is required as unused vein may be easily discarded while insufficient length may prejudice successful surgery. The vein becomes more superficial just above the knee and the finger dissection technique may have to be abandoned in favour of blunt tunnelling with scissors under direct vision with scissor division of the overlying skin. Blind tunnelling may perforate and damage the vein. Dabs of patent blue violet are applied to the superficial surface of the vein before it is lifted from its bed. This enables the vein to be carefully aligned without twists when it is later positioned in the tunnel. When the required length of vein is completely exposed two operators working from opposite ends free the vein from the surrounding fat and stringy periadventitia by a combination of sharp and blunt dissection, ligating each small branch of the long saphenous vein with 3/0 silk ties on the vein side and 2/0 chromic catgut or polyglycolic acid at the other end. The ligatures must not be tied too close to the main vein to avoid constriction.

When there is still some doubt over the length of vein that will be required for the bypass, it is better to leave the vein *in situ* (*see Illustration 5*) and to explore the popliteal artery to determine its suitability (*see Illustration 8*) before proceeding to harvest the vein (*see Illustration 6*).

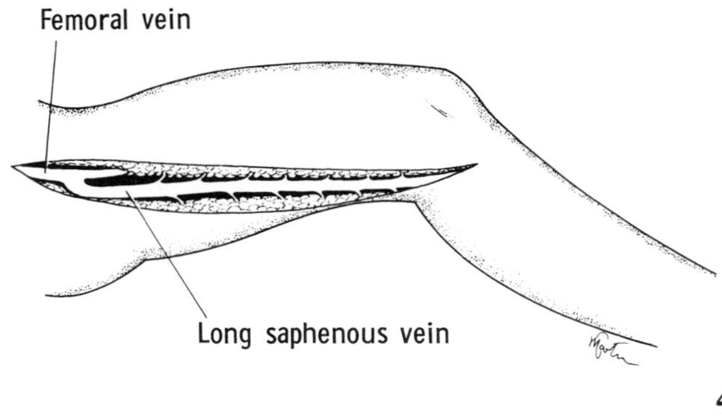

4

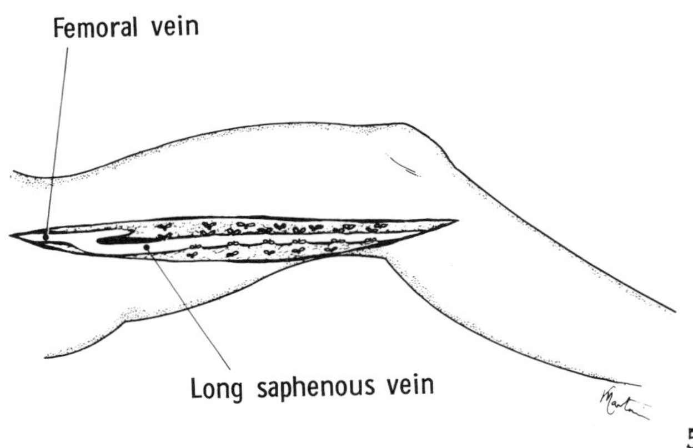

5

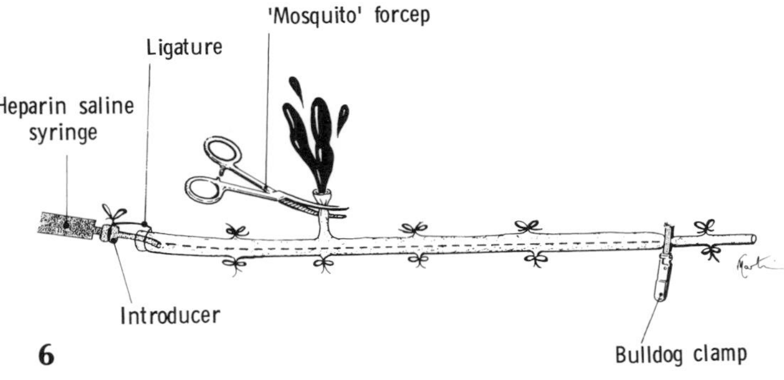

6

6

Vein distension

When the vein has been lifted from its bed, both attached ends are tied off with 2/0 silk ligatures, before the vein is divided and removed. A cannula is tied into the distal end of the vein. Then, 20 ml of 1:400 000 heparin saline solution or heparinized blood are drawn up into a syringe which is attached to the cannula. A bulldog clamp is then placed across the vein and a segment is gently distended by depressing the plunger of the syringe. Side branches that were not ligated when the vein was dissected out are revealed when they emit small jets of perfusate. The stumps of unligated side branches can usually be picked up with accurately placed mosquito forceps and ligated. A small 6/0 polypropylene stitch is used to close any sideholes in the vein where branches have torn off flush with the main channel. Great care must be taken to avoid narrowing the lumen of the graft when picking up small branches or placing a stitch in the side of the vein wall.

When the entire vein has been distended and rendered watertight, adventitial bands are divided with small curved scissors and the outer layers of adventitia are divided longitudinally to allow maximal venous dilatation. Overdistension of the vein must be avoided, since this has been shown to separate and damage endothelial cells, exposing the underlying collagen, which is known to promote platelet adhesion and thrombosis. Devices to prevent overdistension are now marketed, but we do not use them at present, relying instead on gentle pressure to prevent damage.

7

Femoral artery exposure

The common femoral pulse is palpated through the upper end of the incision which is used to expose the vein. Self-retaining Travers' retractors are inserted to hold the wound edges apart and the subcutaneous fat and deep fascia over the pulse are then divided in the long axis of the limb by sharp dissection until the vasa vasorum on the anterior surface of the artery are clearly seen. The common femoral artery is displayed from the inguinal ligament to its division into the superficial femoral and profunda branches. The three main vessels are dissected free and taped with polythene snares; small branches are ligated and divided or controlled by looped silk sutures.

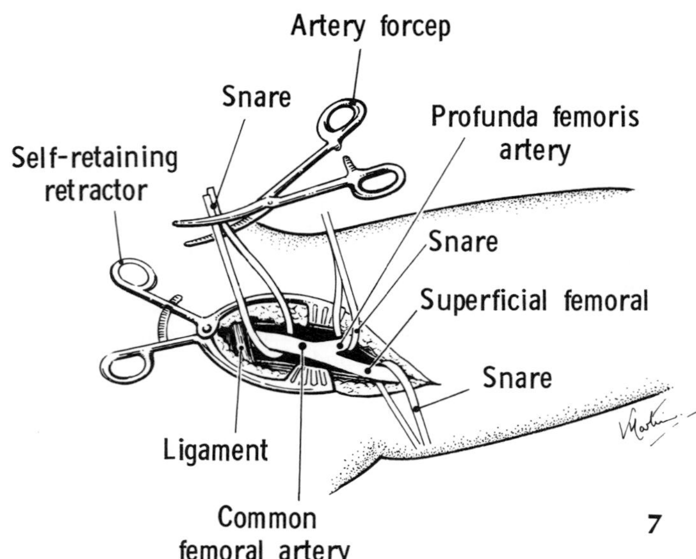

7

8

Low popliteal artery exposure

The segment of popliteal artery between the knee joint and the trifurcation is usually the least diseased and this is the segment of vessel usually chosen for the lower anastomosis. The posteromedial border of the tibia is identified by palpation through the lower end of the incision used to expose the saphenous vein. The deep fascia of the calf is then incised vertically about 1 cm behind this bony attachment. This incision is extended upwards, until the tendons of sartorius, gracilis, semimembranosus and semitendinosus are encountered at about the level of the knee joint, and downwards as far as necessary. A finger pushed in front of the medial head of gastrocnemius which lies beneath the deep fascia separates loose areolar tissue between this muscle and the posterior border of the tibia. This space is enlarged by inserting the twin Browse retractors which open up the lower part of the popliteal fossa. These retractors are 'rake-type' paired self-retaining retractors similar to Travers' but with a long and short blade. The short blades sit against the tibia while the long blades 'hold back' the calf muscles. The popliteal vessels lie anteriorly on the posterior surface of the bone with the vein lying on the medial side of the artery and the nerve lying behind. The vein is gently dissected off the artery which is freed at one point and taped with a plastic snare. A reasonable length of artery is then dissected free and a second snare is placed around the artery. Small branches between the snares should be ligated. A Lahey forceps is then passed behind the artery and the vessel is gently palpated against the rigid forceps. This confirms the presence of a satisfactory lumen and allows the extent of the atheroma to be gauged. The optimum site for the lower anastomosis can then be selected. Control of blood flow from the segment of artery to be used for the anastomosis can often be obtained by gently pulling up the snares and holding them taut over the central pinion of the self-retaining retractor. This avoids cluttering the wound with bulldog clamps which are applied if there is continued bleeding. Access to the upper part of the artery is obtained by dividing the medial head of gastrocnemius and the tendons attached to the upper end of the tibia. If exposure of the tibial vessel is required, the origin of soleus and anterior tibial veins can be divided.

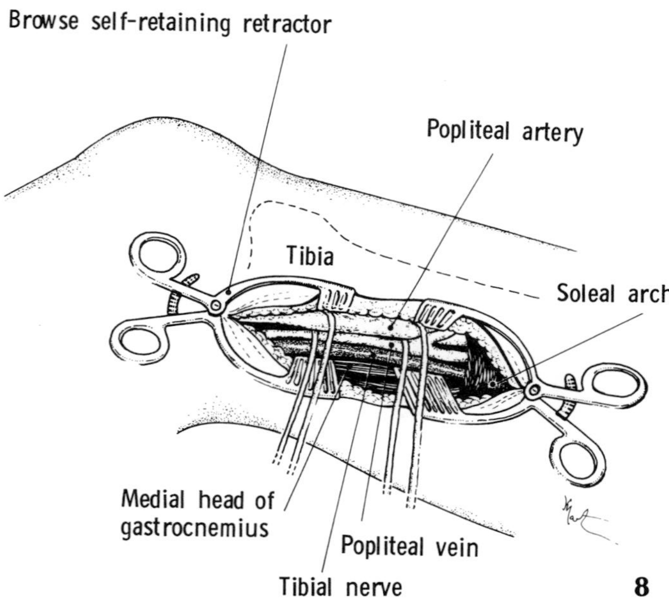

8

High popliteal exposure

Better results are obtained from a short bypass ending above the knee provided the upper popliteal artery is found to have a lumen and is relatively disease-free. The anterior border of sartorius is found and freed above the knee through the incision used to expose the saphenous vein. This muscle is then retracted posteriorly and the upper part of the popliteal fat is exposed. The fat is separated by blunt dissection and the vessels are found lying deeply within the popliteal space. They lie close to the back of the bone and after insertion of the Browse self-retaining retractors are dissected and prepared in an identical manner.

9

The tunnel

A Wilson's or Taylor's tunneller is pushed upward between the heads of gastrocnemius through the apex of the popliteal space, into the thigh medial to the tendon of adductor magnus. The tunneller passes along Hunter's canal deep to sartorius and in front of the superficial femoral artery to emerge in the femoral triangle. The upper end of the saphenous vein is attached to the tunneller or its introducer by a silk suture and pulled back down from the groin to the popliteal space taking great care not to twist the vessel during its passage. This is checked by watching the dye marks previously applied to the surface of the vein, and making sure that they point in the same direction. The proximal end of the vein should lie over the common femoral artery and the distal end should lie over the prepared segment of popliteal artery without tension. The vein should be trimmed at the top end since this is usually its narrowest portion.

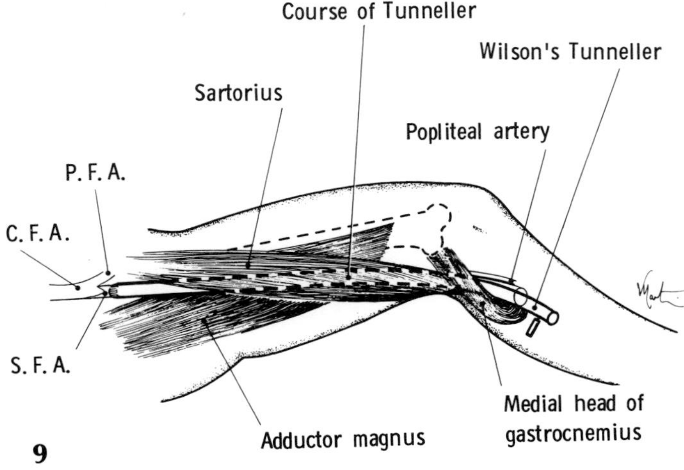

9

The popliteal anastomosis

The upper and lower anastomoses are carried out in an identical manner and may be performed simultaneously if two experienced surgeons are available with adequate assistance. This has the benefit of saving time and reducing the period of distal ischaemia. Heparin 5000 u is given by the anaesthetist and allowed to circulate. This dose is sufficient to prevent thrombosis during 1 h of arterial occlusion in normal-sized individuals, but it may be increased if the patient is very fat. Further increments of 2000 u are given if the anastomosis takes longer than 1 h.

The surgeon who is seated on a stool on the opposite side of the patient occludes the popliteal artery by tensing the snares over the central pinion of each self-retaining retractor. A small arteriotomy is then made in the centre of the prepared segment of popliteal artery using a No. 15 blade on a long-handled scalpel. A small quantity of blood escapes when the lumen of the vessel is entered. Bulldog clamps are applied if bleeding persists, which may occur in a heavily diseased or calcified vessel. The initial arteriotomy is then enlarged using Potts' scissors, angled on the vertical, until the length of the arteriotomy exceeds the width of the vein (usually 1 cm or more). The arteriotomy should finish well short of both snares. They are then released to assess the volume of back- and downbleeding before heparin saline is instilled into the distal and proximal segments via a catheter of appropriate size. The end of the saphenous vein is then tailored to the length of the arteriotomy by cutting it obliquely while ensuring that there is enough vein to reach the distal point of the arteriotomy. The cut end of the vein should be matched for size against the arteriotomy.

10

A double-ended 6/0 polypropylene suture is used for the anastomosis, inserting both needles into the 'heel' of the vein as shown. The needles are then passed out through the proximal end of the arteriotomy on either side of its apex and a knot is tied on the superficial side of the vessel. One needle is then passed back between the attached vein and artery to the far side of the vessel in order to carry out the 'deep side' of the anastomosis.

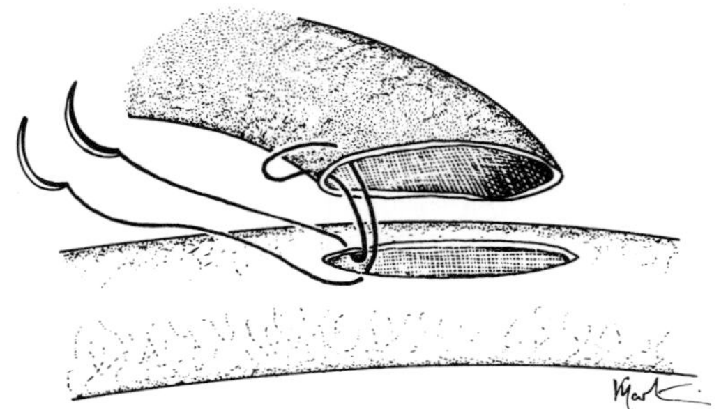

10

11

A standard continuous suture is then begun, entering the vein from out to in and the artery from in to out. Three or four sutures are placed on either side of the 'heel' under direct vision before the backhand side is sutured towards the apex of the graft.

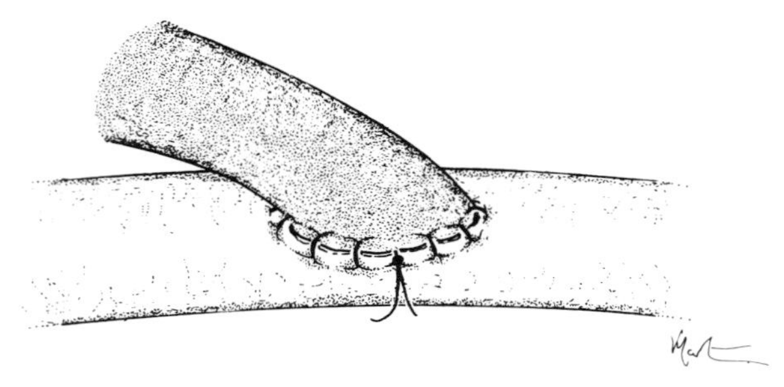

11

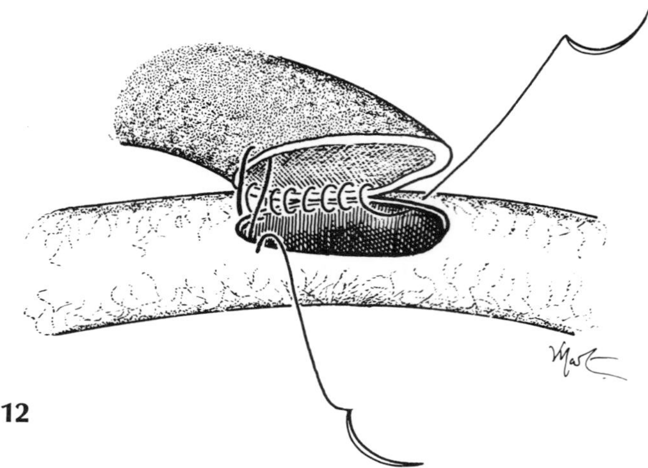

12

12

Carefully placed smaller bites are taken at the apex or 'toe' to ensure that the distal vessel is not narrowed or occluded. This part of the anastomosis must be carefully made to avoid picking up the far side of the vessel and to prevent narrowing.

Alternatively, a number of loops may be inserted under direct vision and pulled tight when the apex has been completed, or the continuous suture may be tied off and a series of carefully placed interrupted sutures put in around the apex.

13

When the 'toe' has been passed, the over-and-over suture is completed on the near side, tying off both ends in the middle of the forehand side.

A bulldog clamp is then placed on the graft just proximal to the suture line and both snares are relaxed to allow the anastomosis to be checked for leaks and to allow the blood to perfuse the distal vessels again.

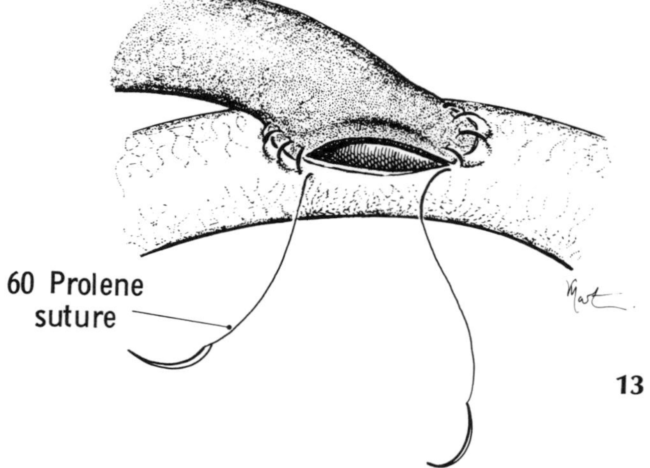

13

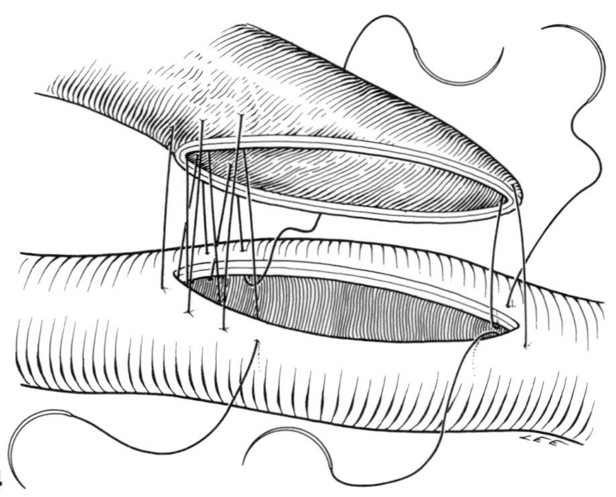

14

14

Alternative anastomosis technique

A parachute technique may be used on both the heel and the apex of the anastomosis inserting a number of 'loose' loops on both sides without tying down a knot. After six sutures have been inserted, the vein may be slid down to the artery while gentle traction is applied to the sutures. The central part of the anastomosis can then be completed in the usual manner on both sides.

15

Upper anastomosis

A small, angled Fogarty clamp is placed across the common femoral artery as close to the inguinal ligament as possible. Bulldog clamps are used to occlude the profunda and superficial femoral vessels. An arteriotomy is made in the common femoral artery which may be extended into the profunda femoris artery in the presence of a localized stenosis near its origin. The inflow is checked by releasing the proximal clamp and the backflow from both superficial and profunda vessels is examined by releasing the bulldog clamps. A few millilitres of heparin saline are instilled into both distal vessels which are then reclamped. The anastomosis is made in an identical manner to that described for the popliteal vessels. When the anastomosis nears completion, the upper clamp is released to expel any thrombus which may have developed in the iliac artery above the clamp, and the final sutures are inserted. The ends are tied together as before. The bulldog clamp is removed from the lower end of the saphenous vein and the clamps on the superficial and profunda vessels are released. The Fogarty clamp is then released and the anastomoses at either end are examined for bleeding. Leaks are occluded by accurately placed single 6/0 polypropylene sutures inserted, if necessary, after the brief reapplication of the upper Fogarty clamp. A reversing dose of protamine 25–50 mg is given by the anaesthetist when it is certain that the vessel will not need to be reclamped again.

Confirmation of patency – operative arteriography

When the anastomoses are dry, the popliteal artery distal to the graft is carefully palpated to confirm the presence of pulsatile flow. The foot pulses are also examined through the sterile plastic bag. A green butterfly needle is inserted into the common femoral artery and an X-ray plate wrapped in a sterile Mayo table cover is placed behind the knee. The common femoral artery is briefly occluded and 20 ml of contrast (Conray or Hexobrix) are injected slowly through the butterfly to outline the graft. A spot film is taken of the popliteal anastomosis and run-off to detect any technical errors which might lead to early occlusion of the graft. We routinely perform operative arteriography after crural bypasses but only perform operative arteriography if in doubt for femoropopliteal bypasses.

Closure

The wound is closed with suction drains inserted near both anastomoses to prevent haematoma formation. The deep fascia and subcutaneous fat are closed with interrupted 2/0 chromic catgut. The skin is closed with 2/0 or 3/0 interrupted nylon mattress sutures or by disposable metal staples if preferred. The wound is covered with sterile adhesive dressings or a thin layer of gauze held in place by zinc oxide tape. Care is taken not to occlude the graft or its outflow by tight circumferential bandaging of the limb.

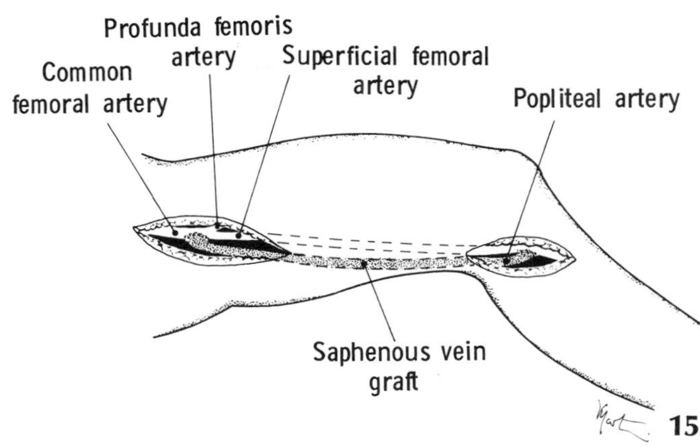

15

Postoperative care

The knee is flexed to 10° or 15° by supporting the lower leg on a soft pillow. The ankle is kept free of the bed clothes by a cradle placed over the feet, and the patient is kept in the recovery ward overnight in order that the pulses can be carefully monitored by well-trained staff. Doppler ankle pressures are used if severe distal disease makes the foot pulses impalpable. Some surgeons prefer to use a continuous pulse volume monitor.

The patient returns to the ward the following day provided that the pulses remain palpable and the Doppler pressures are satisfactory. Any disappearance of a previously palpable pulse or a marked deterioration in Doppler pressure is investigated by urgent digital subtraction angiography, conventional arteriography, or re-exploration and operative angiography. Confirmation of graft occlusion is an indication for urgent reoperation unless the run-off is deemed too poor to allow satisfactory graft function to be maintained. The suction drains are removed after 24 or 48 h if the postoperative course is uncomplicated. The patients should begin to walk on the third or fourth day after operation. Our patients can remain in hospital until the sutures or staples are removed on the tenth day, but many now leave hospital on the fifth or seventh day if they have an uncomplicated postoperative course.

Complications

The main complications are early graft occlusion, haemorrhage, infection, skin necrosis from undermining and leg swelling which is common. A careful technique reduces these problems to a minimum.

References

Harris, P. L., How, T. V. and Jones, D. P. (1987). Prospective randomised clinical trial to complete *in situ* and reversed saphenous vein grafts for femoropopliteal bypass. *British Journal of Surgery* **74**, 252.

Mosley, J.G., Manhine, A. R., Raphael, M. and Marston, J. A. P. (1983). An assessment of long saphenous venography to evaluate the saphenous vein for femoropopliteal bypass. *British Journal of Surgery* **70**, 673.

Senapati, A., Lea Thomas, M. and Burnand, K. G. (1983). A trial of saphenous phlebography compared with surgical dissection as a method of assessing suitability of long saphenous veins for use as a bypass graft. *British Journal of Surgery* **70**, 688.

Cephalic and basilic veins as arterial conduits

PETER A. SCHNEIDER MD, *Vascular Surgeon*
GEORGE ANDROS MD, *Vascular Surgeon*
ROBERT W. HARRIS MD, *Vascular Surgeon*
LEOPOLDO B. DULAWA MD, *Vascular Surgeon*
ROBERT W. OBLATH MD, *Vascular Surgeon*
Vascular Laboratory, Saint Joseph Medical Center, Burbank, California, USA

Introduction

The greater saphenous vein remains the optimal conduit for small-diameter arterial bypass grafts. In the venous circuit, the saphenous vein remains patent at low blood flow rates and it retains this quality when transposed to the arterial system. Its advantages include the highest long-term patency and limb salvage rates, autogenous reconstruction, ease of implantation and low complication rates. We use cephalic and basilic veins as arterial conduits for lower extremity revascularization when ipsilateral or contralateral saphenous vein is unavailable. Long-term follow-up has demonstrated that patency rates are equivalent to that obtained with saphenous vein (Andros *et al.*, 1992).

Decision to use upper extremity veins

Preoperative knowledge of previous saphenous vein excision permits preparation of the patient for alternative vein harvesting in 10% of patients. Intraoperative discovery of an inadequate greater saphenous vein because of phlebitis, varicosities, inadequate size or multiple trunks, occurs in 10–20% of cases. Arm vein can be employed in most clinical situations as a substitute for saphenous vein. Indications include bypass of occlusive disease of the lower limb, upper limb, and the visceral, renal and coronary vessels. Preoperative duplex evaluation of arm veins is beneficial. Past cutdown or phlebitis, usually from intravenous fluid therapy, accounts for the majority of non-usable upper extremity veins. Satisfactory veins can be harvested on the side of permanent pacemaker implantation or previous subclavian catheter insertion.

Preoperative

1

Preserving a potential graft

The characteristics of size, length and superficial position, which make arm veins desirable arterial conduits also predispose them to potentially damaging venipuncture. Education and protection are needed to prevent vein injury. The patients are shown their own cephalic and basilic veins and instructed to prohibit vein puncture for any reason. Venipuncture is limited to the dorsum of the hand. Signs are placed on the patient's room door, hospital bed, hospital chart and nursing records. The arm is wrapped with gauze upon which is written: NO IV's or VENIPUNCTURE.

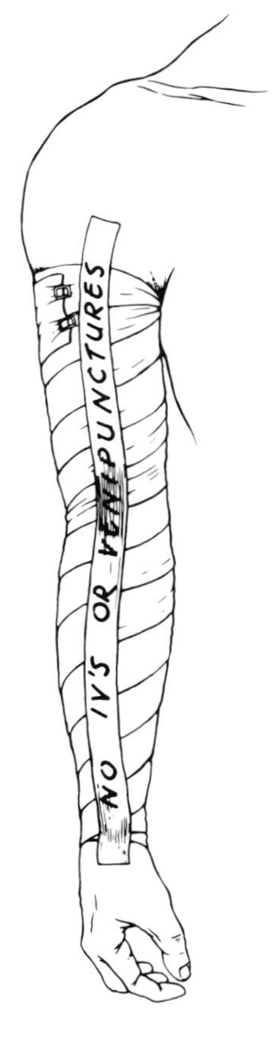

1

2

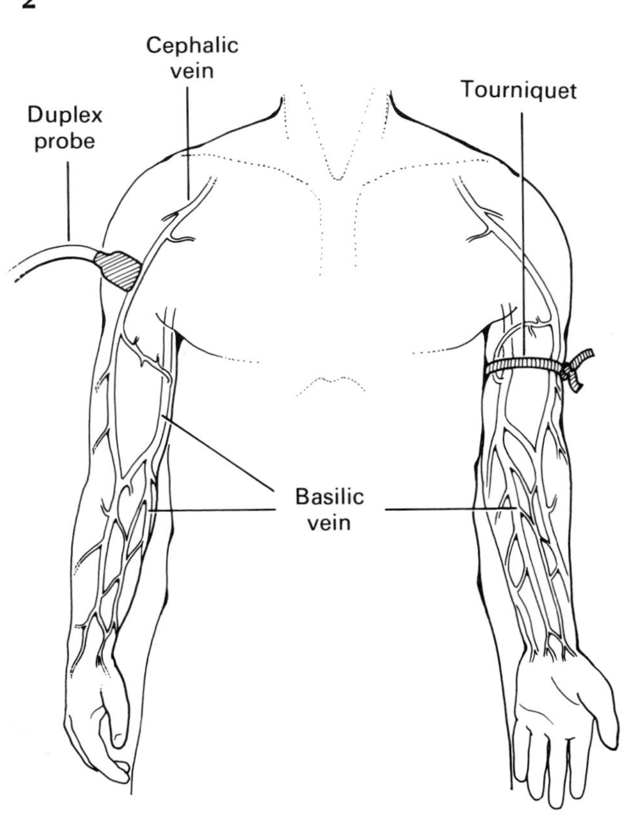

2

Arm vein assessment

Arm veins are evaluated preoperatively on physical examination and with non-invasive ultrasonic techniques. The cephalic and basilic veins are examined in a warm room, by inspection and palpation, employing tourniquets, exercise and dependency. Special attention is directed to the antecubital fossa where variations in venous anatomy are often encountered. Inexact preoperative assessment may result from hair, obesity or tattoos. The latter, however, do not produce vein damage. Preoperative arm vein duplex evaluation has proven valuable in identifying useable veins (Salles-Cunha *et al.*, 1986). An arm vein map is constructed for each patient considered for arm vein harvesting. Arm phlebogram and preparatory cephaloradial arteriovenous fistula are not employed, although their use has been described.

3

Upper extremity venous anatomy

The cephalic vein originates distal to the anatomical snuff box on the radial aspect of the wrist. Coursing medially to the antecubital fossa, it joins the median antecubital vein and then continues proximally (centrally), first on the lateral aspect of the biceps brachii and then in the deltopectoral groove, terminating in the axillary vein.

The median antecubital vein receives one or more deep muscular tributaries and the forearm tributary of the basilic vein; thereafter it continues as the basilic vein to the axilla. In the forearm the basilic vein diameter is more variable than the forearm portion of the cephalic vein. Males and females appear to have equally usable cephalic veins. Cephalic vein diameter is generally 5–6 mm distally and 6–8 mm proximally. The basilic vein proximally (centrally), is usually 7–10 mm. At the proximal end, both veins are very thin walled. The true cephalic vein from wrist to clavicle is only 15% shorter than the greater saphenous.

Choices of arm vein conduits include; 1) cephalic (forearm and upper arm), 2) forearm cephalic-median antecubital-upper arm basilic, 3) upper arm cephalic-median antecubital-upper arm basilic, 4) forearm basilic-median antecubital-upper arm cephalic (rare).

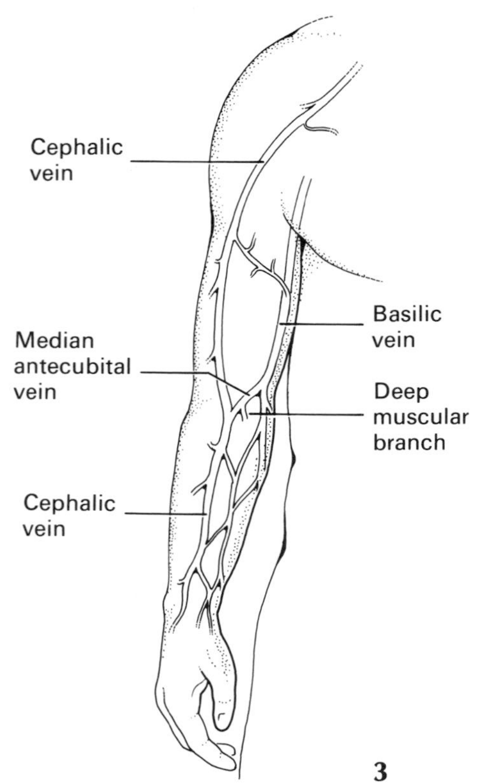

3

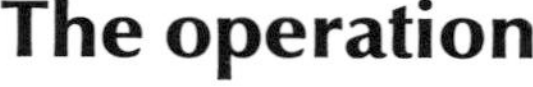

The operation

4

Operative preparation of the arm

Leg bypasses are generally performed under regional anaesthetic. When the decision is made to harvest arm veins, a general anaesthetic is administered. If both arms must be explored for veins, a jugular intravenous line is inserted. The arm is shaved from the wrist to the clavicle, including axilla, and placed on a moveable arm board. The hand is draped out with a towel. If a radial artery cannula is required for blood pressure monitoring, the wrist and hand are excluded from the field and the monitoring extension tubing extends from the towel wrapping the hand. The arm vein duplex map is posted in the operating room.

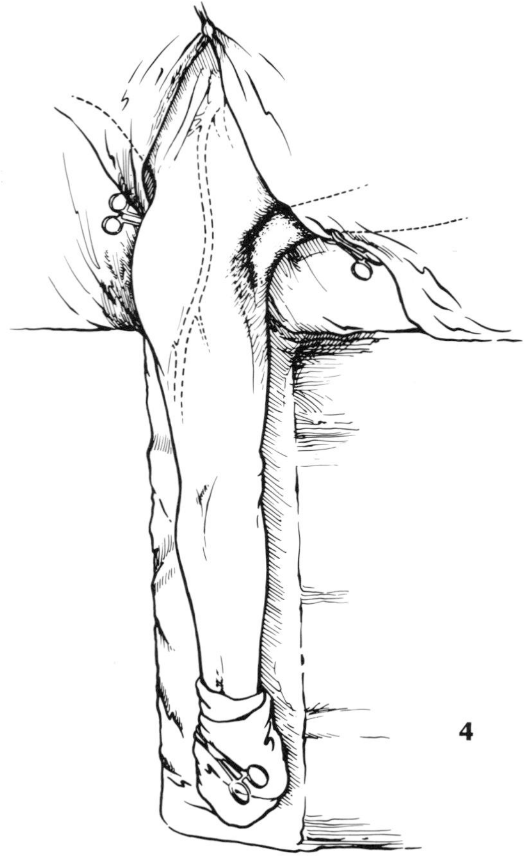

4

5 a–d

Unroofing

The antecubital incision is always transverse and is usually made first. Through the antecubital incision, the upper and lower cephalic and basilic veins can be localized so that longitudinal incisions can be placed directly over the veins. Before excision is undertaken, the entire vein is unroofed. Each incision is started with a scalpel and extended using scissors. Two manoeuvres help to prevent harm to the vein: spreading the scissors between the skin and the vein creates a space (shown as a stippled area) for the scissors' blades when the skin is cut (*b*); only the body of the scissor blade, and not the tip, is used to cut the skin (*c*).

Very few branches arise anteriorly and are easily seen as the vein is unroofed. One 2–3 cm skin bridge is generally placed in the proximal forearm and one in the distal upper arm. The proximal cephalic vein is mobilized up to the deltopectoral groove to its junction with the axillary vein (*d*). The skin is undermined for 5 cm or more to decrease the length of the incision.

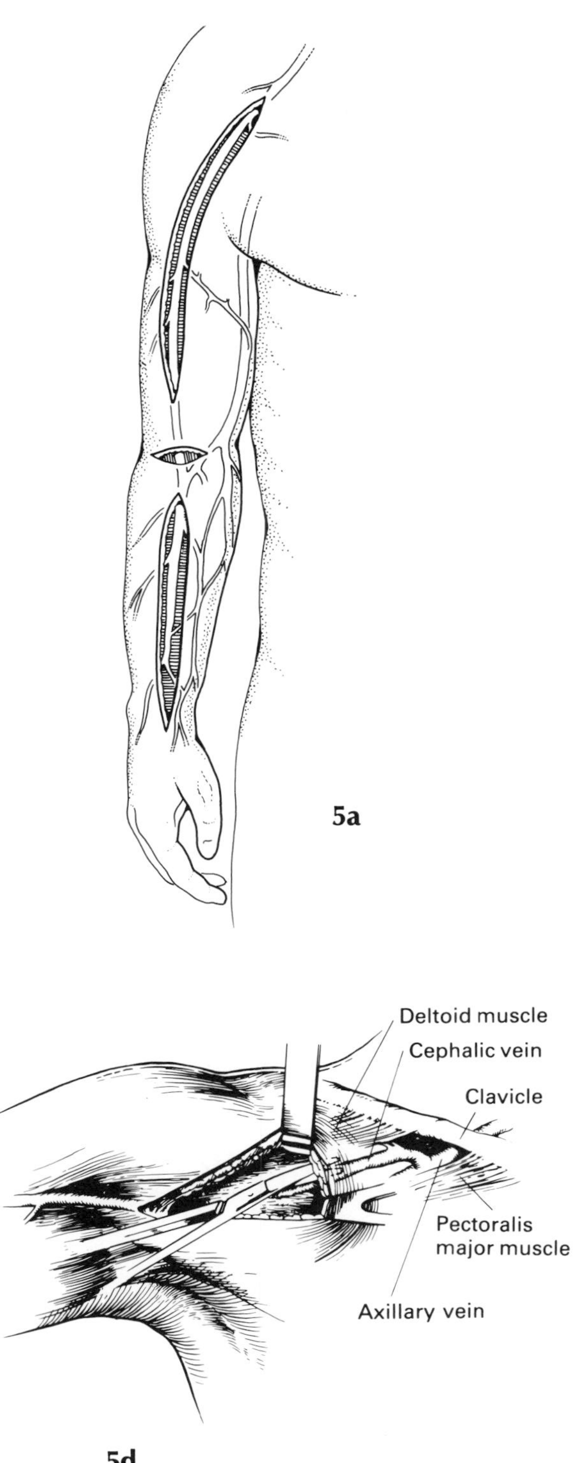

5a

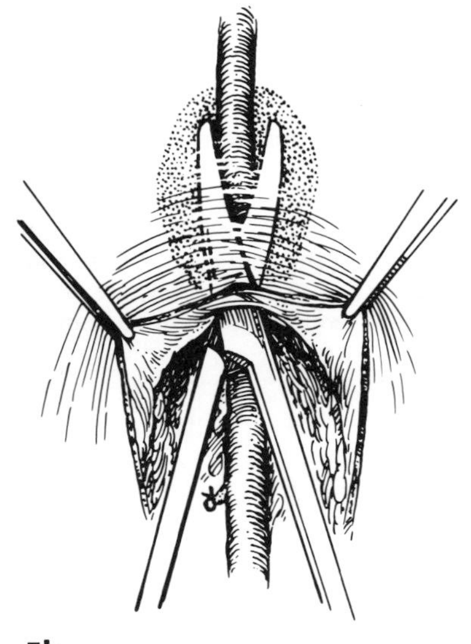

5b

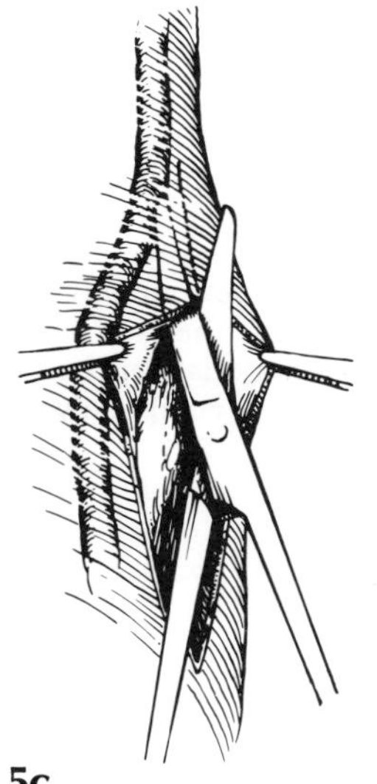

5c

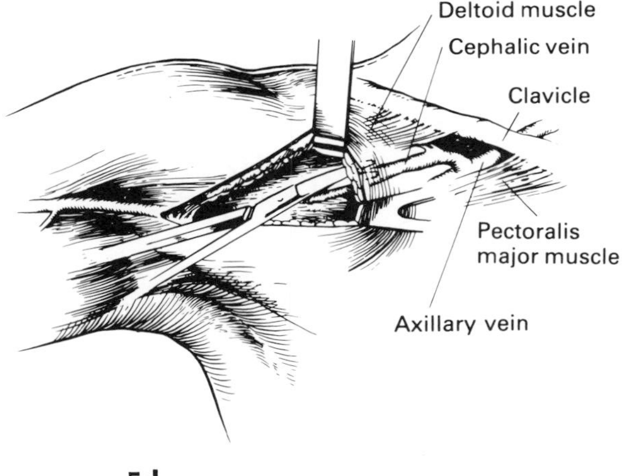

5d

6

The antecubital decision

As the cephalic vein is unroofed proximally along the lateral biceps brachii, it may be found to be scarred or small. If so, the vein is usually inadequate all the way to the clavicle. The course of unroofing is then redirected. The transverse antecubital incision is extended medially along the median antecubital vein. The basilic vein is then unroofed through one long incision to the axilla, terminating the incision at the hairline. The upper arm basilic vein is usually free of disease because of difficulty of performing venipuncture in this area.

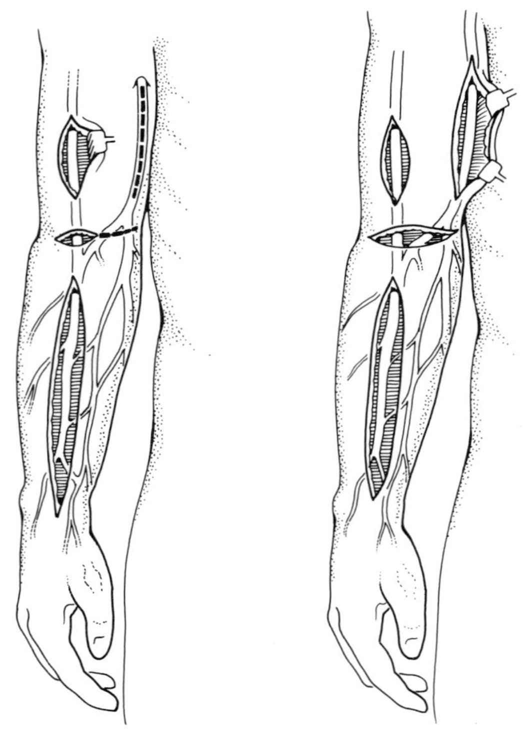

6

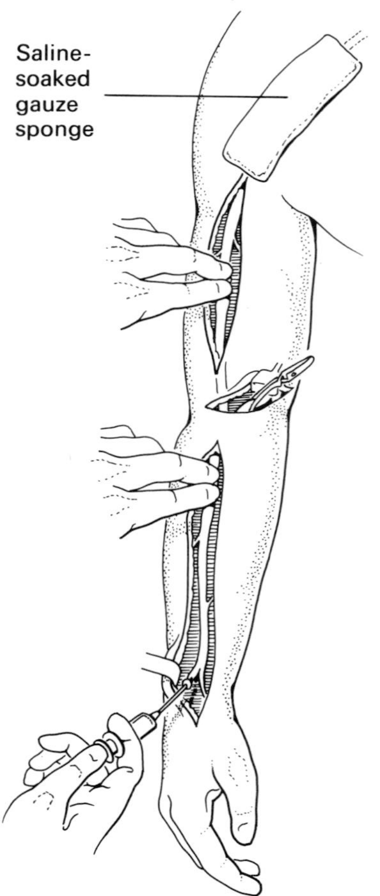

7

7

In situ distension

In situ distension with heparinized saline introduced through a No. 16, 5-cm plastic catheter placed in a side branch is helpful in deciding whether to use the cephalic or the basilic vein. Finger pressure is applied at various sites to permit distension of the segments in question. Some of the vein may be unusable and the decision to use the other arm or alternate graft material can be reached without excising the entire vein or even completely unroofing it.

8a, b & c

Excision

Excision of the unroofed vein is begun at the wrist or the most distal site. The vein is tied as distally as possible under the skin to obtain maximum length. It is divided, gently mobilized and rolled on to a wet gauze sponge; the unexcised portion is covered with wet sponges frequently irrigated with saline (*a*).

The vein and its tributaries are circumferentially dissected (*b*). It is important to tie branches 1–2 mm from the vein to prevent adventitial gathering; 4–0 silk ligatures are used (*c*). The vein is divided so that a 2–3 mm stump extends beyond the tie. Tributaries are haemoclipped distally. The vein is freed under the skin bridges and passed to the next incision. The vein is doubly tied with 2–0 silk at the axillary vein and divided. Venous scarring produced by antecubital venipuncture makes dissection more difficult and risks damage to both the cephalic and basilic veins. If the cephalic vein in the forearm and upper arm are usable, the median antecubital vein is not disturbed. If a segment of vein is diseased, it is excised and a long spatulated venovenous anastomosis is constructed using 7–0 Prolene.

Following excision, reversed venous conduits are filled with heparinized saline. The ease of irrigation is assessed and blood is removed. With a bulldog clamp on the central end, the vein is gently distended to determine length. Easily identified leaking tributaries are ligated with 4–0 silk ties.

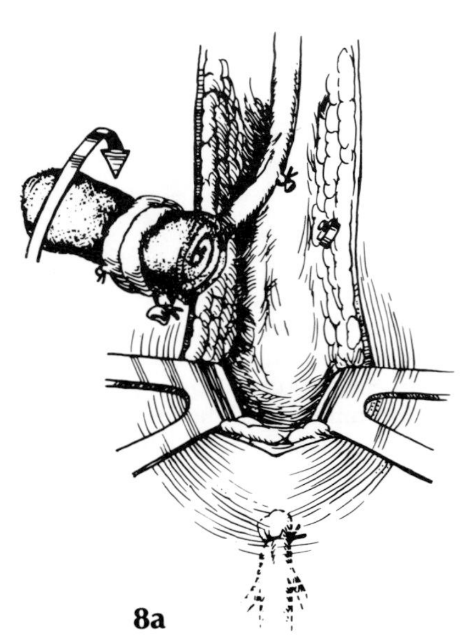

8a

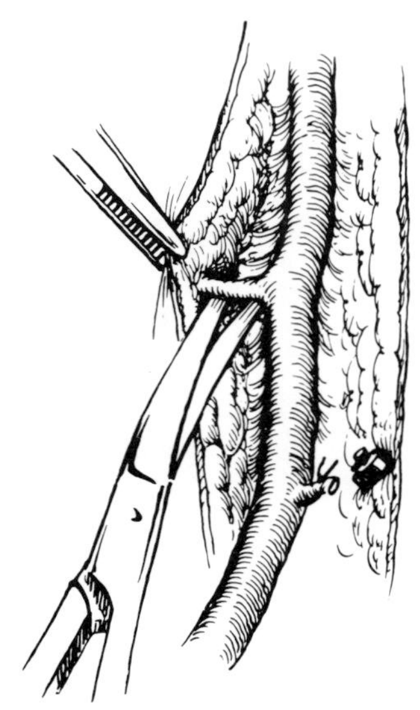

8b

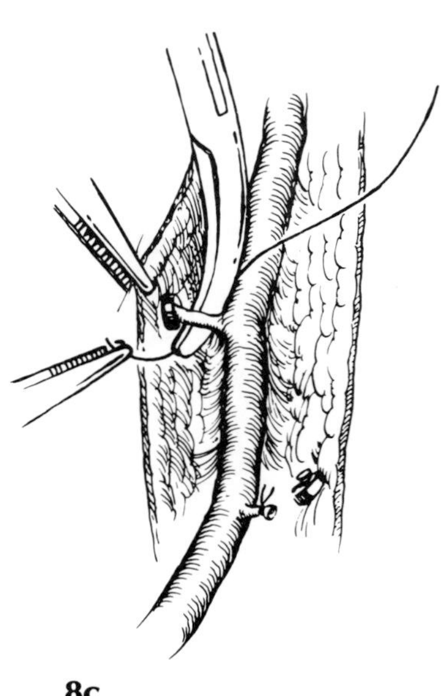

8c

9

Implantation

With the vein reversed, the proximal anastomosis is performed using 6–0 Prolene. Whenever possible, prosthetic grafts are avoided for the proximal anastomosis. Lower extremity grafts maintain long-term patency when originating from the common, superficial or deep femoral arteries and the popliteal artery.

With the proximal anastomosis completed and inspected, the vein graft is allowed to distend with heparinized blood. Constricting adventitial bands are carefully divided. The graft is examined for additional bleeding tributaries. Blood flow from the end of the graft is observed. When a vein segment is placed in non-reversed orientation, valves must be lysed. The valvulotome is placed through the open end of the graft and introduced in retrograde fashion. Valve lysis in arm veins requires greater force than in saphenous veins. Firm counter traction must be held by the assistant. Vein valves can usually be seen through the vein wall. The end of the graft is brought to the distal anastomotic site in a previously formed deep tunnel adjacent to the native artery. By passing the graft when it is distended with blood, the risk of twisting or inappropriate graft length is minimized.

Postoperative anticoagulants are employed in the same way as for saphenous vein conduits begun on the first postoperative day.

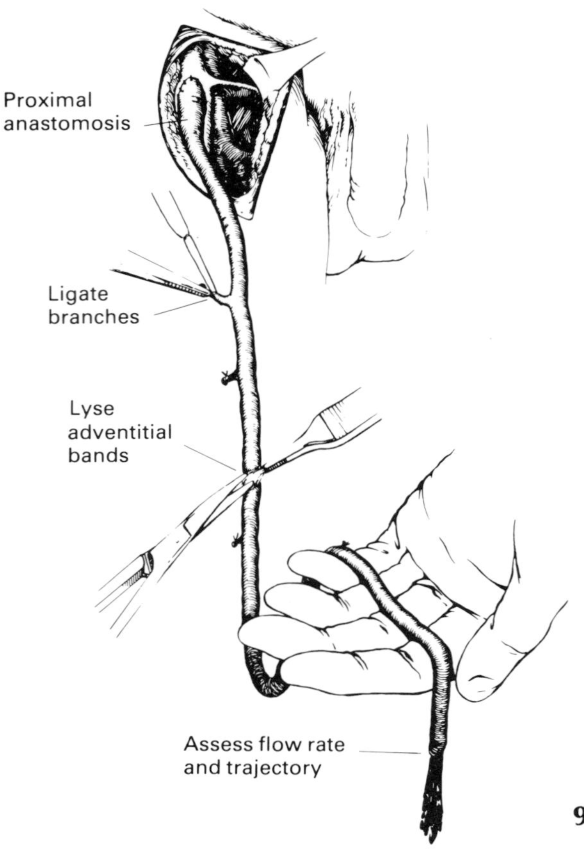

9

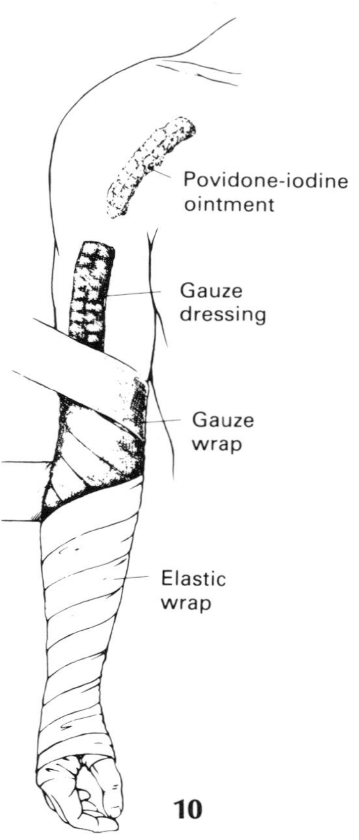

10

10

Wound closure

Subcutaneous tissue is closed with running 3–0 chromic suture and skin is closed with staples. Incisions are covered with povidone-iodine ointment, dry dressings, a gauze wrap and padding over bony prominences. The entire area is wrapped with a 10-cm elastic bandage from the base of the fingers to the axilla. Dressings are removed on the third day and clips removed on the seventh day.

No long-term morbidity has been observed in arms from which veins have been harvested, even when both the cephalic and basilic veins are removed. Surprisingly little postoperative pain or swelling is experienced.

Complications

Arm veins are susceptible to all of the early and later complications encountered with saphenous veins. Haemorrhage and infection are infrequent and are treated as with saphenous vein. Thrombectomy within the first day of operation is difficult and should not be performed *in situ*. The vein wall is too thin to withstand catheter thrombectomy. The entire vein is removed, gently stripped of clot, irrigated with heparinized saline and reimplanted. Balloon embolectomy catheters can be hazardous and are best avoided. Late complications of inflow occlusion, neointimal hyperplasia, vein valve hypertrophy, aneurysmal dilatation and progression of outflow occlusive disease have all been observed and are treated as with saphenous veins.

Acknowledgement

We thank Ms Donna Welch for assistance in preparing this chapter.

References

Andros, G., Salles-Cunha, S. X., Harris, R. W., Schneider, P. A., Dulawa, L. B. and Oblath, R. W. (1992). Arm veins for arterial reconstruction surgery: A twenty-three year experience. In *Long Term Results in Vascular Surgery* Yao, J. and Pearce, W. Eds. Norwalk, CT: Appleton and Lange, pp. 247–258.

Salles-Cunha, S. X., Andros, G., Harris, R. W., Dulawa, L. B. and Oblath, R. W. (1986). Preoperative noninvasive assessment of arm veins to be used as bypass grafts in the lower extremities. *Journal of Vascular Surgery* **3**, 813.

Semi-closed endarterectomy of the superficial femoral artery

F. H. W. M. VAN DER HEIJDEN
Th. THEODORIDES
R. W. H. VAN REEDT DORTLAND
B. C. EIKELBOOM
Department of Surgery, Section of Vascular Surgery, University Hospital Utrecht, The Netherlands

Introduction

In 1946 the Portuguese surgeon Dos Santos, in attempting a thrombectomy of a brachial artery, not only removed the arterial thrombus but the entire intima and a part of the media as well (Dos Santos, 1947). This was the first endarterectomy ever performed; 35 years later the artery was still patent. Following this first success, endarterectomy found many applications and was in fact the start of a new era in vascular surgery. Dos Santos used the technique for desobstruction of the superficial femoral artery (SFA) and was in fact the first surgeon to treat arterial occlusive disease. A few years later Kunlin introduced the technique of femoropopliteal reversed venous bypass which has replaced endarterectomy in most hospitals. A number of recent studies have shown that complication rate, mortality and cumulative patency of SFA endarterectomy are comparable with those of femoropopliteal reversed venous bypass (Heijden *et al.*, 1993).

1

The technique of superficial femoral artery endarterectomy has since the days of Dos Santos been modified by a number of surgeons. Wylie introduced the technique of open endarterectomy (Wylie, 1952) which was later modified by Edwards (1960) who proposed closure of the entire endarterectomized segment by vein patching. Cannon and Barker (1955) introduced the semi-closed technique with the use of a ring stripper. Many other methods of developing a cleavage plane between intima and media have beeen used such as gas endarterectomy (Sobel *et al.*, 1966) and saline endarterectomy (Blaisdell, Kall and Thomas, 1966). They all proved to be inferior to the ring stripper. The shape of the ring stripper has been altered over the years and a number of devices have been used to replace the ring stripper, like a wire loop or spiral dissector (Le Veen, 1965). From all the techniques described above, the semi-closed endarterectomy with use of a ring stripper with a 45 degree angle is preferred.

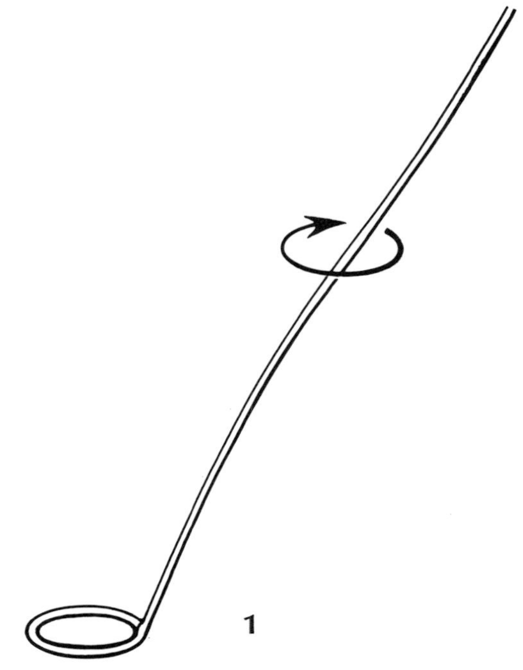

1

2

The operation starts with a groin incision to expose the femoral bifurcation. A curved vertical incision is made over the femoral pulsation below the inguinal ligament. The origin of the superficial and deep femoral arteries are encircled as is the distal part of the common femoral artery.

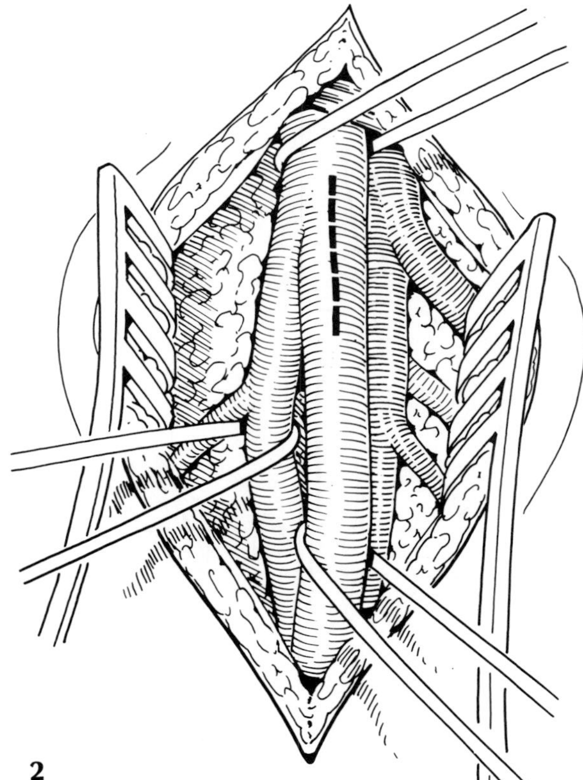

2

3

The distal part of the superficial femoral artery and proximal part of the popliteal artery are exposed through a medial supragenual approach. An incision is made in the lower part of the thigh parallel to the long axis of the leg in the course of the greater saphenous vein which should be spared. The fascia overlying the sartorius muscle is incised longitudinally. The sartorius muscle is retracted medially and posteriorly. The incision is deepened to the vasto adductor membrane which is bluntly dissected and forms the anterior wall of Hunter's canal. The tendon of the adductor magnus is exposed over its entire length and is resected for better exposure of the artery and to facilitate passage of the ringstripper. Care should be taken not to damage the saphenous nerve.

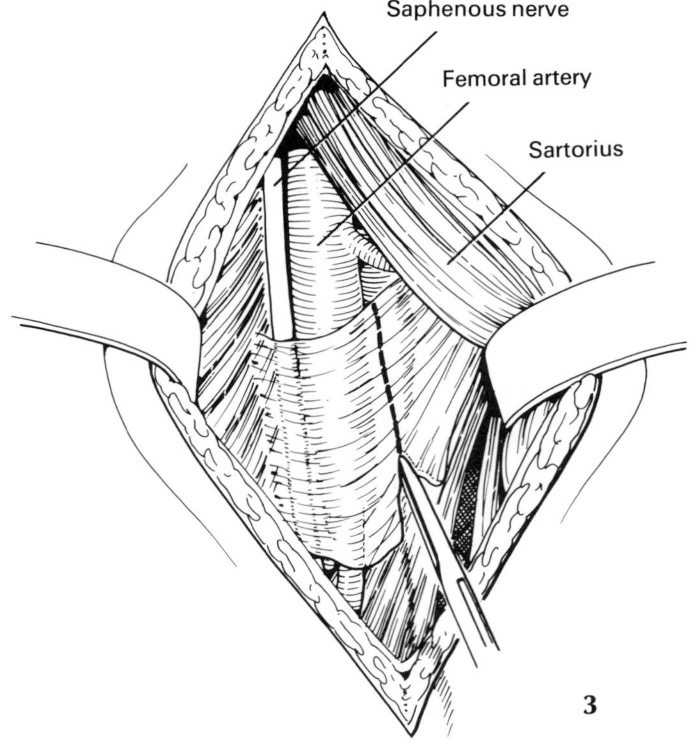

3

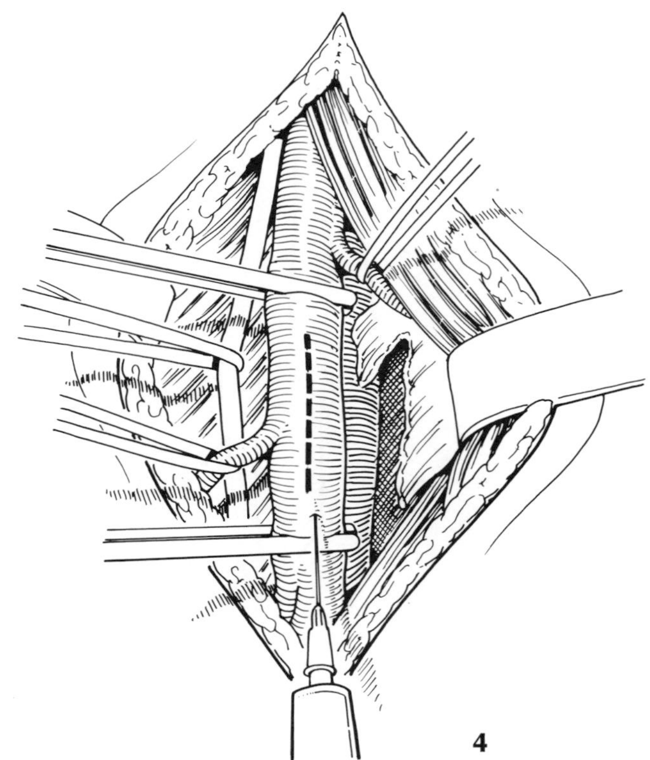

4

4

The artery is further exposed and collateral arteries are temporarily encircled with vessel loops. After intravenous administration of 25 mg heparin, the arteries are clamped. The extent of the atheromatous plaque is judged by palpation to determine the site of the arteriotomy. In order to facilitate the arteriotomy the locally clamped arterial segment can be inflated with saline solution. The arteriotomy is placed at the distal end of the atheromatous plaque up into the relatively normal part of the supragenual popliteal artery.

5

At this site a local open endarterectomy is performed. One of the most critical technical details of endarterectomy is the selection of the appropriate endarterectomy plane. The optimum plane of dissection lies between the diseased intima and the circular fibres of the media. A dissector is used to open up the cleavage plane between the outer layer of the atheroma and the media. This cleavage plane is easily established partly as a result of the pathological process in the diseased artery.

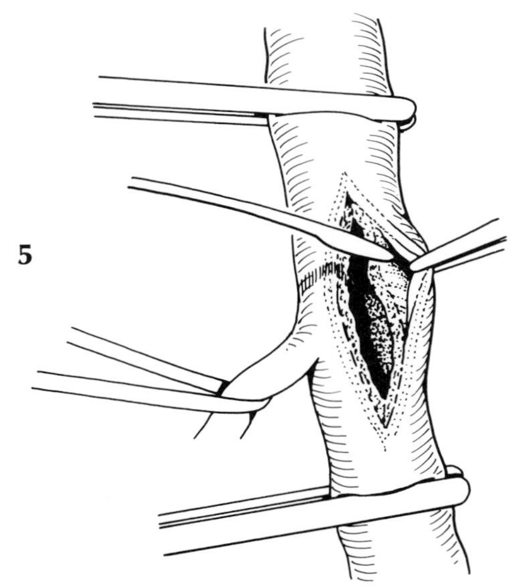

5

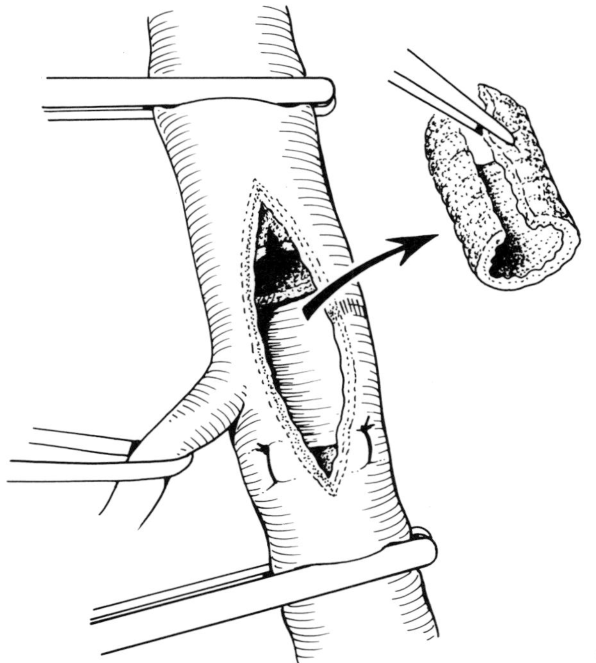

6

6

When the local endarterectomy is completed the endarterectomy core is cut. The distal end of the intima is fixed with tacking sutures to prevent dissection by ante-grade blood flow. The local open endarterectomy is proximally extended just beyond the arteriotomy.

7

A ring stripper is selected which just fits inside the artery. The proximal end of the intima is threaded inside the loop of a ring stripper. One hand should hold the arterial wall and intima core fixed together in order to prevent 'roll-up' of the intima, while the other hand operates the ringstripper.

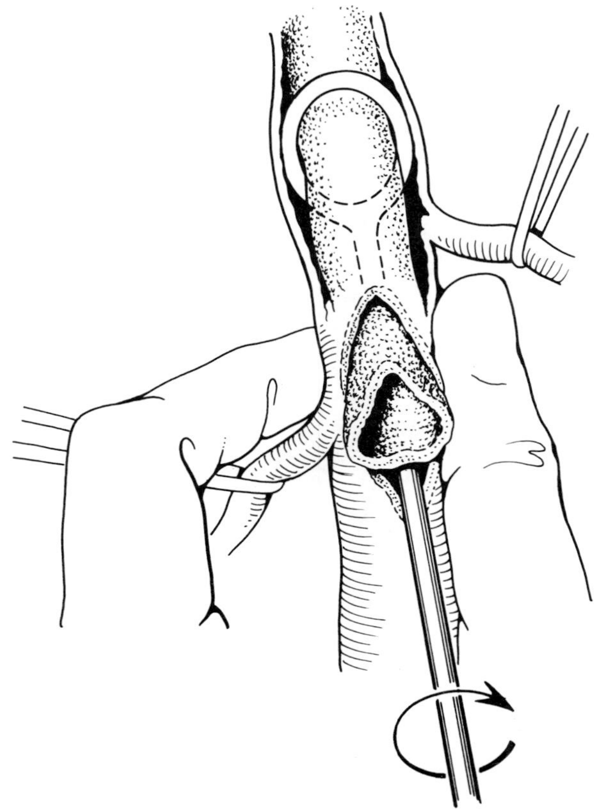

7

8

With a gentle rotating and thrusting motion the cleavage plane is gradually extended up into the groin. The stripper will usually pass the entire length of the superficial femoral artery without difficulty. If passage of the ring stripper cannot be achieved from this site, the stripper can also be introduced via an arteriotomy at the femoral bifurcation.

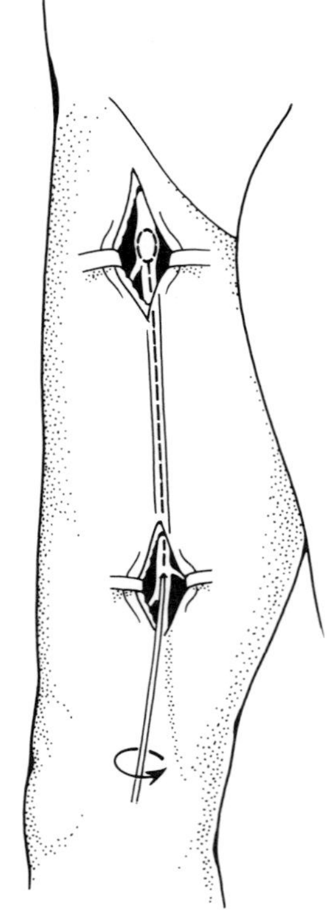

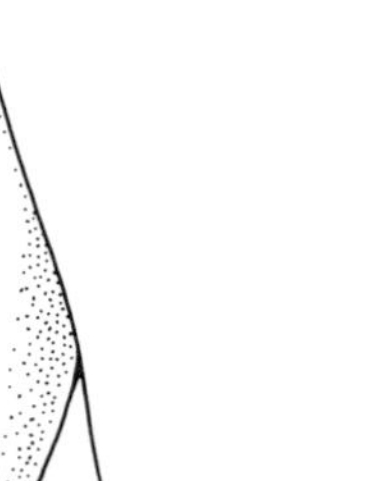

8

9

After palpation of the ring stripper in the groin a longitudinal arteriotomy is made at the femoral bifurcation. The intima core is cut at the origin of the superficial femoral artery. Distally slight traction is given to the intima core and ringstripper, and the entire core can be removed through the distal arteriotomy. The femoral bifurcation is inspected and if necessary an open endarterectomy of the femoral bifurcation is performed. The intima in the deep femoral artery can be fixed with tacking sutures.

10

The superficial femoral artery is then flushed with heparinized saline solution. The diameter of the lumen of the endarterectomized superficial femoral artery is checked by passage of an olive shaped probe with a diameter of about 6 mm.

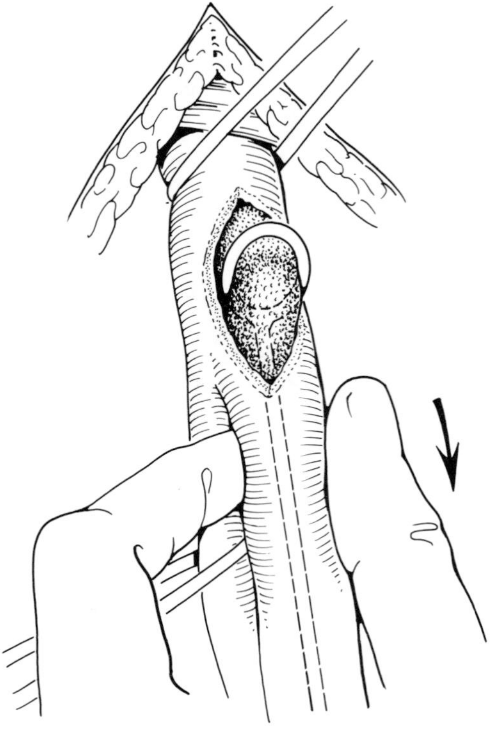

9

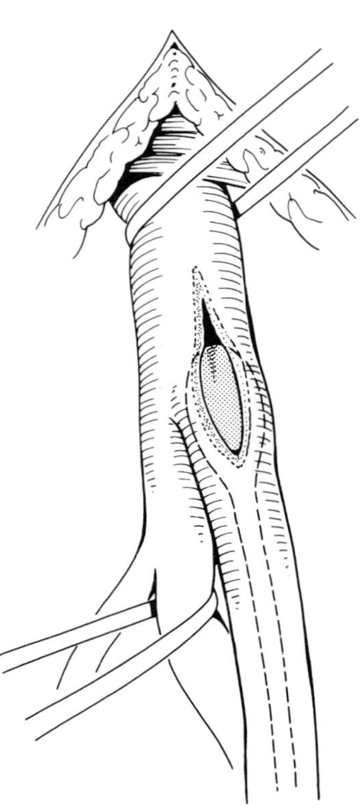

10

11

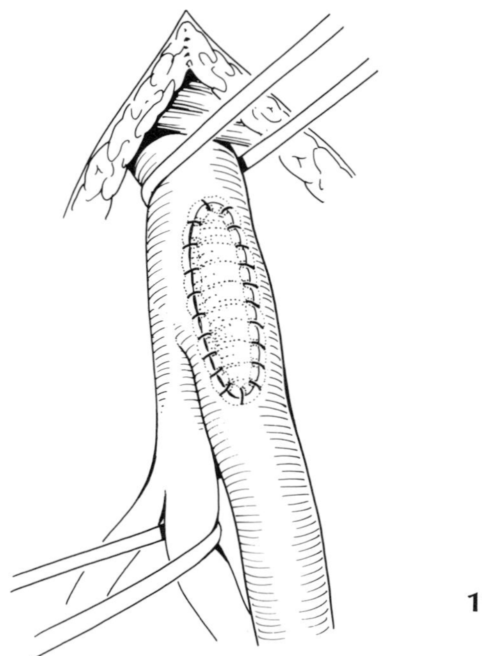

11

Both arteriotomies are closed by vein patches taken from the saphenous vein at the level of the ankle. The arteriotomy at the femoral bifurcation is closed first. Pulsations and flow in the distal superficial femoral artery are judged after declamping in the groin. Finally the distal arteriotomy is closed with a vein patch. At this point of the operation it is essential to perform a completion angiogram in order to detect intimal flaps or incomplete removal of the intima resulting in stenosis of the endarterectomized segment. All patients receive coumadines indefinitely.

Endarterectomy is a technically difficult operation with an intraoperative failure rate of 10% (Vollmar *et al.*, 1968). Failure often results from extensive calcification of the arterial wall which makes it impossible to establish a cleavage plane. Therefore if the preoperative angiogram shows extensive calcification of the artery or involvement of the middle or distal segment of the popliteal artery, femoropopliteal venous bypass should be performed.

While performing the endarterectomy special attention should be paid to the distal end of intima. The distal end of the intima should be fixed with tacking sutures to avoid dissection by antegrade blood flow. An arteriotomy at the level of the femoral bifurcation should always be performed. Blind dissection of the proximal end of the intima core will result in incomplete removal of the proximal intima and leads to residual stenosis. To prevent restenosis both longitudinal arteriotomies must be closed with a venous patch. At the end of the operation a completion angiogram should be performed in order to detect incomplete removal of the intima core. Often reopened collateral arteries are seen on the completion angiogram. Loose intimal flaps seen on the completion angiogram, can be removed with a Fogarty adherent cloth catheter. Although we treat our patients with coumadines following endarterectomy, Schneider showed in a small randomized study that antiplatelet therapy was superior to anticoagulation (Schneider, Brunner and Bollinger, 1979). Therefore postoperative treatment with antiplatelet drugs may be considered as well.

Endarterectomy is a valuable alternative in the treatment of superficial femoral artery occlusive disease. No foreign bodies are being used and the saphenous vein is spared for future use. In case of endarterectomy failure a femoropopliteal above-knee venous bypass remains possible. Endarterectomy should be considered as an alternative in patients with superficial femoral artery occlusive disease resulting in claudication. Furthermore the technique can be applied to restore vascular continuity after removal of an infected femoropopliteal bypass.

References

Blaisdell, F. W., Kall, A. D. and Thomas, A. N. (1966). Surgical treatment of chronic internal carotid artery occlusion by saline endarterectomy. *Annals of Surgery* **163**, 103.

Cannon, J. A. and Barker, W. F. (1955). Successful management of obstructive femoral arteriosclerosis by endarterectomy. *Surgery* **38**, 48.

Dos Santos, J. C. (1947). Sur la desobstruction des thromboses arterielles anciennes. *Mémoires de L'Académie de Chirurgie* **73**, 409.

Edwards, W. S. (1960). Composite reconstruction of the femoral artery with saphenous vein after endarterectomy. *Surgery, Gynecology and Obstetrics* **111**, 651.

Heijden, F. H. W. M. van der, Eikelboom, B. C., Reedt Dortland, R. W. H. van, Graaf, Y. van der, Steijling, J. J. F., Legemate, D. A., Theodorides, Th. and Vroonhoven, Th. J. M. V. van (1993). Long term results of semi-closed endarterectomy of the superficial femoral artery and the outcome of failed reconstructions. *Journal of Vascular Surgery* **18**, 271.

LeVeen, H. H. (1965). Technical features in endarterectomy. *Surgery* **57**, 22.

Schneidner, E., Brunner, U. and Bollinger, A. (1979). Medikamentose Rezidivprophylaxe nach femoro-poplitealer Arterienrekonstruktion. *Angio* **2**, 73.

Sobel, S., Kaplitt, M. J., Reingold, M. and Sawyer, P. N. (1966). Gas endarterectomy. *Surgery* **59**, 517.

Vollmar, J., Trede, M., Chir, B., Laubach, K. and Forrest, H. (1968). Principles of reconstructive procedures for chronic femoro-popliteal occlusions: Report on 546 operations. *Annals of Surgery* **2**, 215.

Wylie, E. J. (1952). Thromboendarterectomy for arteriosclerotic thrombosis of major arteries. *Surgery* **32**, 275.

Popliteal aneurysm and entrapment

NORMAN M. RICH MD, FACS

Professor and Chairman, Department of Surgery, and Chief, Division of Vascular Surgery, F. Edward Hebert School of Medicine, Uniformed Services University of Health Sciences, Bethesda, Maryland, USA;
Co-Director, Vascular Fellowship Program, Walter Reed Army Medical Center

Introduction

The popliteal artery is approximately 20 cm in length extending from the adductor hiatus to the lower border of the popliteus muscle. Identification of the many structures in the popliteal area is considerably different from the medial and posterior approaches. The anatomy can be confusing and those with limited experience are frequently at a higher location on the popliteal artery than recognized. An anatomic surface landmark is the head of the fibula, which is usually at the level of the origin of the anterior tibial artery with the continuation of the tibial-peroneal trunk continuing for approximately an additional 3 cm before dividing into the posterior tibial artery and the peroneal artery. Anatomic classification can be confusing because there is frequent description of a popliteal trifurcation which exists in only a very small percentage of patients. There are numerous anatomic variants which should be recognized appropriately. Aneurysms may be difficult to palpate, particularly in the upper third. Aneurysms contain laminated thrombus which can detach an emboli with movement and muscular action. This is an unfortunate complication. Elongation and kinking can accompany dilatation of the popliteal artery and occlusion may occur.

Popliteal aneurysmectomy has been generally abandoned in place of popliteal aneurysmorrhaphy because of the frequent trauma to the popliteal vein which is closely adherent to the wall of the aneurysm. Thrombosis of the popliteal vein with subsequent lower extremity swelling was a frequent complication when aneurysmectomy was performed. A bypass can be used successfully in the majority of cases; however, decompression of a large popliteal aneurysm may be valuable with an incision into the wall of the aneurysm opposite the vein with extraction of the thrombus. Occasionally, there might still be consideration for proximal Hunterian ligation in the very elderly who are at increased risk, especially when the aneurysm is ruptured.

The medial approach for popliteal aneurysmorrhapy

While general anaesthesia can be used and the patient is monitored as described in the chapter on 'Operation planning', regional anaesthesia may be utilized, particularly in the elderly who are at high risk. The leg is semi-flexed at the knee with support in that position and the foot can be held by a cushion or a heel-ring. The surgeon has the advantage by facing the medial side of the leg.

1

Incision

The incision is usually continuous. It can be placed conveniently over the greater saphenous vein which can be harvested easily. Efforts should be made to prevent undermining skin flaps which may lead to poor healing of the incision. The vein may be obtained at this level or from the groin area and prepared as described in the chapter on 'Reversed saphenous vein for femoropopliteal bypass'.

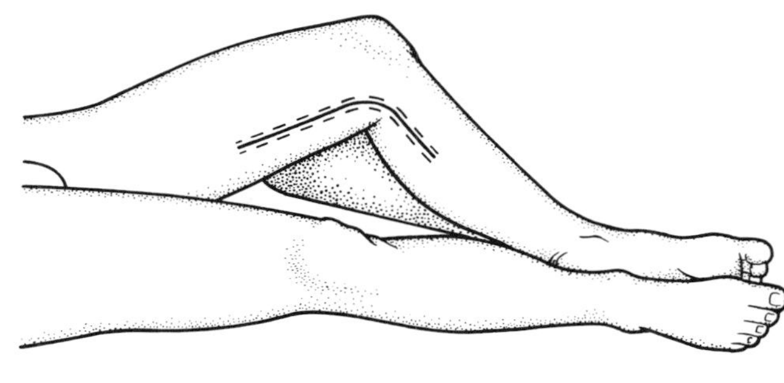

1

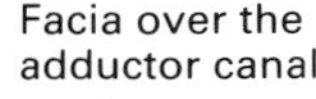

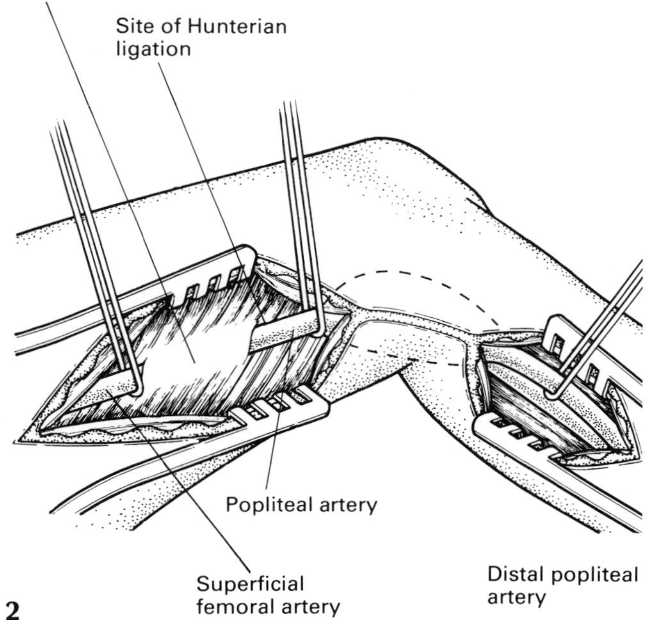

2

2

Approach to the artery

Initially, the popliteal artery is identified as it emerges below the adductor hiatus by separating the sartorius and vastus medialis muscles. Proximal arterial control is obtained by use of a vascular loop (it is also the site of Hunterian ligation which might be considered for a ruptured popliteal aneurysm in the compromised elderly patient). The superficial femoral artery above the adductor hiatus may also be encircled with a vascular tape if this is the intended site of the upper anastomosis.

The popliteal artery distally is approached as described in the chapter on 'Reversed saphenous vein for femoropopliteal bypass'. The sartorius, gracilis, semimembranosus and semitendinosus muscles are encountered and usually do not require division. It is usually not necessary to divide the soleus tunnel. The popliteal artery is separated from the popliteal vein and tibial nerve and a vascular loop is placed for distal control. The anterior tibial artery origin is usually easily identified.

3

Anastomosis for the graft

With the patient's blood heparinized, atraumatic vascular clamps can be applied both proximally and distally. At this stage a ligature of strong suture is used to ligate the popliteal artery just proximal to the aneurysm and the distal popliteal artery is ligated as high as possible. An end-to-side proximal anastomosis of the reversed greater saphenous vein bypass is usually accomplished most easily in the distal superficial femoral artery. The distal anastomosis can either be end-to-side or end-to-end using 5/0 vascular suture.

After completion of the proximal anastomosis and near completion of the distal anastomosis, the arterial clamps are removed to fill the vein and to eliminate any air, followed by completion of the anastomosis.

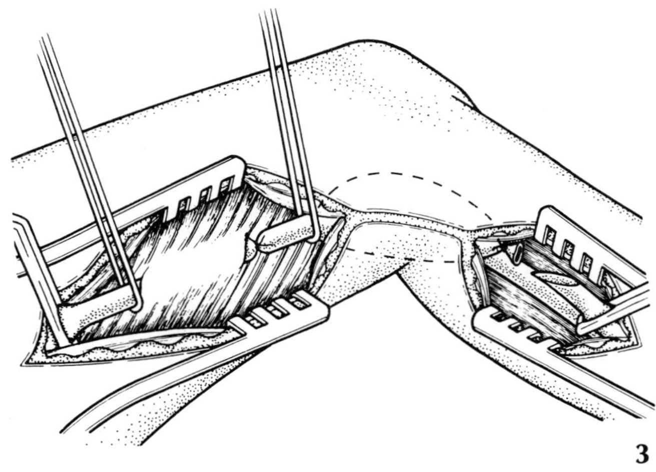

3

4

Tunnelling and the upper anastomosis

There may be variation in the best route for the vein bypass. This may require incision into the aneurysm to evacuate thrombis to prevent tension against the vein. Care must be taken to prevent entrapment of the bypass by the long medial tendons. A subcutaneous route may be elected and satisfactory. The proximal anastomosis may be end-to-end as well as end-to-side. Precise suture techniques are described in the chapter on 'Techniques of anastomosis'.

The incision is closed in layers. The use of suction drains for 12 h is a matter of choice.

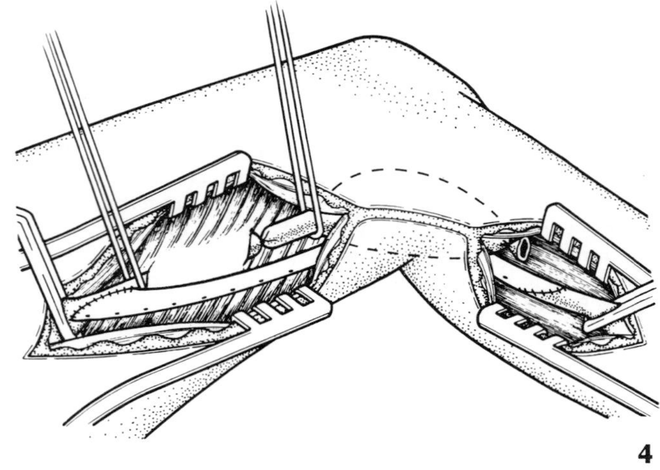

4

Popliteal entrapment and the posterior approach to the popliteal artery

Since the anomalous course of the popliteal artery was first identified in 1879 by a medical student in Edinburgh, a variety of forms of entrapment of the popliteal artery, and vein, have been identified and one classification includes five separate varieties. Most commonly, however, there is an abnormal lateral insertion of the medial head of the gastrocnemius muscle which can entrap and displace the popliteal artery medially (Rich *et al.*, 1979; Bouhoutsos and Daskalakis, 1981). There can also be accessory slips of the medial head of the gastrocnemius muscle, fibrous bands and an assortment of more unusual anatomic variations.

The posterior approach is preferred to identify the anatomic variants easily, which might be missed when utilizing the medial incision to the popliteal neurovascular bundle. Yet, there might be an associated aneurysm with the entrapment, and the medial approach and bypass might also be selected. For the posterior approach, the patient is prone and the ankle is slightly raised to flex the knee. Colour duplex scanning has been shown to be the ideal diagnostic method for this condition (MacSweeney, Cuming and Greenhalgh, 1994).

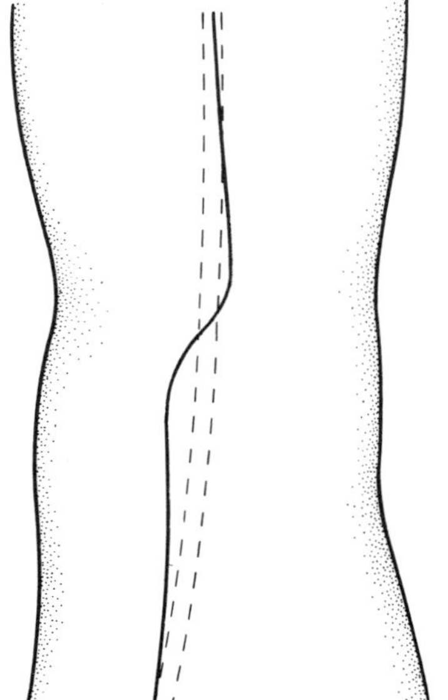

5

5

Incision

The incision is 'S' shaped, being reasonably vertical and midline to follow the course of the artery. At the popliteal fossa the skin crease is included in the incision in an attempt to avoid later skin contracture.

6

The incision is extended through the fascia into the popliteal fossa approaching the neurovascular bundle, and then the artery is separated carefully from the vein and the tibial nerve. Vascular loops are placed proximally and distally on the popliteal artery. Usually, it is necessary to divide the small branch of the nerve to the medial head of the gastrocnemius muscle to aid in exposure. Incision through the fibrous portion of the abnormal lateral attachment of the medial head of the gastrocnemius muscle may be all that is required, or similar incision through fibrous bands or accessory muscles may release the popliteal artery, and possibly the vein from the entrapment. If there is poststenotic dilatation which has progressed to aneurysm formation, bypass or replacement with a reversed segment of autogenous greater saphenous vein may be required. If thrombosis of the artery has occurred, an onlay saphenous vein patch graft with thromboendarterectomy may be successful.

The wound is closed in layers. Drainage is not usually required.

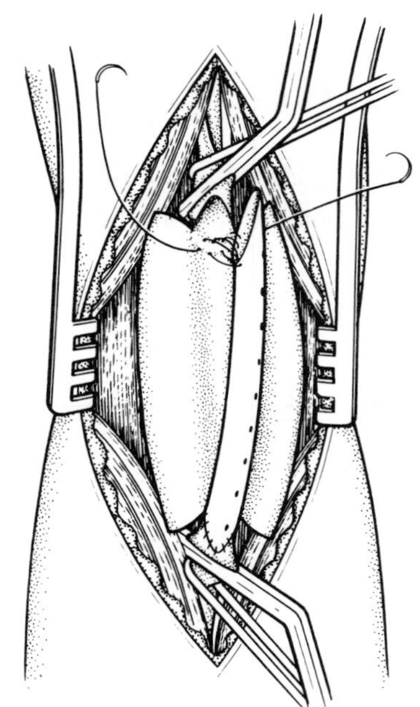

6

Complications

Thrombosis of any arterial reconstruction may be due to technical fault. Re-exploration and removal of the thrombus with a Fogarty catheter is recommended. These problems can be minimized by confirming patency and suture line integrity using on-table angiography at the completion of the reconstruction.

With a popliteal aneurysm care must be taken to see that there is no unnecessary manipulation so as to prevent distal embolization of thrombus from the aneurysm.

Thrombosis of the popliteal vein can occur and this is a reason to avoid unnecessary dissection around the popliteal vein. Elevation of the limb, early inactive calf movements, physiotherapy and compression hose are all adjunctive measures that can be utilized to prevent this complication. If thrombosis occurs, heparin and warfarin therapy should be utilized.

References

Bouhoutsos, J. and Daskalakis, E. (1981). Muscular abnormalities affecting the popliteal vessels. *British Journal of Surgery* **68**, 501.

MacSweeney, S. T. R., Cuming, R. and Greenhalgh, R. M. (1994). Colour Doppler imaging in the timely diagnosis of popliteal artery entrapment syndrome. *British Journal of Surgery* (in press).

Rich, N. M., Collins, G. J., McDonald, P. T., Kozloff, L., Clagett, G. P. and Collins, J. T. (1979). Popliteal vascular entrapment *Archives of Surgery* **114**, 1377.

Sites and approach for tibial anastomoses

CHARLES N. McCOLLUM MD, FRCS

Professor of Surgery, University of South Manchester, Manchester, UK

Introduction

A feature in the development of vascular surgery in recent years has been the increasing willingness to extend arterial bypass to smaller distal arteries in an attempt to avoid amputation. The posterior tibial artery was first used as the 'run-off' vessel approximately 30 years ago (Palma, 1960; Dale, 1963), but these techniques were not widely accepted until recently. Where an adequate vein is available, and with careful case selection, graft patency rates of 50–70% at 1 year have produced worthwhile limb salvage in these cases (Noon *et al.*, 1969; Davies, Davies and Mannick, 1975). However, where the vein is not adequate and a prosthetic substitute has to be used, the results are considerably less encouraging, with graft thrombosis sometimes exceeding 50% within 6 months (Klimach and Charlesworth, 1983). In the absence of a dramatically new material or approach to the bypass of small arterial disease, we can only expect improvement by attention to three main areas. First, the use of saphenous vein could be extended to a greater proportion of patients by one of the techniques for *in situ* vein bypass (Hall and Rostad, 1978; Leather, Powers and Karmody, 1979). Secondly, it may be possible to improve patency by increasing the blood flow within the graft using a distal arteriovenous fistula as suggested by Ibrahim *et al.* (1980) and further discussed in the chapter on 'Adjuvant arteriovenous fistula at the distal anastomosis of a femorotibial bypass graft'. Thirdly, patency may be improved in vascular reconstructions by prescribing platelet inhibitory drugs, although good evidence of their benefit in peripheral reconstruction is only available in patients receiving prosthetic bypasses (Green, Roedershecmer and De Weese, 1982; Goldman *et al.*, 1983).

The quality of popliteal 'run-off' is important in femoropopliteal bypass with the best results obtained when two to three tibial arteries are patent. It therefore seems logical in bypasses below this level to consider implanting the distal anastomosis to more than one calf artery. This approach has recently been described using both inverted Y vein grafts and sequential anastomoses at and below the knee (Edwards *et al.*, 1976; Piccone *et al.*, 1978). The combination of *in situ* saphenous vein bypass with the use of either a natural or a sutured bifurcation might extend the use of vein, improve total graft flow and increase perfusion to the distal calf and foot. By these means it may be possible to prevent the few frustrating amputations that have to be performed in the presence of a patent femorotibial bypass.

Indications and preoperative assessment

The almost exclusive indication for tibial bypass is ischaemic rest pain or frank tissue necrosis or ulceration of the foot. Occasionally, patients with severely ischaemic feet and lower legs may suffer a minor injury which ulcerates and fails to heal. In these cases reconstruction may have to be considered in the absence of typical rest pain. Reconstruction to the proximal posterior tibial artery may, very rarely, be indicated for severe claudication alone, but the author doubts that reconstruction to the other calf arteries, particularly at the distal sites of anastomosis, should ever be performed for this indication. The peripheral distribution of arterial disease in these patients is such that calf claudication is rarely an important feature in the history. Many of the patients undergoing these procedures will be diabetic and some will have thrombangitis obliterans. These conditions are not contraindications but it is unlikely that a successful outcome will result when none of the calf arteries cross the ankle and communicate with the foot. This does not of course prohibit the use of the peroneal artery where one of the other two arteries is reconstituted at or just below the ankle and may then be filled by collaterals.

Most patients requiring arterial bypass to the distal calf are elderly and usually unfit. The preoperative assessment must obviously include careful evaluation of all the factors already described in the chapter on 'Operation planning'. Angiography is almost always required, not only to assist in the selection of distal anastomotic sites, but to confirm the adequacy of the proximal arterial system. Often with a distal distribution of disease typical in these patients it is possible to site the proximal anastomosis at the superficial femoral artery just above the adductor canal, thereby shortening the length of bypass. The quality of image obtained in the distal calf is often poor, and selective angiography to each limb is essential. It is now well recognized that despite the most carefully performed angiography, patent distal arteries may not opacify. Patency can be detected with greater sensitivity using a standard Doppler flow probe to insonate the three arteries at ankle level which also allows assessment of the pedal arch (Simms, 1988). Angiography detects only a mean of 1.3 patent arteries per leg in patients requiring femorotibial bypass, whereas Doppler insonation will detect a mean of 2.2 arteries per leg. It must of course be recognized that those arteries detected by arteriogram may be more suitable for distal anastomosis and that a higher rate of failure may be associated with Doppler detection alone.

Preoperative preparation

Many patients requiring tibial bypass will already have had either an operative or a chemical lumbar sympathectomy. On the basis that a few patients do improve with sympathectomy alone we usually perform a chemical sympathectomy during the period of evaluation. Although sympathectomy may only increase the flow of blood in arteriovenous shunts in the distal limb this may augment the total graft flow following implantation and theoretically improves the chances of subsequent patency (Terry, Allan and Taylor, 1972). Once it has been determined that a femorotibial bypass is possible, the patient is started 2 days preoperatively on the platelet inhibitory combination of aspirin and dipyridamole given orally. At this stage a plan is made as to which arteries should be explored and in what order. Obviously, where two patent calf arteries are known to cross the ankle the selection of distal anastomoses is easy. Finally, on the day before surgery the saphenous vein and, where possible, its natural branches, are marked on the skin to aid the subsequent dissection.

Operative technique

1

Medial incisions and long saphenous vein exposure

The medial incisions are placed over the long saphenous vein to minimize dissection in the subcutaneous fat. The author's preference is for separate incisions with the upper one extending 12 cm below the saphenofemoral junction in order that the first two valves and the upper branches can be seen. Further incisions are made centred 12–15 cm above the knee and 8–10 cm below the knee as these are regions where sizeable branches are usually found. Where there are many branches from the long saphenous vein or where the valve stripper does not pass easily, the incision may be converted to full length without hesitation.

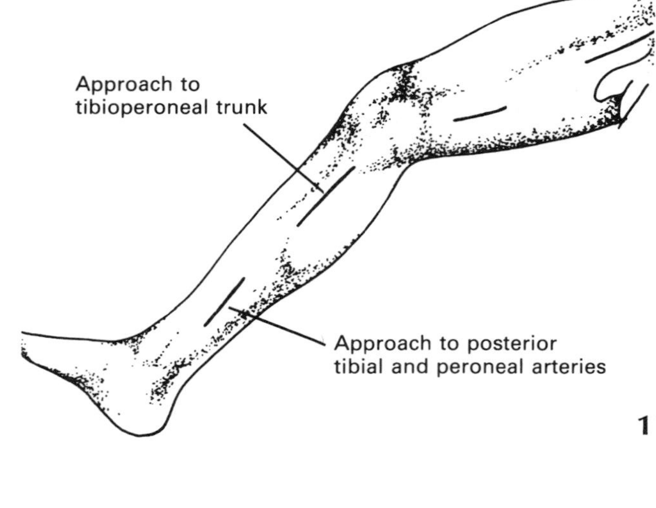

1

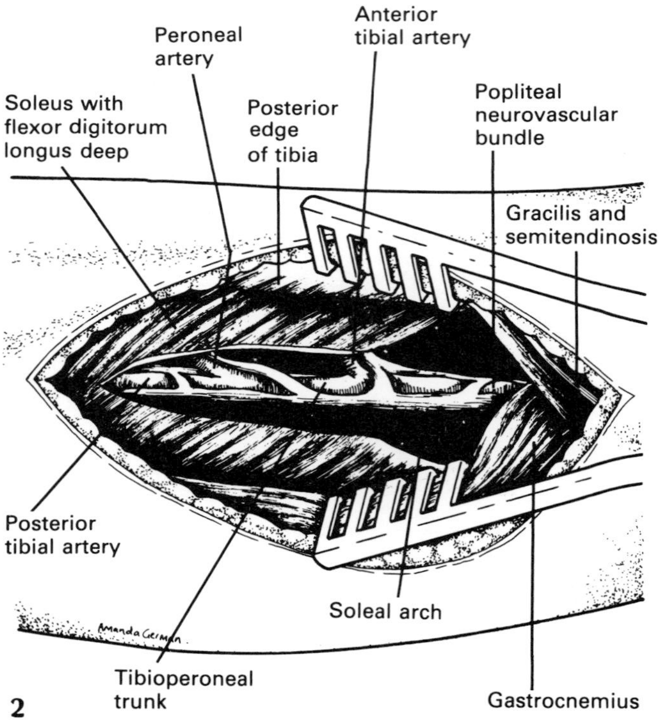

2

2

Exposure of tibioperoneal trunk

The incision used to expose the saphenous vein just below the knee is deepened. The deep fascia is incised 1–2 cm posterior to the upper tibia as shown. The gastrocnemius muscle is retracted posteriorly and in the upper part of the incision the tendons of semitendinosis and gracilis are exposed. Where the distal popliteal artery above the bifurcation of the anterior tibial artery is of adequate quality to receive the graft, these tendons may need to be divided to gain adequate access. The tibioperoneal trunk is found deep to the arch of the soleus which is most easily divided 1 cm posterior to its origin on the tibia. A mass of soleal veins usually obscures the anterior tibial artery which must be exposed by gentle dissection with ligation of the venae comitantes that lie superficial to the artery. It is interesting that with severe ischaemia of the distal limb the soleal veins are often found to be thrombosed. Distal anastomosis of a single stem bypass may be placed anywhere along the tibioperoneal trunk, providing its bifurcation into the posterior tibial and peroneal artery is not severely diseased. It may also be placed directly over the peroneal artery to widen the origin, but with disease of the proximal peroneal and posterior tibial artery, bypass to the distalf calf seems preferable.

3a & b

Exposure of posterior tibial and peroneal arteries distally

The exposure of the posterior tibial and peroneal artery of the lower calf can best be achieved by placing the incision well distally in the medial calf (*see Illustration 1*). The lateral approach to the peroneal artery should ideally be avoided and only be used when a bifurcated graft to both the anterior tibial and peroneal arteries is planned. The incision is centred approximately 10 cm above the medial malleolus even if the calf arteries are patent above this level. The deep fascia is incised 0.5–1 cm posterior to the medial border of the tibia and the incision is deepened posterior to flexor digitorum longus (*a*). The soleus muscle is retracted posteriorly using a self-retaining retractor which engages the posterior tibia. The arteries are still surrounded by the venae comitantes but these are more easily dissected free farther distally. Approximately 5 cm of the healthiest length of artery is mobilized and gently retracted posteriorly. The peroneal artery is exposed by deepening the plane of dissection and incising flexor hallucis longus longitudinally (*b*). This may be done by finding the peroneal vascular bundle in the upper wound and then dividing the overlying muscle over the jaws of a curved clamp passed in the plane just superficial to the vessels. Dissecting the peroneal artery from its venae comitantes is tedious and demands both good light and magnification.

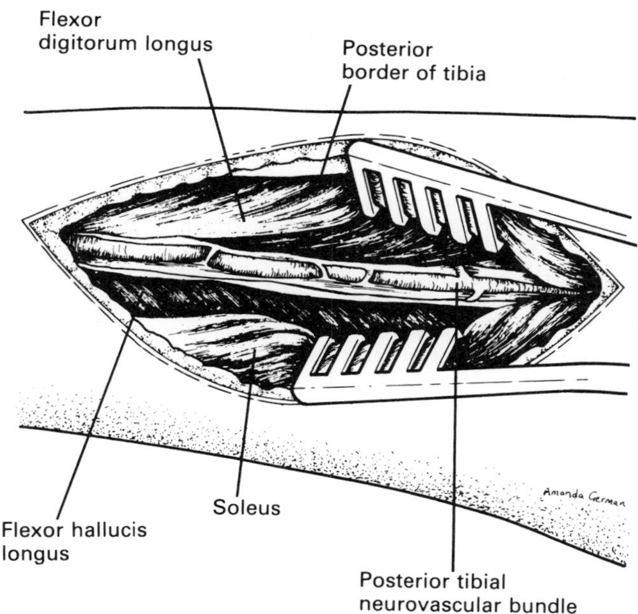

3a

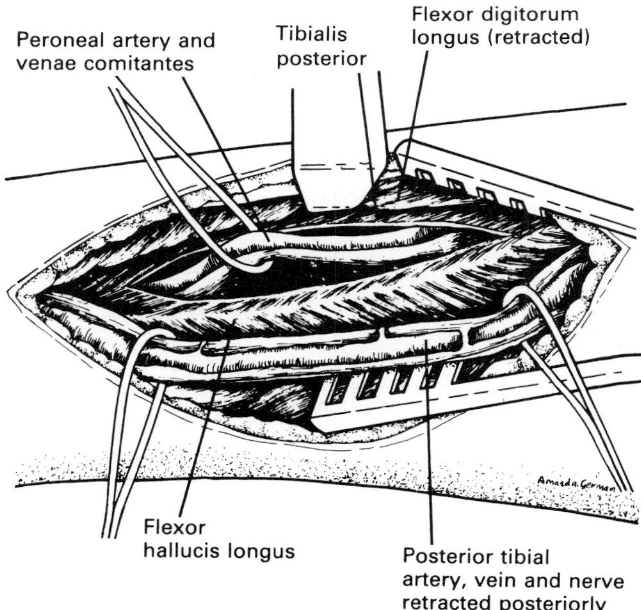

3b

4a, b & c

Anterior and lateral leg incisions

Exposure of the anterior tibial artery

The anterior tibial artery may be easily exposed throughout its length in the anterior tibial compartment (*a*). The incision is placed just lateral to the centre of the anterior tibial compartment and is deepened between tibialis anterior and the two extensor muscles (digitorum longus and hallucis longus) (*b*). In practice, the plane between these muscle groups is not always immediately apparent but it is easy to split the muscles of tibialis anterior. If it is planned to route the graft to the anterior tibial artery from the medial aspect of the leg, a sufficient length should be mobilized and a cruciate incision in the interosseous membrane made 2 cm above the proposed anastomosis (*c*).

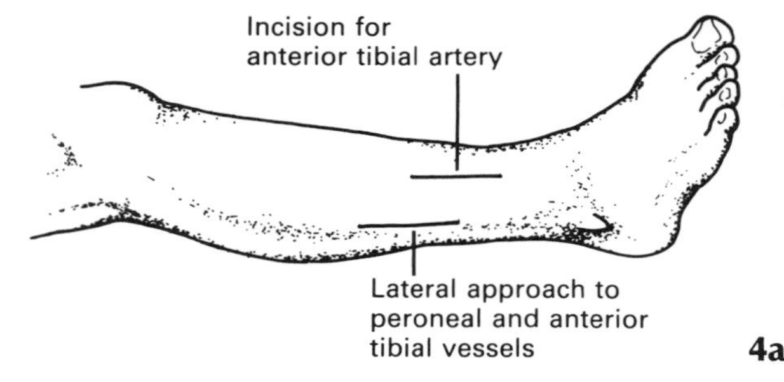

4a

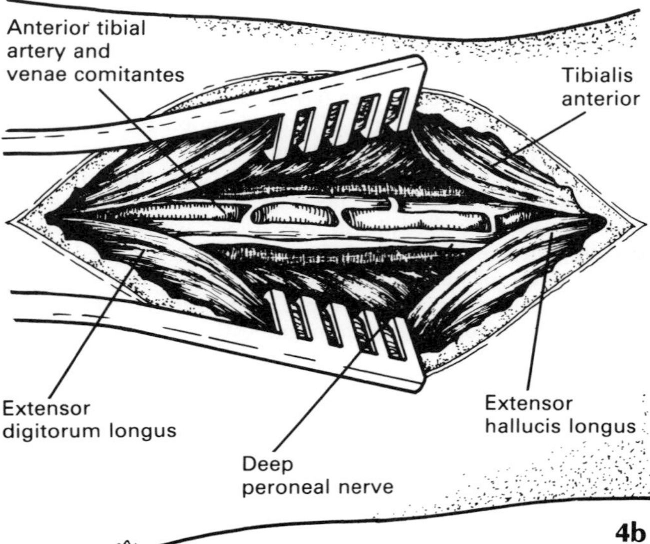

4b

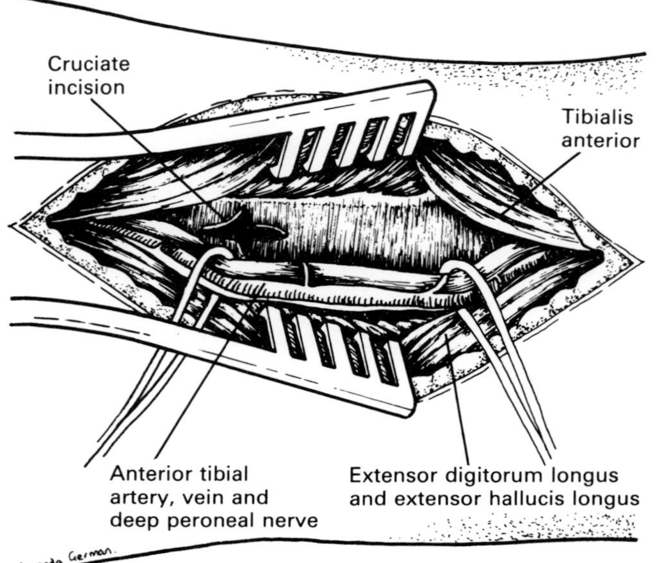

4c

5a & b

Lateral approach to both anterior tibial and peroneal arteries

As previously stated, this approach is rarely required. However, where preoperative Doppler evaluation or angiography indicates that the anterior tibial and the peroneal artery are patent, with an occluded posterior tibial artery, then the lateral approach with a view to a bifurcated bypass to these two vessels may be appropriate. The incision is placed directly over the fibula (*see Illustration 4a*) and deepened between the soleus and the peroneal muscles. The periosteum over the fibula is elevated and a 10–12 cm segment is excised using rib shears (*a*). Incision of the periosteum posterior to the interosseous membrane leads to the peroneal vessels and incision anterior leads to the anterior tibial neurovascular bundle. *Illustration 5b* depicts a suitable layout for a sequential bypass routed from the medial calf with a side-to-side anastomosis to the peroneal artery and an end-to-side anastomosis to the anterior tibial artery.

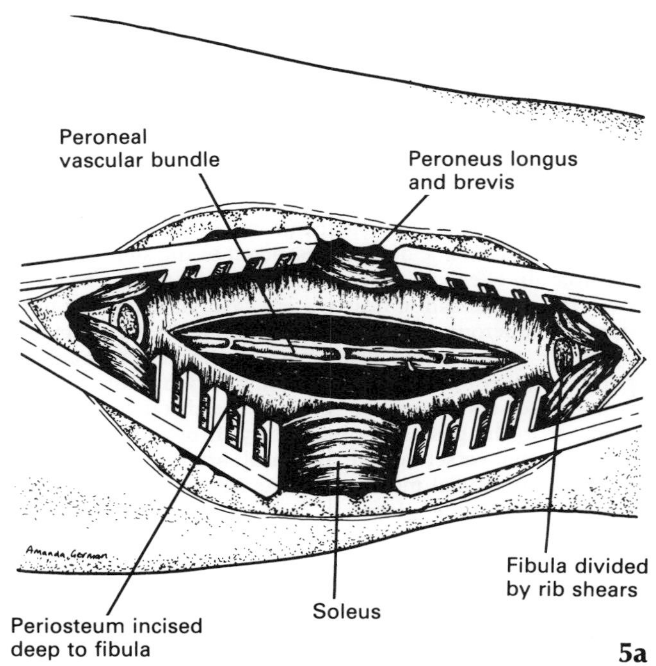

5a

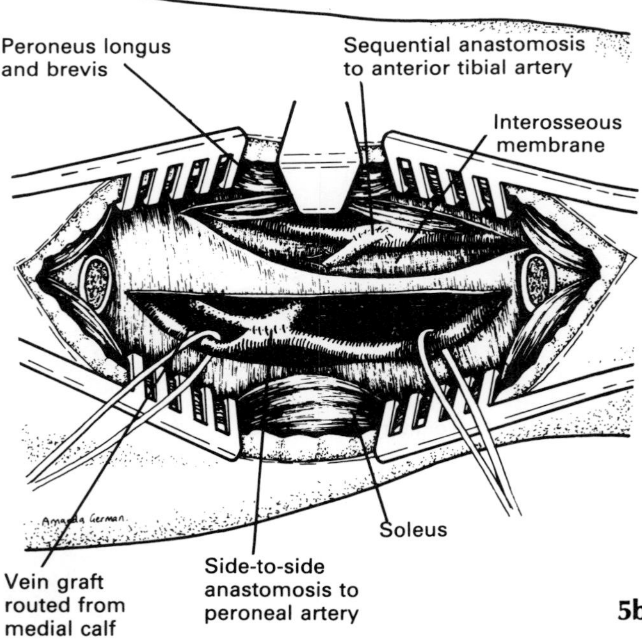

5b

6

Routes for bypass

When performing *in situ* saphenous vein bypasses it is undesirable to mobilize the long saphenous vein from its bed. Clearly, the distal and proximal ends have to be dissected free in order to route them to the proposed site of anastomosis, but this dissection should be restricted to the shortest length possible. In effect, this means that the graft should be routed from the medial calf in nearly every case. In bypassing to the upper tibioperoneal trunk or distal popliteal artery it may be necessary to route the distal part of the vein through the popliteal fossa to avoid excessive angulation. However, this is not necessary when bypassing to the distal tibioperoneal trunk or to the posterior tibial artery throughout its length. Routing the vessel to the peroneal artery when exposed through the medial incision is quite simple in that the graft merely lies in the plane of dissection already developed between soleus and flexor digitorum longus. In the vast majority of cases, we prefer to take the same route for anastomosis to the anterior tibial artery, tunnelling between flexor digitorum longus and flexor hallucis longus and through the interosseous membrane. It is important that the cruciate incision in the interosseous membrane is made at least 2–3 cm above the proposed site of anastomosis, so that the vein can curve laterally around the anterior tibial artery, allowing the anastomosis to be performed on the anterolateral aspect.

Where saphenous vein is being mobilized from its bed, either in a reversed or '*in situ*' orientation, some surgeons prefer to route grafts to the anterior tibial or peroneal artery subcutaneously across the front of the thigh, and then lateral to the knee, passing just anteriorly to the head of the fibula. This route can also be used when a prosthetic graft or human umbilical vein is employed. It is doubtful that it confers any real advantages. However, where the distal anastomosis is to the dorsalis pedis or anterior tibial artery at or just above the ankle, the graft may have to pass from medial to lateral anterior to the tibia. This is far from ideal as necrosis may develop in the overlying skin.

Planning bifurcated grafts

In considering approaches to bifurcated bypass to distal calf arteries it is usually possible to select preoperatively which vessels are most likely to be adequate. In practice there are three possible combinations: posterior tibial and peroneal; posterior tibial and anterior tibial; or peroneal and anterior tibial. Wherever possible the bypass will be routed to anterior or posterior tibial arteries as these cross the ankle but the peroneal artery is available more often as it is relatively spared by atherosclerosis.

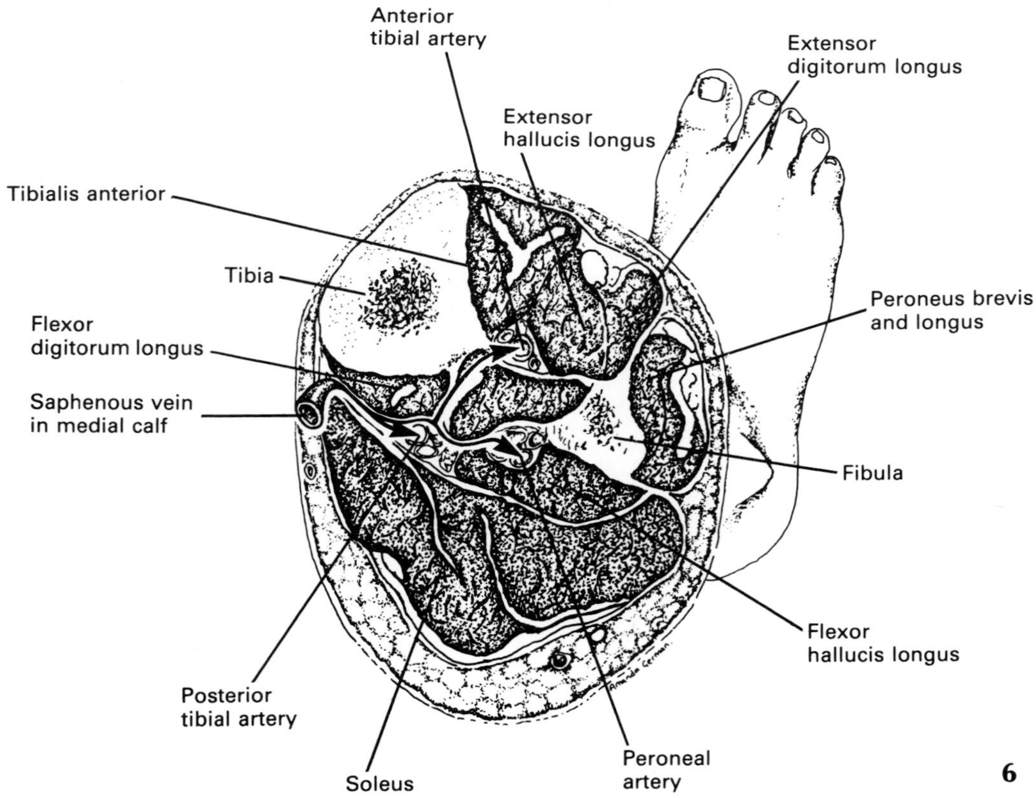

6

Postoperative complications

Patients undergoing femorotibial bypass are usually old, in poor health and may have diabetes. As the major body compartments are not opened, the perioperative mortality should be low, but over the following months and years a substantial number of these patients will die from myocardial or cerebral ischaemia. In contrast, postoperative morbidity often leads to prolonged hospital stay.

Pressure sores are avoided by carefully padding the patient on the operating table and immediately turning the patient and massaging the pressure areas on completion of the procedure. Wound edge necrosis which predominantly affects the distal wounds is related to ischaemia but can be minimized by keeping wound edges moist with saline swabs and releasing the pressure from self-retaining retractors whenever possible. Occasionally, vein grafts may become exposed with the risk of secondary haemorrhage.

Lower leg swelling and oedema occurs in nearly all patients and can be treated symptomatically with leg elevation and gentle elastic compression. Persistent arteriovenous fistulae and anastomotic problems will be reduced to a minimum if intraoperative assessments, including on-table angiography, are used.

References

Dale, A. W. (1963). Grafting small arteries. *Archives of Surgery* **86**, 22.

Davies, R. C., Davies, W. T. and Mannick, J. A. (1975). Bypass vein grafts in patients with distal popliteal artery occlusion. *American Journal of Surgery* **129**, 421.

Edwards, W. S., Gerety, E., Larkin, J. *et al.* (1976). Multiple sequential femoral tibial grafting for severe ischaemia. *Surgery* **80**, 722.

Goldman, M., Hall, C., Dykes, J. *et al.* (1983). Does indium-platelet deposition predict patency in prosthetic arterial grafts? *British Journal of Surgery* **70**, 635.

Green, R. M., Roederschecmer, R. L. and De Weese, J. A. (1982). Effects of aspirin and dipyridamole on polytetrafluorethylene graft patency. *Surgery* **92**, 1016.

Hall, K. V. and Rostad, H. (1978). *In situ* vein bypass in the treatment of femoro-popliteal atherosclerotic disease: a ten year study. *American Journal of Surgery* **136**, 158.

Ibrahim, I. M., Sussman, B., Dardik, L. *et al.* (1980). Adjunctive arteriovenous fistula with tibial and peroneal reconstruction for limb salvage. *American Journal of Surgery* **140**, 246.

Klimach, O. and Charlesworth, D. (1983). Femoro-tibial bypass for limb salvage using human umbilical vein. *British Journal of Surgery* **70**, 1.

Leather, R. P., Powers, S. R. and Karmody, A. M. (1979). A reappraisal of *in situ* saphenous arterial bypass: its use in limb salvage. *Surgery* **86**, 453.

Noon, G. P., Diethrich, E. B., Richardson, W. P. *et al.* (1969). Distal tibial artery bypass – analysis of 91 cases. *Archives of Surgery* **99**, 770.

Palma, E. C. (1960). Treatment of arteritis of the lower limbs by autogenous vein grafts. *Minerva Cardioangiologica* **1**, 36.

Piccone, V. A., Moon, W., Harry, H. *et al.* (1978). Limb salvage by inverted Y vein grafts to below-knee arteries. *Archives of Surgery* **113**, 951.

Simms, M. H. (1988). Is pedal arch patency a pre-requisite for successful reconstruction? In *Limb Salvage and Amputation for Vascular Disease*. Greenhalgh, R. M., Jamieson, C. W. and Nicolaides, A. N., eds. London and San Diego: W. B. Saunders.

Terry, H. J., Allan, J. S. and Taylor, G. W. (1972). The relationship between blood flow and failure of femoro-popliteal reconstructive arterial surgery. *British Journal of Surgery* **59**, 549.

The *in situ* saphenous vein arterial bypass by valve incision

ROBERT P. LEATHER MD, *Professor of Surgery*
DHIRAJ M. SHAH MD, *Professor of Surgery*
BENJAMIN B. CHANG MD, *Assistant Professor of Surgery*
R. CLEMENT DARLING III MD, *Assistant Professor of Surgery*
The Albany Medical College, Albany, New York, USA

Introduction

Technically, the crucial issue in using the greater saphenous vein *in situ*, and the primary reason for its excision and reversal, for femoral to distal arterial bypass, is the elimination of valvular obstruction to arterial flow. All other considerations aside, leaving the saphenous vein *in situ* appears to be the most reliable method of achieving endothelial preservation, provided the valves can be rendered incompetent without injury to this very delicate endothelial cell monolayer. In addition, leaving the vein *in situ* requires interruption of venous side branches, some of which would otherwise become arteriovenous fistulas when the vein is arterialized, and minimal mobilization of its ends for construction of the proximal and distal anastomoses. The objective is to accomplish these manoeuvres with a minimum of operative manipulation of the vein, and especially its endothelial surface with particular avoidance of circumferential longitudinal shear. The simplest, most expedient, and least traumatic method of rendering the bicuspid venous valve incompetent is to cut the leaflets in their major axes, thus bisecting them. This is the essence of the valve incision technique.

The evolution of instruments and constraints of their use to achieve valve incision was guided by an overriding concern toward minimizing the potential for endothelial injury while producing an incompetent valve. Our data show that, particularly with the addition of the intraluminal valve cutter, there was no penalty in performance (Leather, Corson and Karmody, 1984) despite the greater potential for circumferential endothelial abrasion, the most devastating form of injury. In concert with this, our technical methodology for performing the *in situ* bypass has been developed with the primary goal of universal application. An *in situ* bypass can be performed by this technique in virtually all cases, regardless of the vagaries of venous anatomy, while minimizing the extent of exposure of the vein necessary for consistently safe and atraumatic valve incision. The high incidence of venous anomalies (up to 30% of double systems) and smaller veins distally (greater than 50%, <3.5 mm OD) makes the use of a cylindrical transluminal retrograde valve disrupter such as the Hall, Cartier, or LeMaitre strippers hazardous (Moody, Edwards and Harris, 1992; Gruss *et al.*, 1982; Fietze-Fischer *et al.*, 1987; Denton, Hill and Fairgrieve, 1983).

For the same reasons, the use of preoperative venous anatomic assessment either by venography or duplex ultrasonography is not only advisable, but mandatory, particularly if a valve cutter is to be used safely. A duplex ultrasonographic venous map provides the relevant information for the careful planning and execution of this procedure. Without this, attempts to define such anatomic variations surgically will result in excessive dissection, increasing the potential not only of injury to the vein, but also of wound complications. Experience with over 2000 duplex mappings has proven its safety, reliability, and utility in the performance of the *in situ* bypass as well as in vein harvesting.

The operation

1

An incision is made in the groin crease and is extended downwards over the saphenous vein. By sharp dissection, 5–10 cm of the proximal of the vein is identified. Its tributaries are ligated with silk or fine Prolene suture ligature and divided, and the vein is dissected from its bed. The saphenofemoral junction lies at the level which commonly corresponds to the bifurcation of the common femoral artery into the superficial and profunda artery. Hence, detachment of the entire saphenous bulb with, if necessary, a small portion of the anterior wall of the common femoral vein will ensure that the upper end of the bypass reaches the common femoral artery.

Alternately unobstructed profunda femoral or superficial femoral arteries can be effectively used as an inflow source without influencing immediate or long-term patency. It is best approached from the medial aspect (with the surgeon on the opposite side of the table) by incision of the subcutaneous tissue immediately lateral to the saphenous vein and down to the underlying investing myofascia (*B*). Dissection laterally in this fusion plane to the superficial femoral artery is bloodless. The fascia is incised over the superficial femoral artery and, if it is occluded, a segment of 3–5 cm can be excised, thus facilitating exposure of the deep femoral artery. If patent, a plane is developed between the femoral vein and the superficial femoral artery.

1

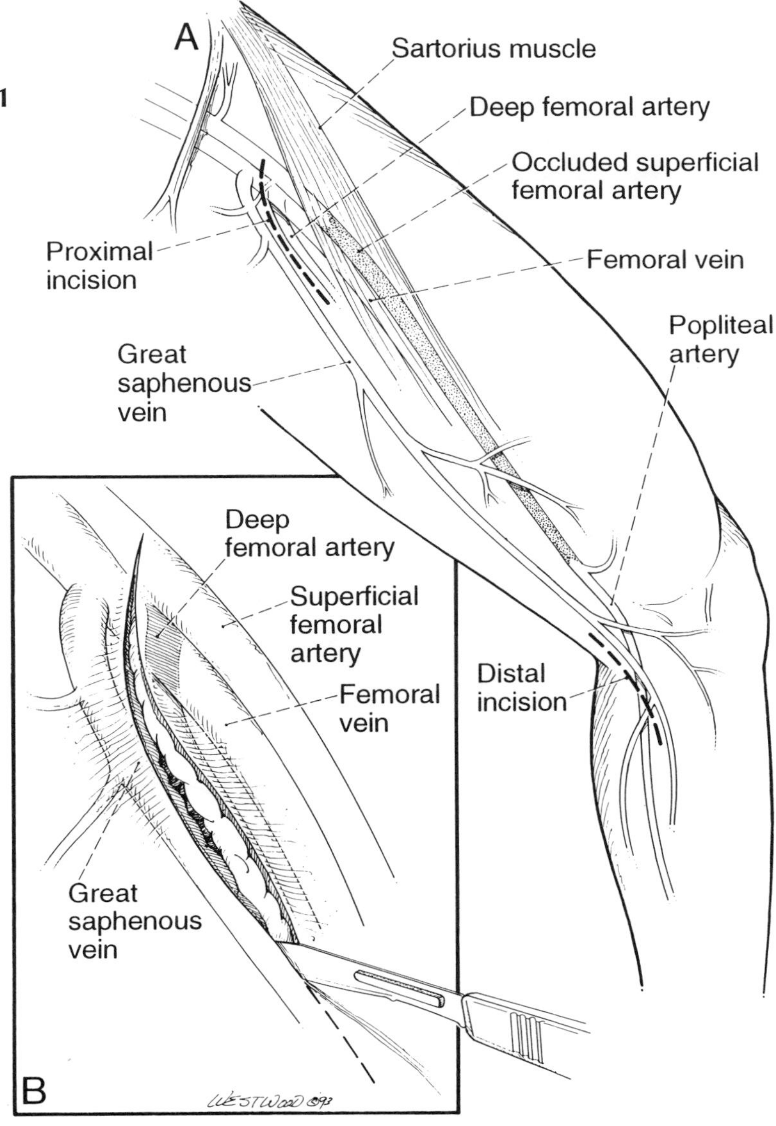

2

The lateral circumflex femoral vein is divided, exposing the proximal deep femoral artery which lies immediately deep to it (profundafemoris artery). Having determined the most satisfactory site of proximal anastomosis, the length of the proximal saphenous vein required to reach it is apparent.

3

The most proximal valve at the saphenofemoral junction is excised by lifting each cusp with a fine forceps and excising it through the base of the leaflet (only the transparent part) with a microscissor. For the one to three proximal valves, a valve scissor engages the valve most efficiently when it is in the closed position. The valve can be kept closed by a pressurized column of fluid introduced through a fine catheter at a controlled pressure of 200 mmHg.

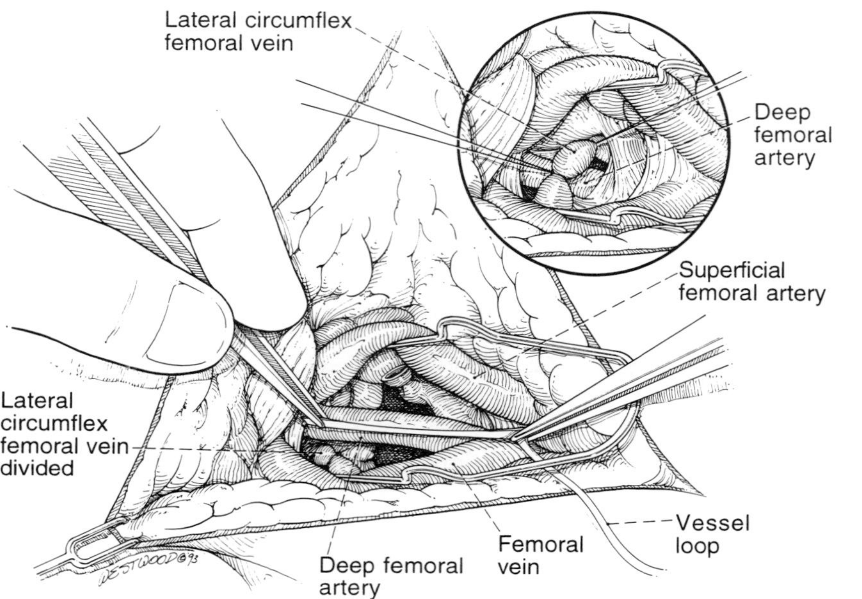

2

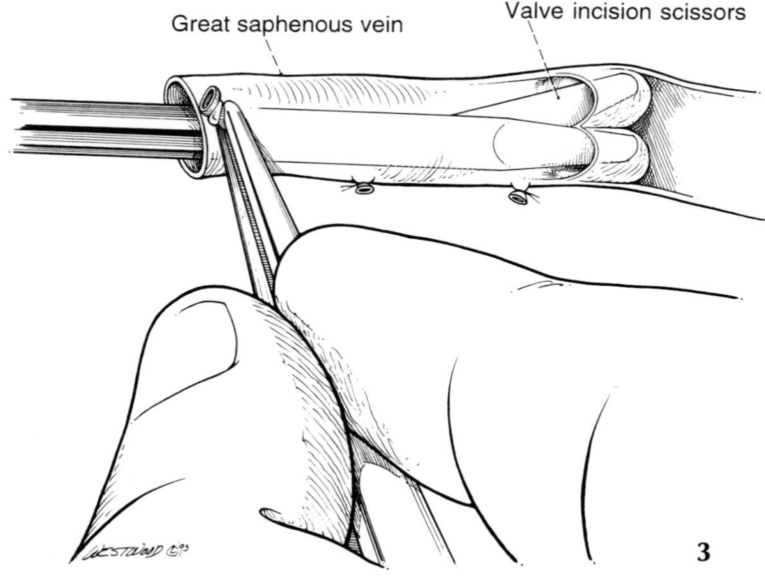

3

4a & b

When the saphenous vein is greater than 3 mm ID (4 mm OD) with a single trunk in its thigh portion, an appropriate size (2 or 3 mm) detachable intraluminal valve cutter is used which divides the cusps up to the level of the knee without the necessity of surgical exposure of the vein (Leather, Corson and Karmody, 1984). A small incision is made posterior to the previously marked vein below the level of the knee joint. A branch of suitable size is located and a 3 French Fogarty embolectomy catheter is passed into the saphenous vein and advanced through the detached proximal end with the knee straightened. The catheter is cut obliquely at the 20 or 30 cm mark and the cutter is prepared as shown in *a*. A 6 or 8 French catheter through which pressurized fluid is delivered into the vein is attached to the upper end of the cutter ('follower') with a 6/0 monofilament suture. The oblique cut end of the Fogarty catheter is used to firmly screw the self-tapping cutter leader before the pressure catheter is attached. The infusion bag is pressurized to 200–300 torr. *Illustration b* shows the orientation of the cutter within the saphenous vein. the fluid pressure distends the vein, sealing leakage from the open end of the vein by a 1 mm silastic vessel loop closing the valves so that they will be efficiently engaged by the cutter blades, and provides a fluid interface on which the cutter 'floats' away from the vein wall. The 'leader' centres the device in the saphenous vein and prevents it from engaging any side branches.

The valves are serially cut to the level of the knee joint by one or two passes of the valve cutter. The cutter is then withdrawn with the traction catheter through the proximal end of the vein and dismounted and the catheter is removed from below.

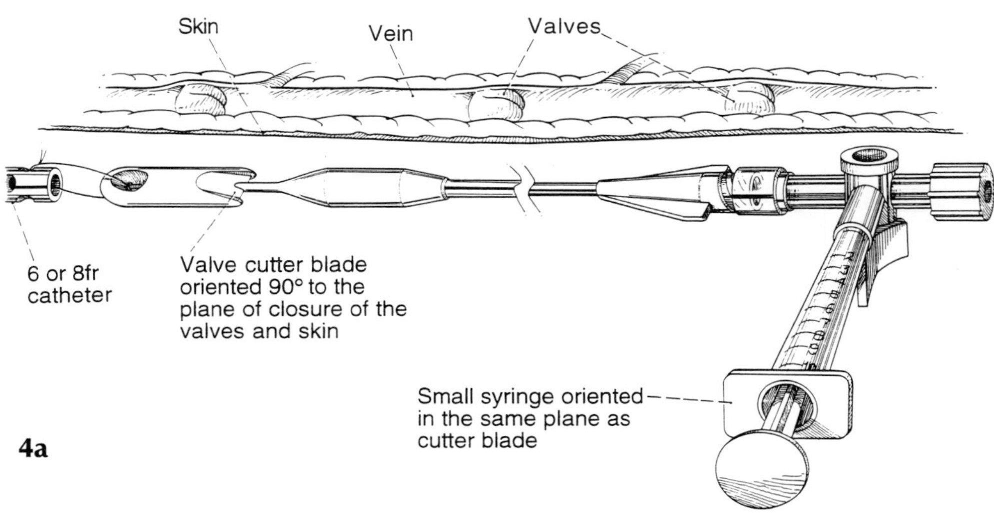

4a

4b

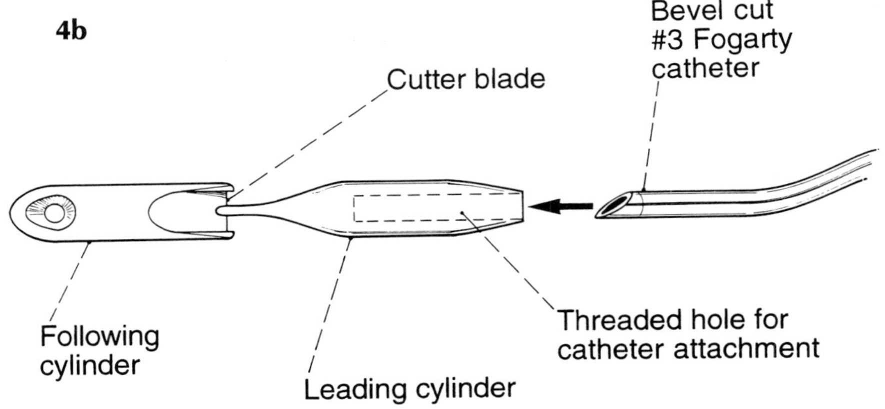

5a, b & c

With clips placed proximally and distally, a deep femoral arteriotomy has been performed at the proposed anastomosis site. The vein is sharply divided from posterior to anterior, and a small tissue bridge will be left connected to a 'handle' for manipulating the vessel (*a*). All work on the vein is done with a 'no touch' technique using 3.5 × magnification loupes to minimize any potential trauma to the vessel. With traction on the handle, the venotomy on the posterior vessel wall is accurately placed and oriented. Anastomosis of the bypass vein to the deep femoral artery is carried out by the 'open parachute' technique, which allows for accurate and atraumatic placement of each individual suture in the heel portion of the anastomosis. A single, double-needle suture of 6–0 or 7–0 Prolene is used (*b*). After placement of as many sutures as the length of suture material allows, the vein is drawn down to the artery. The handle will be excised (*c*). Arterialization of the saphenous vein is completed by continuing the medial suture line clockwise around the arteriotomy to meet the lateral suture line at the midpoint of the arteriotomy.

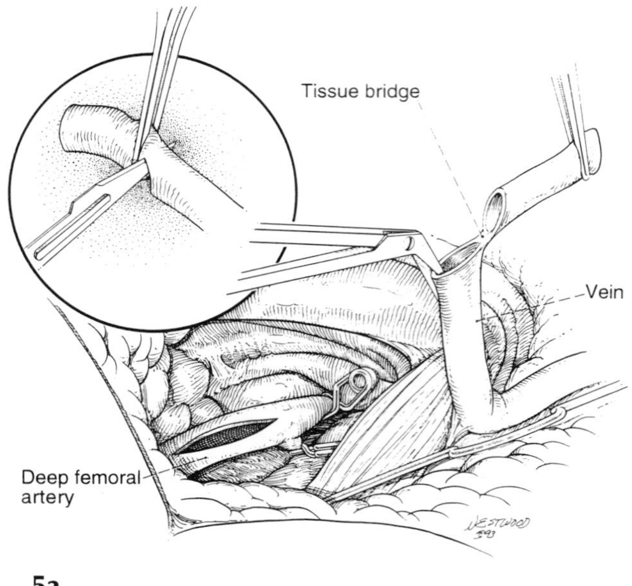

5a

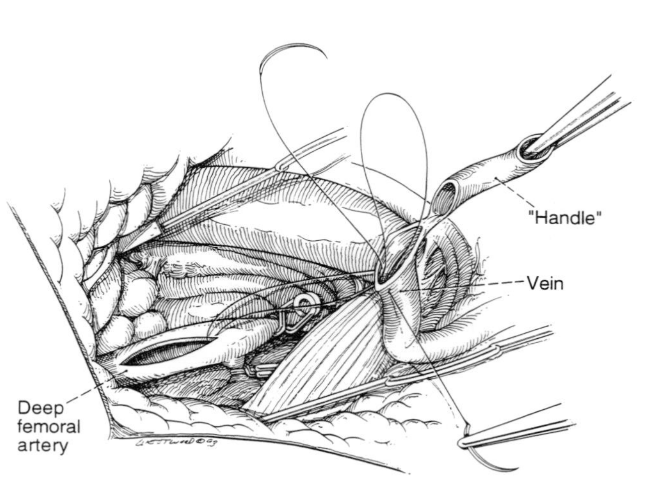

5b

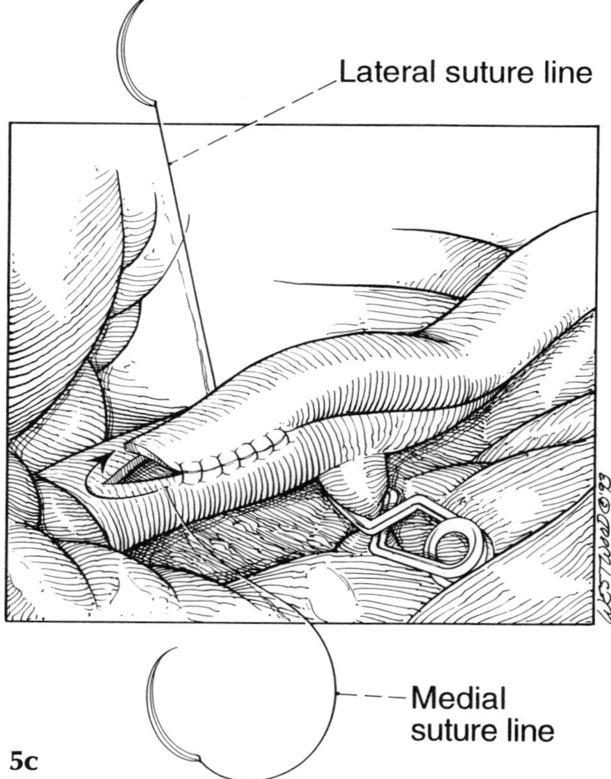

5c

6

Once arterial pressure has been established down to the knee level, the Mills retrograde valvulotome is used for all subsequent valve incisions. This retrograde valvulotome consists of a 20-cm long, 1 mm flexible shaft, a blade at right angles to the shaft and a ball-tip which protects the vein wall. The instrument is passed either through a side branch or through the open end of the vein after it has been distally detached. Before any intraluminal instrumentation is carried out, the mobilized segment of vein is dilated with dextran solution at a controlled pressure of 200 mm Hg. A retrograde valvulotome is introduced through the distal end of the vein, and as it is withdrawn, it cuts one valve leaflet. It is readvanced, rotated 180 degrees, and again withdrawn, cutting the second leaflet.

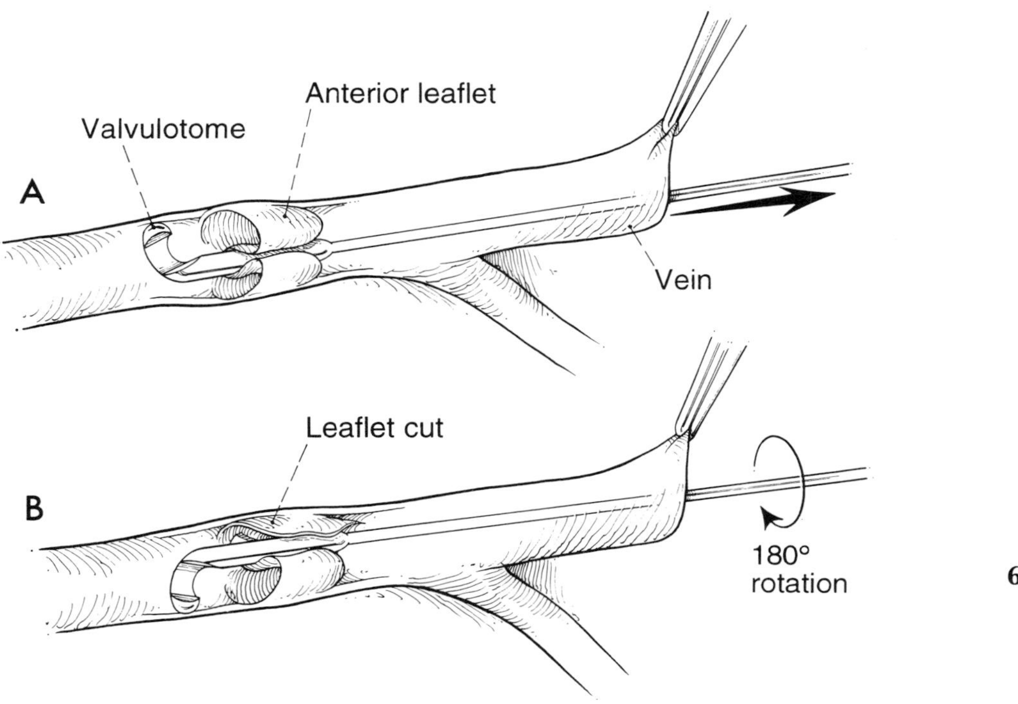

6

7

The simple expedient of assessing flow from the distal divided end of the saphenous vein before construction of the distal anastomosis is very reliable in detecting any proximal haemodynamically significant obstructive lesions. If there is steady, undiminished pulsatile flow, it is unlikely that such a lesion is present proximally with high volume flow in the *in situ* conduit either into a distal fistula or via this distal divided end. A towel is rolled over the entire course of the vein to precipitate closure of any leaflet that has been mechanically placed on the wall and might result in a 'missed valve'. Distal anastomosis is performed using the technique shown in *Illustration 5*. Elimination of arteriovenous fistulae is not a difficult part of the procedure. The position of most of the branches which will become fistulae will be already identified either from the preoperative venogram or during venous exposure for valve incision as discussed previously. Residual arteriovenous fistulae (usually no more than two) are initially determined by the use of intraoperative Doppler probe as shown here. Sequentially the probe placed in the proximal position provides a flow signal when a fistula is present and an obstructive signal when the vein is compressed proximal to this point. After this, an intraoperative arteriogram (considered to be mandatory) is carried out.

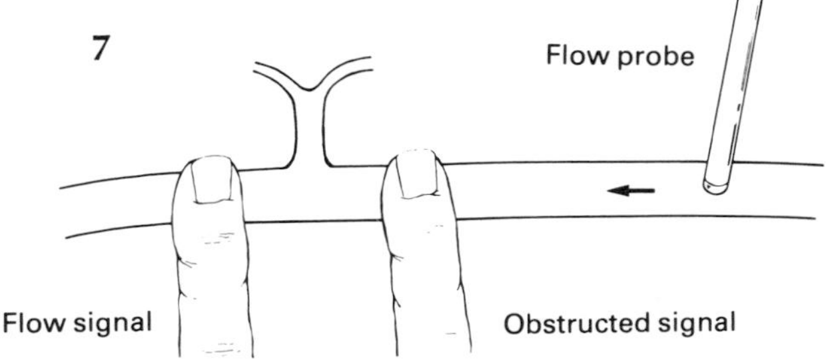

8

On the completion arteriogram, remaining fistulae can be readily identified and the technical accuracy of the distal anastomosis can be seen. A 22-gauge plastic sheath is inserted into the proximal part of the vein and contrast is injected. A needle grid shown numerically allows rapid location of the fistulae. The perforating vein which connects directly with the femoral vein is shown at the third needle position. Note that the valve in the vein is directed towards the deep system. A subcutaneous vein which forms a fistula beyond the fifth needle is not of haemodynamic value and can safely be left if desired. Most such fistulae subsequently become occluded because of the formation of true phlebitis within the vein wall.

The distal anastomosis must also be examined on the arteriogram. Its adequacy should be confirmed in this way as well as by Doppler ultrasound of the flow at this point.

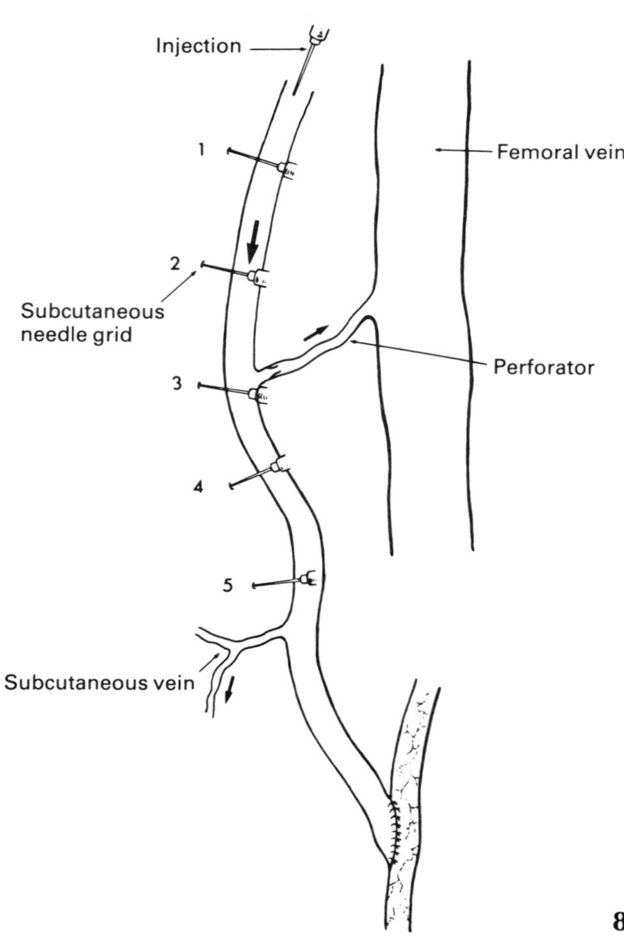

8

Complications

Occasionally, pathological difficulties within the saphenous vein may occur during the operative procedure. These consist of platelet deposition at the site of injured endothelium, unyielding valves because of previous fibrosis, a missed valve cusp, or laceration of the vein wall. Vein wall lacerations are easily identified because of leakage of blood and haematoma formation of the vein wall. When platelet deposition occurs within the vein, this will be seen on the operative angiogram as a foamy filling defect and the Doppler ultrasound will reflect a diminished flow signal. These difficulties, though rare, must be diagnosed and managed intraoperatively if early failure of the bypass is to be avoided.

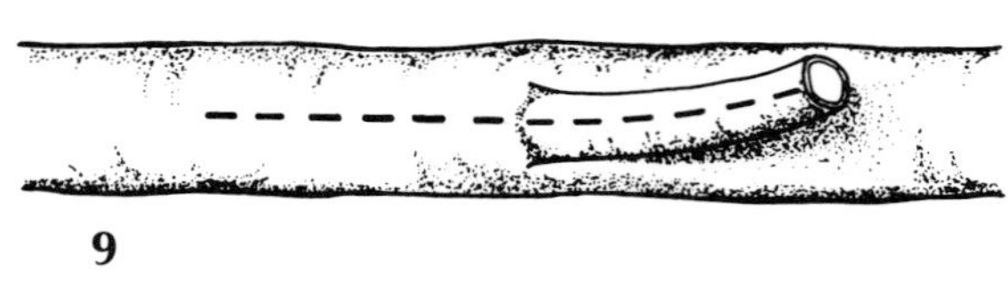
9

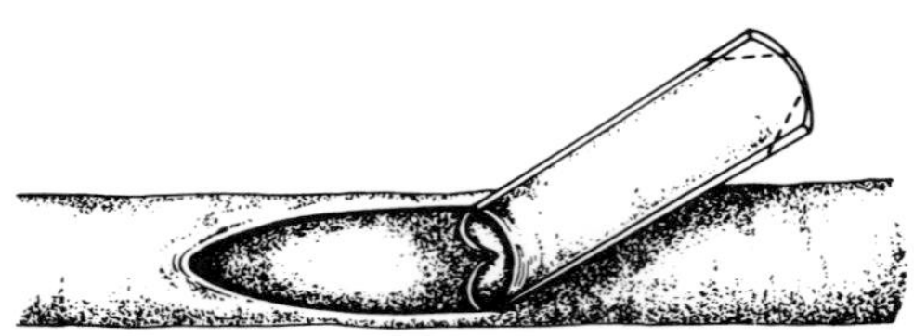
10

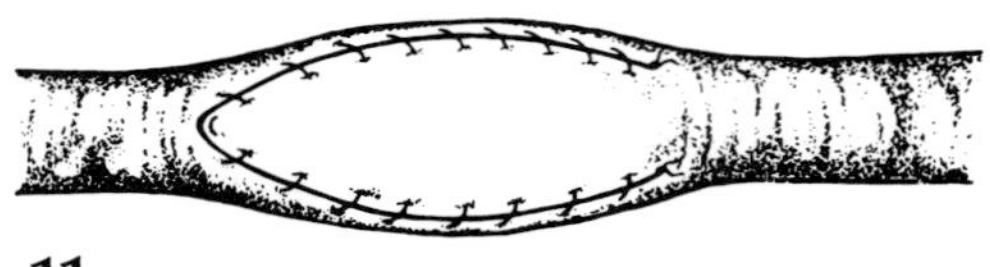
11

9, 10 & 11

When such problems occur, they can usually be treated by the technique of vein branch angioplasty. The vein is opened in order to visualize its endothelial surface. Platelets can be removed through the venotomy and/or missed valves dealt with. The venotomy is subsequently closed by patch angioplasty using a venous branch opened in continuity with the diagnostic venotomy.

This technique is in keeping with and preserves the complete *in situ* nature of the entire procedure (Corson *et al.*, 1984). It is stressed that at the termination of the procedure, the predicted physiological criteria resulting from the bypass should be confirmed in the distal limb by non-invasive methods, e.g. Doppler ultrasound, systolic pressures and wave form analysis. In this respect, the intraoperative arteriogram should also be helpful. The patient should not leave the operating suite until the surgeon is satisfied that these criteria have been met.

References

Corson, J. D., Leather, R. P., Shah, D. M. and Karmody, A. M. (1984). *In situ* vein branch angioplasty. *Surgery, Gynecology and Obstetrics* **159**, 283.

Denton, M. J., Hill, D. and Fairgrieve, J. (1983). *In situ* femoropopliteal and distal vein bypass for limb salvage: Experience of 50 cases. *British Journal of Surgery* **70**, 358.

Fietze-Fischer, B., Gruss, J. D., Bartels, D. *et al.* (1987). Prostaglandin E1 as an adjuvant therapy in the event of femoropopliteal and crural great saphenous vein *in situ* bypass surgery. *VASA* **17**, 23. (suppl).

Gruss, J. D., Bartls, D., Vargas, H. *et al.* (1982). Arterial reconstruction for distal disease of the lower extremities by the *in-situ* vein graft technique. *Journal of Cardiovascular Surgery,* **23**, 231.

Leather, R. P. (1993a). Overview: history and evolution of techniques. In: Rutherford R. B., eds. *Seminars in Vascular Surgery.* Philadelphia: W. B. Saunders **6**, 3.151.

Leather, R. P. (1993b). The current Albany approach. In: Rutherford R. B., eds. *Seminars in Vascular Surgery* Philadelphia: W. B. Saunders **6**, 3.159.

Leather, R. P., Corson, J. D. and Karmody, A. M. (1984). Instrumental evolution of the valve incision method of "*in-situ*" saphenous vein bypass. *Journal of Vascular Surgery* **1**, 113.

Moody, A. P., Edwards, P. R., Harris, P. L. (1992). *In situ* versus reversed femoropopliteal vein grafts: Long-term follow-up of a prospective, randomized trial. *British Journal of Surgery* **79**, 750.

The use of the vein cuff and PTFE

JUSTIN H. MILLER MB BS, FRCS, FACS

19 High Street, Unley Park, South Australia, Australia

Introduction

The cuff (or 'sleeve' as it is often, but less correctly called) is a cylinder of vein interposed between a polytetrafluoroethylene (PTFE) tube and small artery. It was introduced in 1981 (Miller *et al.*, 1984) to facilitate the anastomosis of large (6 mm diameter) stiff PTFE grafts to small (often <2 mm diameter) tibial arteries.

Since 1978 attempts have been made to eliminate this mechanical mismatch problem with variations of the 'Linton patch' (Linton and Wild, 1970), which had the basic problem of accommodating four rows of sutures in a narrow opened vein (6–10 mm wide). In 1979 Siegman (1979) suggested linking a Dacron tube to a small artery by a cylinder of vein and this technique was adapted to join PTFE to tibial vessels with encouraging results (Morris *et al.*, 1993).

Its application has now become very widespread, gradually replacing all direct PTFE anastomoses, such as those to the popliteal and profunda femoris arteries. In selected cases, it is also used at the proximal common femoral inflow anastomosis.

Likewise, a recent innovation has been to facilitate the side-to-side anastomosis between the PTFE and an artery, such as sequential ilio-profunda-popliteal reconstructions, or sequential composite PTFE-vein femoro-popliteal-tibial grafts.

While the main advantage of the cuff over direct anastomosis remains its technical facility, evidence is accruing that it leads to improved long-term patency (Tyrrell, Grigg and Wolfe, 1989). This may well be that it alters the mechanical or elastic mismatch at the distal anastomosis and thereby reduces neointimal hyperplasia (Suggs, Henriques and DePalma, 1988; Tyrrell, Clark and Wolfe, 1989). Another major advantage is that the presence of the cuff facilitates later thrombectomy, thereby extending the life of the graft and limb by reoperation (Morris *et al.*, 1993). The cuff mimics vein at the cuff/artery anastomosis, leading to preservation of the original outflow artery on occlusion of the graft. Moreover, the cuff has less fibrotic reaction than PTFE directly in contact with artery, thereby minimizing the amount of dissection required to control the vessel.

Indications

Femorodistal bypass

It is emphasized that autogenous saphenous vein is still the preferred conduit in all forms of femorodistal grafting. However, PTFE remains a satisfactory alternative when vein (for numerous reasons, not the least of which are multiple previous operations in the same limb) is not available.

The cuff is indicated in all situations where PTFE is to be anastomosed to tibial arteries and is strongly recommended when the anastomosis is to the below-knee popliteal artery, a situation hitherto considered to be a contraindication to the use of any prosthesis. The use of the cuff for the above-knee popliteal artery is not essential but is useful in situations where extensive atheroma makes direct suturing difficult. In the sequential bypass (femoro-popliteal-tibial), the cuff facilitates the side-to-side anastomosis of PTFE (or composite PTFE-vein).

Aortofemoral or cross-over bypass surgery

Aortofemoral surgery often requires the distal end of the graft to be anastomosed to the profunda femoris vessel. Mismatch of the graft vessel diameters requires the use of a long tapering graft down the profunda femoris. The cuff is ideal in this situation, reducing the extent of the dissection required and actually reducing the operating time for the anastomosis. The cuff is equally applicable when a cross-over femoro-profunda graft is required (Miller *et al.*, 1991). When an inflow operation is combined with a distal bypass (aorto- or ilio-profunda-popliteal graft), a cuff applied to the profunda greatly facilitates the side-to-side anastomosis between that vessel and the PTFE graft.

Special considerations for infrainguinal PTFE grafts with cuff

The total experience in femorodistal bypass grafting has been with 6-mm PTFE, initially with the standard graft, but mostly with thin-walled grafts since 1984. More recently many have found it particularly useful with external supported ringed PTFE. With the profunda femoris as outflow vessel, 8-mm tubing has been used.

Infection

Contrary to accepted belief, the risk of infection (from foot necrosis, nearby wound breakdown after failed surgery or removal of infected graft) has not been a problem. This is provided that the new PTFE graft lies in a new non-devitalized tract, that the suture line of PTFE to cuff is properly buried in living tissue and that the graft remains patent (and this aided by the cuff) (Miller, 1993). Apart from this, prosthetic grafts are at higher risk of infection than vein and the use of preoperative intravenous antibiotics is essential. The agent selected should have good activity against *Staphylococcus aureus* as well as any local cultured organisms, and should be continued for 48 h postoperatively.

Dissection

Anastomosis with prosthesis needs a good blood supply. Local tissue ischaemia should be avoided by minimal and gentle dissection at anastomotic sites. Approaches to arteries should not transect lymph channels and should avoid collaterals. This is especially so in the groin. A less extensive exposure is required for the cuff than a direct anastomosis with PTFE. Often in the presence of difficult atheroma at the inflow common femoral artery anastomosis, deliberate use of the cuff will simplify the operation compared with direct anastomosis.

Graft length

PTFE is more unforgiving than vein and in judging the length of the graft it is better to err on the side of making the graft too slack rather than too tight. A rule of thumb is to extend the leg fully, distend to arterial pressure and cut the graft to the exact length plus 1 cm. See *Illustration 5b*.

Graft site

Subcutaneous placement of PTFE is preferred to subfascial. However, when the distal anastomosis is to popliteal artery immediately below the knee joint the preference is to run the graft through the popliteal fossa between the heads of gastrocnemius muscle even when using Ringed PTFE. It is possible the cuff allows flexibility of the anastomosis. Because of the narrow popliteal canal PTFE and artery tend to lie parallel just prior to the anastomosis and it is the authors' habit to make a 'double tier' of the distal cuff (see *Illustration 6a and b*) to avoid the 'cervix' effect of the heel. A minority of surgeons favour running the graft subcutaneously around the medial condyle (even laying it on the anterior shelf) reasoning that this relates to the true centre of movement of the joint. Grafts to the anterior tibial and peroneal arteries are placed on the lateral side of thigh and leg although recently a medial approach to the peroneal artery is favoured even if a segment of fibula has been resected for access.

Clotting

PTFE is intolerant to either stasis of blood within the graft or slow flow, and this must be carefully avoided as follows:

1. Adequate peroperative systemic heparinization is essential. There is little evidence regarding the exact dose to be used but our experience has been to use a bolus of 5000 u of heparin, supplemented by 1000 u/h if the clamp time exceeds 1 h. The advantage of this regime is that it almost never requires reversal with protamine.
2. Heparinized saline (5000 u/1000 ml) is used liberally to irrigate the graft and artery. Once the proximal anastomosis is completed, heparinized saline is forcibly refluxed upstream into the proximal artery of supply prior to clamping of the graft (*see Illustration 5a*). Although there is little evidence of its value in an effort to reduce platelet adherence, the author uses heparinized rheomacrodex as well as saline.
3. Postoperative systemic heparinization is not used routinely, but it is recommended for at least 48 h or until maximum perfusion is manifest by pulses and reactionary warmth in the foot in redo situations, or when there is poor distal run-off.
4. After thrombectomy, the author frequently infuses heparin directly into the graft via a 16 gauge epidural catheter, maintaining moderate therapeutic levels as measured systemically. This has the advantage over intravenous application in that heparin concentrates inside the lower graft and run off (especially with poor outflow) preventing local thrombus formation before overflowing systemically and risking bleeding from wounds and elsewhere. The dosage needed is much lower than that necessary to achieve the same effect intravenously.

Preliminary clearing of the outflow with fibrinolysis after graft occlusion

1. After occlusion a PTFE graft with vein cuff behaves like vein in that the original outflow tract is retained. Should this not happen (e.g. from progression of disease beyond the graft), it is preferable to clarify outflow with fibrinolysis rather than proceed to a more distal bypass immediately. The original outflow may be restored completely (e.g. retaining an above-knee segment of artery) or partly (e.g. extending to below-knee popliteal rather than tibial artery). It is also probable that streptokinase augments perfusion by clearing thrombus in the very small vessels in contrast to the Fogarty which can only risk damage to the lining of the larger tibial arteries.
2. A radiological catheter (5 French) is introduced via a sheath by downhill puncture in the ipsilateral common femoral artery (or by traversing the aortic bifurcation by uphill puncture in the opposite femoral artery) and manipulated into the proximal ostium of the graft and down to within 1 or 2 cm of the distal anastomosis. If this is not possible it is better to introduce the catheter through a small incision over the upper graft under local anaesthetic. Repeated attempts at percutaneous puncture directly into the graft are more likely to cause multiple holes which leak. It is important that the entry point is a snug fit in the graft otherwise blood will track back from the outflow artery once connection is established and leak into the tissues. This is best achieved by exposing the surrounding incorporated tissue of the graft but not baring its wall and making the entry point with an 18 G needle.
3. Streptokinase at an hourly rate of 5000 units plus 600 u heparin is perfused via an intra-arterial pump (e.g. IMED). Alternatively urokinase (120 000 u/h plus heparin), although more expensive causes less allergic reaction, and does not develop resistance. The distal tree is checked via the catheter at 6–8 h intervals and perfusion continues until the run off is optimal. Systemic monitoring is with usual blood coagulation studies, the most important of which is the fibrinogen level. For optimal benefit the lytic agent must be perfused directly into thrombus before it overflows into the general circulation (if necessary by advancing the catheter into clot in native artery). Overdose in the general circulation declares itself by bleeding from the puncture site and rapidly falling fibrinogen level (<1 g/l). Correction is by Fresh Frozen Plasma or intravenous aminocaproic acid (5 g i.v.). The distal native arterial tree is mostly restored to the original state but usually the distal and almost always the proximal anastomosis will require surgical intervention.

Preparation of the patient: choice of vein for the cuff

The whole limb (or both, if veins are scarce) is prepared in the usual way, and the outflow artery is exposed to establish operability. The vein is chosen from the following sites:

1. Long saphenous vein on the shelf of the medial malleolus, unless as in very critical limb ischaemia the site is unlikely to heal. This can be a problem if there is no boost to the local blood supply by the operation.
2. The lateral saphenous vein in the groin incision. (The main trunk makes an excellent and even better cuff but would be more appropriate in some other capacity, e.g. as a sequential composite graft.) Saphenous vein seems to have the right muscular strength; others such as arm veins can be used but are generally too fragile.
3. The beginning of the short saphenous vein behind the lateral malleolus.
4. In the lower edge of a below-knee approach to the popliteal artery. This segment of long saphenous vein is often spared after coronary artery surgery or previous femoropopliteal bypass. Sometimes an *in situ* vein graft is abandoned at an early stage because the vein is too small at this site; however, it is still adequate for a cuff.

Procedure

The usual order is to suture the cuff on the outflow vessel, then to make the proximal inflow anastomosis, place the graft, cut to length and then join the PTFE to the cuff as the final procedure. Completing the distal anastomosis before the proximal, as is often done with reversed vein graft, is not recommended. PTFE is not as tolerant of stagnant blood as is vein. To shorten operating time it is usually possible for a second operator to execute the proximal anastomosis, while the cuff is being made.

1a, b, c

Cuff and inflow anastomosis

Most consider that a cuff is not necessary at the upper inflow anastomosis, and this is certainly true if it is beyond the take-off of the profunda femoris. However, a direct anastomosis to the common femoral vessel does constitute a risk to the integrity of the flow of the profunda artery, especially if there is a chance of early graft occlusion and need for removal, e.g. desperate attempts at limb salvage by femorotibial grafting. To minimize this risk the following steps can be taken:

1. Bring a direct anastomosis wholly on to the superficial femoral vessel by enlarging the outlet of the common femoral artery with a vein patch, so that no PTFE intrudes into the main vessel (*a*). This is most effective.
2. This patch can be varied to resemble that described by Taylor at the outflow end (Taylor *et al.*, 1992) making sure the vein extends up to the common femoral artery and down enough to cover the heel of the PTFE (*b*). A wide piece of vein is necessary for this manoeuvre to be effective.
3. Sometimes in very complex atheromatous situations it is more expeditious (in the interests of minimal dissection and avoidance of lymph nodes) to simply let in a cuff in any soft spot free from plaque (*c*). The cuff helps avoid what experience has shown to be a bad combination (especially in the groin) – endarterectomy and direct suturing of PTFE.

Concomitant profunda disease at the inflow anastomoses

The decision as to whether to combine a profundaplasty with a distal bypass is always difficult. There are times however when the need cannot be ignored. With vein, the two procedures combine well by using the hood of the proximal anastomosis as the vein patch for the profundaplasty (Greenhalgh, 1980). The combination of cuff and PTFE can be utilized in a similar and simple manner:

1. Simple orifice stenosis is easily handled by siting the cuff partly on the soft profunda and partly on the common femoral artery without endarterectomy. It is often possible to incorporate the lateral circumflex artery orifice as well.
2. When extensive endarterectomy is necessary (e.g. common femoral orifice coralline atheroma), the combined patch and cuff is useful (*see Illustration 61*). Here the cuff can be sited over the junction of endarterectomized profunda and normal intima, so that any tendency to lift will be in the mid-portion of the cuff.

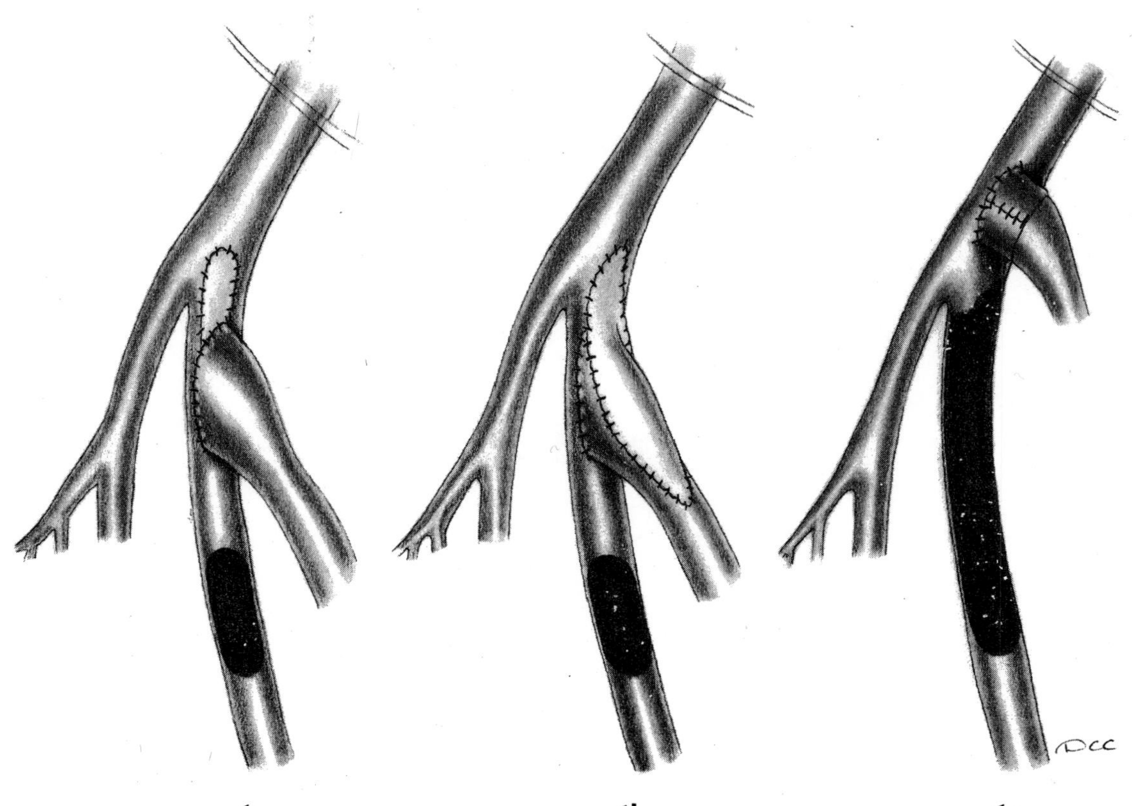

1a 1b 1c

2a–d

Technique of creating the cuff

This is the standard technique for any anastomosis, and despite the many modifications which have been suggested, it remains essentially unchanged since it was first developed in 1981.

A total of 3–4 cm of saphenous vein with a diameter of 2–4 mm is opened up longitudinally (*a*). A larger diameter makes an even better cuff, but this is an extravagant use of vein. An arteriotomy (*b*), 1–1.5 cm in length, or approximately twice the diameter of the graft, is made in any soft portion free of plaque. Siting is critical, avoiding 'exploratory arteriotomy' and preferably leaving plaque with potential to lift at the cephalic end. The sleeve is then sutured with continuous Prolene sutures (6/0 for popliteal, 7/0 for tibial) to the inferior edge of the arteriotomy (*c*). Some surgeons prefer the traditional method of commencing at the distal apex (or 'toe') using the parachute technique to view the lumen first (*d*). In either case, it is essential to stitch the artery from within out, so that the vein fixes the intima against the medial coat.

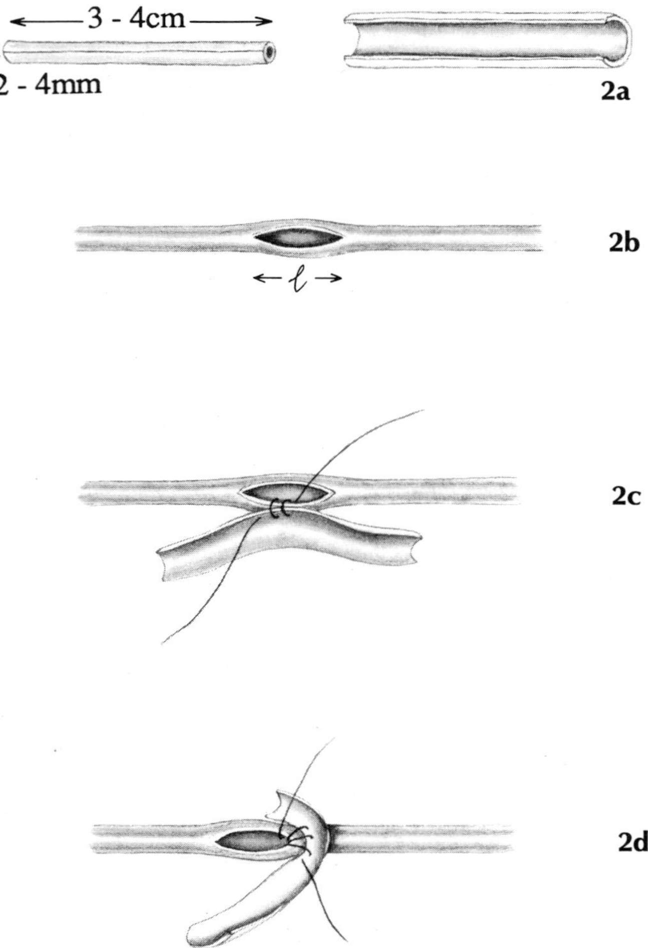

3a–d

Suturing the apices

In the middle portion of the arteriotomy, the bite of artery should be larger than that of vein, so as to take the vein well down into the artery to fix the intima (*a*). As the apex is approached, this bite should be reduced so as to prevent the vein intruding into the lumen. The interval between sutures should be small and they should be left loose to be tightened later (with a nerve hook if necessary) (*b*). The heel is treated in the same way as the apex. As each suture is placed at both ends, the lumen of the vessel beyond should be clearly visible. This is to preserve outflow in both directions, so that in the event of graft occlusion, artery patency is preserved (*c*). This is vital at the level of the tibial artery or distal profunda femoris. Suturing is continued on the upper edge until the two separate sutures meet (*d*), when they are tied together. A sealing corner suture is made by passing one needle out–in through the vein and then in–out through the other edge of the vein, where it is tied to the free length of the suture. Alternatively, if dealing with narrow fragile vein, one might choose to carry on suturing vein to vein. See *Illustration 6a* and *b*.

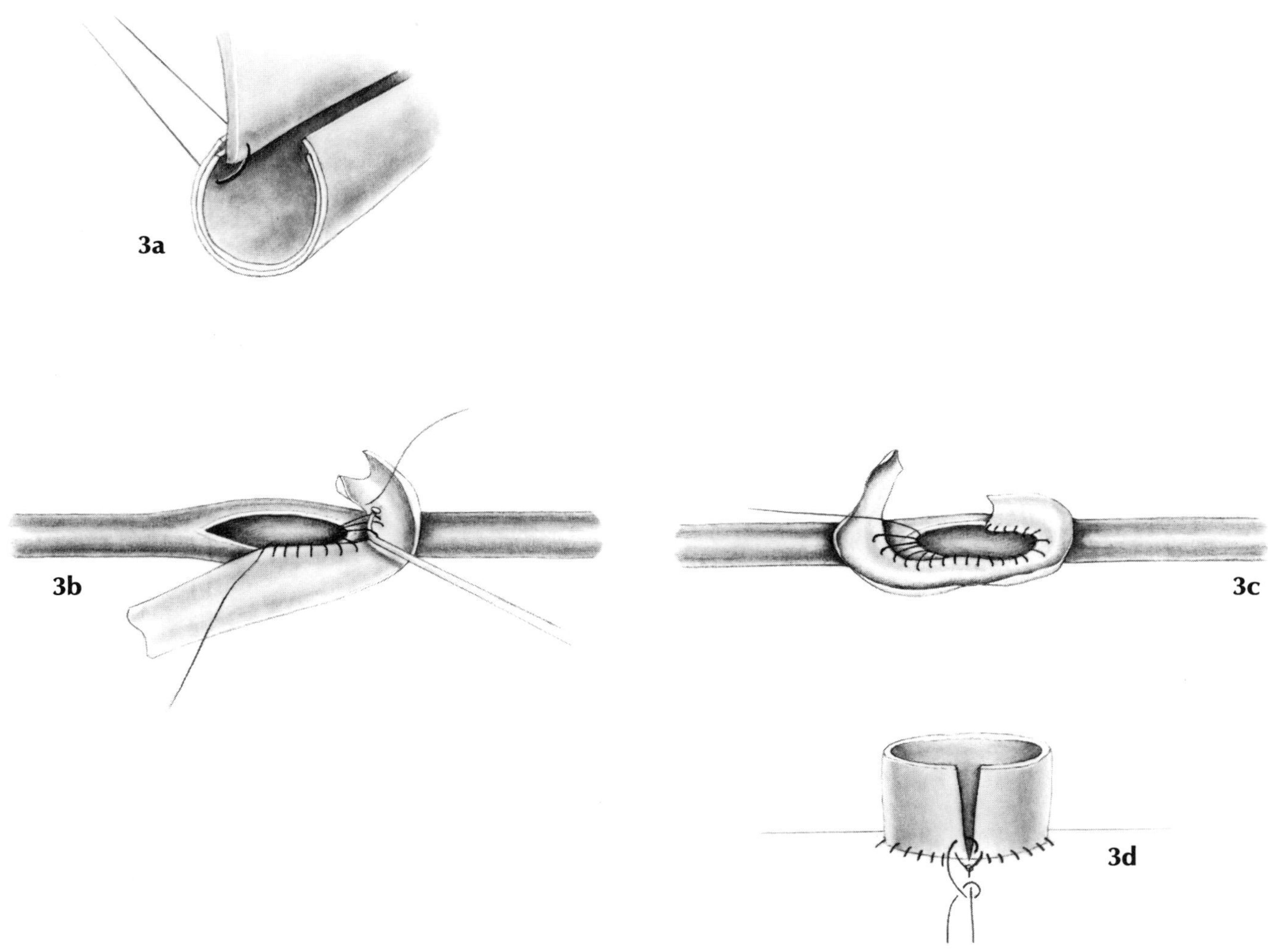

4a–d

The vein ends are squared off, leaving a little extra for suturing. One thread is cut or used as a stay. The remaining suture is used to approximate the square ends of the vein carefully with frequent bites until the corners meet, where the suture is tied to itself, clipped and used as a stay suture for the next part of the procedure (*a*). The upper anastomosis is then made and the graft is placed in its appropriate tract. Heparinized saline is forcibly refluxed upstream (see *Illustration 5a*) and the graft is clamped distally.

The PTFE is cut at the appropriate angle with a blade (conveniently along a clamp). The angle at which it is cut will determine its circumference, which should equal the circumference of the cuff. This in turn should be twice the length of the arteriotomy ($c = 2l$). If half the circumference ($c/2 = \pi d/2$) of a 6-mm tube cut at right angles = 9.4 mm, then $c/2$ cut at an angle of 60° = 10.8 mm (9.4/sin 60), $c/2$ cut at 45° = 13.3 mm, and an 8-mm tube cut at 60° = 14.5 mm (*c*).

The circumference of the cut PTFE should now approximate to that of the sleeve. If there is to be a disparity in length, it is better that the cuff diameter exceed that of the PTFE, so that 'tenting' takes place in the vein rather than the PTFE (this makes extra suturing easier). See *Illustration 6g and i*. By squaring off the tip of the PTFE with a blade, its circumference can be shortened (*d*). It is a simple matter to join the PTFE and cuff end-to-end (*d*). A parachute technique using 6/0 Prolene is appropriate.

Prior to the completion of the anastomosis, backbleeding from both directions is checked to flush out any thrombus. After a final irrigation both proximally and distally, the suture line is completed and the clamps released. A peroperative arteriogram is performed through a 21-gauge butterfly needle inserted into the PTFE near the distal anastomosis and facing upstream. This allows the minimum amount of contrast to be used to display the distal anastomosis. This is important with tibial artery outflow, where excessive contrast can be harmful.

4a **4b**

θ = 60° d = 6mm $\frac{c}{2}$ = l = 10.8mm
45° d = 6mm l = 13.3mm
60° d = 8mm l = 14.5mm

4c

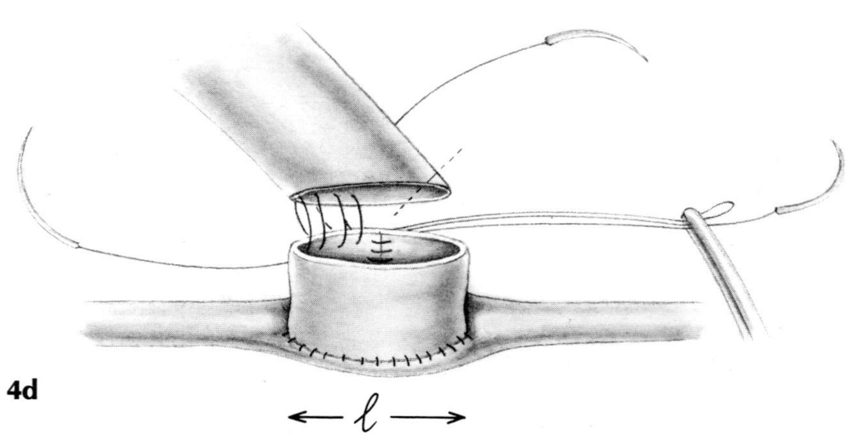

4d

5a–d

Care of the graft and prevention of clotting

Considerable care is taken to ensure that the graft is of the correct length and that at no stage is there any stationary blood, either in the graft or the well of the cuff and artery, where blood is inclined to accumulate during the execution of the proximal anastomosis. After the proximal anastomosis is made, the graft is placed in its selected tract by a tunneller or sponge-holding forceps. Heparinized saline is then forcibly refluxed upstream through the graft and inflow artery with a 20-ml syringe and malleable cannula (e.g. Oschner), and the graft is clamped distally (*a*). This has the effect of ironing out any kinks or malrotation and of ascertaining the optimal length under arterial pressure at the moment the graft is cut (*b*). It also makes absolutely sure that there is no stagnant blood in the graft.

Just prior to completion of the anastomosis, the downflow is checked. A cannula is gently inserted between the loose continuous suture and the cavity of the cuff, and then the graft is flushed with heparinized saline with the arterial clamps removed (*c*). The suture is tightened and the graft clamp is released. This variation in the technique is important with tibial arteries, where backbleeding is often negligible. The perfect tibial clamp is yet to be designed, and therefore clamping and unclamping should be kept to a minimum. Some surgeons make use of the pneumatic tourniquet technique to avoid this clamping (Bernhard *et al.*, 1991).

Most suture line bleeding stops within 5 min with gentle swab pressure. 'Tents' from excess vein to PTFE cause 'spurters', which may require individual suturing with the graft reclamped. At no stage should there ever be stationary blood in the PTFE graft. If clamping longer than 1 min is required for any reason, heparinized saline solution should be refluxed back up the graft (clamped distally) to the proximal anastomosis via the scalp vein needle used for the arteriogram (*d*).

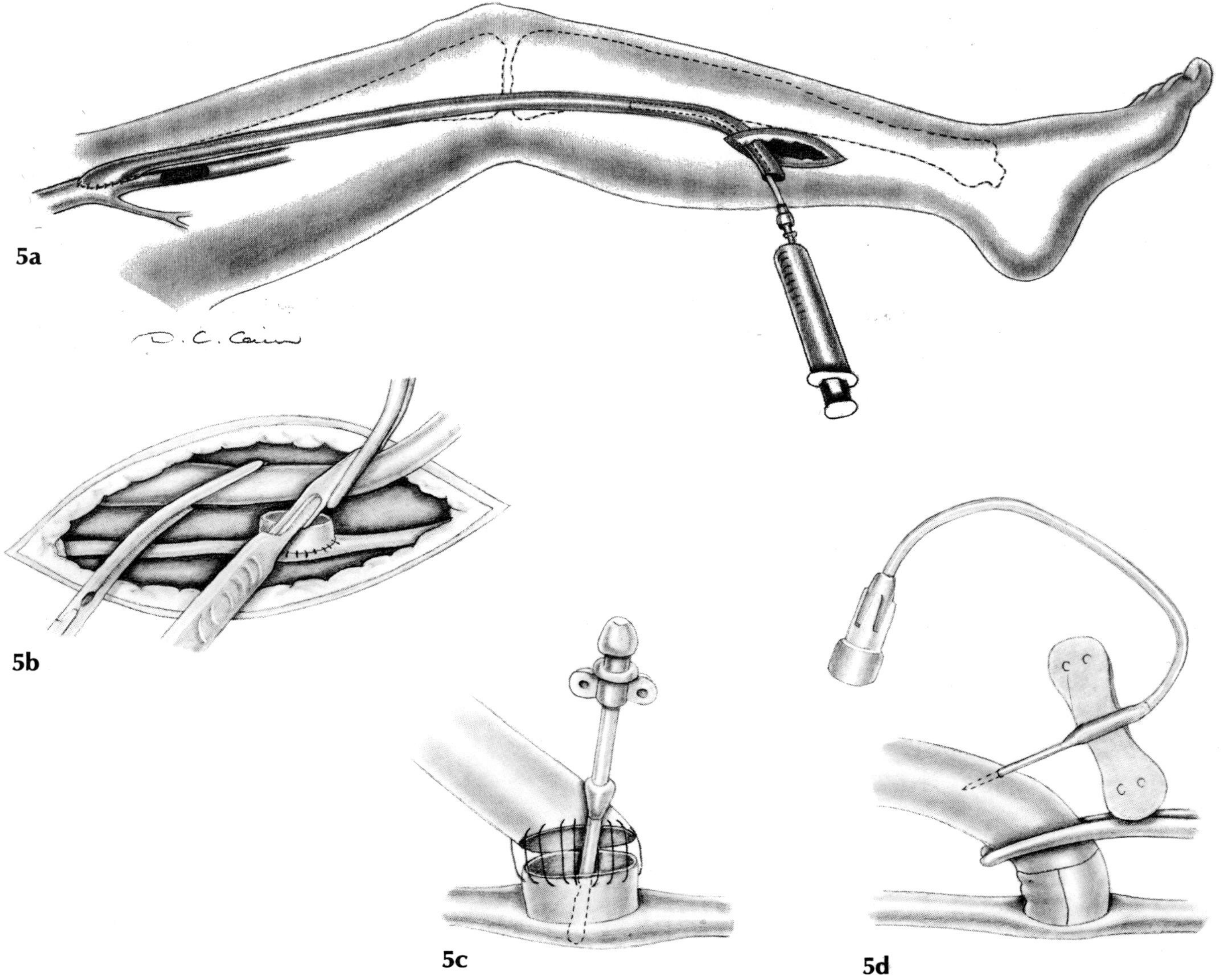

5a

5b

5c

5d

6a–l

Pitfalls and variations

If the vein is too narrow the sutures to both artery and PTFE get uncomfortably close especially at the vein–vein join. This overcrowding of sutures can be avoided (with suitable length of vein) by continuing suturing to the free edge of the vein initially crossing the apex (*a*) and finishing on the near side (*b*) as a 'double tier'. This makes a smoother and more haemodynamic PTFE-cuff join which the author often deliberately uses when traversing the popliteal fossa to a below-knee popliteal artery insertion.

When the vein is too short, stretching it under tension (*c*, *d*) predisposes to necrosis and bleeding at a later date. It is better to cut another piece of vein and suture this in place, tedious though this might be (*e*). A common mistake is to cut the PTFE too acutely (e.g. 30°) in an effort to reduce the angle of insertion to cuff-artery complex (*f*), making the circumference of PTFE longer than cuff. They can then only be matched by 'tenting' the PTFE causing crowding of sutures in more fragile vein (*g*), risking tearing and bleeding. This is corrected by cutting the PTFE more obtusely (e.g. 45°–60°) (*h*) so that 'tenting' occurs in a vein and tougher PTFE takes the crowding of sutures (*i*).

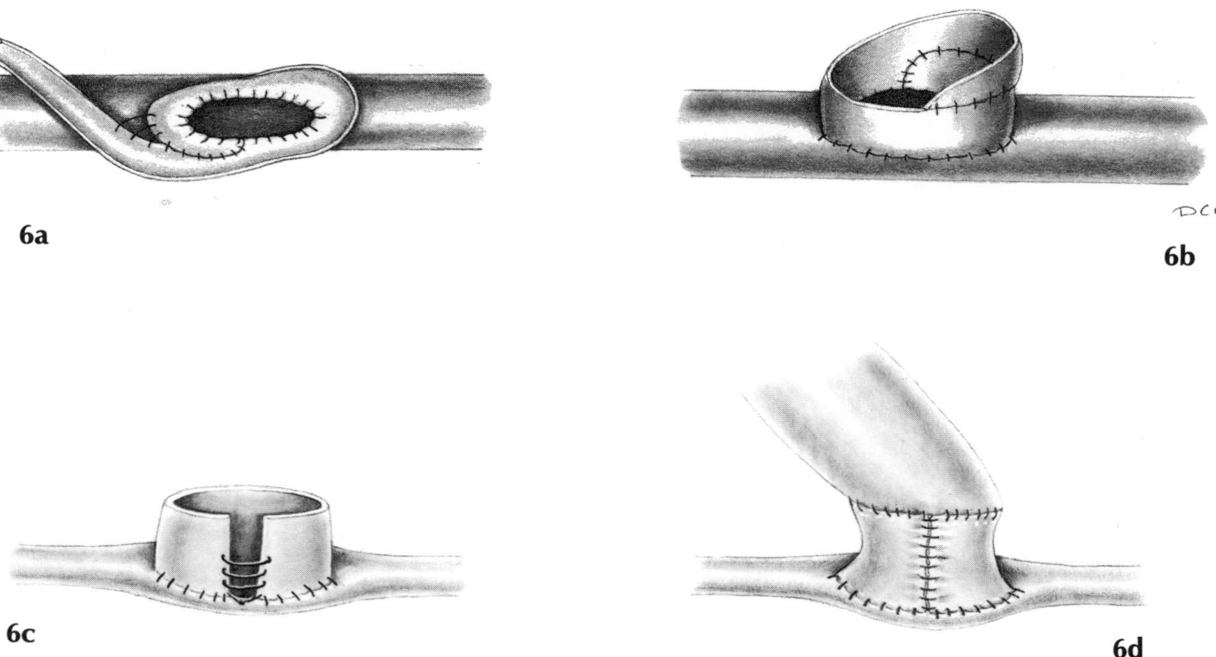

6a

6b

6c

6d

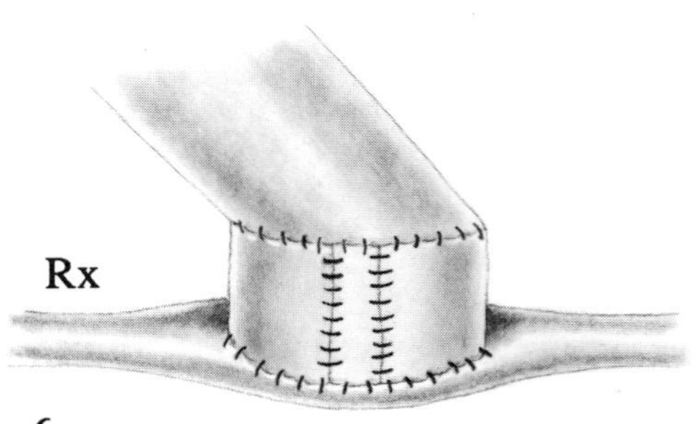

6e

If the arteriotomy is too long, the resultant cuff becomes aneurysmal (*j*). To compensate, part of the vein is sutured in as a patch leaving sufficient as cuff to accommodate the cut PTFE. It is usual to place the cuff component at the downstream end so as to provide for the vital distal outflow lumen (*k*), unlike Tyrrell and Wolfe (1991), who prefer it as a 'collar' on the upstream end for haemodynamic reasons. The use of this procedure is sometimes made in concomitant profundaplasty. The patch component widens the proximal profunda, and the cuff accommodating the PTFE isplaced distally over uninvolved vessel (*l*).

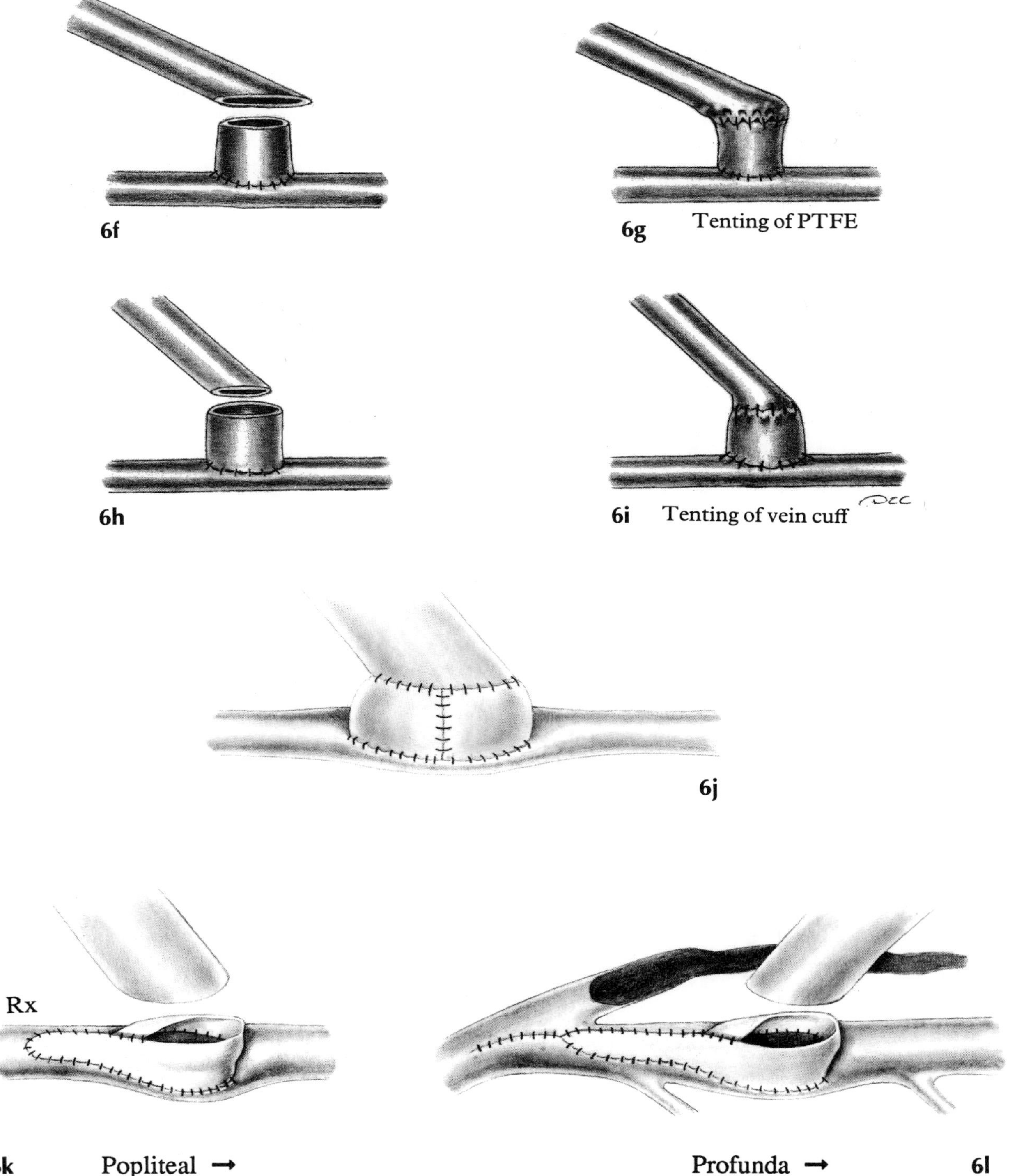

6f

6g Tenting of PTFE

6h

6i Tenting of vein cuff

6j

6k Popliteal →

Profunda → **6l**

7a, b & c

Sequential composite femoro-popliteal-tibial graft

The accepted method for composing a femoro-popliteal-tibial graft by making use of a short segment of vein is to make a direct anastomosis of the PTFE to the popliteal artery and run a jump graft from the PTFE to the tibial vessel (Finn *et al.*, 1980), or to join the PTFE distal outflow anastomosis and the vein inflow anastomosis sequentially to the popliteal artery. There are two problems, however. Technically, the proximal portion of the vein is narrow (at the best 4 mm, otherwise it would have been used in its entirety as a complete vein graft) and therefore likely to be narrow immediately at the heel. Secondly, in the long term, neointimal hyperplasia may develop as a consequence of the compliance mismatch.

By applying a cuff to the intermediate popliteal anastomotic site first (*a*), the PTFE and the vein can be joined using the sleeve as an intermediary (avoiding the direct vein–PTFE join or the vein to thick-walled artery). The critical heel of the small-diameter vein is first parachuted on to the mid-distal point of the sleeve, and then the wider heel of the PTFE on to the proximal or cephalic side of the sleeve. The apical opened-out part of the vein becomes a long patch on the PTFE (*b*). Alternatively, a single tube of PTFE can be anastomosed side-to-side to the popliteal artery via the cuff (*c*). A direct side-to-side anastomosis between the PTFE and the artery is very difficult.

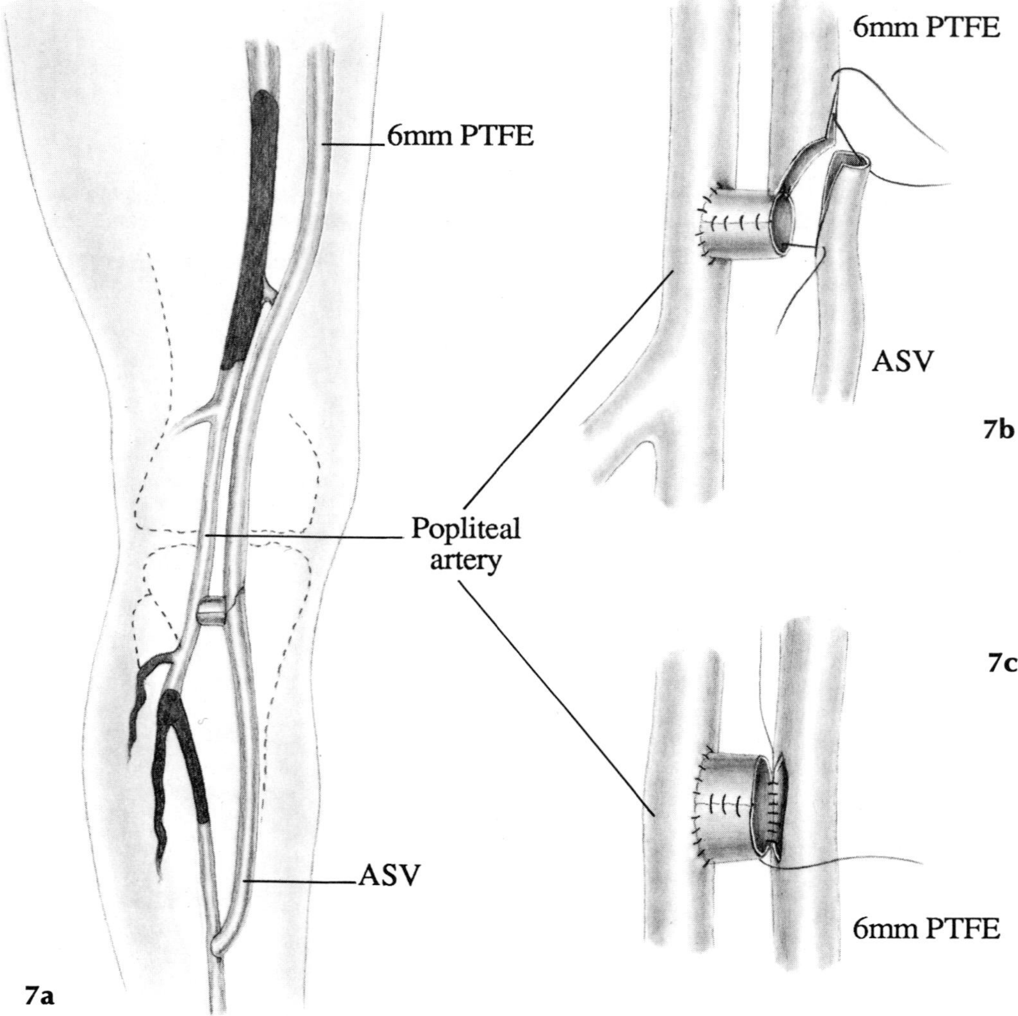

8a, b & c

Sequential composite aorto (ilio) profunda popliteal graft

An aorto (or ilio) profunda popliteal graft is constructed in the same way using a cuff on profunda femoris as an intermediary to link 8 mm PTFE to 6 mm PTFE or the narrow end of reversed saphenous vein. It is possible to use the proximal portion of the reversed vein in continuity as the cuff component. The vein is simply opened as though it were being used for the hood of a conventional proximal anastomosis (*a*), sutured all the way around the arteriotomy as for the cuff (*b*), but is continued down the open vein suturing vein to vein, widening the proximal vein as a funnel especially opposite the heel (*c*) (Vladimirovich, 1985). With more romantic than geographical insight this manoeuvre is known as a 'Hungarian wrap'. It is equally as effective in the femoro-popliteal tibial situation.

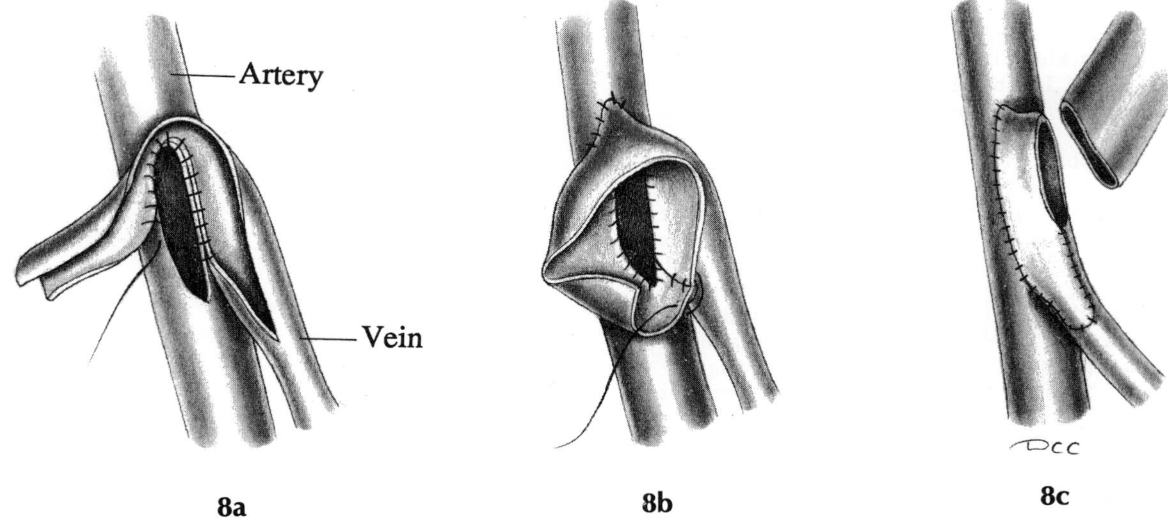

8a 8b 8c

9a & b

Late thrombectomy of occluded PTFE graft and cuff

When a PTFE graft occludes (often years later), the presence of a cuff facilitates the thrombectomy. Usually, the original outflow artery remains open and shows up on the arteriogram. If not, it can sometimes be cleaned out by local infusion of streptokinase via the graft. Failing this, the main body of the graft can be thrombectomized and extended with a fresh piece of PTFE to a new site lower down via a cuff. It is unlikely that simply clearing the graft at its midpoint with a Fogarty catheter will have any lasting outcome. Both ends must be exposed and cleaned under direct vision. Similarly, lysis of the popliteal trifurcation is preferable to Fogarty exploration.

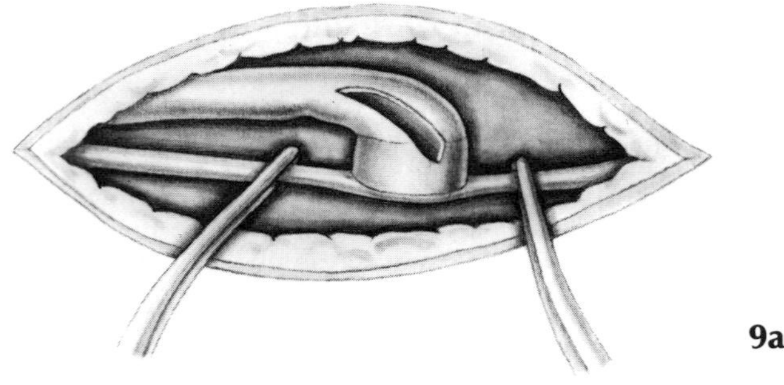

9a

Clearing the distal anastomosis

The junction of the PTFE and cuff is exposed by sharp dissection, as are both the upstream and downstream arteries, sufficient to control backbleeding using straight clamps and without formal taping. It is best not to bare the original vein-to-artery stitching. An arteriotomy is made across the PTFE and cuff (*a*).

Thrombus is then lifted from within the vein–artery cavity. This results mostly in backbleeding from either end. It is not usually necessary to pass a Fogarty catheter, but this can be decided upon using the arteriogram. Very occasionally, a vessel full of clot can be cleared from here, but it is more likely that the artery lining will be damaged. On rare occasions, neointima may line the junction of the PTFE and vein cuff, possibly extending to the arterial lumen. This will endarterectomize cleanly (it is quite distinct from atheroma), leaving natural endothelium. No attempt should be made to clear out above with a Fogarty catheter at this stage.

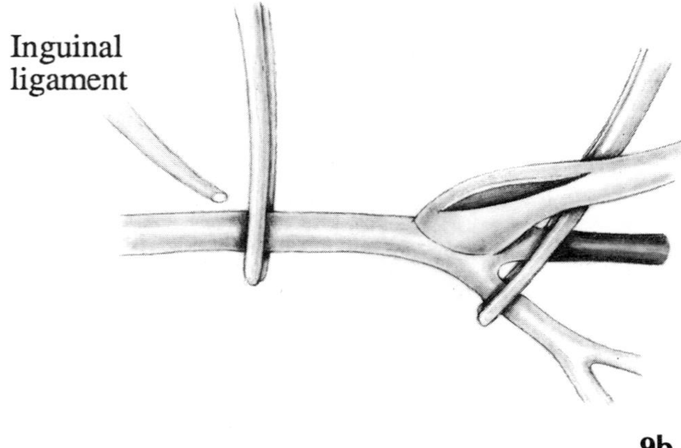

9b

Clearing the upper anastomosis

The upper graft is exposed by sharp dissection and followed up to the anastomosis. It is preferable to avoid laying bare the previous sutures. The common femoral artery is then similarly dissected just under the inguinal ligament, separating the femoral vein to the lateral side and the femoral nerve laterally. This should be virgin territory. Taping, which risks damaging the backwall, is not necessary; a Bainbridge DeBakey clamp directed backwards will suffice. Profunda backbleeding is controlled using a similar clamp across the superficial femoral and profunda artery complex (*b*). Again it is preferable that the profunda femoris is not taped.

The hood of the PTFE is opened and the cavity is cleared of fibrin. This is facilitated if there has been a previous cuff. The downflow is then checked and, if found to be inadequate, a Fogarty catheter or sound may be gently passed to ascertain the need for a patch above the anastomosis. It may be necessary to have profunda backbleeding during the final stages of cleaning. A view is obtained using a blunt paediatric sucker and irrigation. A common mistake is to shift to a new anastomosis more proximally. Ultimately, this only prejudices the profunda circulation, lengthens the graft and leads to a lower patency rate. It is possible to use the original anastomosis over and over again.

10a–e

The graft is then cleared through both openings. A No. 4 Fogarty catheter is passed from below upward to extract the main thrombus (*a*, *b*). Often there is surprisingly little. This procedure should be carried out with care unless a thin layer of fibrin is disturbed. The passage of the catheter from above downward is to make sure there are no kinks. Finally, a large malleable cannula (e.g. Oschner) is introduced from above and the graft is vigorously flushed downwards with heparinized saline (*c*).

The upper opening is then closed (after checking downflow). Sometimes, a protruding mound ('cervix') presents from the original heel of the PTFE graft. If so, it is preferable to add a patch of PTFE or vein (*d*). It is best not to clamp just beyond this suturing, in case clot accumulates. Instead, heparinized saline (or rheomacrodex) should be refluxed against the bloodstream as described (*see Illustration 5a*), and a clamp attached just above the distal opening. This allows any debris to separate and prevents it from going down the outflow vessel. A brisk outflow when the clamp is released ensures the flow is not impeded.

Finally, the bottom opening is closed. Usually, a patch is required (preferably vein), especially if there is a protuberance of the original PTFE heel. The apex of the patch parachutes nicely into the previous cuff (*e*).

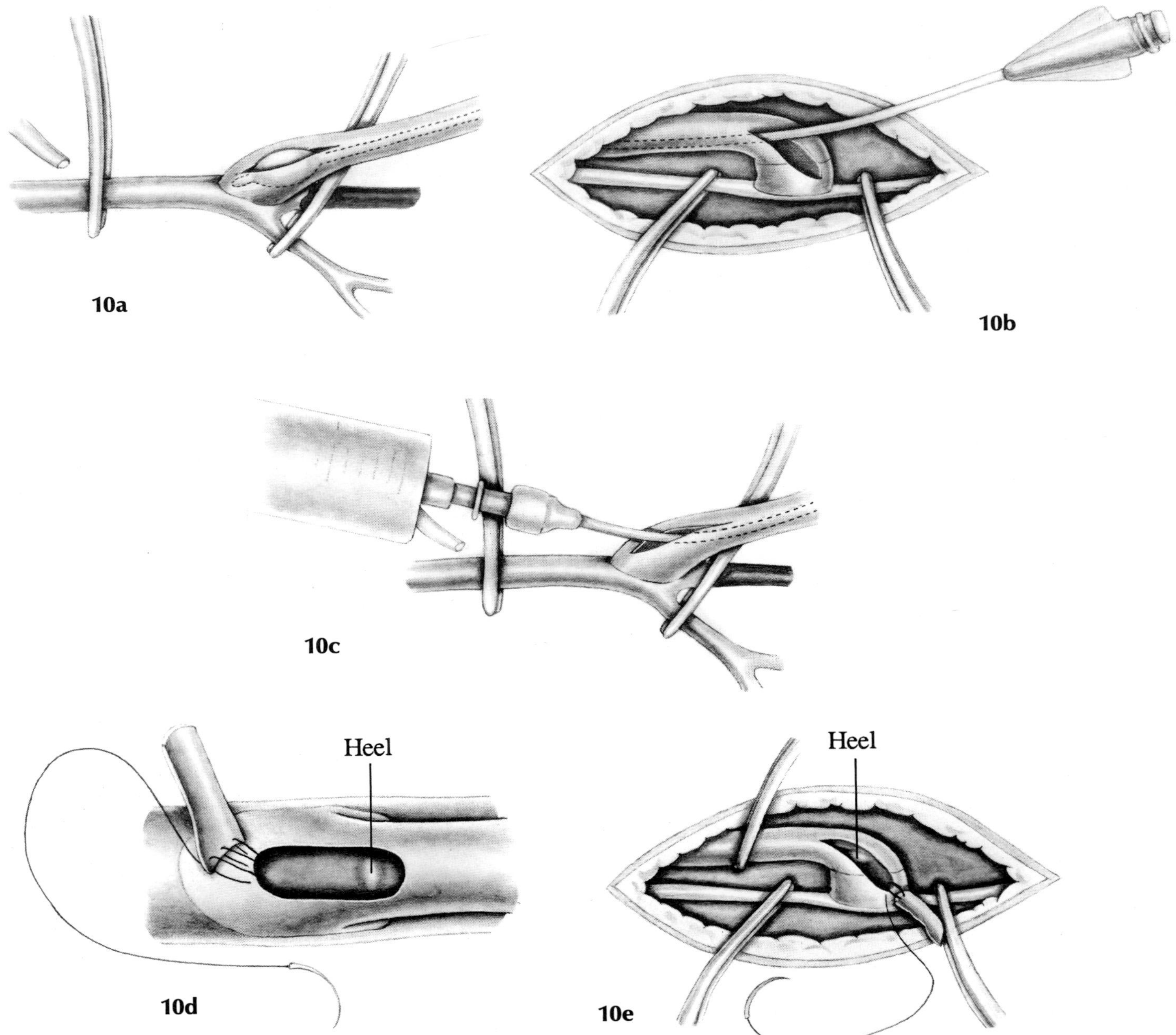

10a 10b 10c 10d 10e

10f

After thrombectomy, it is recommended that immediate full heparinization and long-term anticoagulation be instituted. It is the author's practice to run heparin (750–1000 u/h) directly into the graft via a 16 gauge epidural catheter introduced through the lower end of the upper wound (*f*) maintaining a level of 2 × N APPT (50–60 therapeutic >32) as measured systemically, until distal perfusion is optimal (as manifest by a 'hot foot'), if necessary for several days. The catheter can be used for a distal arteriogram (with digital subtraction angiography) and causes no bleeding on ultimate withdrawal.

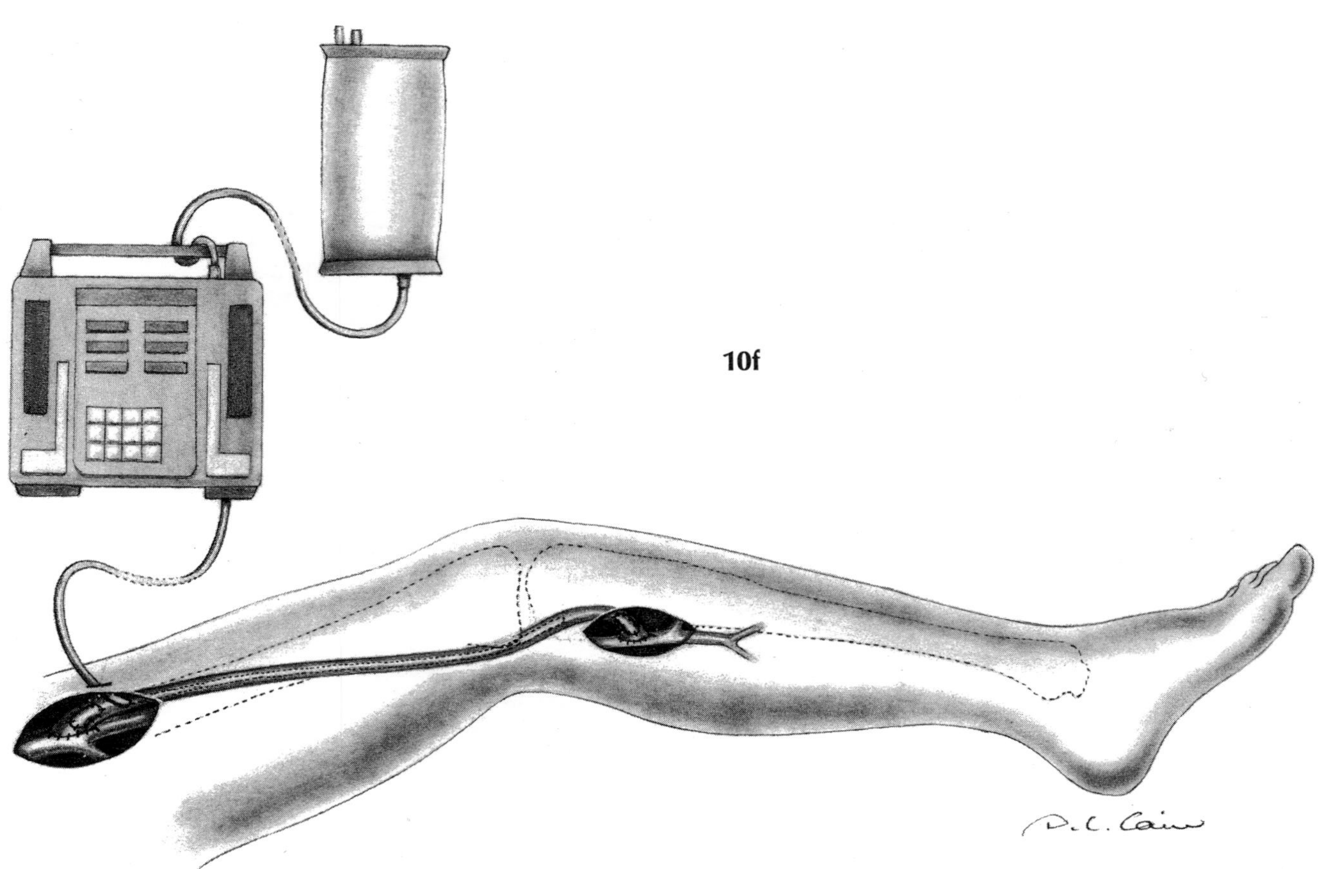

10f

Acknowledgements

The illustrations for this chapter were drawn by Deirdre Cain.

References

Bernhard, V. M., Parent, F. N., Hunter, G. C. and McIntyre, K. E. (1991). The pneumatic tourniquet as an alternative to clamps for anastomoses below the knee. *Journal of Cardiovascular Surgery* (Suppl.) **32**, 65.

Finn, W. R., Flanigan, D. P., Verta, M. J., Bergan, J. J. and Yao, J. S. T. (1980). Sequential femoro-tibial bypass for severe limb ischaemia. *Surgery* **88**, 357.

Greenhalgh, R. M. (1980). Profunda femoris reconstruction with and without distal bypass. In *Operative Techniques in Vascular Surgery* 1st edn. Bergan, J. J. and Yao, J. S. T., eds. London and Orlando: Grune and Stratton, p. 189.

Linton, R. R. and Wild, W. L. (1970). *Surgery* **67**, 234.

Miller, J. H. (1993). Partial replacement of an infected arterial graft by a new prosthetic polytetrafluoroethylene segment: A new therapeutic option. *Journal of Vascular Surgery* **17**, 546.

Miller, J. H., Foreman, R. K., Ferguson, L. and Faris, I. (1984). Interposition vein cuff for anastomosis of prosthesis to small artery. *Australia and New Zealand Journal of Surgery* **54**, 283.

Miller, J. H., Allen, D., Berce, M. B., Benveniste, G. B., Faris, I. F., Ferguson, L. J., Jury, P. J., Raptis, S. and Quigley, F. (1991). Profunda femoris artery as outflow using PTFE with vein cuff. *Journal of Cardiovascular Surgery* (Suppl.) **32**, 96.

Morris, G. E., Raptis, S., Miller, J. H. and Faris, I. B. (1993). *European Journal of Vascular Surgery* **7**, 329.

Siegman, F. A. (1979). Use of venous cuff for graft anastomosis. *Surgery, Gynecology and Obstetrics* **148**, 930.

Suggs, W. D., Henriques, H. F. and DePalma, R. G. (1988). Vein cuff interposition prevents juxta-anastomotic neointimal hyperplasia. *Annals of Surgery* June, 717.

Taylor, R. S., Loh, A., McFarlane, R. J., Cox, M. and Chester, J. F. (1992). Improved technique for polytetrafluoroethylene bypass grafting: long term results using anastomotic vein patches. *British Journal of Surgery* **79**, 348.

Tyrrell, M. R. and Wolfe, J. H. N. (1991). New prosthetic venous collar anastomotic technique: combining the best of other procedures. *British Journal of Surgery* **78**, 1016.

Tyrrell, M. R., Clark, G. H. and Wolfe, J. H. N. (1989). Consideration of the mechanical properties of the distal anastomosis of PTFE may improve patency rates. *Journal of Cardiovascular Surgery* (Suppl.) **30**, 91.

Tyrrell, M. R., Grigg, M. J. and Wolfe, J. H. N. (1989). Is arterial reconstruction to the ankle worthwhile in the absence of autogenous vein? *European Journal of Vascular Surgery* **3**, 429.

Vladimirovich, K. V. (1985). Plasty of proximal anastomosis in femoro-popliteal reconstruction with a small autovenous graft. *International Congress of Angiology, Athens* (Abstracts), 50.

Repair of the failing femorodistal graft

JOHN H. N. WOLFE MS, FRCS

Consultant Vascular Surgeon and Honorary Senior Lecturer, St Mary's Hospital Medical School, London, UK; Consultant Vascular Surgeon and Honorary Senior Lecturer, Royal Postgraduate Medical School, Hammersmith Hospital, London, UK

PETER R. TAYLOR MA, FRCS

Consultant Vascular Surgeon, Guy's Hospital Medical School, London, UK

Introduction

In recent years the number of bypass grafts performed to the more distal arteries in the lower limb has increased considerably. Despite experience and improved operative techniques, the failure of these arterial grafts continues to be a problem of considerable magnitude. Reported failure rates of femoropopliteal and femorocrural grafts range between 20 and 50% at 5 years. Brewster and colleagues (1983a) showed that 65% of graft failures occurred within the first post-operative year, and that 79% of grafts occlusions occur within 2 years of operation.

Graft failures can be divided into three groups, based on the postoperative time interval:

1. *Immediate failures.* These occur within 1 month and are almost invariably attributable to errors of surgical technique or judgement. Such failures can be minimized by careful objective intraoperative assessment with Doppler probes and arteriography (Whittemore *et al.*, 1980).
2. *Early failures.* This group accounts for the majority of graft failures and spans the time period from 1 month to 1 year following operation. This group may benefit particularly from graft surveillance techniques (Wolfe and McPherson, 1987).
3. *Late failures.* These occur after 1 year and are usually secondary to progression of the original atherosclerotic disease process. Although graft surveillance may be useful, the failure rate at this stage is only 25% per annum for vein grafts and 7% per annum for prosthetic grafts (Berkowitz *et al.*, 1981).

Techniques of graft surveillance

1. *Serial ankle Doppler pressure measurements.* Initial reports using this technique were encouraging (Taylor and Fox, 1977). However, more recent studies show that if this method is used alone, many graft stenoses are missed (Wolfe *et al.*, 1987; McShane *et al.*, 1987; Moody *et al.*, 1989).
2. *Serial intravenous digital subtraction angiography.* This is a reliable method for detecting graft stenoses, providing that the patient has a good cardiac output. However, patient compliance remains a drawback despite the introduction of non-ionic contrast medium.
3. *Serial duplex Doppler assessment.* This non-invasive method can detect graft stenoses before they become haemodynamically significant. Graft flow measurements are inaccurate (Grigg *et al.*, 1988), but changes in peak systolic velocity of 50% or more within a 2-cm length of graft suggest the presence of a stenosis (Grigg, Nicolaides and Wolfe, 1988).

If patients are monitored regularly for the first year, approximately 20% of grafts will develop stenoses (Wolfe *et al.*, 1987; Cohen *et al.*, 1986). However, not all stenoses will be haemodynamically significant. Our current policy is to monitor their progression. When the change in velocity suggests a 50% reduction in diameter (equivalent to a 75% reduction in cross-sectional area), we intervene, since we believe that the graft is at risk of occlusion from a haemodynamically significant stenosis. Whittemore *et al.* (1980) have shown that the results of thrombectomy are much worse compared with those of graft repair before occlusion. Not all stenoses progress to become significant, and in approximately half no progression is seen so that intervention is not indicated. Difficulties in imaging may be encountered when the graft is very deep to the skin, such as the area immediately adjacent to a popliteal anastomosis. Distal grafts to the crural vessels are more superficial and reliable recordings can be obtained. Colour flow Doppler imaging may be useful in this regard since the deeper grafts are more easily identified (Buth *et al.*, 1991). This policy of graft surveillance leads to a number of re-operations on arterial bypass grafts. These secondary procedures can be classified into the following three categories: (1) inflow problems, (2) graft problems, and (3) outflow problems.

Secondary procedures

Inflow problems

1a & b

In the presence of ipsilateral iliac artery occlusion, vein grafts may remain patent even though clinically they do not pulsate (*a*). In these patients an appropriate procedure is performed to improve the inflow of the graft. This may include a femorofemoral cross-over graft, iliofemoral cross-over graft (*b*), unilateral iliofemoral graft or an aortobifemoral graft. The upper end of the graft is anastomosed, end-to-side, to the new graft using the usual anastomotic technique. There is no purpose in interposing parent artery between the two grafts. Clamp injury may damage the common femoral artery, but in our experience this is rare (Grigg, Nicolaides and Wolfe, 1988).

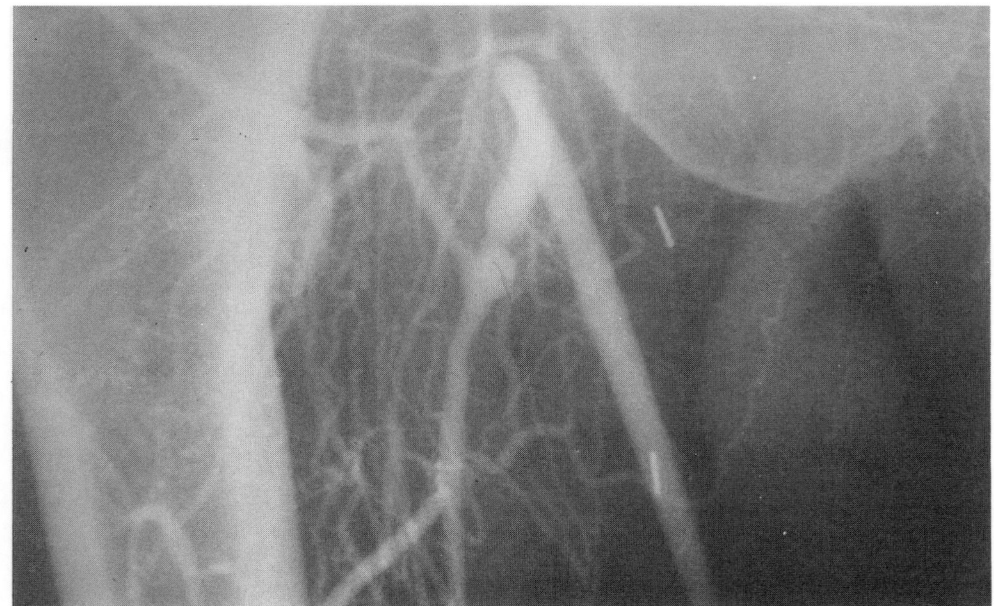

1a

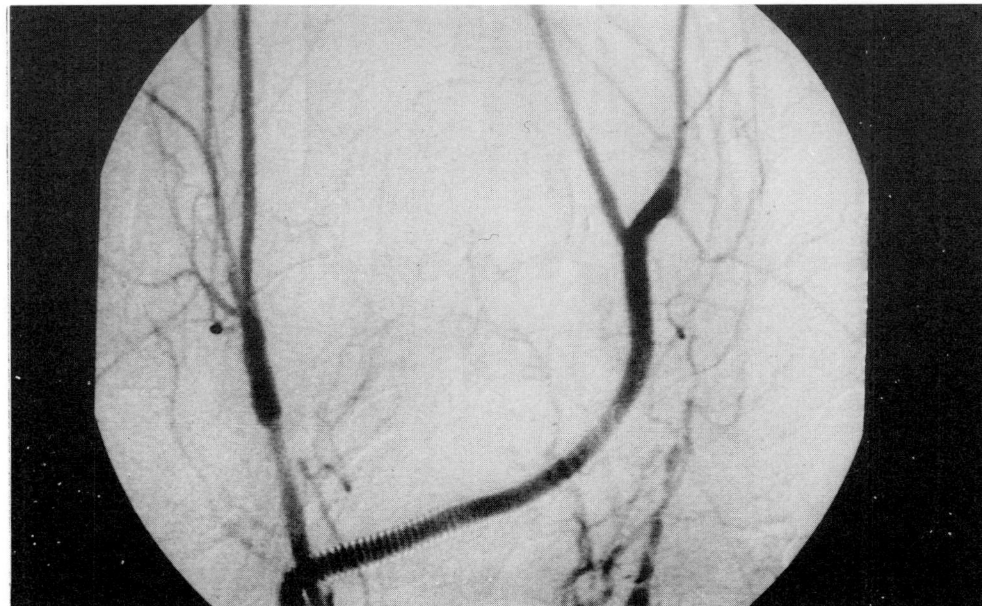

1b

2a & b

A more common problem is aggressive myointimal hyperplasia occurring at the site of femoral endarterectomy performed to facilitate the proximal anastomosis (*a*). This can be repaired with a vein patch (*b*) across the stenosed segment.

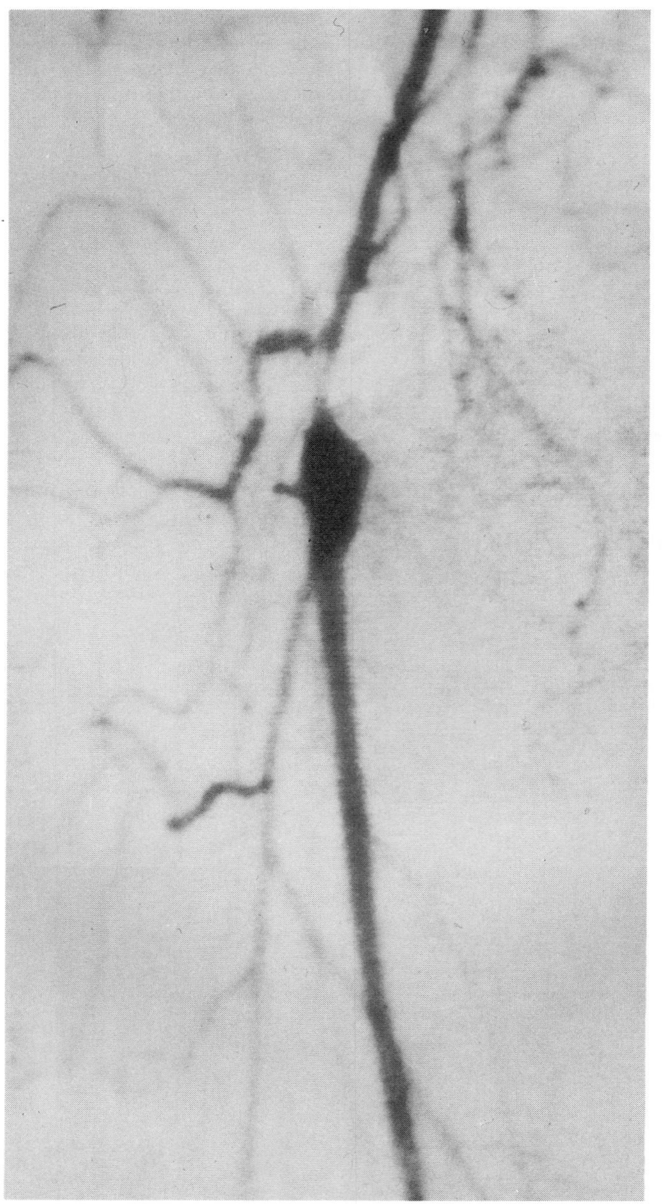

2a

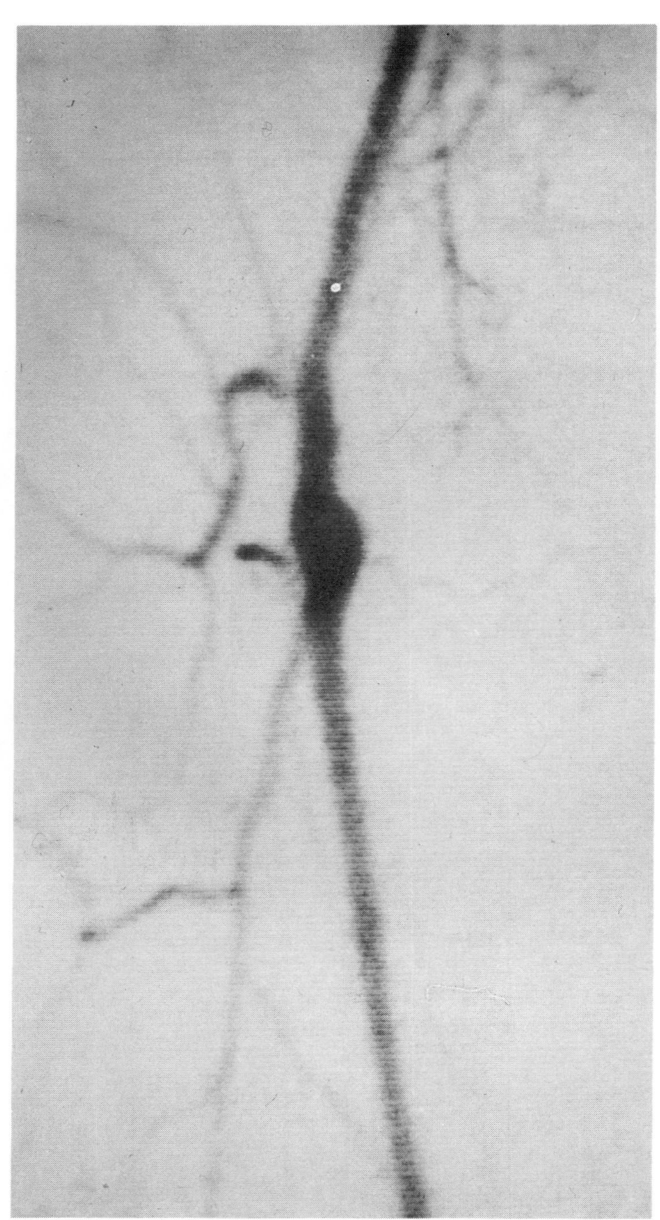

2b

Graft problems

3 & 4

Short fibrotic stenoses occurring in vein grafts are frequently related to valve cusps. These can be treated by either vein patch (taken from either the arm or the short saphenous vein) or percutaneous balloon angioplasty. However, balloon angioplasty is not as successful as surgery (Whittemore *et al.*, 1980); Cohen *et al.*, 1986; Brewster *et al.*, 1983b; Veith *et al.*, 1984), and assessing the discrepancy in results between three centres it became apparent that stenoses >2 cm should be treated surgically (Taylor *et al.*, 1990). The use of a 2.5 mm cardiac balloon may improve results since it is more difficult to disrupt vein grafts with these small, softer balloons. We now rarely perform patches, preferring to interpose a short vein segment (*vide infra*).

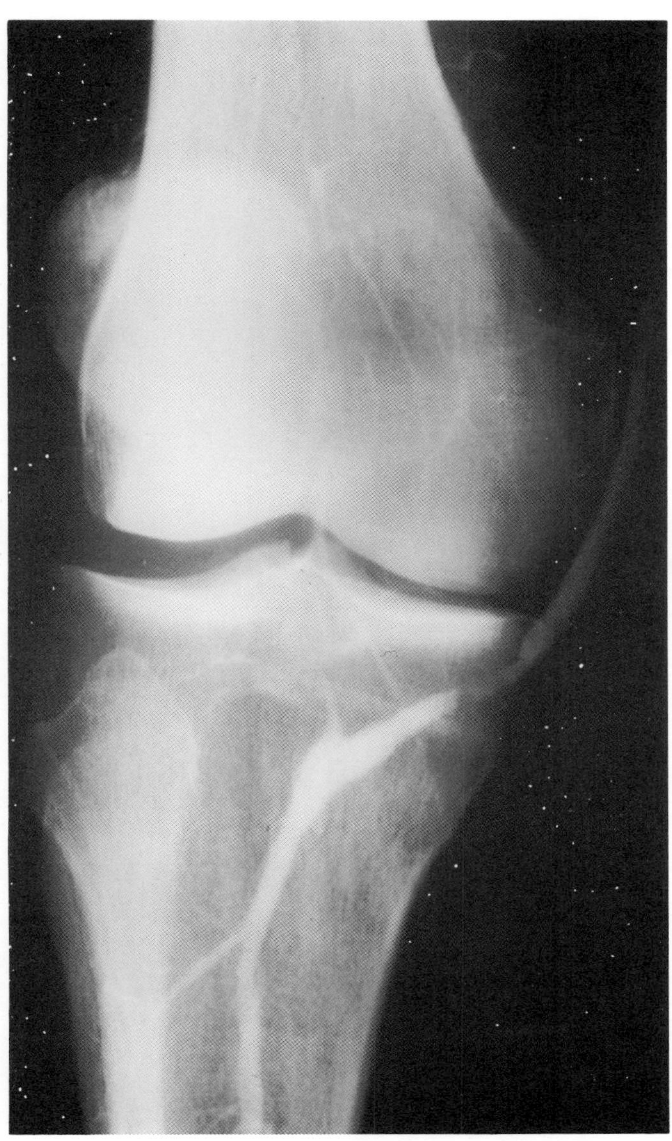

3

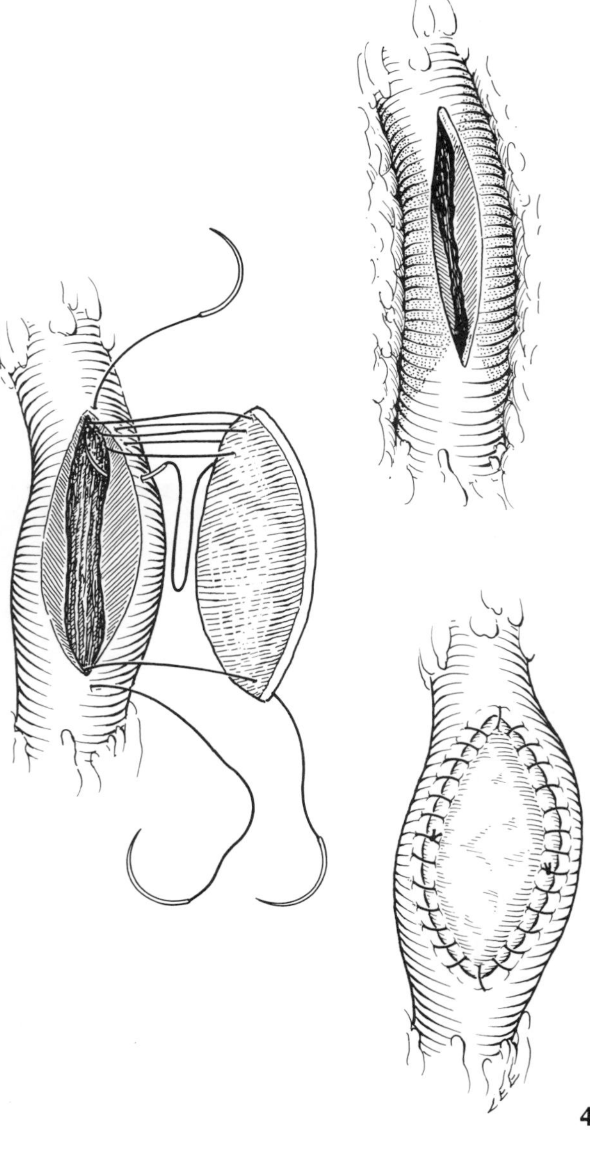

4

5a & b

Longer stenoses should be treated operatively by using a 'jump' graft to bypass the stenosed segment. End-to-end venovenous anastomoses give better flow characteristics and the use of a long oblique anastomosis using 7/0 Prolene protects against stenosis. When long or multiple segments of graft are affected by a stenotic process, surgery is of little value.

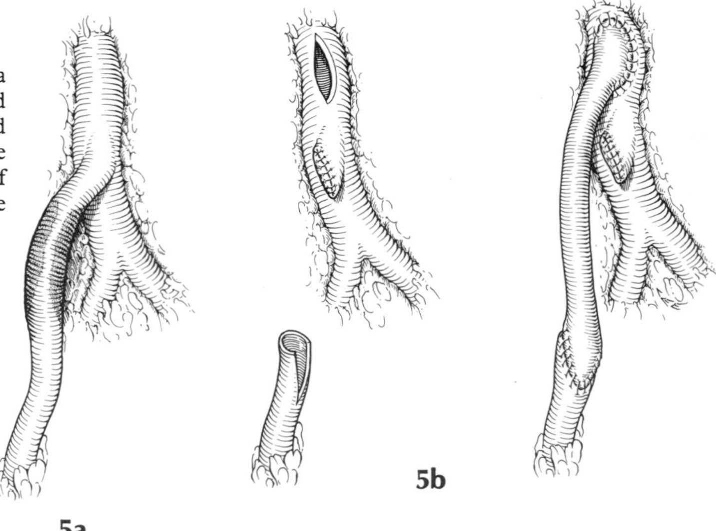

5a

5b

6

The right femoropopliteal graft is older but the left has developed a long segment of stenosis and myointimal hyperplasia. It is unlikely that intervention will assist this graft.

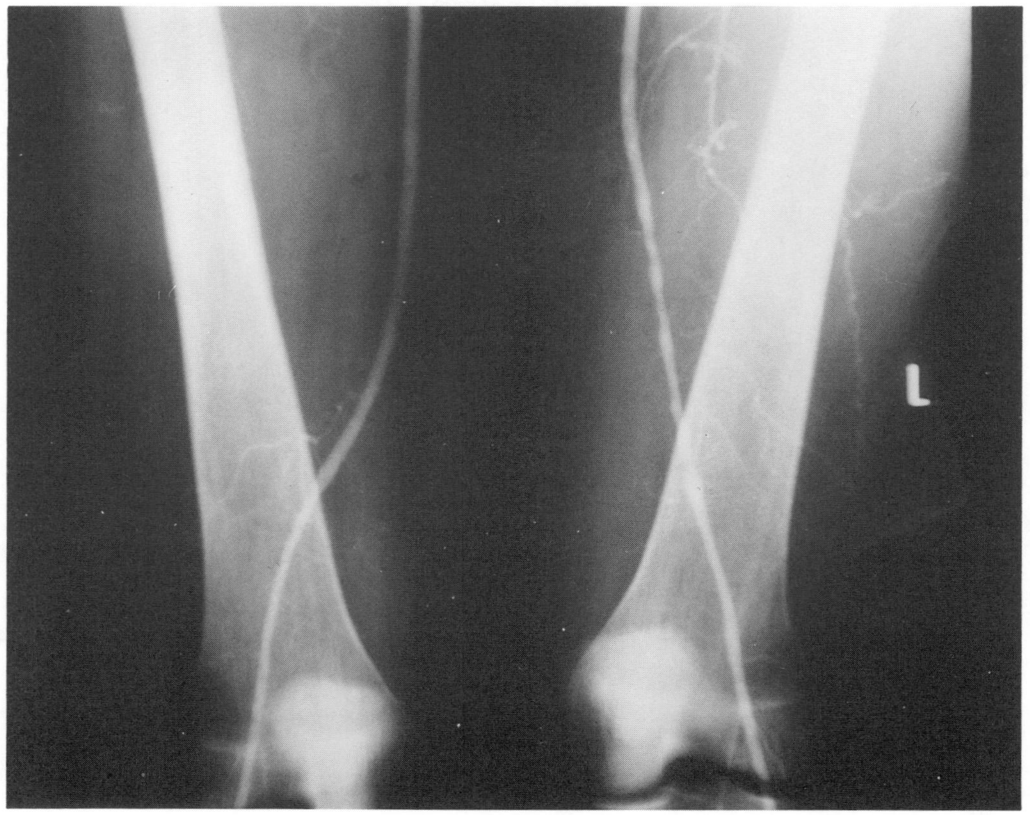

6

Outflow problems

7a, b & 8

We have had some success with balloon angioplasty in treating 'web' stenoses close to the distal anastomosis, but others are more sceptical (Thompson *et al.*, in press). More commonly we perform a bypass 'jump' graft from the graft to a crural vessel distal to the stenosis using arm vein or short saphenous vein. The graft is tunnelled subcutaneously. The dissection of the distal vessel is relatively straightforward providing the previous operating field can be avoided.

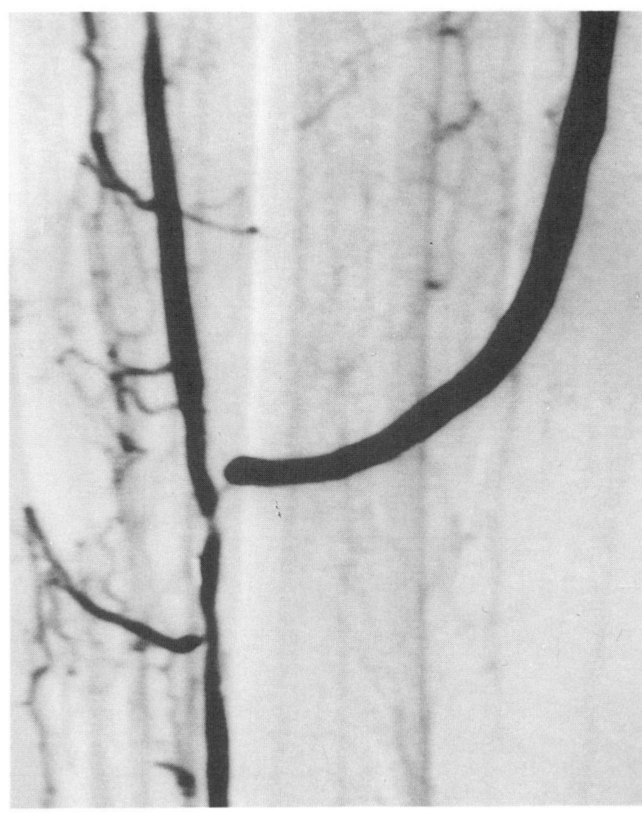

7a

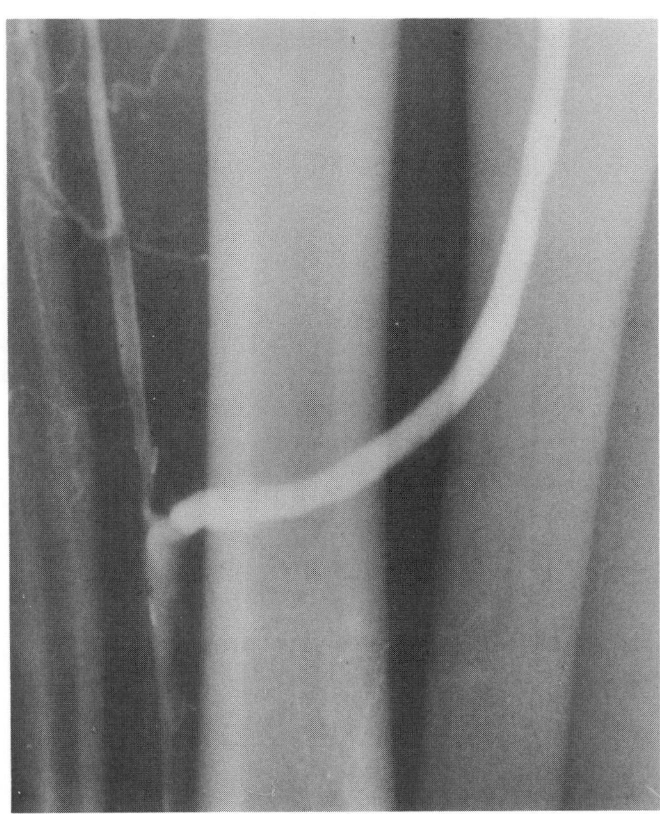

7b

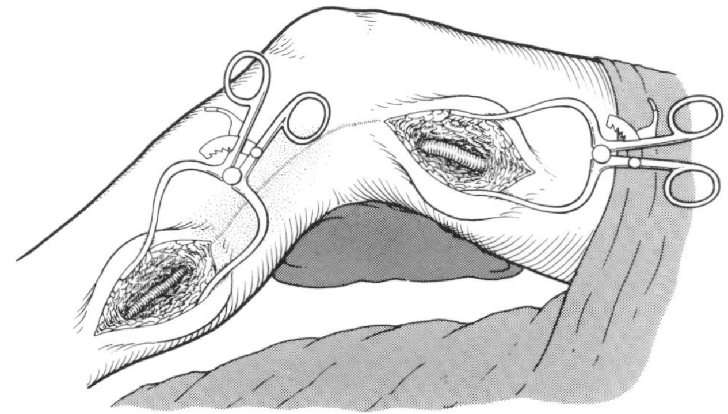

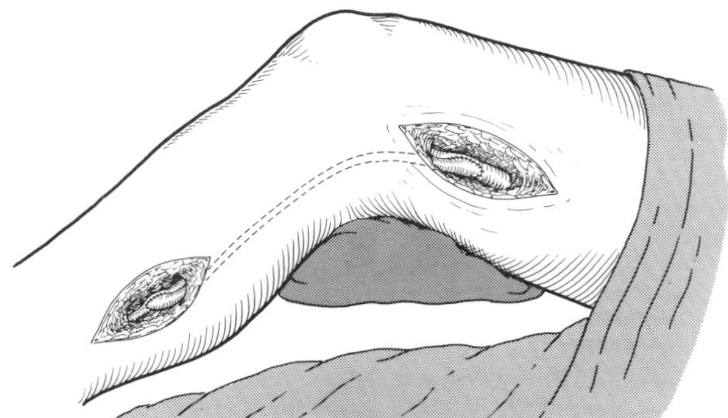

8

9

Except under rare circumstances, no attempt should be made to dissect out the previous anastomosis. The dense scar tissue resulting from the previous operation makes this a procedure fraught with hazard. When it is necessary to dissect a graft from this scar tissue, it can be extremely difficult to visualize or palpate, and a hand-held Doppler probe placed within a sterile operating glove may be invaluable in localizing the graft.

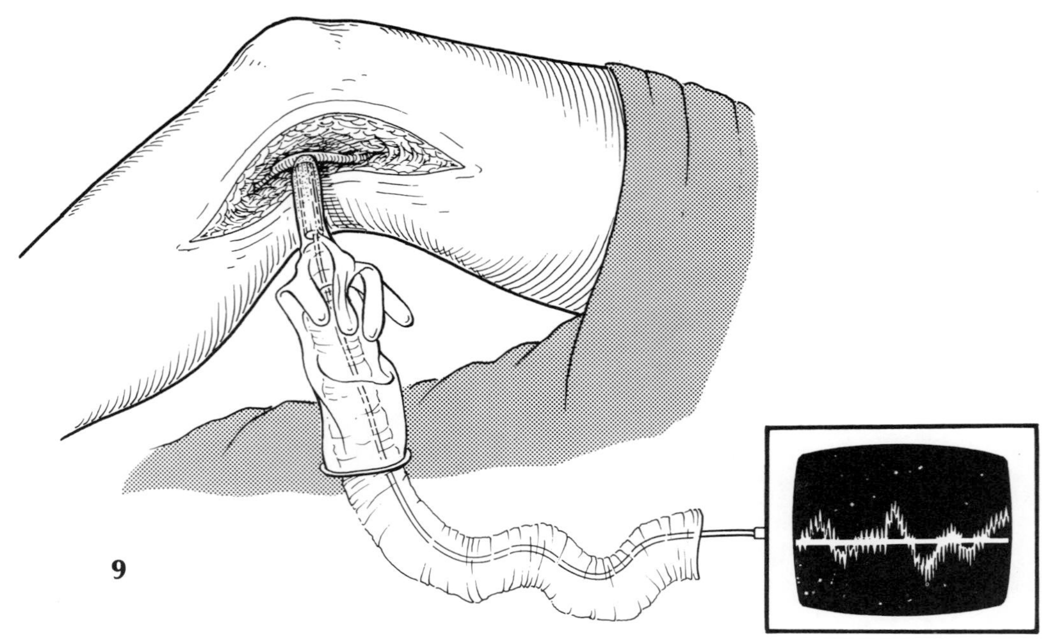

9

References

Berkowitz, H. D., Hobbs, C. L., Roberts, B., Freiman, D., Oleaga, J. and Ring, E. (1981). Value of routine vascular laboratory studies to identify vein graft stenoses. *Surgery* **90**, 971.

Brewster, D. L., La Salle, A. J., Robison, J. C., Stranghorn, E. C. and Darling, R. C. (1983a). Factors affecting patency of femoro-popliteal grafts. *Surgery, Gynecology and Obstetrics* **157**, 437.

Brewster, D. C., La Salle, A. J., Robison, J. G. *et al.* (1983b). Femoro-popliteal graft failures: Clinical consequences and success of secondary reconstructions. *Archives of Surgery* **118**, 1043.

Buth, J., Disselhoff, B., Sommerling, C., *et al.* (1991). Colour flow duplex criteria for grading stenoses in infrainguinal vein grafts. *Journal of Vascular Surgery* **14**, 716.

Cohen, J. R., Mannick, J. A., Couch, N. P. and Whittemore, A. D. (1986). Recognition and management of impending vein graft failure. *Archives of Surgery* **121**, 758.

Grigg, M. J., Nicolaides, A. N. and Wolfe, J. H. N. (1988). Femoro-distal bypass graft stenoses. *British Journal of Surgery* **75**, 737.

Grigg, M. J., Wolfe, J. H. N., Tovan, A. and Nicolaides, A. N. (1988). The reliability of duplex haemodynamic measurements in the assessment of femoro-distal grafts. *European Journal of Vascular Surgery* **2**, 171.

McShane, M. D., Gazzard, W.H., Clifford, P. C., Hacking, C. N., Fairhurst, J. J., Humphries, K. N., Birch, S. J., Webster, J. H. H. and Chant, A. (1987). Duplex ultrasound assessment and femoro-distal grafts – correlation with angioplasty. *European Journal of Vascular Surgery* **1**, 409.

Moody, P., DeCossart, L. M., Douglas, H. M., *et al.* (1989). Asymptomatic strictures in femoropopliteal grafts. *European Journal of Vascular Surgery* **3**, 389.

Taylor, P., Gould, D., Harris, P., *et al.* (1990). Balloon dilatation of graft stenoses – reasons for failure. *British Journal of Surgery* 7, 371.

Taylor, R. S. and Fox, N. D. (1977). Ultrasonic prediction of graft failure. *Journal of Cardiovascular Surgery* **18**, 309.

Thompson, J., McShane, M., Gazzard, V., Webster, J. and Chant, A. (in press). Intervention for graft stenoses: Experience following 206 femoral-distal reconstructions. *British Journal of Surgery*.

Veith, F. J., Weiser, R. K., Gupta, S. K., Ascer, E., Scher, L. A., Samson, R. H., White Flores, S. A. and Sprayregen, S. (1984). Diagnosis and management of failing lower extremity arterial reconstructions prior to graft occlusion. *Journal of Cardiovascular Surgery* **25**, 381.

Whittemore, A. D., Clowes, A. W., Couch, N. P. and Mannick, J. A. (1980). Secondary femoro-popliteal reconstruction. *Annals of Surgery* **193**, 35.

Wolfe, J. H. N. and McPherson, G. A. D. (1987). The failing femoro-distal graft. *European Journal of Vascular Surgery* **1**, 295.

Wolfe, J. H. N., Thomas, M. L., Jamieson, C. W., Browse, N. L., Burnard, K. G., and Rutt, D. L. (1987). The early diagnosis of femoro-popliteal graft stenoses, a prospective one year follow up. *British Journal of Surgery* **74**, 268.

The use of glutaraldehyde-stabilized umbilical vein for lower extremity reconstruction

HERBERT DARDIK MD, FACS

Chief, General and Vascular Surgery, Englewood Hospital & Medical Center, Englewood, New Jersey, USA; Clinical Professor of Surgery, Mt. Sinai Medical Center, New York City, USA

Introduction

Significant developments in the technology for performing lower limb revascularization procedures have eclipsed the historical importance and continued current value of synthetic materials for lower extremity bypass. Autologous venous tissue is the bypass material of choice and should be employed wherever possible. My personal experience supports this view with availability and utilization of autologous tissue for arterial conduits in the majority of cases, exceeding 80%. Is there any role for synthetics in lower limb bypass procedures, particularly those terminating at infrapopliteal levels? The answer, in my opinion, is decidedly yes.

Based on our experience with more than 1200 glutaraldehyde-stabilized umbilical vein graft implantations in the lower extremity, we have recognized the special technical requirements essential for the successful implantation of this graft material. The results of vascular surgical reconstruction depend on many factors including precise selection of cases, classification and staging of the disease process, and judicious application of appropriate therapeutic modalities. We previously discussed some of these factors with regard to selecting patients for vascular reconstruction of the lower extremities (Dardik *et al.*, 1975; Dardik, Ibrahim and Dardik, 1979). However, once the appropriate patient and a particular procedure have been selected, the technical expertise and the intraoperative judgement exercised by the surgeon are essential to achieving long-lasting success.

Graft selection

The glutaraldehyde-stabilized umbilical vein graft (Biograft®, Biovascular, Inc., St. Paul, Minnesota) is an appropriate choice of graft material in the absence of a suitable autologous saphenous vein or if circumstances militate against its use, such as limited life expectancy of the patient. Our experience over the past 20 years with glutaraldehyde-stabilized umbilical veins has convinced us of its excellent qualities and applicability for lower extremity bypass reconstructions, yet being aware of its deficiencies, notably the increasing likelihood for biodegradation after implantation for 5 or more years (Dardik *et al.*, 1988). Recent experience has shown a dramatic decrease in this problem, suggesting that the improved methods for manufacture, storage and preparation of the currently employed UV graft are responsible.

The most important factor governing graft selection is the required length. This is determined by intraoperative measurement of the distance between the proximal and distal anastomoses with the extremity in full extension. It is obviously prudent to add an additional few centimetres to compensate for any error in measurement and to allow for better trimming of the graft at the anastomotic areas. In the absence of a single long graft long enough to reach from the proximal to the distal site, composite grafts are perfectly acceptable, whether they are constructed at the time of surgery or presutured by the manufacturer. We generally employ grafts with 5 mm diameters for all types of reconstruction although tapered 6 to 5 or other variations may be appropriate in select circumstances.

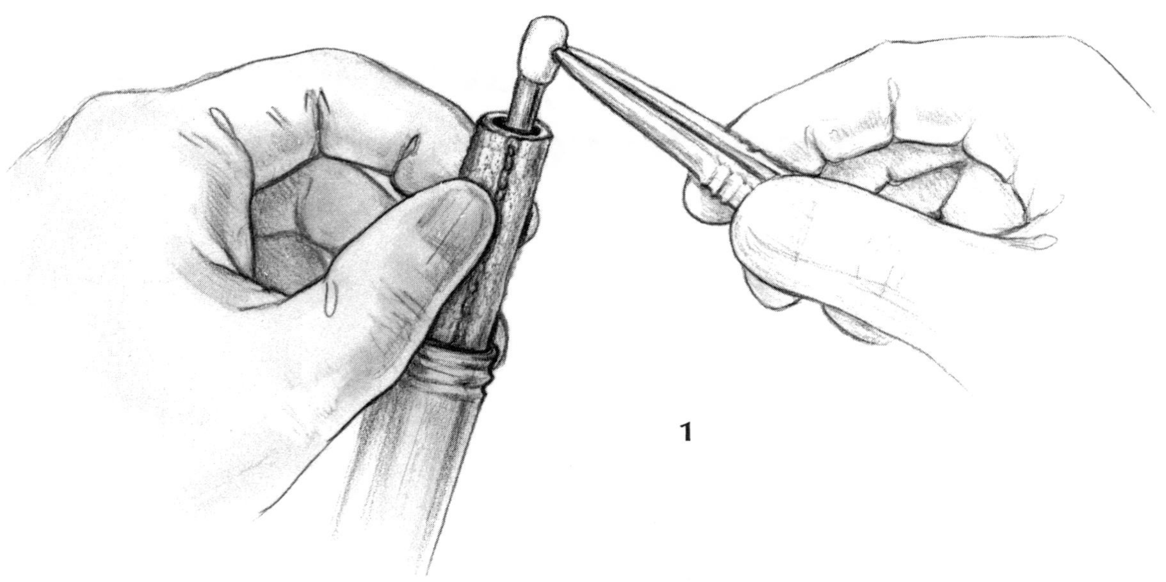

1

Graft preparation

Irrigation

All umbilical vein grafts must be thoroughly washed prior to implantation. Our current method is to soak the graft for 3 to 5 minutes in a low molecular weight dextran solution followed by a brief rinse with dilute heparin solution. It is possible that these manoeuvres are superfluous in that alcohol and aldehyde residues are extremely low but total omission of the irrigation process has not yet been attempted.

1 & 2

The graft is first removed from its container in an area away from the irrigation basin and is gently compressed manually from above downwards in order to milk out excess fluids.

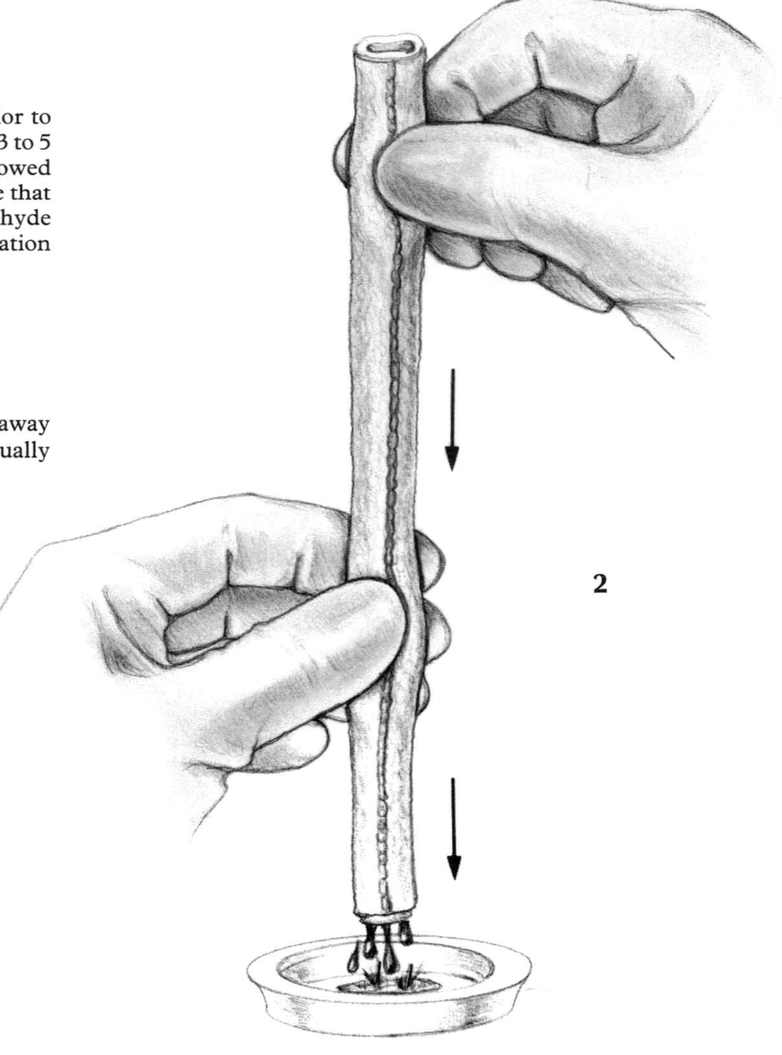

2

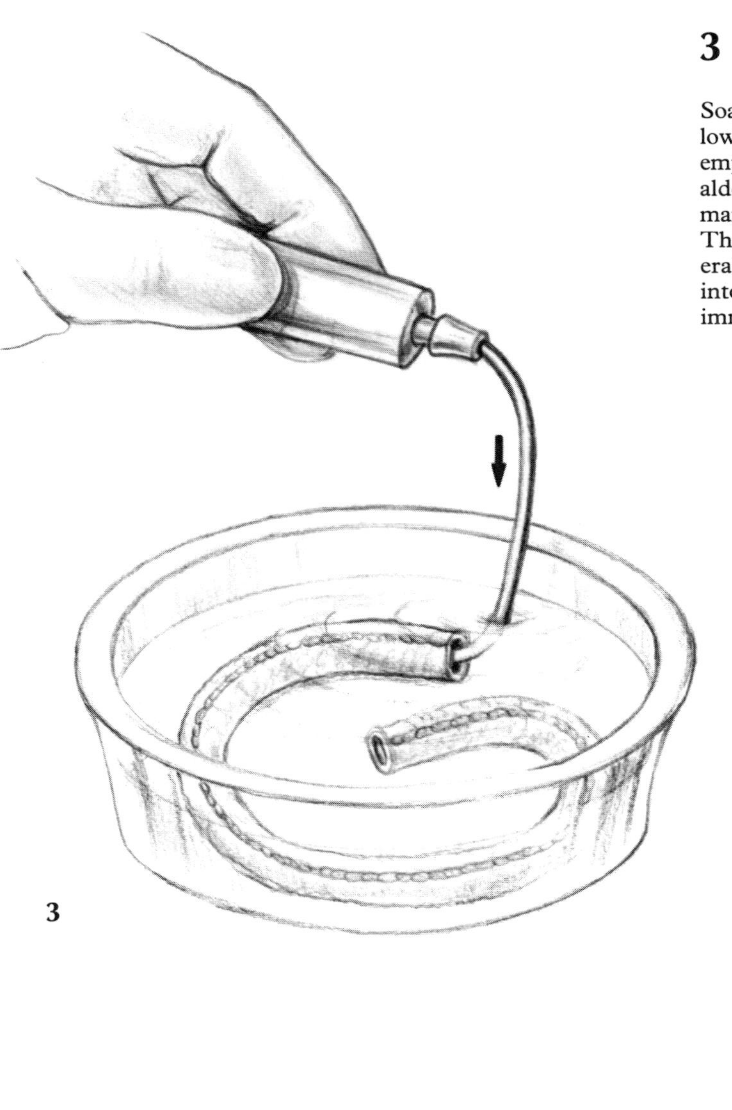

3

3

Soaking the graft in a basin containing 500 ml of heparinized low molecular weight dextran (LMWD) is the method employed to dilute and wash out residual alcohol and glutaraldehyde. It is important to avoid airlocks in the graft by manual irrigations at intervals during the 3 to 5 minute soak. This is done most conveniently by the scrub nurse with several 50-ml aliquots of dilute LMWD solution injected directly into the graft via a soft rubber catheter as the graft is immersed in the soaking basin.

4

4

After the actual irrigation or soaking is completed, several millilitres of diluted heparin solution are instilled directly into the graft and simply flushed from its lumen. The use of undiluted concentrated heparin is no longer practised.

The operation

Anaesthesia/analgesia

The anaesthetic management of patients requiring lower limb revascularization should be performed by physicians skilled in caring for the diverse medical problems that are indigenous to this patient population. Although general anaesthesia is frequently employed and is even desired by many patients, our preference is for epidural anaesthesia. This method is very effective, is acceptable to patients after an explanation of the procedure, and it avoids many of the potential debilities associated with inhalation anaesthesia. Postoperative injections of analgesics into the epidural space provided prolonged pain-free periods, thereby avoiding many of the undesirable effects of systemic analgesics. Patient controlled anaesthetic techniques are also important alternatives.

Instrumentation, sutures and anastomoses

5a–e

Standard metallic vascular instruments are *not* used to clamp the graft. The umbilical vein graft is fragile and subject to intimal fracture and splitting if excessive pressure, whether manual or instrumental, is applied. We have devised a special clamp ('D' clamp) and to date it appears to function very well in securing vascular occlusion with minimal, if any, trauma. Although special clamps or intraluminal balloon tamponade can be employed, we still prefer either reclamping of the host arterial system or simple digital compression of the graft for vascular control.

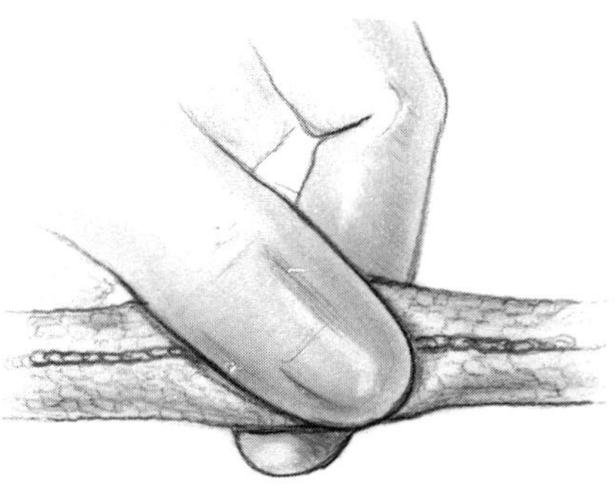

5a Digital control

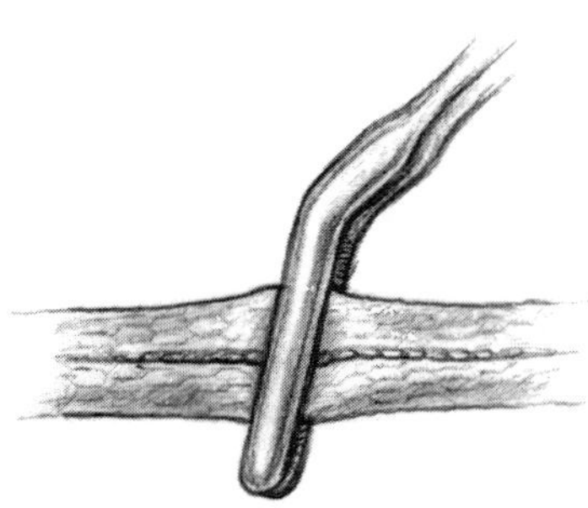

5b "D" clamp

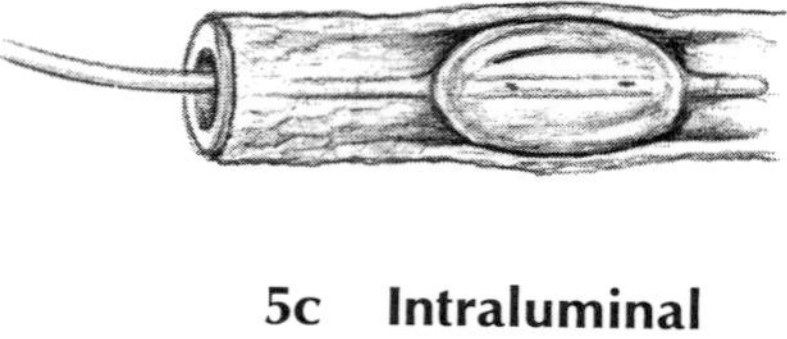

5c Intraluminal

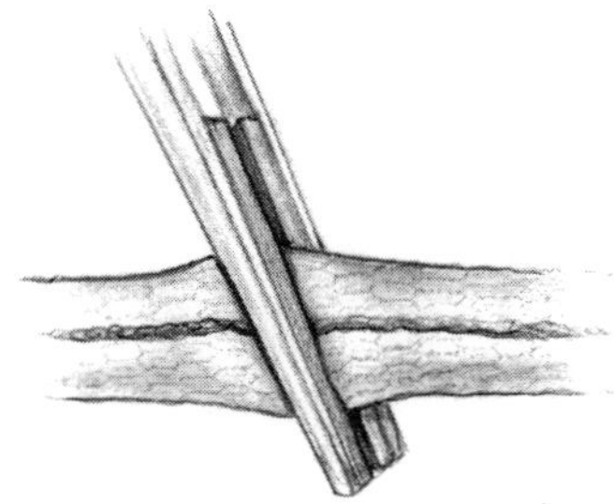

5d Fogarty atraumatic clamp

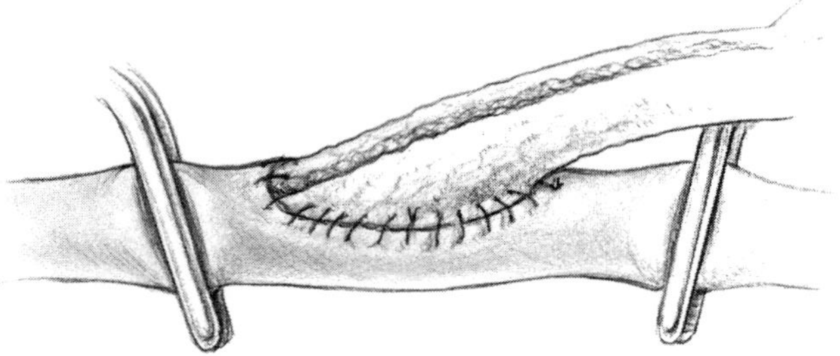

5e Reclamp host artery

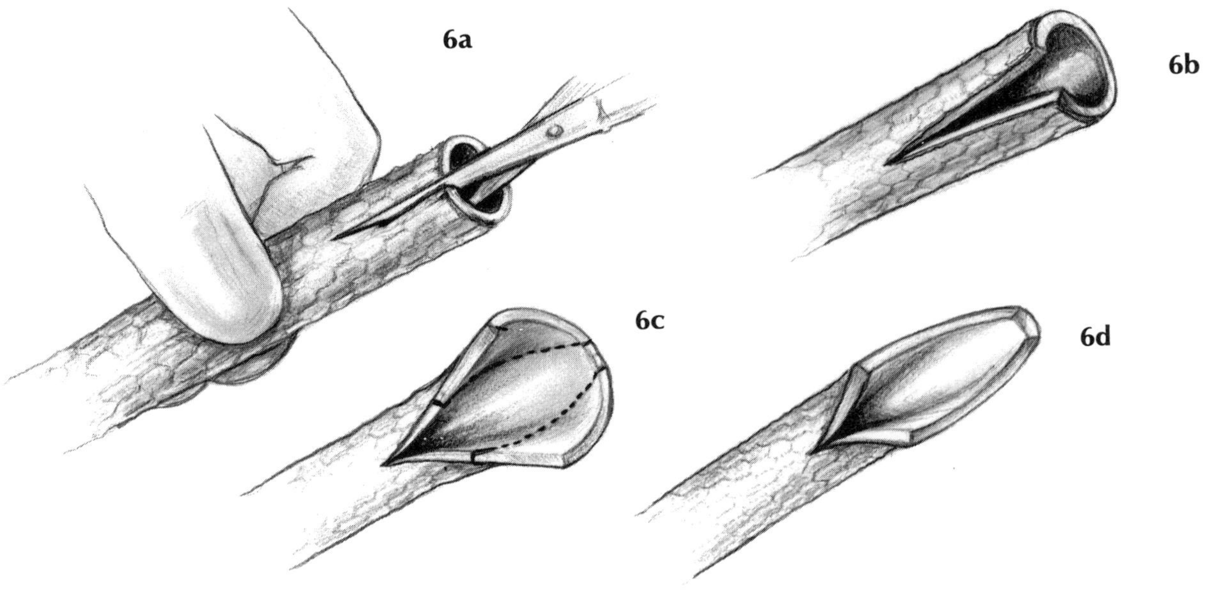

6a–d

Proper trimming of the graft is important and should be done with sharp scissors. The distal end of the graft should have a squared-off taper to avoid sutures tearing through at this point. All arteriotomies should be long, ranging from 20 to 25 mm.

Monofilament polypropylene has been our choice for suture material, but any of the standard types can be used. Number 6/0 is generally employed, but in the distal areas and particularly for the peroneal artery and construction of adjunctive arteriovenous fistulae, 7/0 is recommended to avoid or minimize bleeding through needle holes.

7

Over the past decade, it has become our preference to perform the distal anastomosis first. We have encountered no problem from the graft or the presutured composite anastomosis. Nevertheless, it is perfectly feasible to do the proximal anastomosis first if this is the surgeon's preference. Although we have employed diameters of 4–6 mm, we prefer the 5-mm diameter graft for all reconstructions in the lower extremity.

Umbilical vein grafts are now prepared so that the wall thickness varies from less than 1 mm to slightly more than 1 mm. Thus the surgeon will need some experience to become accustomed to the management and suturing of this wall. It is interesting that no matter how thick the wall may be at the time of implantation, it becomes thinner within a short time thereafter because of resorption of extracellular fluid and compression from intraluminal forces.

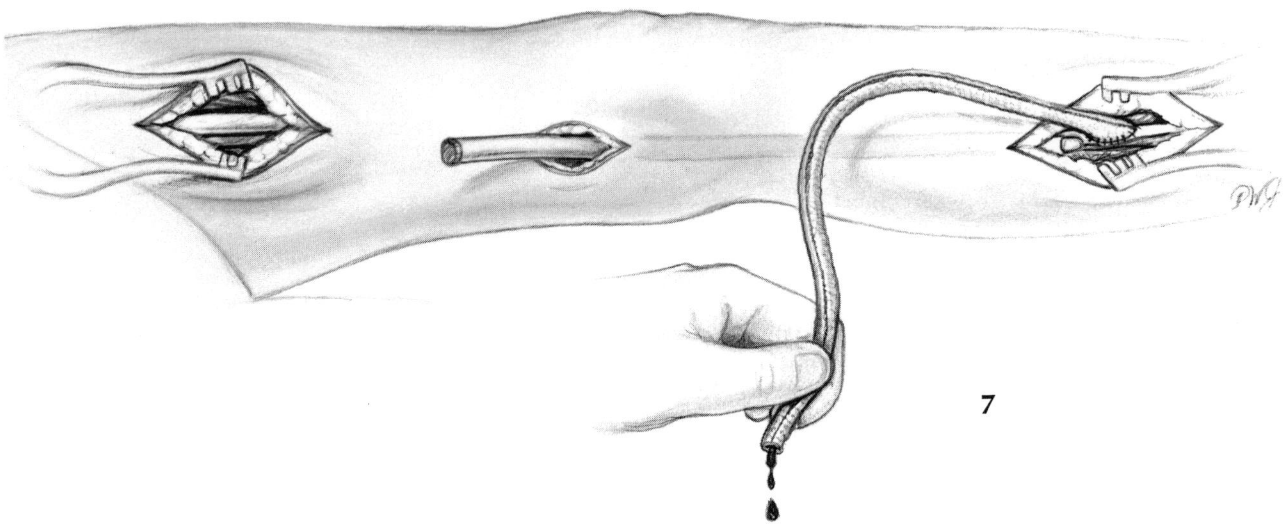

8–11

Interrupted suture technique is advocated at both the proximal heel and distal toe of the distal anastomosis. This avoids shearing of the tissue as well as purse-stringing of the anastomosis. This may help to minimize compliance mismatch. Just prior to completion of the final suture line, calibrated dilators are passed beyond the anastomosis to overcome any clamp compression effects.

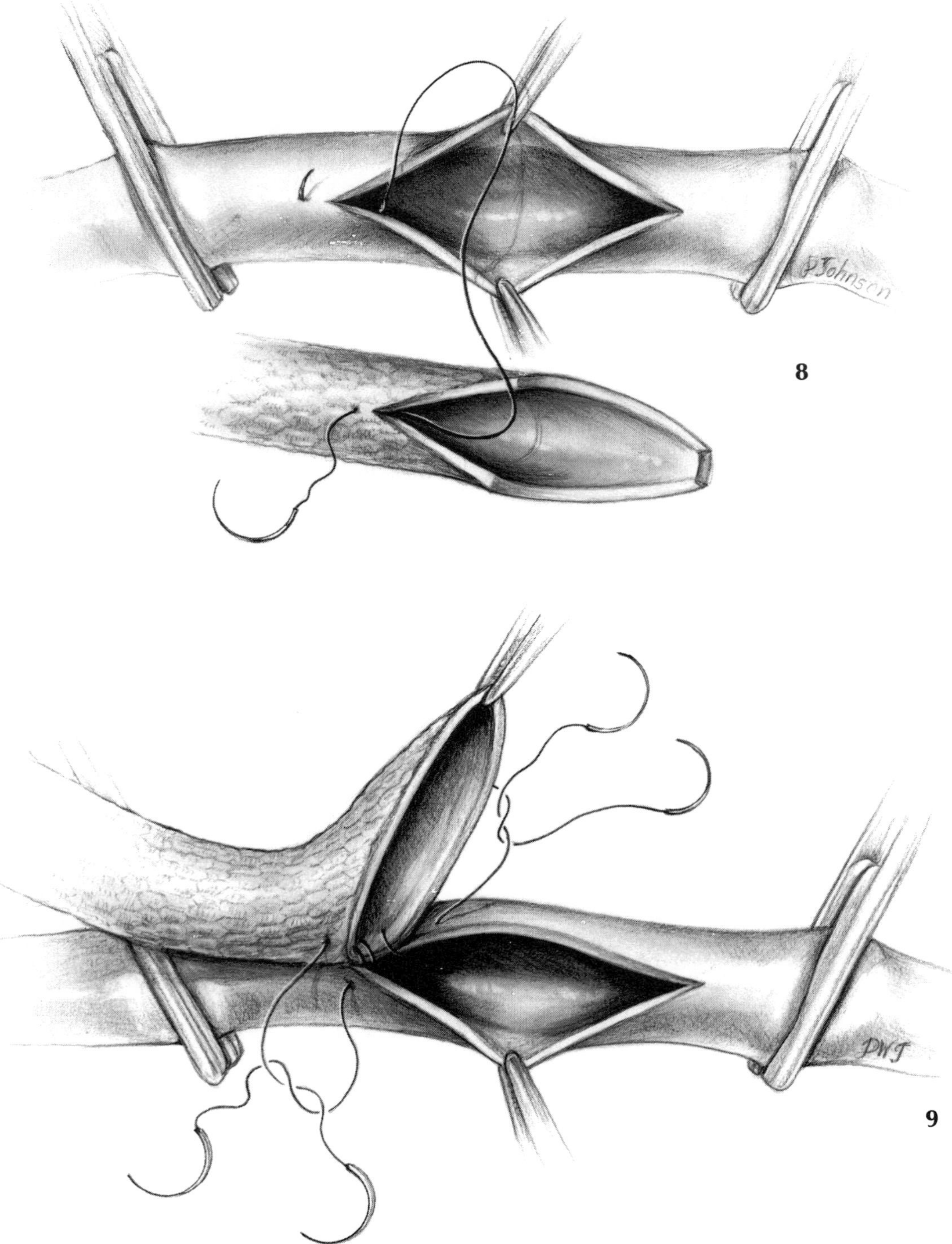

8

9

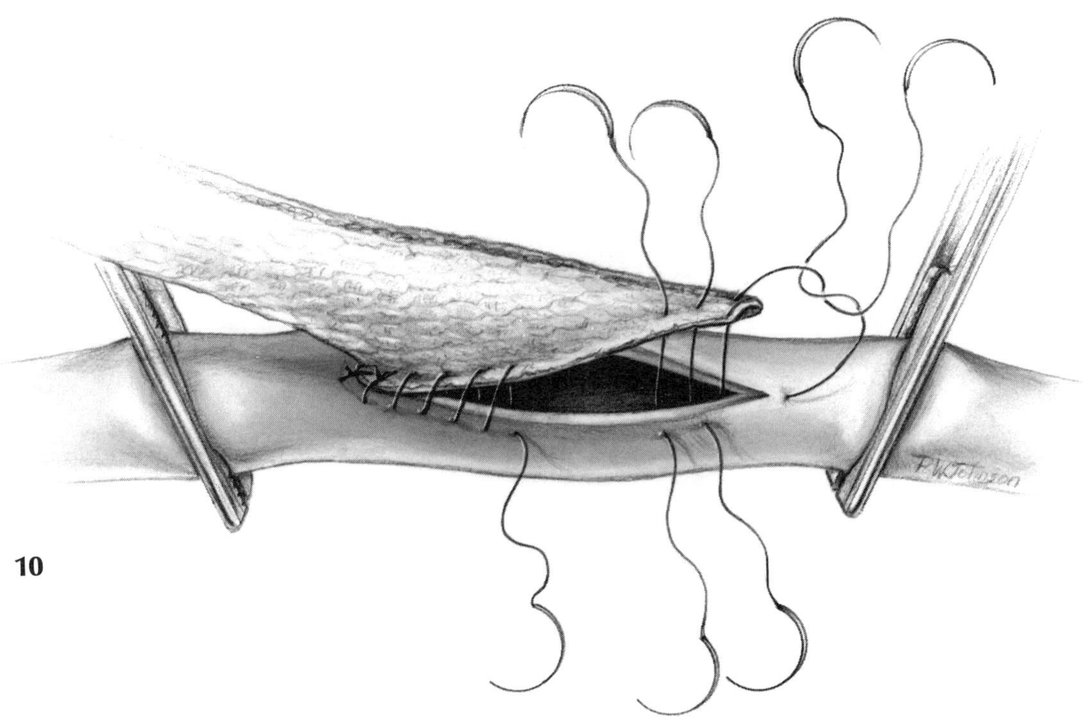

10

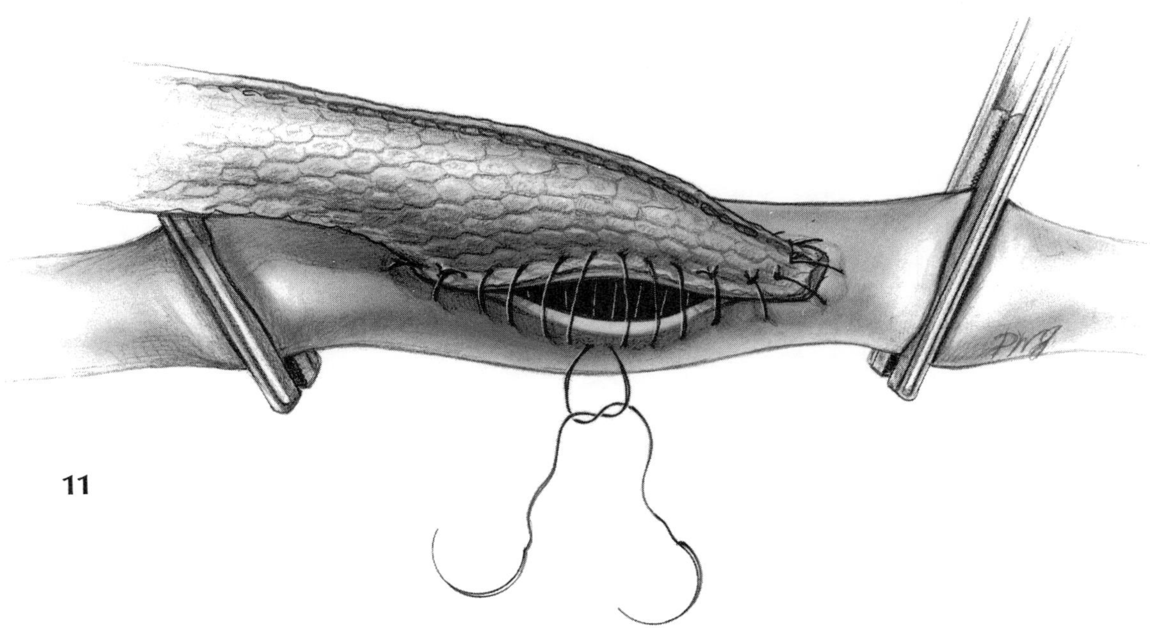

11

12–15

The proximal anastomosis is performed with a continuous technique. The 'parachute' method is particularly helpful at the heel and toe areas.

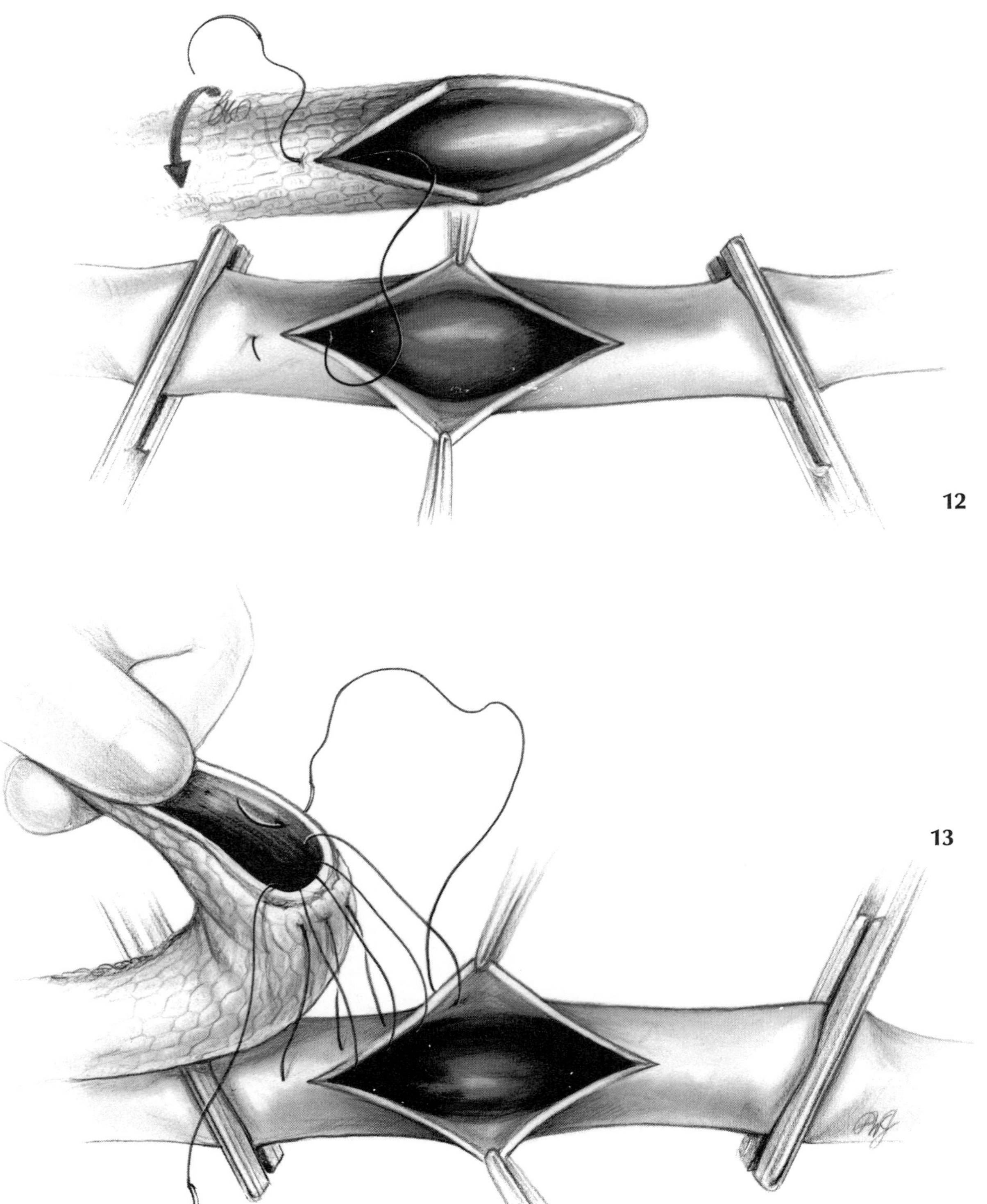

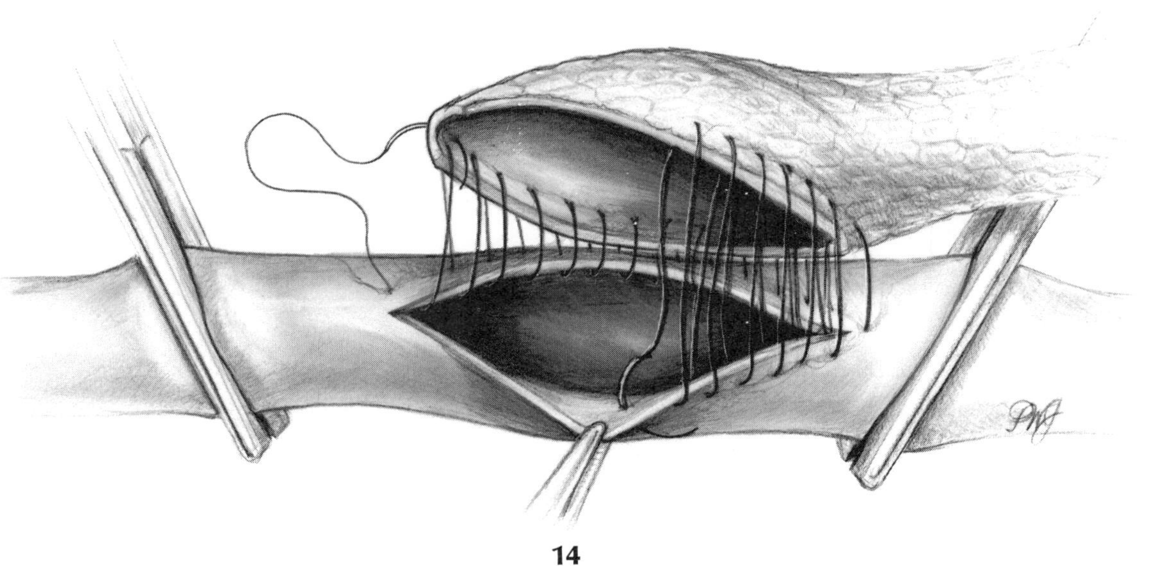

14

15

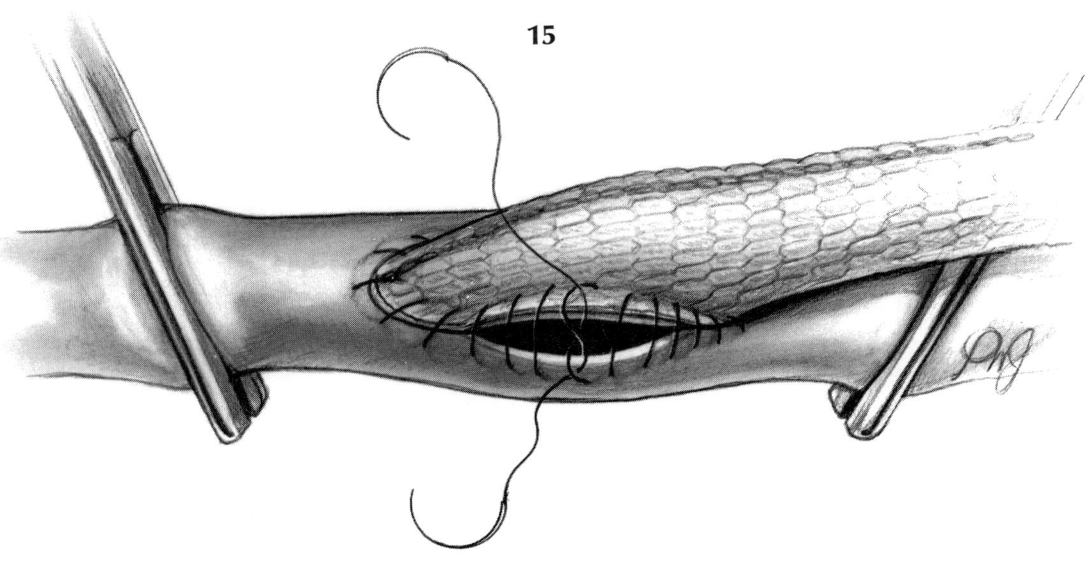

16

The mesh is incorporated with each suture, but it is not particularly critical if one or more areas are missed. What is important, however, is that each needle bite should penetrate the actual intimal component of the graft, which can be recognized as a slightly deeper beige-coloured tissue compared with the major outer component of the graft. Anastomotic aneurysms and intramural dissection can be prevented by precise suturing technique. For the same reasons, it is also essential to avoid needle penetration of the intima of the opposite wall when taking an outside-in bite, particularly at the beginning of the suture line at or adjacent to the acute angle. Both inside-out and outside-in needle passage are acceptable provided the above cited precautions are taken. The only exception for overlooking 'missed intima' would be on one or two needle passages of a continuous suture line or a distal anastomosis where the downstream flow direction precludes intimal lifting and mural dissection. It is not critical if the mesh does not cover the entire suture line because a desmoplastic response provides adequate support at the anastomosis.

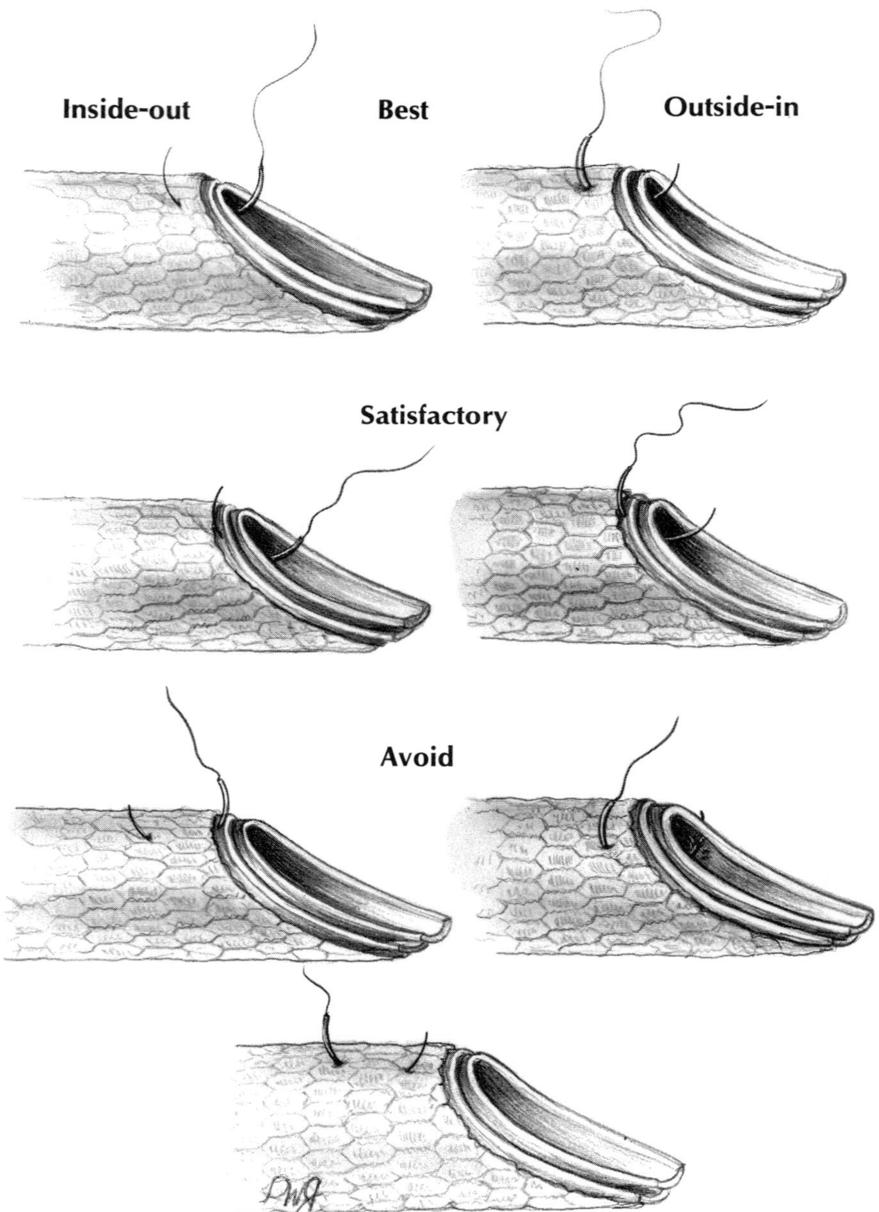

16

Tunnelling

Tunnels are established in the anatomical location for all popliteal reconstructions, as well as for bypasses to the proximal posterior tibial artery. Subcutaneous tunnels are established medially for many distal posterior tibial artery reconstructions, and laterally for most peroneal and anterior tibial artery reconstructions.

17 & 18

Tunnels are generally established before the patient is heparinized. This is performed with a slightly curved blunt instrument consisting of a metallic obturator and outer plastic sheath. The obturator is withdrawn after placement of the entire apparatus and the graft brought through the plastic sheath component with a long alligator-type forceps, the first anastomosis having usually been completed or initiated. The graft is positioned slightly taut, and then the outer plastic tunnel is withdrawn over the graft and grasping forceps. Passing the graft through a tunneller is essential to avoid friction between the outer Dacron mesh and the host tissues which could cause damage to the graft. Once a subcutaneous graft has been seated, wound retractors must be positioned to avoid pressure on the graft, particularly above a lower leg exposure. Cloth or styrofoam padding is very helpful in this regard. It is also essential that tunnels be initiated and completed in the subcutaneous position, since it is possible to perforate the fascia blindly at the knee level and create a constriction by which the graft can be compressed. For this reason all subcutaneous tunnels are established with the aid of an auxiliary anterolateral incision in the lower third of the thigh. The incision is brought down to the fascia and the tunnel is initiated by finger dissection, pushing the subcutaneous layer off the fascia. The tunnelling instrument is then passed from this site upwards to the inguinal incision and downwards to the site of distal arterial exposure.

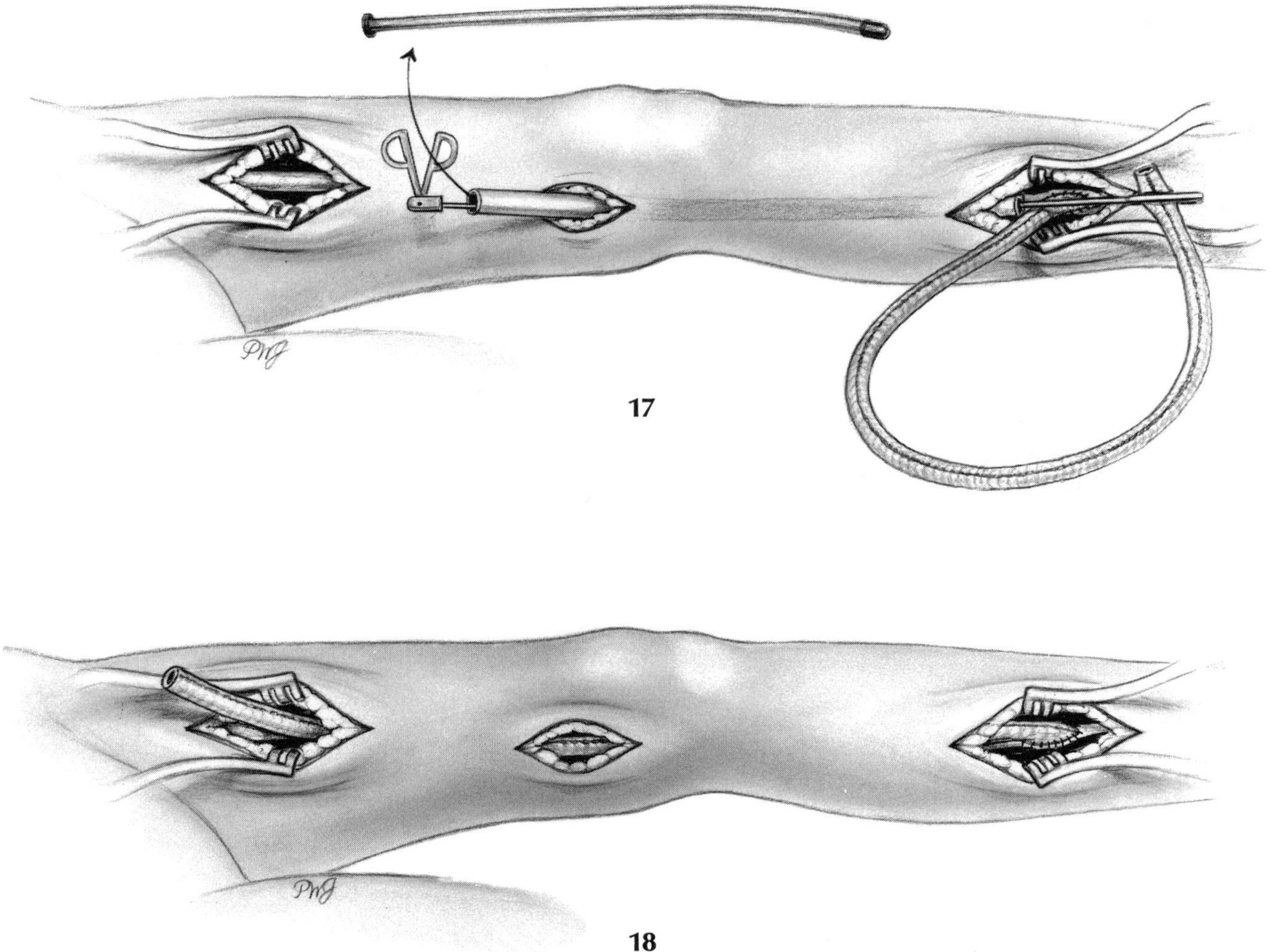

17

18

Intraoperative adjuncts

Heparin usage and monitoring

All patients are heparinized systemically at least 5 min before securing vascular control and performing the first anastomosis. We usually start with 2500–3000 units and add increments of 1000–2000 more units depending on the estimate of anticoagulation by the activated clotting time test. This test is useful to monitor adequacy of heparinization and need for reversal. Reversal of heparin anticoagulation, if required, is performed at the conclusion of all anastomoses and is accomplished with protamine sulphate in increments of 10–20 mg. Generally, none is required. During the operative period we irrigate the local anastomotic area with dilute heparin solution (50 mg per 500 ml). Dilute solution is also instilled into the distal circulation when the distal arteriotomy is established, but this should be done with the utmost caution and perhaps even omitted if the patient has extensive disease, particularly calcification.

Electromagnetic flowmeter recordings

Electromagnetic flowmeter recordings can be performed but are not essential. We have found that the information provides data suggesting the prognosis for early graft patency; it cannot be considered as an absolute monitor of the technical expertise with which the reconstruction was performed, nor can it provide assurance that the disease will not progress. Nevertheless, if flow is augmented to at least twice the baseline value with papaverine hydrochloride, the prognosis for early graft patency and function is good for most of these patients (Dardik *et al.*, 1978).

Completion arteriography

Completion arteriography is, in our opinion, mandatory before concluding the operation. It is performed simply by nicking the mesh and placing a No. 19 scalp vein needle directly into the graft. Contrast medium is injected as the X-ray cassette, placed under the distal anastomotic and run-off area, is exposed. This not only allows for the detection of any potential intraoperative defects, but also provides a definitive view of the run-off circulation for classification and gives some measure of the prognosis for the durability of graft function (Dardik *et al.*, 1978). Run-off and pedal arch structure can be analysed and correlated with the subsequent fate of the graft and stability or progression of the atherosclerotic process. Separate injections are required for popliteal bypasses in order to demonstrate the distal anastomosis on one film and the pedal circulation on the other.

19

A simple, inexpensive device consisting of a double hydraulic syringe system and a holding fixture has been devised for intraoperative arteriography to avoid exposure of personnel to repetitive radiation (Dardik *et al.*, 1980). Completion angiography has thus become safer, less time-consuming and more reliable in obtaining high-quality angiographic studies.

Completion sonography

Assessment of the distal anastomotic area (and other sites as dictated by the clinical situation) with duplex sonography prior to wound closure provides excellent physiologic data and serves as a baseline for subsequent surveillance studies. Combining the duplex with completion angiography yields predictive information and, in some instances, the stimulus for revision or additional surgical manoeuvres.

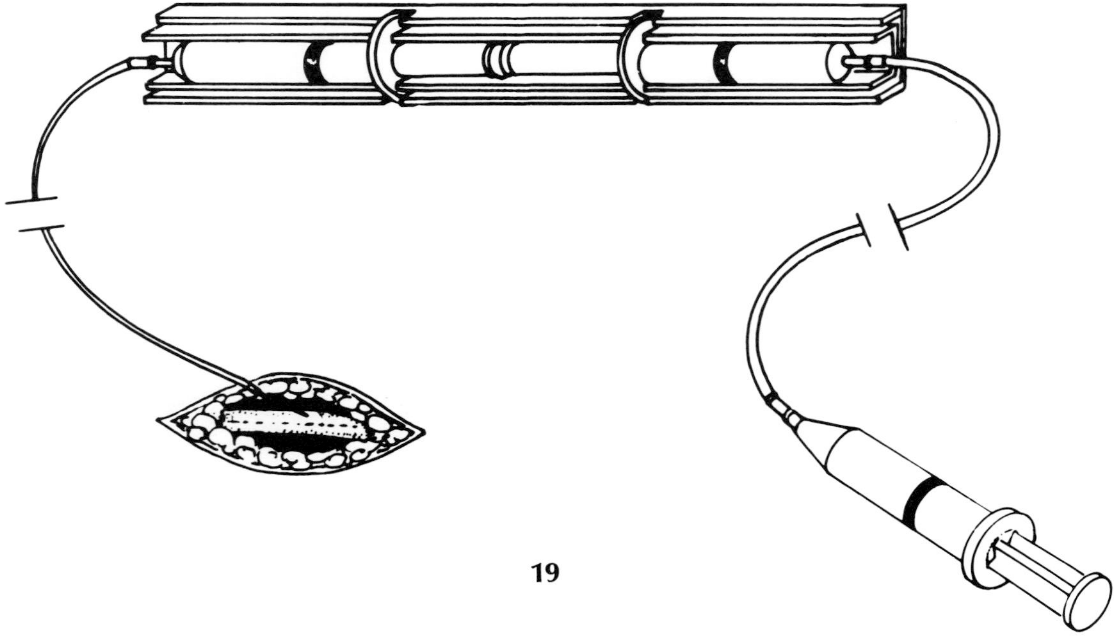

19

Distal arteriovenous fistula

If reconstruction to a crural vessel is required, and a prosthetic graft material deemed necessary, we believe that an adjunctive distal arteriovenous fistula (dAVF) should be created in order to promote the likelihood for a reasonable result that would otherwise not be possible under these circumstances; that is, where haemodynamic factors by themselves will result in early bypass failure (Dardik *et al.*, 1983). The theoretical basis for using distal arteriovenous fistulae as adjuncts to crural reconstructions in order to maintain graft patency and distal perfusion is based upon the need to reduce the vascular overload being presented to the distal circuit and, at the same time, to keep graft flow over the critical thrombotic threshold level (Dardik, 1985).

20

Establishing a vent (dAVF) results in an increased flow in the graft, most of which is then directed into the high capacitance venous circulation. The amount of blood that can be accepted by the arterial run-off, albeit limited, will perfuse distally and reverse the ischaemic state (Dardik *et al.*, 1991).

Variations in dAVF construction are possible but will need to be assessed by prospective randomized studies. These include ligation of the cephalad component of the vein (Jacobs *et al.*, 1993), dAVF distal to the distal anastomosis (Paty *et al.*, 1990), dAVF proximal to the dAVF (Harris, 1989) and saphenous vein takedown with valve lysis (Ascer, personal communication).

Postoperative management

Unless contraindications exist or occur, all patients are maintained on intravenous heparin or converted as soon as possible to maintenance warfarin. Low molecular weight dextran is also infused (500 ml/24 h) for the first 3 days (Rutherford *et al.*, 1988).

Knee immobilization is employed routinely to prevent inadvertent flexion of the hip and knee, particularly as the patient awakens and is unable to follow instructions to keep his extremities straight. We employ the immobilizer for approximately 4 days but suggest that the patient continue using it during the entire period of hospitalization and even for another week at home. It is not required while walking. Weight-bearing and walking are usually instituted after the third postoperative day; crural reconstructions are postponed for an additional day. The progress of those patients with gangrenous foot lesions will obviously determine the rate at which weight-bearing and walking will progress.

Reoperative surgery

Early thrombosis, usually due to technical mishap or poor run-off, is best managed on the basis of the post-reconstruction completion arteriogram. Those with poor run-off must be considered as distinct failures. The only possibility of graft salvage in these cases depends on the ability to use one of several adjunctive techniques including angioplasty, sequential bypass or distal adjunctive arteriovenous fistula. Cases which have failed as a result of technical error or otherwise unanticipated postoperative thrombosis should be returned immediately to the operating room for thrombectomy and correction of the underlying cause of failure. We usually explore the graft distally and, after heparinizing the patient, remove thrombus via an opening in the graft that can, if necessary, be extended across the anastomosis. If all thrombus cannot be easily

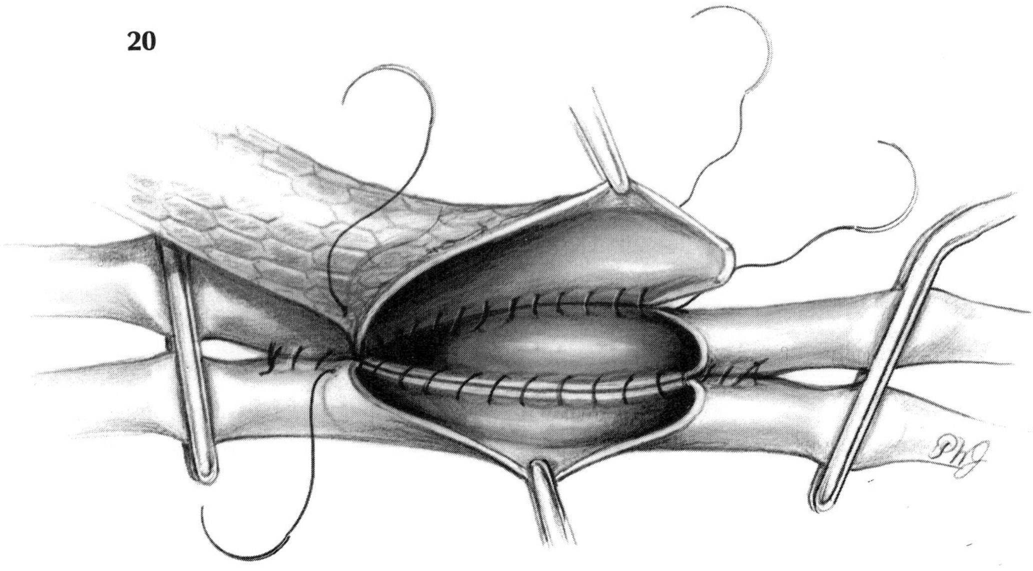

removed in this manner, we do not hesitate to open the upper wound and either massage the thrombus to release it or open the graft at this level for extraction of all thrombus. The most important aspect of umbilical vein graft thrombectomy is extreme gentleness. It is best to try to extrude all thrombus by gentle external massage or direct irrigation of the graft via proximal and distal arteriotomies before proceeding to balloon catheter extraction. Over-inflation of balloon catheters must be avoided. While passing balloon catheters it is also important to make sure that there is no friction between the catheter and the inner vessel wall. This can be avoided by intermittent gentle irrigations of the graft lumen with heparinized solution. Incisions for exploring the grafts are vertical at the proximal and distal anastomotic areas and can usually be closed primarily. In the body of the graft, patching is usually required for vertical incisions. Transverse incisions can be employed but provide limited exposure.

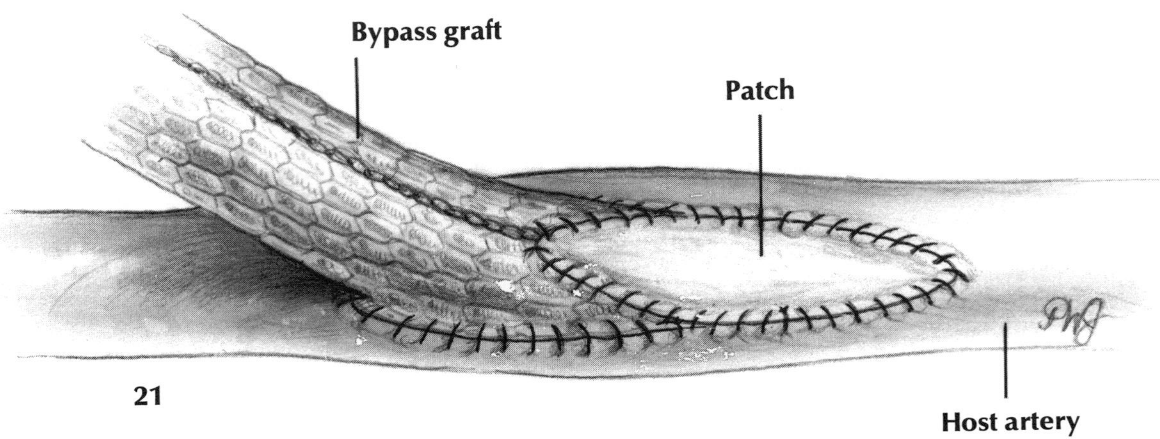

21

Vein patch angioplasty should also be employed at the distal anastomosis if the arteriotomy is carried across the anastomosis into the host run-off artery.

If there is any concern about the structural integrity of the graft or if there is difficulty with the dissection, one should not hesitate to replace the graft with a new one. Late graft closures present a slightly different problem, in that the dissection may be very difficult, particularly at anastomotic areas. Lytic therapy may be employed in selected cases but success is a function of the run-off as well as the time interval between thrombosis and initiation of lytic therapy (Dardik *et al.*, 1984). When surgery is required, manoeuvres similar to those described for early thrombectomy are performed but it is often necessary to abandon the procedure and proceed directly with replacement of the graft either in the same site or at a different level. Ultimate success for either thrombectomy or placement of a new graft in patients suffering late closures will of course depend upon the cause of graft closure. In most instances, the cause is progressive downstream obstruction, and construction of an adjunctive arteriovenous fistula should be considered. For remediable lesions, such as anastomotic stenosis or inflow lesions, an aggressive approach is indicated and appropriate.

Conclusions

The glutaraldehyde-stabilized umbilical vein graft has enabled surgeons to use an on-shelf material than can be reliably employed for reconstruction of the small vessels of the leg as well as of medium-size vessels. Because of this, operating time can be decreased, as can surgical dissection. Patients lacking suitable autologous saphenous veins, as well as those with limited life expectancy or requiring expeditious performance of the operation, can be considered as potential candidates for this graft. Precise surgical technique is required to avoid injury to this material which should only be used by surgeons truly expert in vascular methodology. It is not for the novice or 'occasional' vascular surgeon. The glutaraldehyde-stabilized umbilical vein graft can function well as a vascular conduit at all levels in the lower extremity, provided that the surgeon employs the highest level of judgment for managing the disease process on an individual patient basis. Finally, concern for aneurysm formation and the consequences have been vastly exaggerated. The clinical impact of biodegradation is low and when compared with patency and limb salvage data where prosthetics are employed, superior performance by the umbilical vein grafts is clearly evident.

References

Dardik, H. (1985). The use of an adjunctive arteriovenous fistula in distal extremity bypass grafts with outflow obstruction. In: *The Ischemic Leg*. Kempczinski, R. F., ed. Chicago, Illinois; Year Book Medical Publishers.

Dardik, H., Ibrahim, I. M. and Dardik, I. (1979). The role of the peroneal artery for limb salvage. *Annals of Surgery* **189**, 189.

Dardik, H., Dardik, I., Sprayregen, S. *et al.* (1975). Patient selection and improved technical aspects in small-vessel bypass procedures of the lower extremity. *Surgery* **77**, 249.

Dardik, H., Ibrahim, I. M., Koslow, A. *et al.* (1978). Evaluation of intraoperative arteriography as a routine for vascular reconstructions. *Surgery, Gynecology and Obstetrics* **147**, 853.

Dardik, H., Smith, M., Ibrahim, I. M. and Dardik, I. (1980). Remote hydraulic syringe actuator: Its use to avoid radiation exposure during intraoperative arteriography. *Archives of Surgery* **115**, 105.

Dardik, H., Sussman, B., Ibrahim, *et al.* (1983). Distal arteriovenous fistula as an adjunct to maintaining arterial and graft patency for limb salvage. *Surgery* **94**, 478.

Dardik, H., Sussman, B., Kahn, M. *et al.* (1984). Lysis of arterial clot by intravenous or intraarterial administration of streptokinase. *Surgery, Gynecology and Obstetrics* **158**, 137.

Dardik, H., Miller, N., Dardik, A. *et al.* (1988). A decade of experience with the glutaraldehyde-tanned human umbilical cord vein graft for revascularization of the lower limb. *Journal of Vascular Surgery* **7**, 336.

Dardik, H., Berry, S., Dardik, A. *et al.* (1991). Infrapopliteal prosthetic graft patency by use of the distal adjunctive arteriovenous fistula. *Journal of Vascular Surgery* **13**, 685.

Harris, P. L. (1989). Adjuvant arteriovenous fistula at the distal anastomosis of a femorotibial by-pass graft. In: Greenhalgh R. M., ed. *Vascular Surgical Techniques: An Atlas*. London; W. B. Saunders, 306.

Jacobs, M., Reul, G., Gregoria, I. D. *et al.* (1993). Creation of a distal arteriovenous fistula improves microcirculatory hemodynamics of prosthetic graft bypass in secondary limb salvage procedures. *Journal of Vascular Surgery* **18**, 1.

Paty, P. S. K., Shah, D. M., Saifi, J. *et al* (1990). Remote distal arteriovenous fistula to improve infrapopliteal bypass patency. *Journal of Vascular Surgery* **11**, 171.

Rutherford, R., Jones, D. N., Bergentz, S. E. *et al.* (1988) Factors affecting the patency of infrainguinal bypass. *Journal of Vascular Surgery* **8**, 236.

Adjuvant arteriovenous fistula at the distal anastomosis of a femorotibial bypass graft

P. L. HARRIS MD, FRCS

Consultant in Vascular Surgery, Broadgreen Hospital, Liverpool, UK;
Lecturer in Clinical Surgery, University of Liverpool, Liverpool, UK

Introduction

An arteriovenous fistula is constructed at the distal anastomosis of a long prosthetic femorotibial graft in order to increase the velocity of blood flow through the graft above the thrombotic threshold level.

Indications

(1) Patients with critical ischaemia whose only alternative is a major amputation.
(2) Prosthetic grafts inserted into a single tibial vessel.
(3) Poor run-off due to disease in the distal tibial or pedal vessels, determined by:
   (a) pedal angiography pre- or intraoperatively;
   (b) direct observation of vessels at operation;
   (c) objective assessment of peripheral resistance or impedance;
   (d) failure of the bypass graft despite adequate inflow and perfect operative technique.

Special requirements

(1) Some arterial run-off is essential; the procedure is of no value if the venous system alone is perfused.
(2) The deep venous system should be patent and free from post-phlebitic damage.
(3) The construction of a fistula using superficial veins is associated with a high incidence of impaired wound healing and skin necrosis due to localized venous hypertension and should be avoided.
(4) Unrestricted inflow to the graft is essential. Aorto-iliac stenosis must be identified by appropriate non-invasive tests or biplanar angiography and must be corrected before or concurrently with the femorodistal bypass procedure.
(5) Adjuvant arteriovenous fistula is not advisable for patients with severely impaired myocardial function.
(6) The use of loupe magnification (x 2.5) is recommended.
(7) Heparin anticoagulation is essential during surgery and oral antiplatelet therapy postoperatively.

The operation

Common ostium fistula

1

The selected tibial artery and its largest concomitant vein are approached as described in the chapter on 'Sites and approaches for tibial anastomoses'. A suitable length of these vessels is dissected and controlled with narrow latex slings. Clamps must not be applied to these vessels.

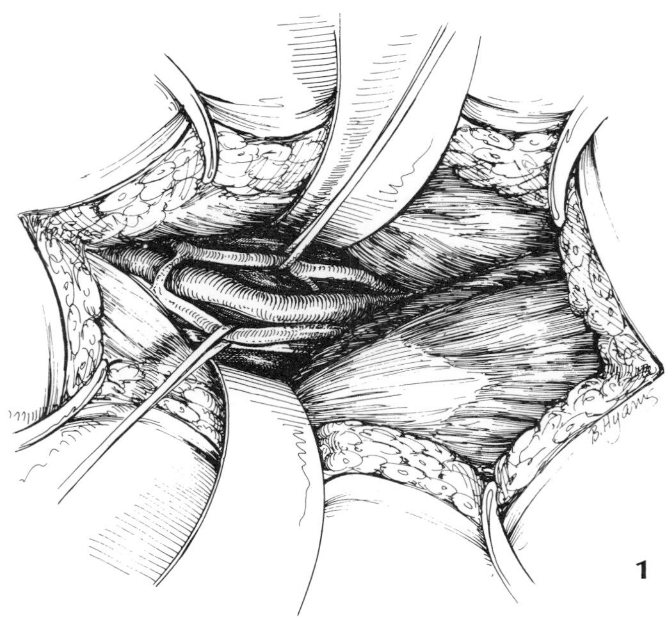

1

2

Longitudinal incisions approximately 15 mm in length are made in the artery and vein. Small catheters (not shown) are inserted into the artery distally and the vein proximally to control bleeding, permit perfusion of heparinized solutions, and to stent the anastomoses during construction. The adjacent walls of the vessels are sutured together using a double ended 7/0 polypropylene suture.

2

3

The distal end of the prosthetic graft is anastomosed to the 'common ostium' using 7/0 polypropylene sutures. Human umbilical vein is shown in the illustration as an example.

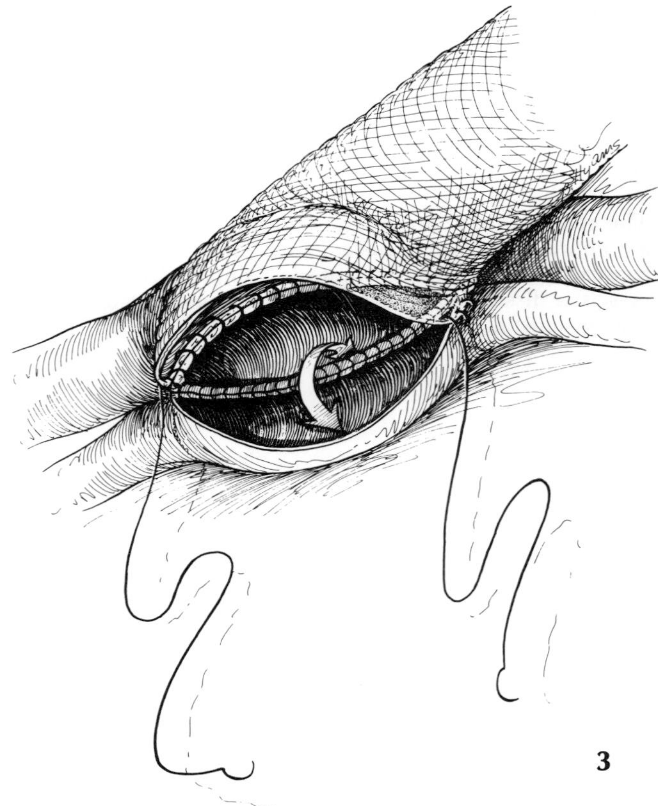

3

4

By reducing the length of the venotomy relative to that of the arteriotomy and constructing the fistula as shown, it is possible to simplify the graft to artery anastomosis at the toe and heel.

This slight modification of technique may help to reduce the risk of technical error at these critical points.

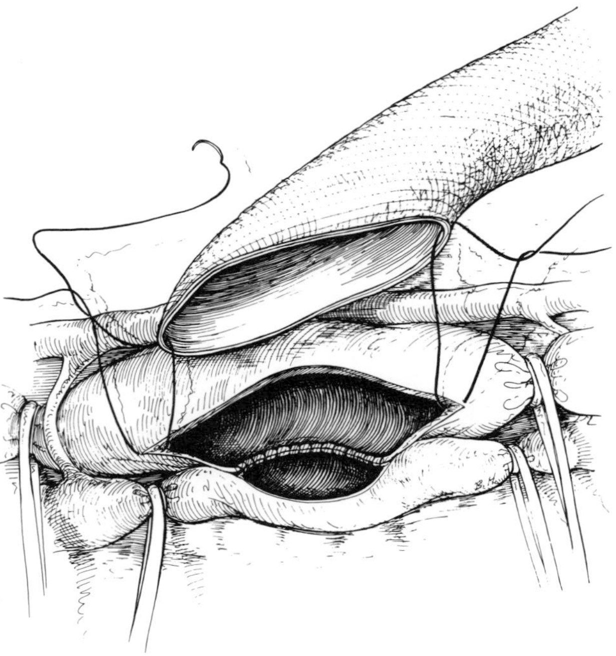

4

5

On completion the presence of a palpable thrill over the anastomosis indicates satisfactory functioning of the arteriovenous fistula. It is helpful to record bloodflow through the graft with an electromagnetic flow probe to assess the effect of the fistula. A mean flow greater than 200 ml per min is to be expected. Experimental studies indicate that less than 20% of the total flow through the graft passes distally into the artery, the remainder being shunted into the veins. There is no evidence that a fistula constructed at this site ever results in a 'steal' of blood from the distal arterial circulation in clinical practice.

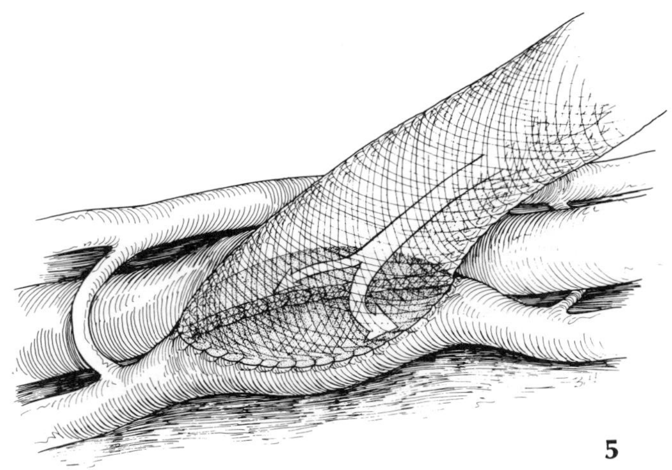

5

Alternative method

Pre-anastomotic fistula

6

Construction of a side-to-side arteriovenous fistula at a point 0.5–1 cm upstream of the graft-to-artery anastomosis, as shown, has the following potential advantages:

(1) The intervening section of artery acts as a resistance which limits the volume of the shunt. The optimum size of shunt is one which results in a sufficient increase in blood flow through the graft to allow the thrombotic threshold to be exceeded with a small margin of safety. The 'common ostium' type of shunt sometimes results in flows considerably in excess of this with possible detrimental effects.
(2) The construction of the graft to artery anastomosis and the fistula separately is less complicated and therefore subject to fewer technical errors.
(3) The simpler form of construction may improve the flow characteristics at the graft-to-artery junction with less turbulence.

In practice the patency rates of grafts with common ostium and pre-anastomotic adjuvant fistula are similar.

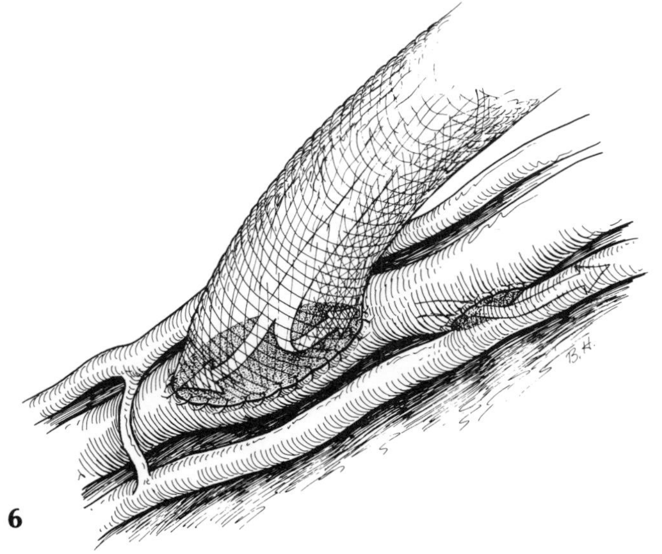

6

7

Remote postanastomotic arteriorvenous fistula

The construction of an arteriovenous fistula at a point downstream to the graft to artery anastomosis carries the advantage of drawing a larger volume of blood flow into the recipient artery than the methods previously described.

However, this disposition can result in a very much reduced perfusion pressure in the arteries distal to the fistula. For this reason a postanastomotic fistula should be sited as remotely as possible in the limb. Another concern regarding this technique is that the fistula may not be of sufficient size to achieve the primary aim of accelerating blood flow in the graft above thrombotic threshold levels.

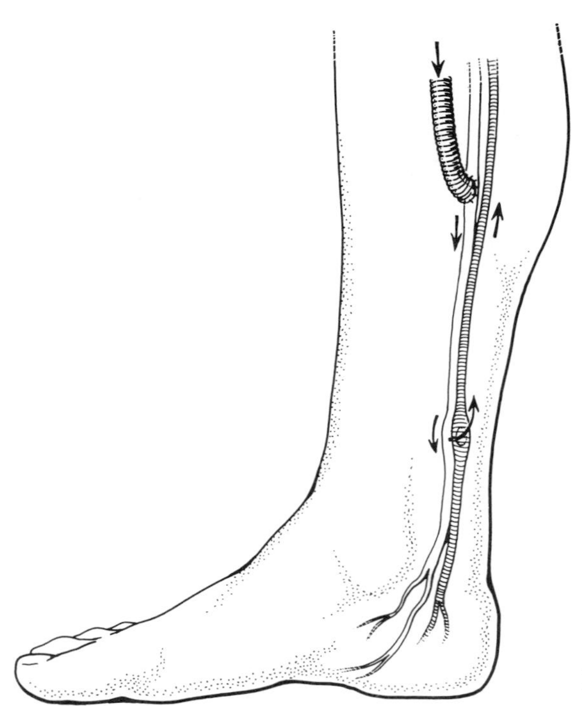

7

References

Harris, P. L. and Campbell, H. (1983). Adjuvant distal arteriovenous shunt with femoro-tibial bypass for critical ischaemia. *British Journal of Surgery* **70**(6), 377.

Dardik, H., Sussman, B. and Ibrahmin, M. *et al.* (1983). Distal arterio-venous fistula as an adjunct to maintaining arterial and graft patency for limb salvage. *Surgery* **94**(3), 478.

Above-knee amputation

HERO VAN URK MD

Chief, Vascular Surgery, University Hospital, Erasmus University, Rotterdam, The Netherlands

Introduction

Although the ratio of above-knee amputations to below-knee amputations has changed over the last decades in favour of the latter, the actual number of above-knee amputations has not decreased dramatically.

Whenever possible, an above-knee amputation should be avoided if it is possible to perform either a below-knee or through-knee amputation. The functional results of rehabilitation of patients with a below-knee prosthesis is infinitely better than those with an above-knee prosthesis.

In almost all cases where this operation is indicated, the superficial femoral artery is occluded, leaving the profunda femoral artery (or its remaining branches) as the only remaining blood supply for the thigh muscles. Usually, this arterial supply is further compromised, resulting in insufficient oxygenation of the distal part of the muscles. Hence the principle of preserving as much leg length as possible no longer applies once the decision to perform an above-knee amputation has been taken.

1

Conventional knee mechanisms extend 8–10 cm into the thigh portion of the prosthesis. Therefore, if a thigh amputation is performed too far distally, this may cause problems with prosthetic fitting and unequal knee height. This difficulty has caused some reluctance on the part of surgeons to perform through-knee amputations, but the most recent prosthetic techniques have overcome this. Nevertheless, a too distal diaphyseal amputation may result in an excessively long stump, which is of no benefit to the patient; such a stump end has poor weight-bearing abilities, in contrast to the mid-diaphyseal or through-knee amputation.

On the other hand, an amputation which leaves the limb too short, is equally to be avoided. About 10 cm below the minor trochanter is the upper limit of an amputation. A shorter stump will lead to a flexion–abduction contracture, which poses a problem both cosmetically and functionally. Disarticulation in the hip is preferred in such cases, usually after a high above-knee amputation has failed to heal properly.

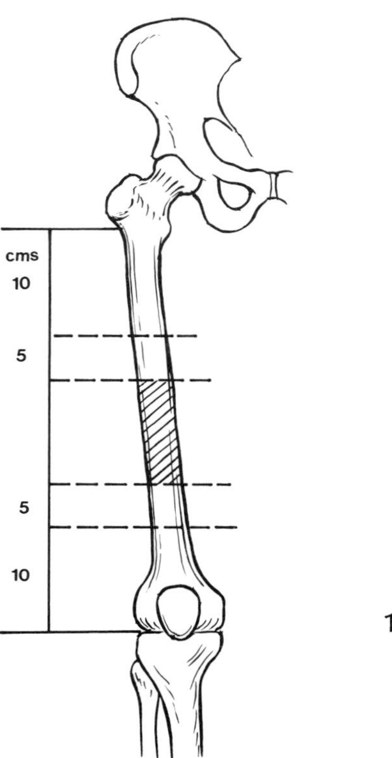

1

The operation

2

The patient is placed in the supine position. Usually, general anaesthesia is preferred, but epidural anaesthesia or a regional block can be given to elderly patients with a critical medical condition.

If gangrene of the foot or lower leg is present, the foot can be packed in a plastic bag. In cases of wet gangrene, the author prefers to administer antibiotics intravenously the evening before the operation. If there is dry necrosis or rest pain only, antibiotics are started just after induction of anaesthesia and continued for 24 h postoperatively.

After suitable skin preparation and draping, the intended skin incision is marked with a sterile marker pen, having the dorsal flap slightly shorter than the anterior flap. The apex of the angle between the anterior and posterior flaps is approximately at the level of transection of the shaft of the femur. On both sides this point is in the mid-medial and mid-lateral line of the thigh or slightly more to the dorsal side.

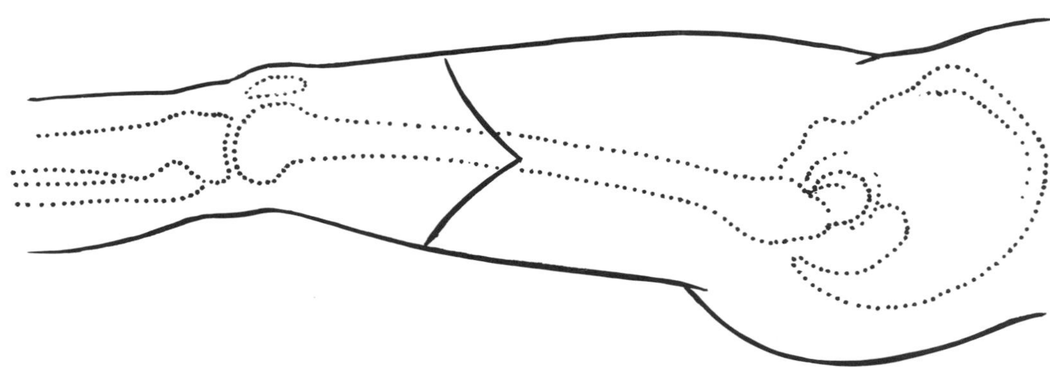

2

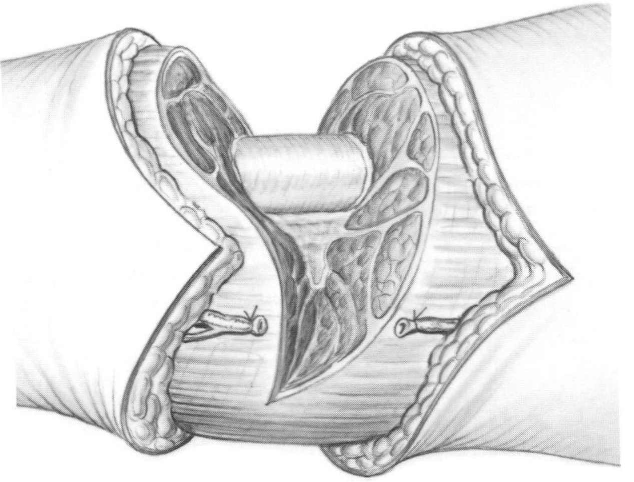

3

3

An incision is made through the subcutaneous tissue and the fascia femoris. If still intact, the greater saphenous vein is transected and ligated. In cases where an *in situ* saphenous vein bypass has previously been performed, this conduit is likely to be thrombosed, but, if not, special care should be taken to avoid blood loss from this source.

After completion of the skin and fascia incisions, the skin usually retracts somewhat on both sides. The muscle incision should be in the same line as the skin incision, because of the tendency of muscles to retract even more than skin.

The anterior and lateral muscles are divided first. When the medial muscles are incised, care should be taken to locate the superficial femoral vessels first. After separate ligation of artery and vein, the deep femoral artery and the sciatic nerve are exposed. In order to minimize neuroma formation, the sciatic nerve is identified anteriorly to the hamstring muscles and is pulled down and divided after ligation of the arteria concomitans. The author prefers not to ligate the sciatic nerve itself, because this is thought to cause more neuroma formation and/or phantom pain.

There seems to be no guaranteed method of avoiding neuroma formation, but the nerve should always be allowed to retract well upwards between the surrounding muscles. It may be of some value for pain relief in the immediate postoperative period to inject the nerve with a local anaesthetic like Marcaine® (bupivacaine).

4

When all muscles have been divided and all bleeding points are clamped and ligated proximally, the periosteum of the femur is incised circumferentially. The periosteum is then pushed upward 3–4 cm. The femoral shaft is divided with a saw, the level of the bony amputation being 4–5 cm more proximal than the musculocutaneous flap.

After the muscle flaps have been bevelled, accurate haemostasis is obtained. In diabetic patients with calcified small vessels, all bleeding points need to be ligated, preferably with absorbable material, because electro-cautery may not be sufficient in such cases.

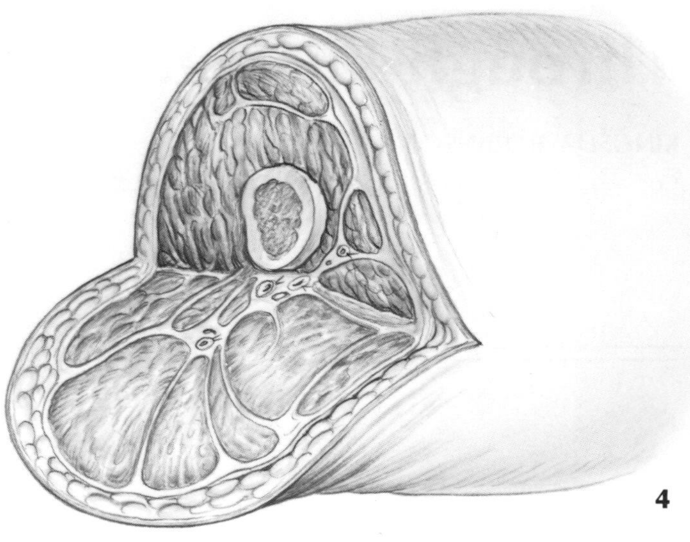

4

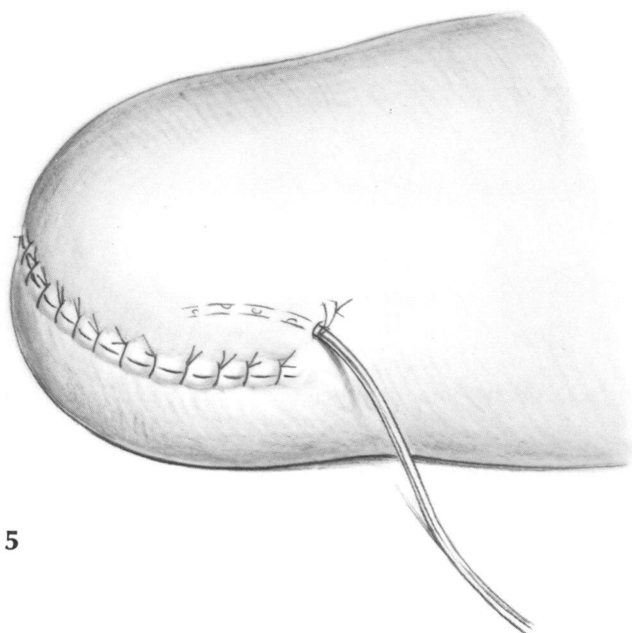

5

5

In order to prevent retraction of the muscles causing the overlying skin to press directly against the femoral stump, a myodesis is desirable in most cases and especially when the muscles are hypotrophic. Three to five holes are drilled in the distal femoral cortex with a thin (2–2.5 mm) drill.

Using absorbable sutures, the fascia of the anterior quadriceps flap can be fixed over the top of the femoral stump to the dorsal side of the cortex, together with the dorsal muscles.

The wound is then closed by approximating – with minimal tension – the anterior fascia to the posterior fascia, using interrupted sutures. One or two suction drains are left deep in the wound. No subcutaneous sutures are necessary and the skin is closed in one layer, preferably with interrupted monofilament nylon sutures.

Postoperative care

6

Sterile dressings are applied, followed by synthetic orthopaedic padding and, finally, a cotton stretch bandage. This dressing can be left in place for several days unless the patient complains of increasing pain, which may be caused by swelling of the stump.

In some clinics, elevation of the stump on a pillow for the first 24–48 h is advised. The author prefers to keep the stump flat on the bed to prevent a flexion contracture. Exercises can be started after the first few postoperative days. Lying in a prone position for several short periods during the day may be helpful in the prevention of a flexion contracture.

Cotton elastic bandages are applied and regularly changed in order to aid shrinkage of the stump. In contrast with below-knee amputations, no temporary plaster cast is used; instead, a prosthesis is fitted directly when the stump is free of oedema after application of the elastic dressings. Unfortunately, only a small proportion of vascular patients are able to follow a complete rehabilitation programme, and the number of elderly patients who are eventually able to walk again is disappointing.

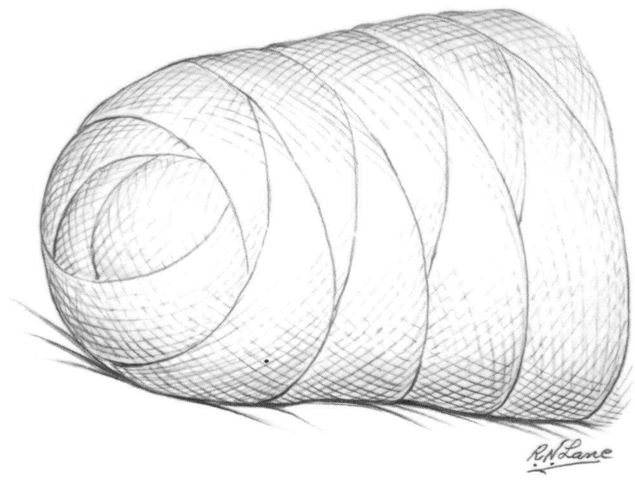

6

Through-knee amputation

KINGSLEY ROBINSON MS, FRCS
Consultant Surgeon, Westminster Hospital, London, UK

Introduction

The through-knee amputation is the quickest major lower-limb amputation that can be performed as no bony structure needs to be divided and ligation of the single large popliteal artery and its accompanying veins controls nearly all the bleeding that can be encountered. Only the long saphenous vein usually requires an additional ligature. The large size of the femoral condyles means that ample skin must be provided for adequate and lax skin cover, otherwise skin necrosis can be produced by tension across the edges of the articular surface. It is also important that the patella retains its normal position on the front of the knee rather than being drawn down where it may be subjected to weight-bearing stresses and produce extreme discomfort. The procedure is so atraumatic and speedy that it can be carried out as a debriding procedure prior to a definitive higher amputation. The absence of noise, because no saw is required, is a great asset when operating on patients under regional anaesthesia.

1

Lateral and medial sagittal flaps centred on the tibial tubercle anteriorly and the fold at the flexion line in the popliteal fossa constitute the most satisfactory skin flaps. The classical skin flap is a long anterior flap with a transverse scar across the popliteal fossa, and if this incision is used the patient is best placed prone with the distal part of the leg flexed to provide access to the anterior structures. This is an unsatisfactory position for the severely ill patient with vascular disease and a supine position with the hip flexed is entirely satisfactory if sagittal flaps are utilized. The skin incision is cut at one with the subcutaneous fat but the fascia lata and aponeurotic fibres of the lower leg muscles need not be incised.

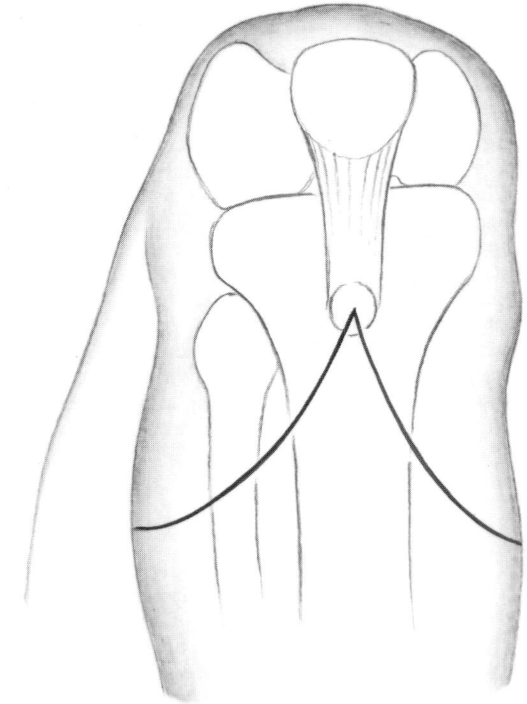

1

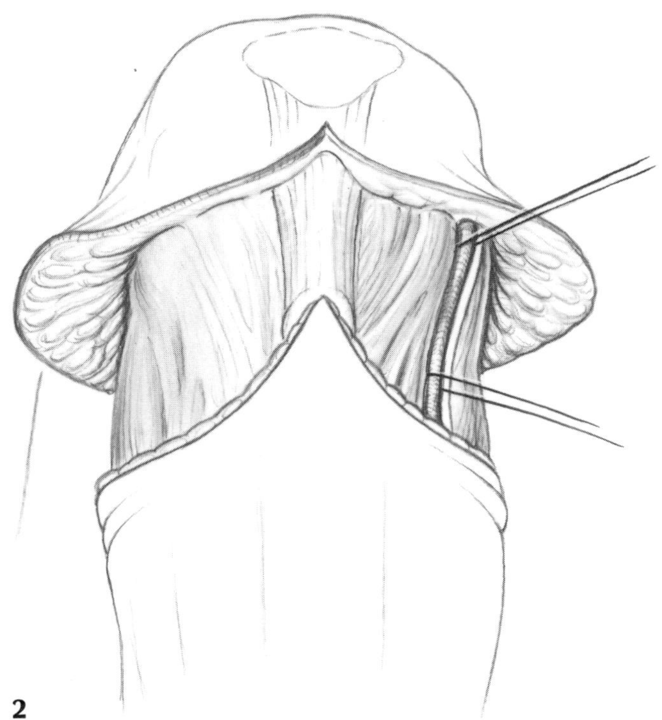

2

2

The skin flaps are elevated by brushing upwards with a wet swab and the patella tendon is defined and its insertion into the tibial tubercle. At this stage the long saphenous vein will be ligated with fine catgut or vicryl, care being taken to avoid inclusion of the saphenous nerve.

3

Retraction on the medial and lateral flap will be necessary to obtain exposure of the tibial plateau. The patella tendon is then divided, erasing it from the patella tubercle to obtain a maximum length and held in a tissue forcep. The patella tendon can be elevated to provide additional retraction and exposure of the fat pad that is anterior to the synovial membrane covering the cruciate ligaments. The joint capsule is incised transversely to each side of the patella tendon exposing the condyles of the femur and if correctly placed the genicular cartilages should be left attached to the tibial plateau. Further flexion of the knee allows clear exposure of the cruciate ligaments. The hamstring tendons and the medial ligament of the knee joint can then be divided as can the lateral ligaments and biceps femoris tendon, allowing further flexion when the cruciate ligaments themselves can be divided leaving as much length as possible attached to the femur.

4

The posterior part of the knee joint capsule can then be incised. Access to the popliteal artery and its veni comitans can either be obtained through the back of the knee joint capsule with some traction on the tibia or, alternatively, a finger can be hooked around the medial head of the gastrocnemius which can then be erased from the point of origin above the femoral condyle when the popliteal artery has been ligated and divided. The two elements of the sciatic nerve can also be transected under tension with the proximal end allowed to retract as far as possible. The lateral head of the gastrocnemius can also be divided.

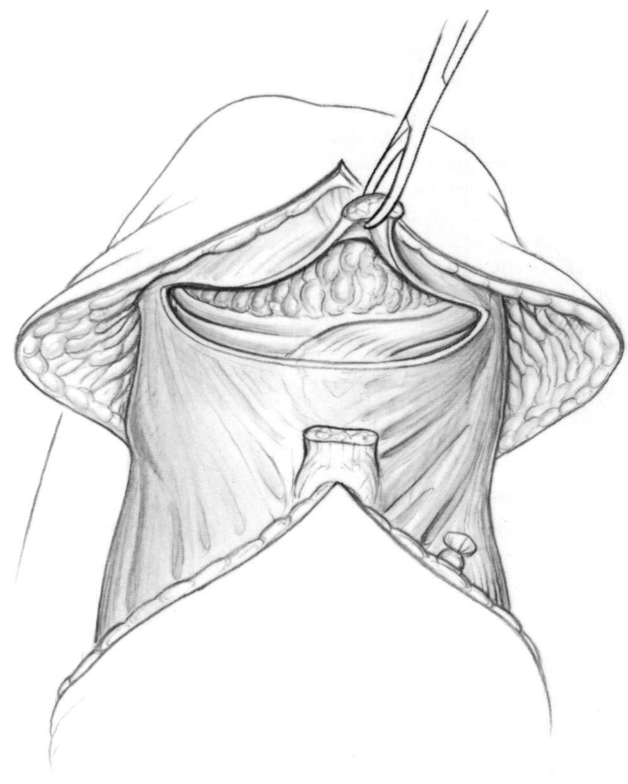

3

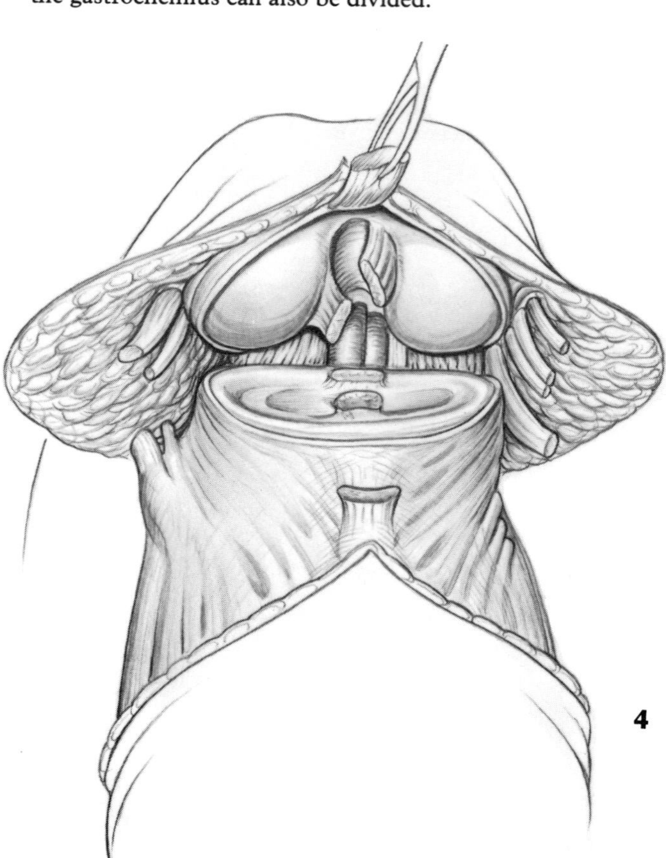

4

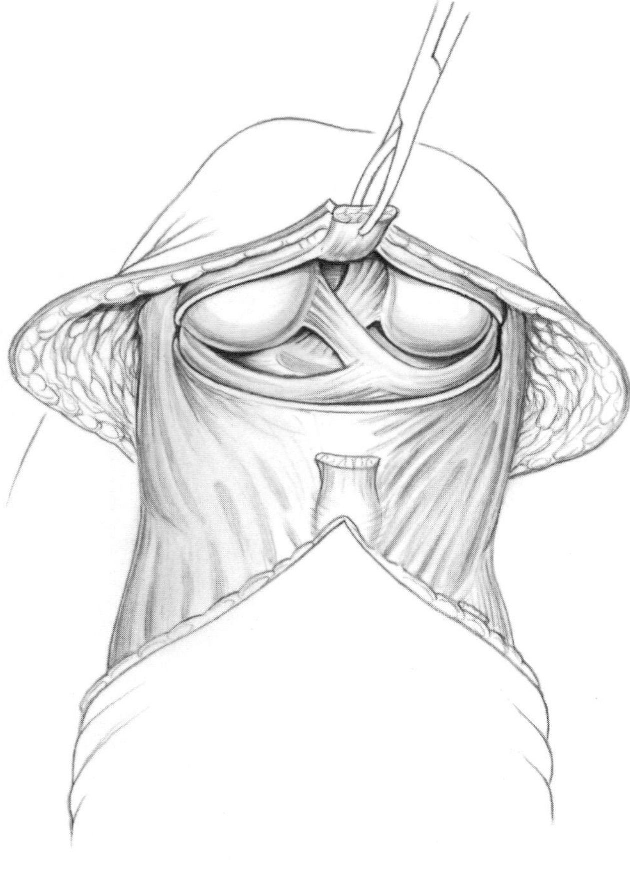

5 & 6

When all these structures are completely divided the specimen is freed. The hamstring tendons and biceps tendons are marked with artery forceps and preserved and haemostasis secured. Myoplasty is effected by anchoring the biceps femoris tendon and the semimembranosis gracivis and semitendonosis tendons being attached to the residue of the cruciate ligaments. These sutures have to hold the tendons against considerable tension when the muscles are active and must be at least 1 chromicatgut or 0 vicryl. At this stage the patellar tendon is also sutured into the intercondylar notch securely attached to the residue of the cruciate ligaments, and care must be taken not to pull the patellar tendon down too far and to allow it to remain in its anatomical position in relation to the anterior surface of the femoral condyles. At this stage there should be an appreciable excess of skin in the flaps and the skin can usually be closed in a single layer. In case of continuing synovial fluid production a Redivac drain is best placed across the condyles and, leaving the stump well above the condylar area, the skin is closed as a single layer of subcutaneous fat using vertical interrupted mattress sutures.

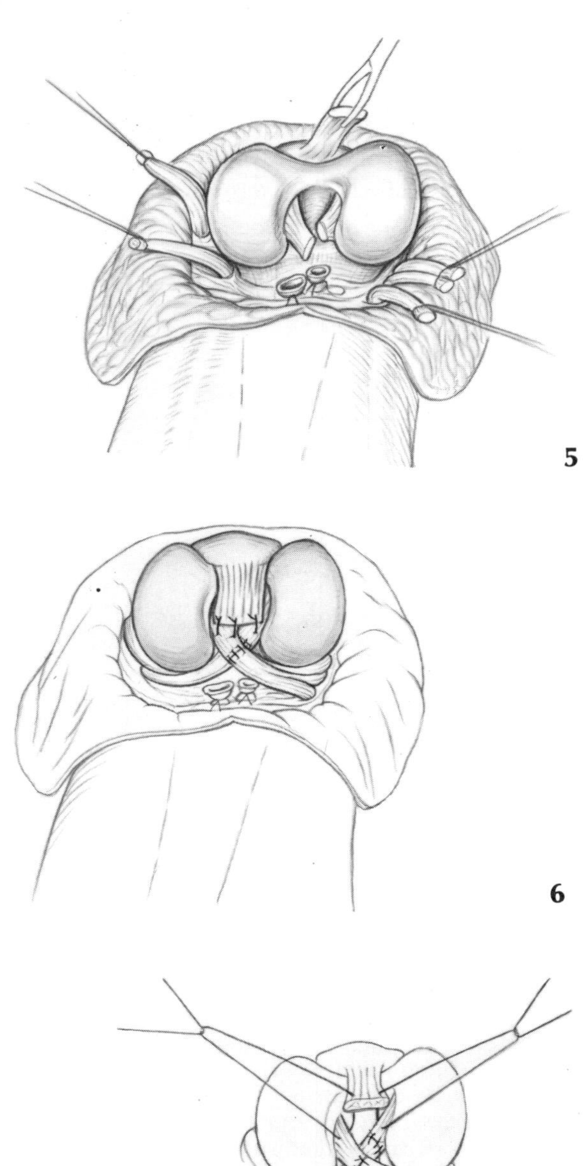

5

6

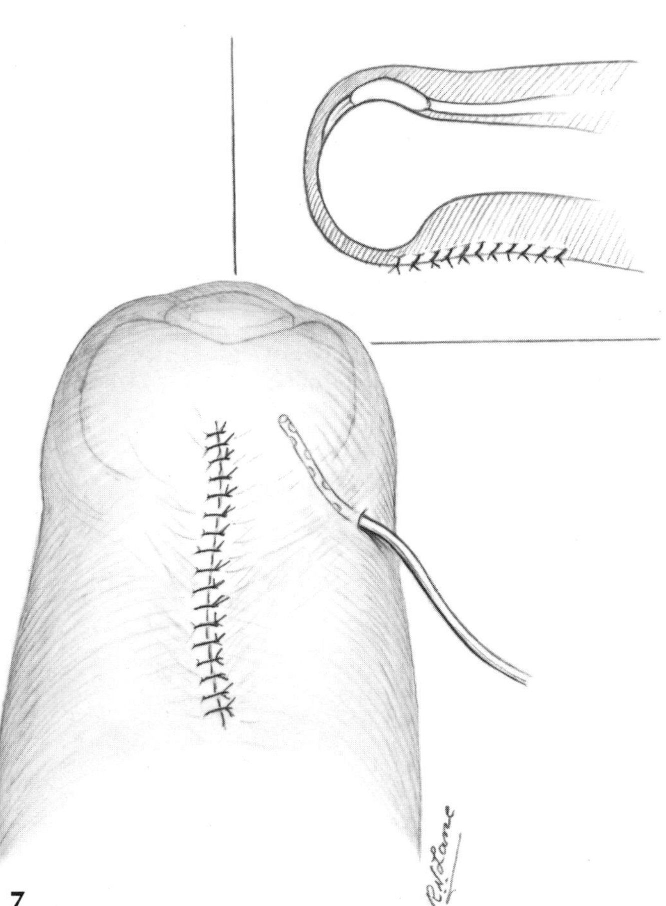

7

7

When the suture line is complete it will be found that the scar lies entirely within and above the femoral intercondylar notch and the skin area related to the inferior surface of the femoral condyles is free of any sutures or scar tissue. This allows the stump to be used for terminal weight-bearing, a great advantage in prosthetic design as ischial weight-bearing can be avoided. Many patients with bilateral through-knee amputations learn to crawl on the stump ends and may be mobile without any prosthesis at all. If the patient finds this mode of progression satisfactory, provision of knee bootees can be of some value.

Posterior-flap below-knee amputation

CHARLES N. McCOLLUM MD, FRCS

Professor of Surgery, University of South Manchester, Manchester, UK

Introduction

In modern practice, over 80% of all lower limb amputations are for peripheral vascular disease with the vast majority performed by vascular surgeons. These amputations are usually necessary because the severity of distal disease prevents arterial reconstruction, acute or severe ischaemia is prolonged, or our reconstructions fail. Nevertheless, the purpose is to relieve pain and to restore mobility to a patient who would otherwise have been immobilized either by pain or by developing gangrene. Amputation surgery therefore requires to be of the highest standard with gentle handling of ischaemic tissues to achieve primary healing. The type of amputation will be tailored to the individual needs of the patient and to their ability to regain full mobility. The surgeon must work in close cooperation with his limb-fitting service, as there is little point in achieving excellent primary healing rates if the resulting stump will only accommodate a difficult or clumsy prosthesis.

In major lower limb amputation, below-knee amputation has substantial advantages for rehabilitation over both through-knee and above-knee amputation. Only 20 years ago it was rarely performed in arterial disease because the anterior flap suffered necrosis and the amputation had to be revised to above-knee. The use of a longer posterior flap was advocated by Kendrick in 1956, but the modern posterior flap technique was popularized a decade later by Burgess (1968; Burgess *et al.*, 1971). Although the proportion of below-knee to above-knee amputations was 6:1 in Kendrick's series, the tragedy of vascular surgery over the following 20 years was that this ratio was progressively reversed, with many vascular surgeons rarely performing below-knee amputation.

Selection for below-knee amputation

Where an amputation is essential, or arterial reconstruction is not possible or has failed, it requires to be performed in such a way as to ensure the greatest chance of the patient returning to full mobility and independence and with the objective of achieving primary healing. Perhaps one reason that above-knee amputation became so frequent was that primary healing could almost be guaranteed. In below-knee amputation, particularly when operating in an ischaemic calf, the technique is critical to achieve primary healing. On our vascular surgical service, above-knee amputation is now reserved for those patients with crippling disability, such as hemiplegia, where mobilization is impossible. As a result, we have only performed 24 such procedures over the last 5 years, with 6 of these being revisions of below-knee amputations. Over the same interval, we have performed 61 below-knee amputations with an in-hospital mortality of 6.5% and revision to above-knee in just under 10%. These results can be achieved even where there is no recordable arterial pressure at the ankle by Doppler as the long posterior flap is based on the collateral blood supply to the calf.

Blood supply to the posterior flap

1

In the majority of patients for amputation, the popliteal artery and the posterior calf arteries are completely occluded, otherwise arterial reconstruction would be possible. An example of a typical arteriogram in a patient where distal reconstruction may not be possible is shown in *Illustration 1* where the superficial femoral artery is patent down to the mid-popliteal with complete occlusion of the distal popliteal and all calf arteries. An almost invariable feature of such cases is a fan of collaterals, including the sural artery, arising with its apex in the suprageniculate vessels. These collaterals fill either from thigh collaterals if the sugrageniculate popliteal is occluded or from the suprageniculate arteries themselves. They then ramify distally, posterior to the gastrocnemius with branches entering the gastrocnemius. These vessels may represent the main source of supply of the lower limb as there are very few collaterals passing down in the tissues anterior to the knee. Clearly collateralization to the anterior skin will be poor, as there is no easy communication between the posterior compartment of the calf and the peroneal or anterior compartments, other than in collaterals within the skin itself.

As these posterior calf collaterals may also be the main source of supply for the lower leg, including the soleus muscle and the anterior and peroneal compartments, there may be considerable 'steal' of blood from the posterior calf compartment. The available blood supply to the posterior flap is, therefore, improved on amputation of the lower leg, providing all tissue anterior to the gastrocnemius is removed. It is for this reason that I emphasize that the soleus muscle should be completely removed up to a level just above the division of the bone.

Preoperative preparation

As the mean age of these patients is over 70 and the early postoperative mortality in the range of 7–14%, these patients require careful assessment for anaesthesia and close postoperative supervision (Hayes and Middleton, 1981; Harrison, Southworth and Callum, 1987; Sethia *et al*., 1986; Robinson, Hoile and Coddington, 1982). Associated cardiovascular or respiratory disease and diabetes add to the risks. Often, these patients have become debilitated and malnourished through prolonged opiate therapy for rest pain, or may have already undergone arterial reconstruction or previous attempts at conservative amputation. Despite this, amputation should not be delayed, because the patients will usually continue to deteriorate with pain, spreading infection or gangrene.

Once the decision to amputate has been made the leg should be elevated to reduce tissue oedema and antibiotics started if there is evidence of infection or gangrene. Diabetes should be carefully controlled by soluble insulin infusion and the patient rehydrated. Where malnutrition is a problem, fine-bore gastric feeding may be started, even though amputation should be scheduled within 24 h. The level of amputation is carefully explained and consent obtained for below-knee amputation only, unless there is spreading gangrene and the viability of the calf muscles is in doubt.

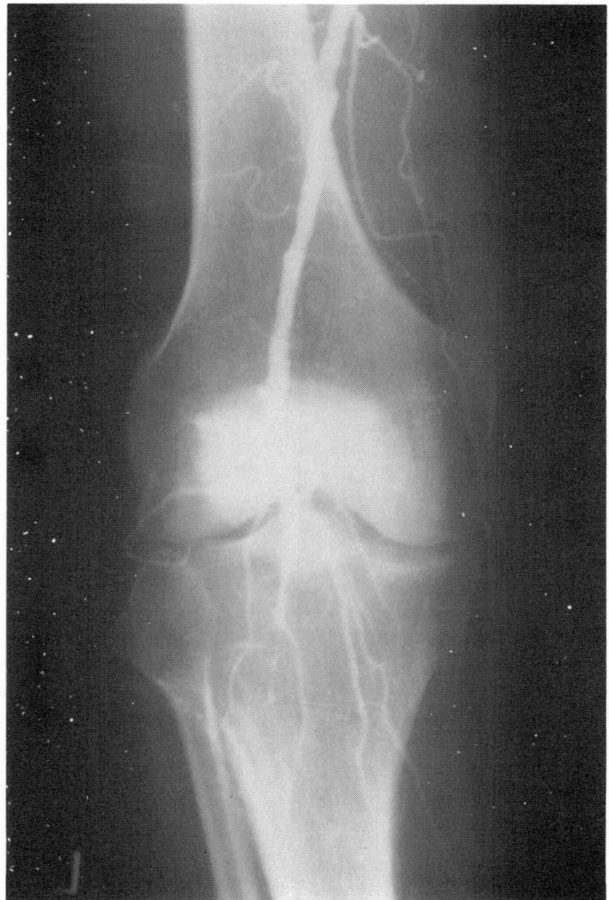

1

Selecting amputation level

Much has been written about methods of assessing tissue perfusion for the selection of the most distal amputation site likely to heal. This is critical, as the more distal the amputation the greater the proportion of patients who achieve complete rehabilitation, whereas the more proximal the amputation the higher the chances of primary healing. Methods described to measure this objectively include Doppler segmental pressures, pulse volume recording, zenon-133 clearance studies, photoplethysmography, muscle pH measurements, thermography and $TCPO_2$ measurements. Of these, transcutaneous oxygen tension measurement appears the most promising, with the potential that laser Doppler may be equally valuable in the future. Planning is still difficult, as healing may occur in the face of low $TCPO_2$ levels unless skin heating to overcome vasospasm or high inhaled oxygen concentrations are administered (Spence and McCollum, 1985; Franzech *et al.*, 1982; Rattiff *et al.*, 1984). Furthermore, in below-knee amputation, it is impossible to predict how much the $TCPO_2$ of the skin flap will improve once the distal tissue dependent on the same collaterals has been removed, although some improvement in the flap has been acknowledged (Katsamouris *et al.*, 1984). For most vascular surgeons, there is still no clear indication as to which technique should be used routinely because development has not yet reached the standard that they can be applied generally. From our own results, clinical judgement alone may be used, because reamputation at a higher level was required in less than 10% of patients despite performing below-knee amputations on all patients with viable posterior calf skin. When an adequate posterior flap cannot be fashioned due to ulceration or gangrene, the 'skin flap' technique may be appropriate, but in my opinion requires a better blood supply (Robinson, Hoile and Coddington, 1982).

The operation

In most cases, general anaesthesia is used, although epidural or spinal local anaesthesia may be appropriate for individual cases. Prophylactic antibiotics are given before incision, or earlier for spreading infection.

2

The skin is marked 8–12 cm below the tibial tuberosity where the anterior skin incision is made and the bone divided. The medial and lateral limits of the anterior incision are then marked, as this will form the base of the posterior flap. This base should be more medially placed by only extending the anterior incision medially 1–2 cm posterior to the border of the tibia, but the lateral incision should extend just posterior to the line of the fibula. The posterior flap will be cut to size later in the procedure.

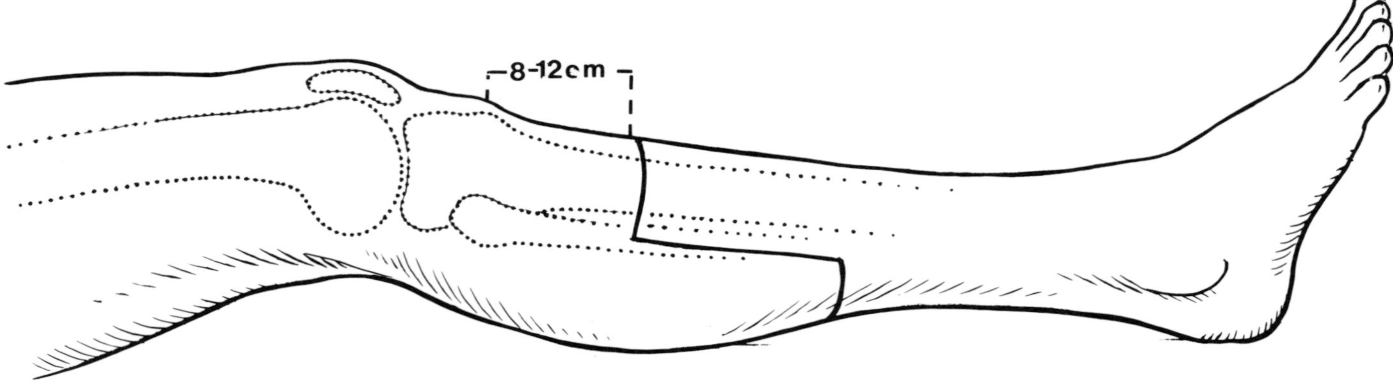

2

3

The anterior skin incision is made down to the tibia and through the anterior tibial compartment to the neurovascular bundle. Once this has been ligated the fibula can easily be cleaned of its periosteum and divided using rib shears 3–4 cm above the proposed level of tibial division.

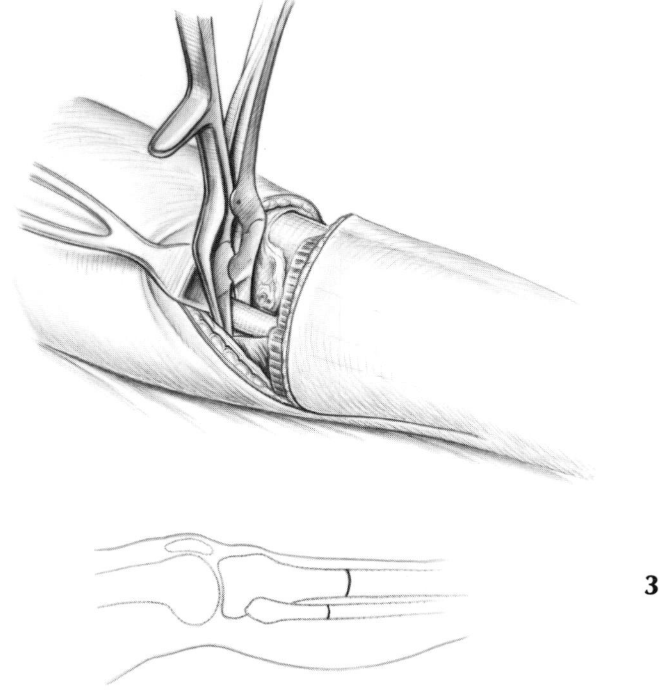

3

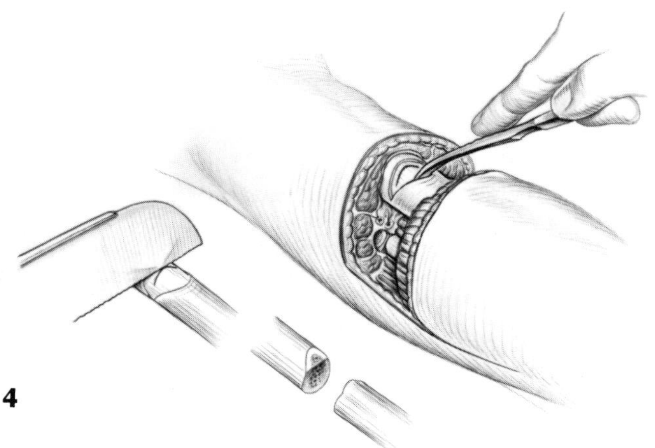

4

4

Using minimal retraction, so as not to disturb the precarious blood supply to the anterior skin, the periosteum on the tibia is then divided and elevated on its anterior surface, only far enough for the anterior bevel on the tibia to be cut. The tibia is then divided transversely and grasped firmly so that it can be pulled gently forward and the cut end of the fibula brought forward from the bulk of the muscle.

5

The posterior flap is cut with long medial and lateral incisions and rapid separation of the calf muscles from the posterior surface of the tibia and fibula. The posterior flap is divided distally to provide excessive length so that it may subsequently be trimmed to fit with absolutely no tension. The cut end of the tibia is rounded by filing and all sawdust and filings rinsed away with saline.

5

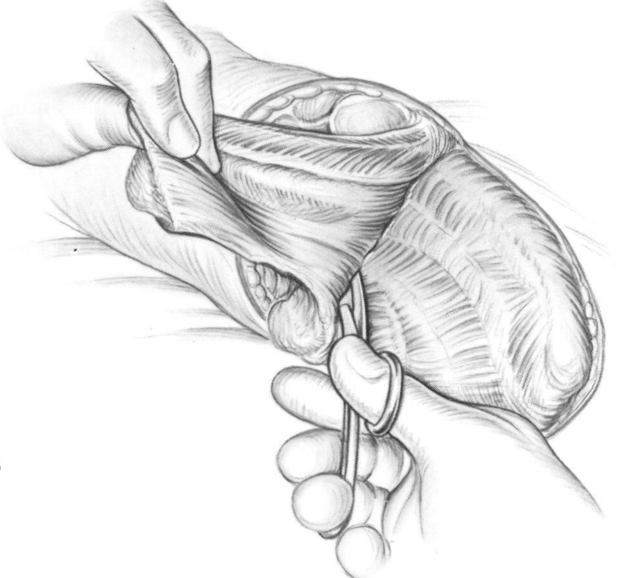

6

6

The plane between the gastrocnemius and the soleus is easily identified on the medial aspect of the flap and can simply be developed by blunt dissection. This plane is virtually avascular, demonstrating that the posterior flap is supplied by the sural arterial and not from the tibial vessels. The soleus is firmly adherent to the tendon of the gastrocnemius in the lateral part of the flap, but this may easily be divided leaving no soleus on the flap.

7

Once fully mobilized, the soleus is pulled distally and divided transversely at the level of the tibia, ligating the posterior tibial vessels and securing haemostasis at this stage. This procedure greatly reduces the bulk of the posterior flap so that the flap may be shortened without undue tension, improving the shape of the stump, preventing 'dog ears' and reducing the disproportion in thickness between the anterior and posterior tissues.

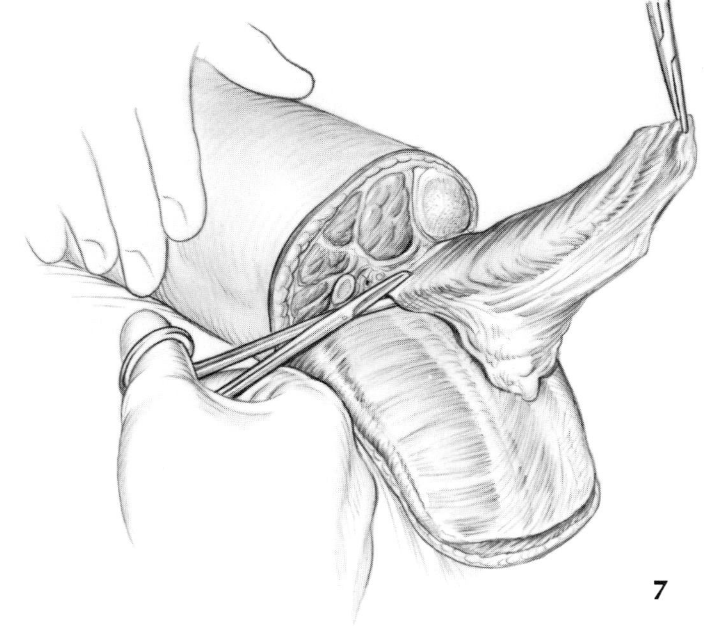

7

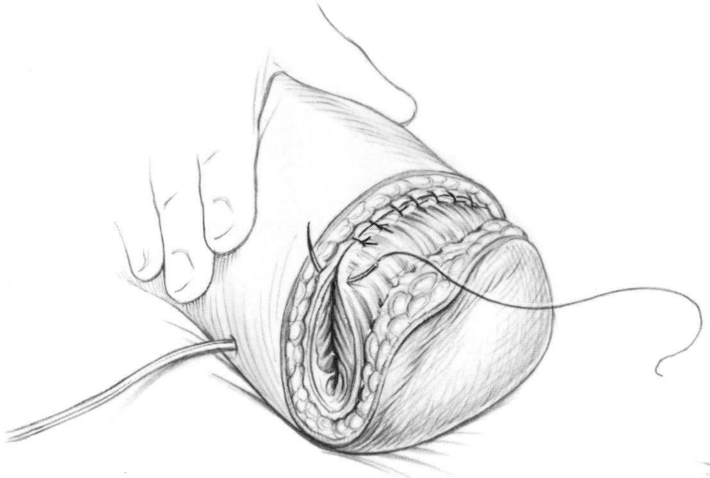

8a & b

The gastrocnemius tendon and deep fascia are divided first and sutured anteriorly, ensuring complete muscular cover of the bone end. Only then is the skin folded up and divided to an exact fit with no tension.

8a

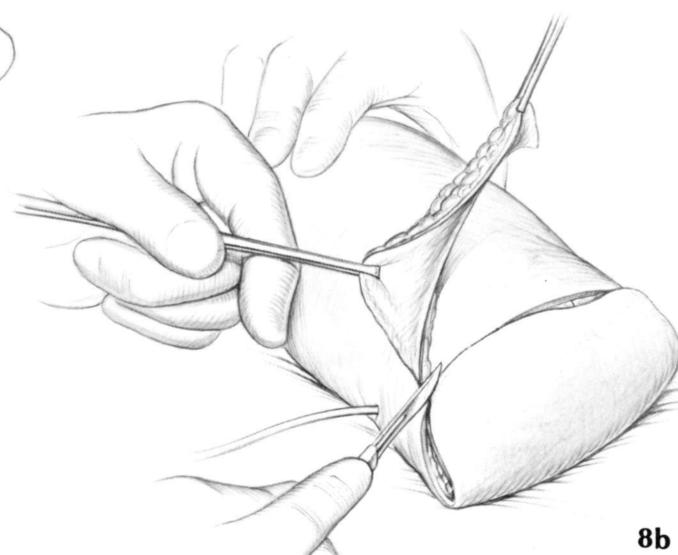

8b

9

Three or four 4/0 prolene sutures are loosely placed, but the main skin aposition is achieved with 0.5-inch wide steri- or suture-strips. I routinely use a redivac drain and the stump is then wrapped in a generous layer of wool, held in place by a gentle crêpe bandage applied to exert as little pressure as possible on the stump.

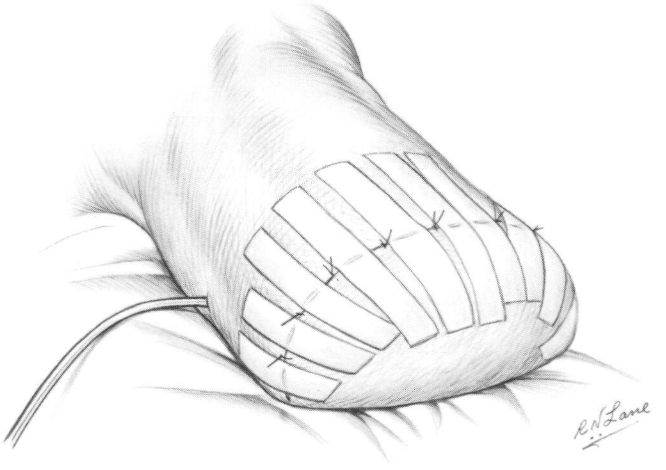

9

Postoperative care and rehabilitation

The patient is encouraged to mobilize the knee from the first postoperative day, with elevation initially and vigorous physiotherapy to ensure complete extension of the knee joint. As the suture strips maintain skin aposition the skin sutures may be removed after 5 or 6 days. The suture strips are left until wound healing is adequate, which may be anything between 8 and 20 days. Physiotherapy ideally starts prior to amputation and is designed to relieve any contractures that may be developing as a result of rest ischaemia. The emphasis is on the rapid recovery of a full range of movement in the knee joint so that the patient can 'drive' a patella tendon-bearing prosthesis. In this respect, knee extension must be complete so that mobilization with a pneumatic limb starts in the second week and a temporary prosthesis may then be fitted within 3–4 weeks.

References

Burgess, E. M. (1968). The below knee amputation. *Bull. Pros. Res. BRP* **10**, 9.

Burgess, E. M., Romano, R. L., Zettl, J. H. and Schrock, R. D., Jr (1971). Amputations of the leg for peripheral vascular insufficiency. *Journal of Bone and Joint Surgery* **53A**, 874.

Franzech, U. K., Talke, P., Bernstein, E. F. *et al.* (1982). Transcutaneous PO_2 measurements in health and peripheral arterial disease. *Surgery* **91**, 156.

Harrison, J. D., Southworth, S. and Callum, K. G. (1987). Experience with "skew-flap" below knee amputation. *British Journal of Surgery* **74**, 930.

Haynes, I. G. and Middleton, M. D. (1981). Amputation for peripheral vascular disease: Experience of a district general hospital. *Annals of Surgery* **63**, 342.

Katsamouris, A., Brewster, D. C., Megerman, J., Cina, C., Clement Darling, R. and Abbot, W. M. (1984). Transcutaneous oxygen tension in selection of amputation level. *American Journal of Surgery* **147**, 510.

Kendrick, R. R. (1956). Below knee amputation for arteriosclerotic gangrene. *British Journal of Surgery* **44**, 13.

Malone, J. M. and Godstone, J. (1986). Lower extremity amputation. In *Vascular Surgery: A Comprehensive Review*, 2nd ed. Moore, W., ed. London and San Diego: Grune and Stratton.

Rattiff, D. A., Clyne, C. A. C., Chant, A. D. B., *et al.* (1984). Prediction of amputation wound healing: The role of transcutaneous PO_2 assessment. *British Journal of Surgery* **71**, 219.

Robinson, K. P., Hoile, R. and Coddington, T. (1982). Skew flap myopastic below-knee amputation: A preliminary report. *British Journal of Surgery* **69**, 554.

Sethia, K. K., Berry, A. R., Morison, J. D., Collin, J., Murie, J. A. and Morris, P. J. (1986). Changing pattern of lower limb amputation for vascular disease. *British Journal of Surgery* **73**, 701.

Spence, V. A. and McCollum, P. T. Evaluation of the ischaemic limb by transcutaneous oxymetry. In *Diagnostic Techniques and Assessment Procedures in Vascular Surgery*. Greenhalgh, R. M. ed. London and San Diego: Grune and Stratton.

Skew-flap below-knee amputation

KINGSLEY ROBINSON MS, FRCS
Consultant Surgeon, Westminster Hospital, London, UK

Introduction

This technique is designed to make the best use of the blood supply to the below-knee skin in patients with peripheral vascular disease to form a stump which is shaped to be suitable for prosthetic use at the conclusion of the surgical operation, and which has a standardized technique that is reproducible in the hands of different surgeons, so that a stump with the same characteristics can be consistently produced.

1

The length of the stump is determined by the line of bone section which is measured from the articular surface of the tibial plateau and according to the patient's build is between 10 and 14 cm below this level. The level should be judged to be just above the maximum convexity of the calf muscle mass and not shorter than a point that allows 4 cm of stump to protrude beyond the hamstring tendons when the knee is flexed to 90°. The line of bone section is drawn on the skin overlying the tibia and a circumferential equator line is extended around the limb at this point. It is important to use a fully waterproof marking device, and if the skin marking is performed in the anaesthetic room, a waterproof fibre-tip cartridge writer is ideal and the skin can be subsequently prepared with a spirit-based antiseptic without removing the marks. A point 2 cm lateral to the subcutaneous tibial crest is marked on the equator line and a vertical mark parallel to the axis of the limb is extended upwards for 2 cm. This point represents the junction of the anteromedial and posterolateral skin flap. To identify the diametrically opposite point on the back of the limb a tape is passed around the equator line and cut to that length. This tape folded in half will then indicate the posterior junction of the flaps. If the same tape is then folded to obtain a quarter length, this will indicate the midpoints of each flap along the equator line from which the quarter circumference length can be drawn on the skin to indicate the length of the skin flap at its maximum extent. A semicircular line then connects the three marks to form the skew flaps. The skin is incised together with the subcutaneous fat, the periosteum over the tibia and the anterior tibial compartment and peroneal compartment fascia.

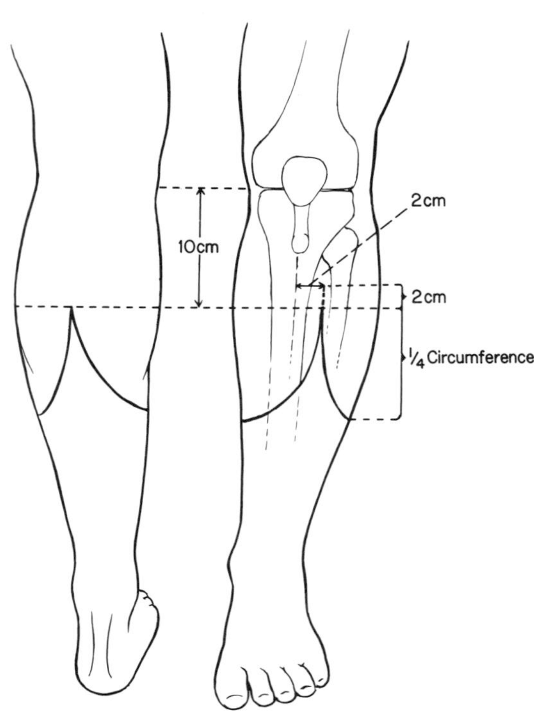

1

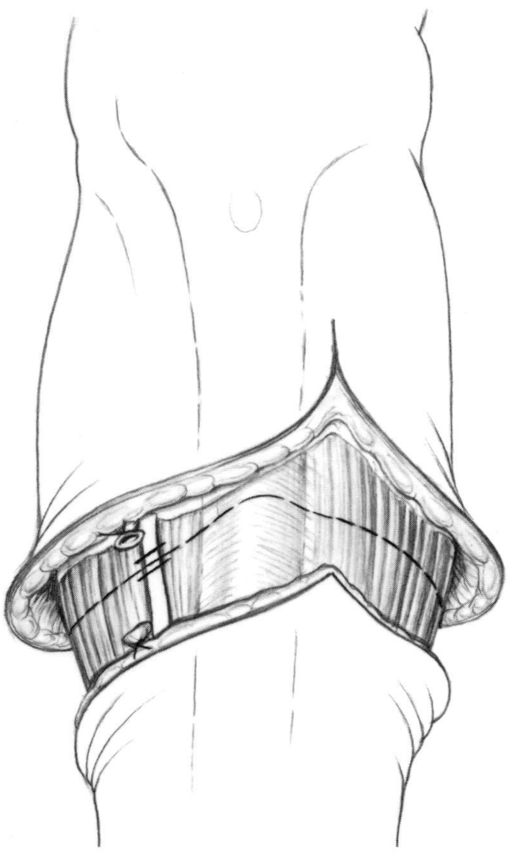

2

2

When the skin incision has been completed and the skin retracted, the long saphenous vein and the short saphenous vein need to be secured with artery forceps and ligated with fine catgut or vicryl 3/0, while the saphenous nerve and sural nerve are separately divided under some tension to allow the ends to retract. Very few bleeding points require attention at this stage and the skin flaps can be elevated to expose the anterior aspect of the tibia and the peroneal and anterior tibial muscle compartments. The tibial periosteum and the anterior tibial muscles are divided along the line of the equator mark on the skin, the upward extension of the skin incision providing access to the anterior tibial compartment with moderate retraction.

3

The dissection is carried through the anterior tibial peroneal muscles, a few muscle fibres at a time, either with a scalpel or diathermy point, until the anterior tibial nerve and the musculocutaneous nerve are revealed in each compartment, allowing them to be drawn down under tension and cut transversely with a scalpel so that they can retract clear of the area of the stump end. The anterior tibial artery and its venae comitans are revealed close to the interosseous membrane and can be divided between haemostats and ligated with a fine vicryl or catgut suture. The anterior surface of the fibula and the lateral surface of the tibia are now exposed together with the interosseous membrane. The latter is divided in the line of the dissection and a periosteal elevator is used to clear all surfaces of the tibia at this same level. The fibula can similarly be cleared and retraction will expose an adequate length to allow the fibula to be divided 2 cm proximal to the line of bone section marked on the skin.

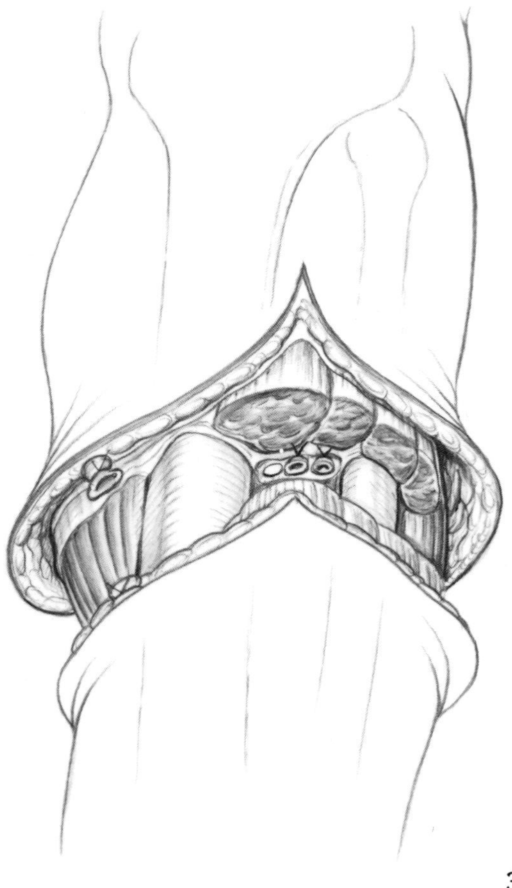

3

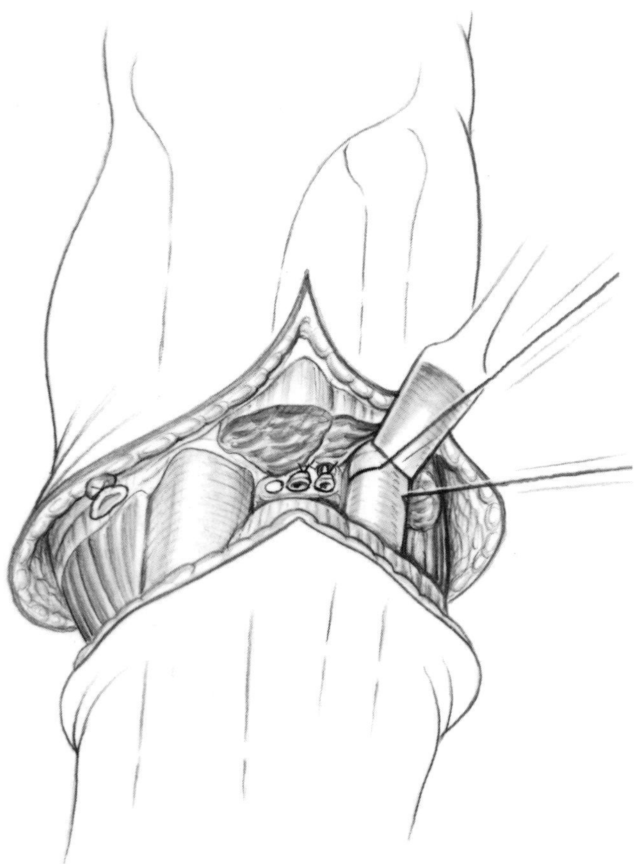

4

4

The fibula is divided first. Bone forceps should not be used for this purpose because the fibula will fragment into sharp pieces and may split along its whole length. A Gigli saw is convenient for dividing the bone, although a cantilever power-saw is much easier to manage. Sometimes the nutrient vessels of both the fibula and tibia are encountered at this level and may produce some bleeding that has to be controlled with a pack until better access is obtained after the bones are divided. Once the fibula is divided, the tibia can be transected.

5

The tibia is most conveniently cut with a cantilever power-saw while copious irrigation is maintained to avoid any heat damage to the bone ends and to remove the bone dust and fragments. The cantilever power-saw will permit a gentle anterior curve to be described as the bone is transected, but if a hand saw is used, a sloping cut is made through the anterior half of the bone and then a transverse cut through the remaining half to produce a partial bevel which can then be rounded by subsequent filing. Once the tibia is completely divided, the distal fragment is stabilized by inserting a sharp bone hook into the medullary cavity and applying some traction.

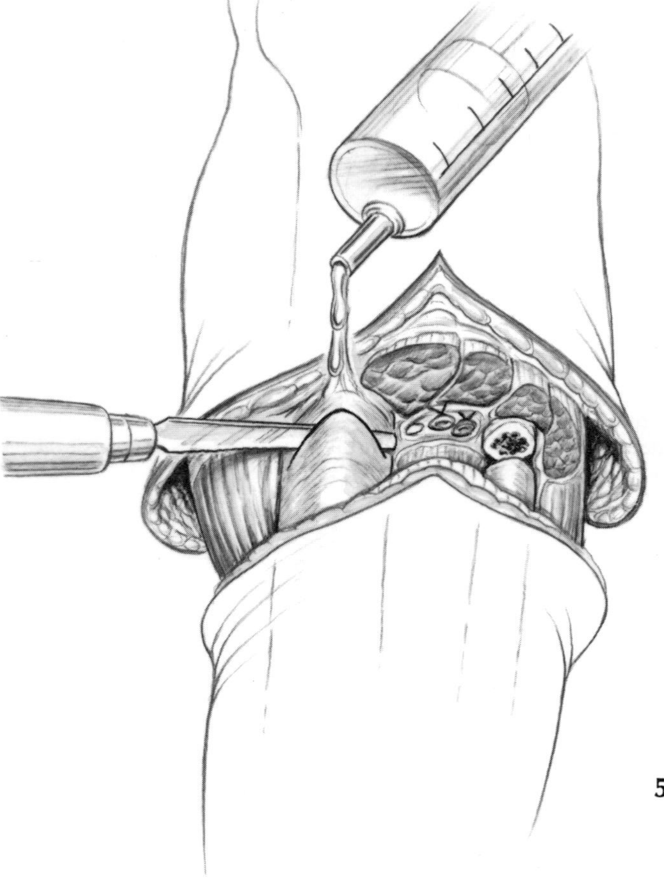

5

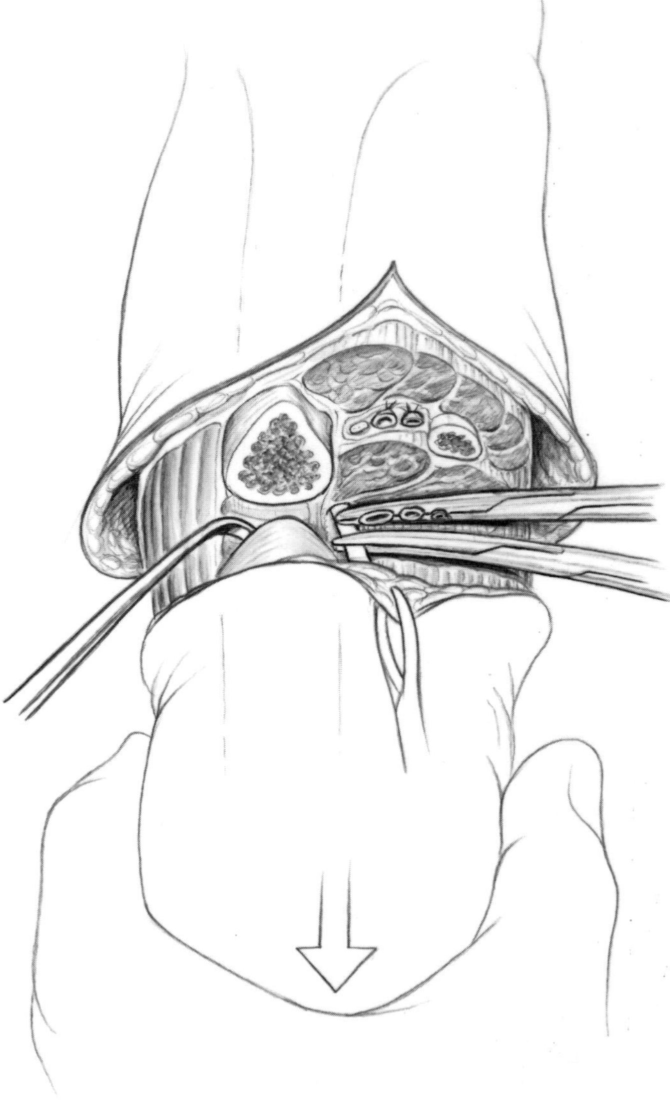

6

6

While downward traction is maintained on the distal fragment of the tibia, the tibialis posterior muscle is clearly visible and can be divided a few fibres at a time until the neurovascular bundles and the posterior tibial nerve are revealed beneath it. The most convenient technique to handle the neurovascular bundles is the application of a large artery forcep of the Robert's type with enough length being allowed for a second forcep to be applied behind the first so that the posterior tibial nerve can be extricated, and both the peroneal and posterior tibial arteries and their venae comitans can then be separately secured and the temporary proximal forcep removed. The posterior tibial nerve, the largest encountered in the dissection, is drawn down strongly and cut across with the scalpel and allowed to retract well away. Some bleeding from its concomitant artery may be encountered and this is never a problem. The skin flaps are separated from the distal part of the limb by a blunt dissection and drawn down to allow access to the full thickness of the gastrocnemius soleus muscle mass which is extricated from the distal portion of the limb, the very distance at least equal to the vertical thickness of the formed stump. If the assistant presses firmly across the upper part of the calf muscles, a degree of control of the remaining vessels is obtained and the gastrocnemius muscle mass can be transected at the chosen distal level with a minimum of blood loss.

7

At this point the myoplastic flap to be formed from the gastrocnemius soleus mass is formed. The muscle tongue is pulled out with tissue forceps and a slope is cut from the line of bone section to the distal end of the flap leaving only aponeurosis for the last few millimetres. This will transect the soleal venous sinuses and numerous small arteries which will require individual transfixion and underrunning with sutures to obtain full haemostasis. The use of diathermy ligaclips and simple ligatures is rarely successful and an underrunning suture will save a considerable amount of time.

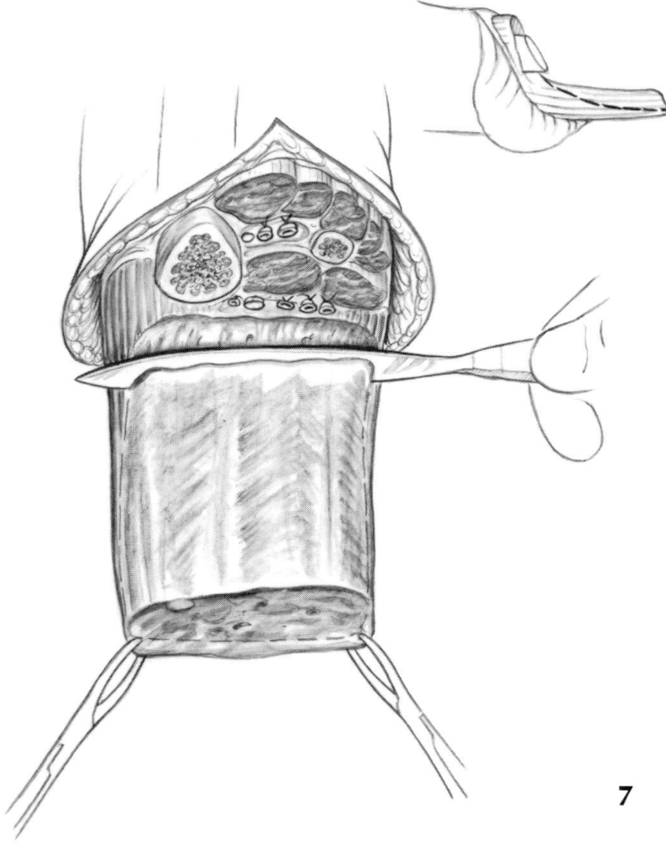

7

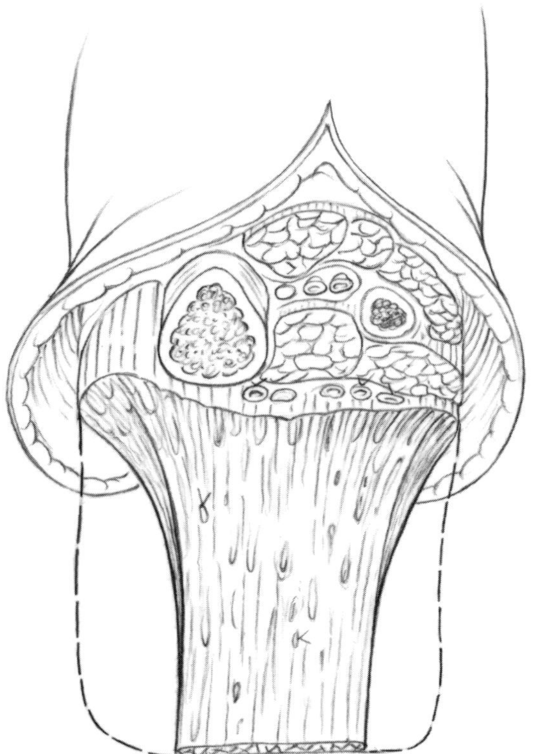

8

8

Once haemostasis is obtained and the tapering flap has been constructed, the dimensions of this are then checked by folding it forward to approximate its distal end to the anterior tibial periosteum and the anterior tibial fascia. This will demonstrate how much bulk the folded muscle mass will produce at the medial and lateral aspects and, following accurate trimming of the distal end of the flap, the sides of the muscle mass must then be reduced to make sure that there is no widening when the muscle flap is folded over.

9 & 10

A large scalpel is used to trim away the excess muscle tissue and the trimming process may have to be extended above the line of bone section into the peroneal muscle group and on the medial side of the gastrocnemius. Some further venous sinuses may require underrunning and ligation. At this stage attention is paid to the bone ends which are then carefully shaped with a coarse rasp and then a fine bone file to produce a rounded corner with a smooth surface in all dimensions. Similar attention must also be paid to the fibula end so that there is no excess scar tissue formed by trauma due to movement of bone fragments in the muscle tissue. A careful wash out is required to remove all the calcium fragments and a suction drain is placed in relation to the bone ends and passed through the skin laterally and secured with a stitch. The myoplastic flap is now finally folded over.

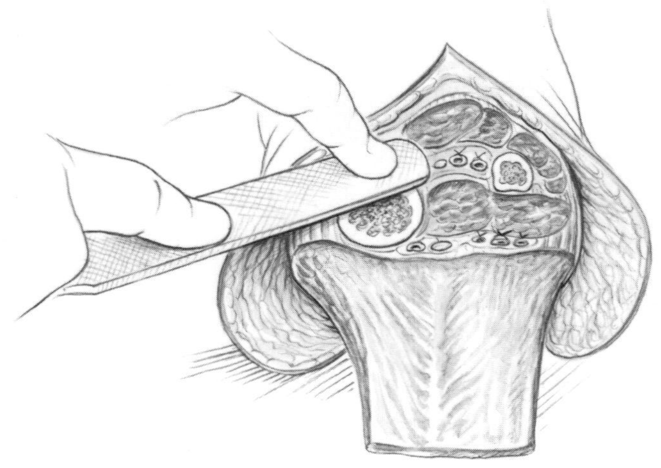

9

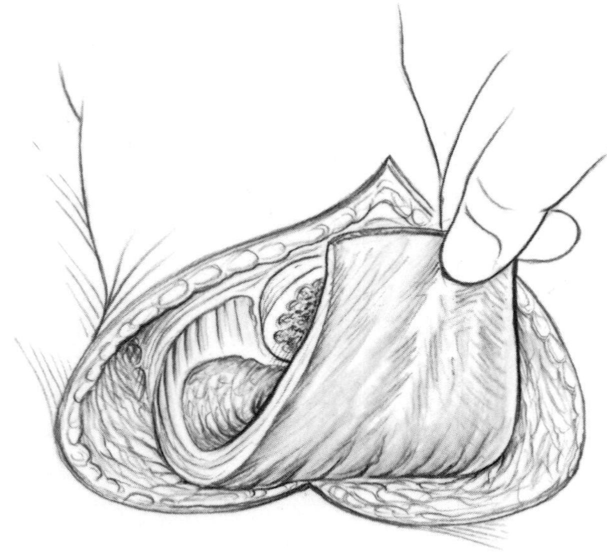

10

11

The folded flap is carefully opposed to the anterior tibial fascia and the anterior tibial periosteum. A continuous suture of '1' chromic catgut or '0' vicryl is used to run along the whole anterior aspect of the stump and to complete the myoplasty. The skin flaps remain partially attached to the gastrocnemius soleus mass and a small degree of separation may be required to allow them to come into comfortable apposition and the skin and subcutaneous fat are sutured with interrupted stitches – usually vertical mattress sutures of 3/0 nylon – to approximate the skin edges along the line of the skew flaps. It is recommended that the anterior and posterior sutures are inserted first and then a central stay stitch to allow any fine adjustment in the alignment of the flaps to be obtained before closure is complete. The application of steristrips to the skin between each interrupted suture may relieve tension loading on the sutures.

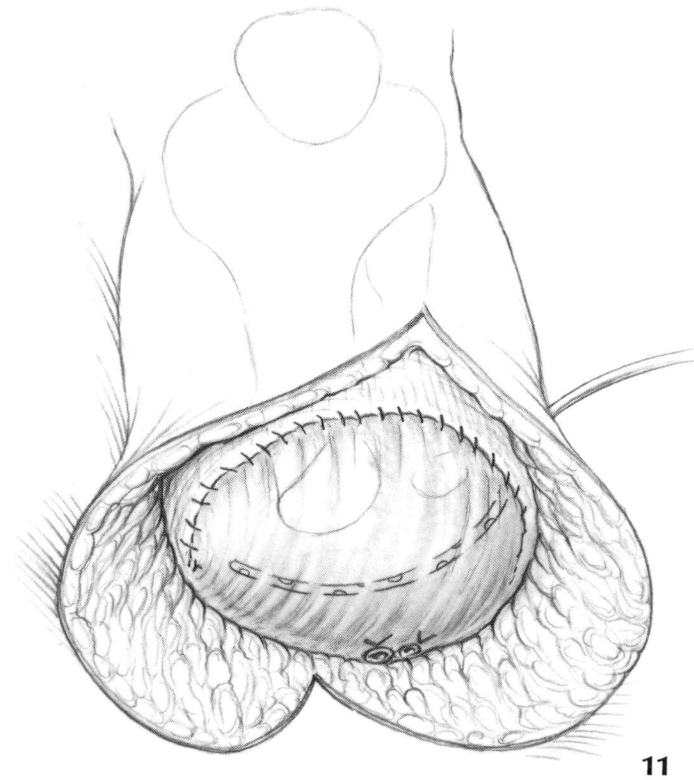

11

12

12

At completion, the stump is usually well-rounded, parallel-sided and symmetrical, with the suture line just clear of the anterior tibial crest and the tibia and fibula bone ends. The soft tissues are not excessive or redundant and the patient may be allowed to apply stress to the stump between 2 and 4 days from the completion of the operation. Definitive stump bandaging is not recommended and our current practice is to use finely fluffed cotton gauze without any cotton wool or padding applied to the stump, and a spiral of 4″ crêpe bandage keeps the fluffed gauze in place without applying any pressure or constriction to the stump itself. At the first dressing change, a netalast elastic net is used to retain the dressing, and as soon as possible the dressing is discarded altogether.

Toe and foot amputations

FRANK J. VEITH MD

Professor of Surgery and Chief of Vascular Surgical Services, Albert Einstein College of Medicine and Montefiore Medical Center, New York, USA

SUSHIL K. GUPTA MD

Associate Professor of Surgery and Associate Chief of Vascular Surgery, Albert Einstein College of Medicine and Montefiore Medical Center, New York, USA

ENRICO ASCER MD

Associate Professor of Surgery, Albert Einstein College of Medicine, New York, USA;
Vascular Surgeon in Charge, North Central Bronx Hospital, New York, USA

KURT R. WENGERTER MD

Assistant Professor of Surgery and Assistant Attending Vascular Surgeon, Albert Einstein College of Medicine and Montefiore Medical Center, New York, USA

Introduction

Performance of successful toe or partial foot amputation can be a critical part of limb salvage surgery in many patients who have gangrene and/or infection with or without ischaemia from arterial occlusive disease. These amputations within the foot include ablation of one or more toes, toe amputation with a portion of the adjacent metatarsal bone, partial (medial or lateral) transmetatarsal amputation, complete transmetatarsal amputation and a variety of unnamed or free-style partial foot amputations or debridements designed to remove necrotic or infected tissue and allow healing of enough of the foot to permit functional weight-bearing on the residual part of the extremity.

General principles

Before considering the specific techniques for these amputations within the foot, several principles must be emphasized. The first is that with normal or near-normal arterial circulation to the foot and adequate debridement or excision of infected and necrotic tissue, remarkable healing of the residual foot can be obtained. Moreover, even a small remnant of the foot can be effectively used for bipedal ambulation in sick, old patients, with one or more other disabilities. Salvage of less than half the foot with its plantar skin intact will permit more effective ambulation than a below-knee amputation if the patient has had a contralateral major amputation or a stroke. In this regard, we have found it possible to remove a major portion of the heel, including the Achilles tendon and the weight-bearing part of the os calcis, and still have the patient use the foot effectively in walking. Similarly, loss of the toes, metatarsals and most of the tarsal bones, leaving a foot remnant one-third the length of normal, does not preclude effective bipedal ambulation, which is not achieved in more than 30% of our patients undergoing below-knee amputation because of their frequent intercurrent disabilities.

A second principle relates to the importance of confirming adequate arterial circulation to permit successful performance of amputations within the foot. Simple toe amputations will occasionally heal with somewhat diminished ankle–brachial pressure indices and pulse volume recordings, but they almost never will when the ankle–brachial index is less than 0.6 and forefoot waves are flat or less than 5 mm in amplitude. Moreover, complex partial foot amputations and particularly some of the free-style transtarsal amputations to be described require near-normal arterial circulation to the foot. If a normal pedal pulse is not palpable or non-invasive tests do not indicate direct or straight-line arterial flow to the foot, the amputation within the foot should not be undertaken until arteriography and successful revascularization of the foot have been performed.

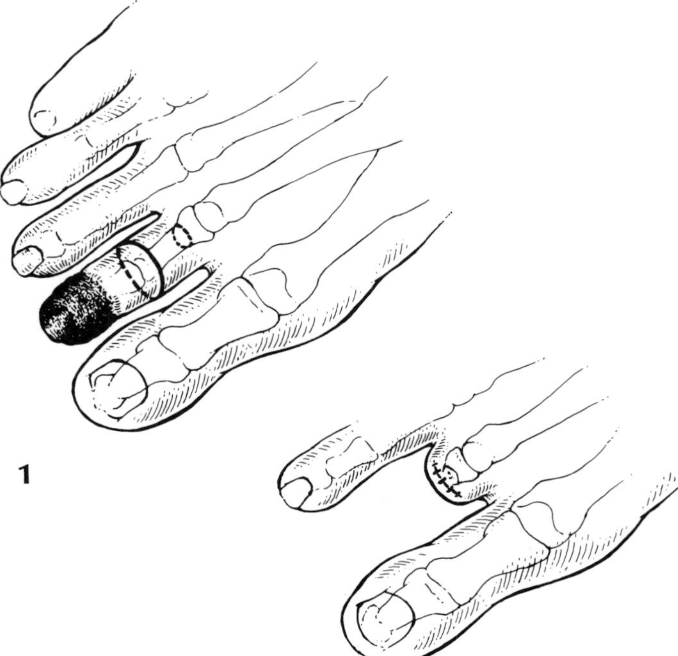

1

A third set of principles relate to the decision to close the skin primarily or leave the wound open. Although this decision requires careful judgement, there are certain guidelines which the surgeon should follow. If infection is evident or tissue viability is in question, the wound must be left open. Skin closure should never be under tension. Any wound that is closed must be reopened if wound edges become dusky or tension develops because of oedema. Open wounds are best kept moist with saline. This can be accomplished effectively by incorporating impermeable plastic within the saline-soaked dressing.

Fourthly, control of infection and normal or near-normal circulation are necessary for successful healing by secondary intention. Adequate debridement of infected and necrotic tissue is also essential and may require several trips to the operating room. Split thickness skin grafting can hasten healing once a clean granulating wound is obtained. Even on weight-bearing surfaces, such skin grafts can help to save feet.

Fifthly, there are no absolute barriers to debridement. Infected or necrotic tissue must be removed even if it requires exposure of joint interiors between the tarsal bones or even the ankle. With good circulation, adequate debridement and postoperative care healing can be achieved. A rongeur is a most useful instrument to perform adequate debridement of infected or necrotic tissues within the foot. This includes soft tissue, tendons, cartilage and bone.

A sixth and final principle is adherence to the use of minimally traumatic technique to handle all remaining tissue. Crushing of tissue and grasping of the skin with forceps must be avoided. Haemostasis should be complete but no adjacent tissue should be ligated or coagulated with blood vessels.

Specific amputations within the foot

1

Simple toe amputation

This is performed by making a circular incision in the skin of the toe as close to the proximal interphalangeal joint as possible, thereby assuring adequate skin length to permit closure by primary or secondary intention. The actual position of the skin incision is determined by the amount of remaining viable skin left on the toe. Care is taken to make the incision in viable skin. The soft tissues are then sharply divided down to the proximal phalanx. A flap of soft tissue is raised to provide access to the base of the proximal phalanx and the bone is divided using a bone-cutting forceps or rongeur without entering the metatarsal-phalangeal joint. If the skin is clearly viable and uninfected and closure without tension can be performed, a few monofilament sutures are placed in the skin to close the wound in a transverse plane. If any of these conditions cannot be fulfilled, the wound is left open to heal by secondary intention. If the metatarsal-phalangeal joint is entered, all of the cartilage, the entire proximal phalanx and much of the head of the metatarsal bone should be removed with a rongeur. Care is taken to remove all bone spicules and tissue fragments using the same instrument.

2

Removal of one or more toes with a portion of the corresponding metatarsal bone

If all the phalanges and all of the associated metatarsal bone are amputated, the procedure is often described as a 'ray' amputation. The 'ray' amputation is frequently required for quite severe osteomyelitis in association with diabetic gangrene. However, more frequently, the degree of infection dictates only that the head of the metatarsal needs to be excised with the toe, as is described here.

The skin incision is performed at the distal-most limit of viability. This incision is deepened to bone. The formation of flaps with so-called racquet handle incisions is kept to a minimum, but proximal extension of the incision is acceptable to provide proximal exposure of the metatarsal shafts. A periosteal elevator is used to expose the metatarsal-phalangeal joint and the distal portions of the metatarsal bones. These are transected in their midshaft with bone-cutting forceps or a vibrating saw. Sharp or projecting bone fragments are smoothed with a rongeur, and the same instrument is used to facilitate excision of deep soft tissue that may be non-viable or infected. The presence of dark thrombosed small blood vessels in the soft tissues indicates both infection and non-viability, and all such tissue must be excised. Haemostasis is obtained, and the wound edges are then loosely approximated or left open according to the principles already outlined.

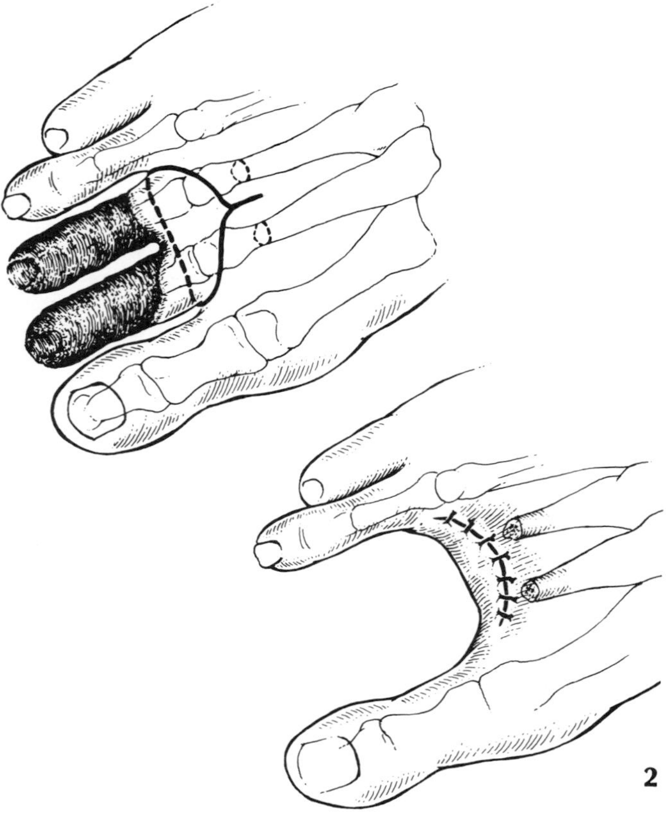

2

3

Partial (medial or lateral) transmetatarsal amputation

These procedures are useful when gangrene involves the proximal portions of one or two toes medially or laterally with or without involvement of the adjacent webspace or webspaces. Again the skin incision is made to preserve as much viable skin and soft tissue as possible. The incision is deepened to bone and the thickest possible flaps are raised using sharp dissection with a scalpel supplemented by a periosteal elevator. The metatarsal bone or bones are then transected through their shaft with bone-cutting forceps or a vibrating saw as far proximally as is necessary to permit the skin and soft tissue to fall together over the bone ends without tension. The interior of the wound is carefully inspected for bone spicules and tissues of questionable viability. These include remnants of divided tendon and joint capsule. All these elements which require debridement are sharply excised by grasping them with a rongeur and transecting them with this instrument or cutting them with a scalpel while they are held in tension by the rongeur. This particular technique with a rongeur is useful in all debridements and excisions of necrotic tissue within the foot. It is the most effective way to assure smooth bone ends and minimally traumatic removal of all tendonous and ligamentous remnants which tend to have a poor blood supply.

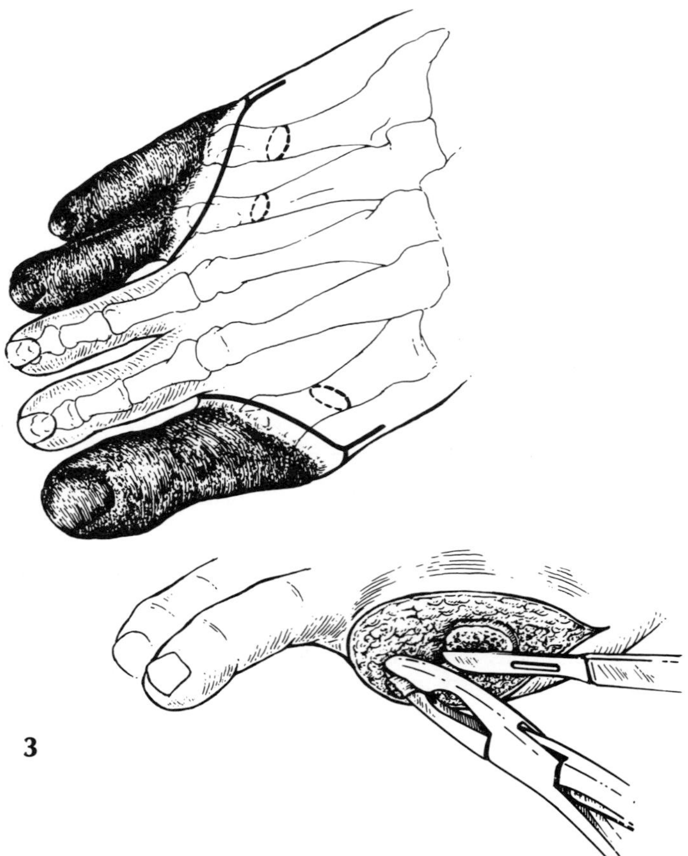

3

4

Transmetatarsal amputation

This operation is indicated when gangrene involves all the toes including one or more webspaces. It produces a very functional foot without the need for a prosthesis or special shoe. If only the distal portion of four or five toes are necrotic, several simple toe amputations are performed in preference to a transmetatarsal amputation. Although the resulting foot remnant after multiple toe amputations may be less pleasing aesthetically, it has the advantage of preserving the important weight-bearing and step-off functions of the metatarsal heads. In addition, leaving the webspaces intact preserves important collateral circulation to skin edges and maintains skin bridges which minimize tension on the suture line.

Transmetatarsal amputation is performed by making an incision through the distal-most viable skin. Because of its greater thickness and tolerance to weight-bearing, preservation of plantar skin is particularly important. Accordingly, if possible, the end of the foot remnant should be covered with a relatively longer plantar flap. However, if viable plantar skin is limited, closure can be achieved by leaving more of the dorsal skin. If closure of viable skin without tension or residual infection is not possible, the wound may be left open to heal by secondary intention with or without skin grafting. Although this may require a protracted hospital stay, the resulting foot remnant can provide excellent function. Occasionally, if a portion of the wound is questionable, the rest of it may be closed loosely by adhesive strips and the questionable part left open and treated with wet dressings.

After the plantar flap is developed superficial to the tendons of the toe flexors to the level of bone transection, the forefoot is plantar flexed and the dorsal incision is carried down to the metatarsal heads. With continued plantar flexion, all tendons are incised as far proximally as possible. The forefoot is then dorsiflexed and the plantar tendons divided as far proximally as possible. The metatarsal shafts are then transected by already described techniques that will permit approximation of wound edges without tension. The rongeur–scalpel techniques described above are then used to provide smooth bone ends and to debride devitalized tissue and tendon ends. Haemostasis is secured and the wound approximated completely or partially, or left open depending on the pathology and principles already discussed.

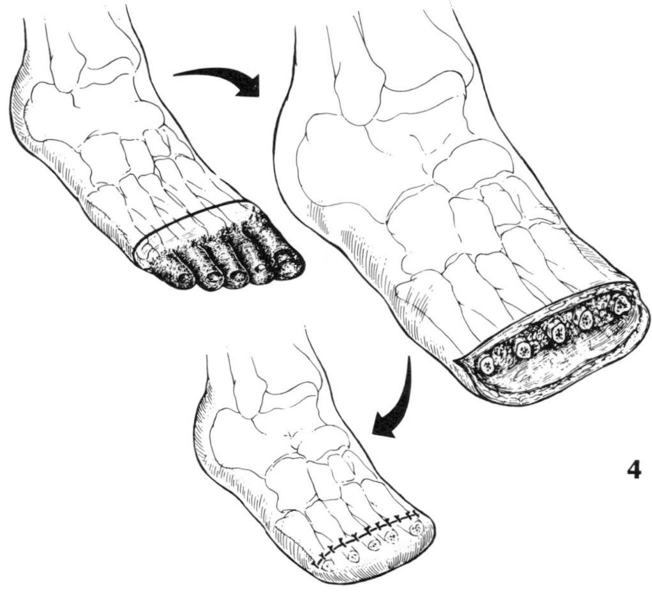

4

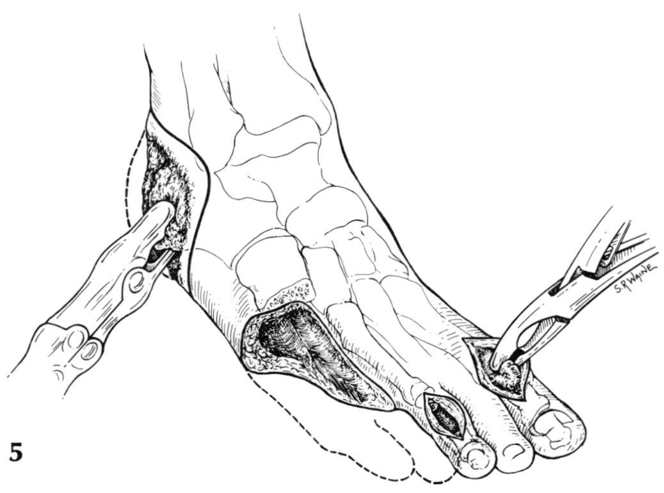

5

5

Freestyle foot amputations (transtarsal amputations, heel amputations, excision of metatarsal-phalangeal joint and excision of toe bones)

The first two of these procedures facilitate removal of necrotic or infected tissues that are more extensive than those treated by the standard procedures already described. The other two procedures preserve the soft tissue of the toes and permit excision of bones that are involved with osteomyelitis, thereby facilitating healing of toe or foot lesions. In all four instances excision of involved bone and soft tissue is accomplished by the rongeur–scalpel techniques already described and wounds are left open to heal by secondary intention with or without skin grafting. If transtarsal amputation is performed the Achilles tendon should be divided by dorsiflexing the foot remnant and cutting the stretched taught tendon with a No. 11 blade inserted alongside the tendon via a 3-mm skin incision.

Conclusions

All of these foot amputations can be valuable in preserving bipedal gait in patients with extensive gangrene and/or infection. In general, as much viable foot as possible should be preserved. Although multiple operations may be required and normal or near-normal arterial circulation is usually a prerequisite, the foot has a remarkable ability to heal and, by using the techniques described in this chapter, functional remnants of foot can be preserved despite the presence of surprisingly extensive gangrene and infection.

Acknowledgements

This work was supported in part by the Manning Foundation, The Anna S. Brown Foundation and the New York Institute for Vascular Studies.

Basic principles in the surgical management of vascular trauma

JOHN V. ROBBS ChM (CT), FRCSEd

Chief, Vascular Service and Head, Division of Surgery, University of Natal Medical School, Durban, South Africa

Introduction

Trauma to the major arteries and veins may present the most taxing technical problems encountered by the operating surgeon. This entails not only access to the major vessels in certain areas, but also control of haemorrhage and the sometimes exacting exercise of accurately restoring continuity of the involved vessels. There are few areas in surgery less forgiving of imperfect technique. The major thrust of this chapter will be towards management of arterial injury.

Mechanisms and pathology of arterial injury

1a, b & c

An understanding of the mechanisms of injury and pathology encountered is essential in order to treat these injuries rationally. In Table 1, mechanisms of injury, each of which results in a specific type of pathology, are summarized. The pathology encountered is illustrated in *Illustration 1a–f.* Following penetration by a sharp instrument or a low-velocity missile (for example, from a small-calibre hand gun) the tissue damage is essentially confined to the track of the penetrating agent. Low-velocity missiles may, however, compound the injury by fragmentation of soft-nosed bullets or fragments of bone; ricochet may also be responsible for more extensive damage.

High-velocity missiles are defined as those in which the muzzle velocity exceeds 2000 feet/s (approximately 600 m/s). Under these circumstances, there is a highly significant energy release during passage through the tissues which causes a cavitation effect resulting in a great deal of soft tissue damage around the track. In addition, extraneous material such as clothing is drawn into the wound.

Penetrating trauma may result in a lateral perforation of the artery with formation of a false aneurysm. Total transection with or without loss of substance of the vessel may also occur and the artery frequently develops spasm at its severed ends (*b*) with resultant thrombosis. Simultaneous lateral perforation of artery and adjacent vein may result in the formation of an acute arteriovenous fistula, with or without an associated false aneurysm (*c*).

Table 1 Mechanisms of vascular injury

Penetrating	Stab
	Missile
	high-velocity (600 m/s or 2000 m/s)
	low-velocity
Blunt	Direct
	Indirect
Blast	Shotgun
	Bomb
Iatrogenic	

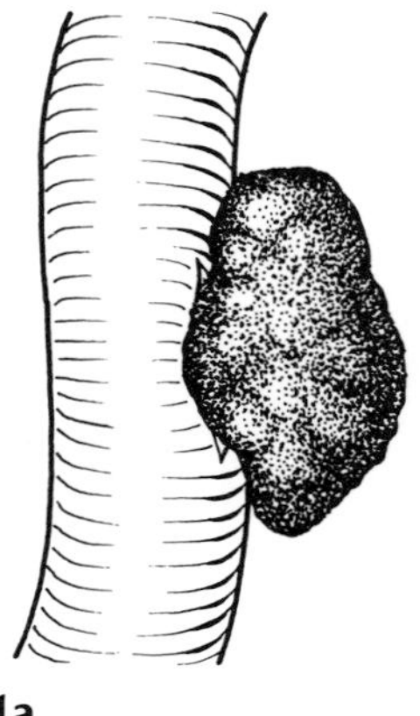

1a

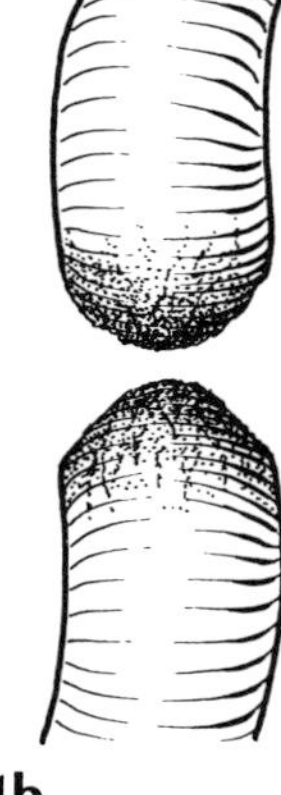

1b

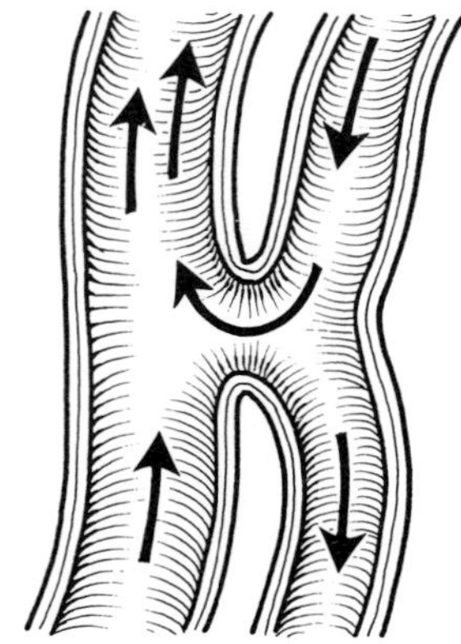

1c

1d &e

Direct blunt trauma is exemplified by a direct localized blow to the vessel against a rigid bony structure. Indirect injuries are caused by distraction which may occur with joint dislocation or acceleration–deceleration trauma with its associated shearing forces at areas of fixity of the artery. An example of the latter is the aortic disruption found at the isthmus or aortic valve ring in road traffic accident victims. The intima and media of the vessel wall are less elastic than the overlying adventitia and when the vessel is subjected to the type of forces described, it tends to disrupt from the less elastic layers on the inside towards the adventitia in proportion to the degree of violence. If the adventitia remains intact with an intimomedial tear in smaller calibre vessels, superimposed thrombosis occurs due to a combination of exposure of blood to the thrombogenic raw surface and the elevation of a distally based flap (*d*). In larger vessels such as the aorta, thrombosis does not occur to any great extent but an aneurysm tends to form at that site. Obviously with this type of trauma, if the forces are great enough all layers disrupt through part or all of the circumference, with perforation of the artery.

Shotgun blast injuries result in extensive soft tissue destruction which is contaminated by multiple small pellets which remain firmly embedded in the tissues. This is particularly noticeable when birdshot has been used. In addition, there are frequently multiple sites of perforation within the neurovascular bundle.

Bomb explosions may produce similar multiple penetrating wounds and soft tissue trauma but, in victims close to the explosion, high-velocity fragments may result in extensive cavitating injury and the situation may be compounded by surface flash burns.

Iatrogenic vascular injuries warrant separate consideration. The most frequently encountered is catheter trauma associated with diagnostic radiological procedures. Laceration at the arterial puncture site may occur with the formation of false aneurysm or free haemorrhage. However, in smaller vessels (as in children), or the brachial artery in adults, thrombosis may occur at the site of the puncture due to the associated intimal damage. In atherosclerotic vessels, dislodgement of plaque and the formation of a flap with subsequent thrombosis or even distal embolization of atheromatous debris may occur (*e*). Passage of the catheter between the layers of a diseased vessel with subintimal injection of contrast resulting in superimposed thrombosis is also occasionally seen following diagnostic radiological procedures.

Excessive inflation of the balloon of an embolectomy catheter may result in significant arterial injury. This applies particularly when the balloon is filled with fluid, thus creating a hydraulic system which is capable of transmitting extremely high pressures. The types of lesions caused range from intimomedial tears or stripping with subsequent thrombosis to transmural rupture with perforation. It is strongly recommended that air be used to inflate the catheter balloon during its use.

Intra-arterial injection of lipid-soluble substances may be responsible for injury to the arterioles by fixing in the intimal tissues with superimposed intense spasm and thrombosis. In clinical practice this is occasionally seen following inadvertent injection of sodium pentothal or diazepam which are both widely used for premedication purposes during anaesthesia or invasive diagnostic procedures. A similar spectrum of pathologies is seen in drug abusers following intra-arterial injection of a variety of agents. These lesions are not amenable to direct arterial reconstructive surgery.

1f

Arterial spasm

This is always associated with trauma to an artery whatever mechanism may have been responsible and whatever the underlying pathology may be. In addition, the lack of intraluminal pressure in the arterial tree distal to the site of injury results in marked diminution in calibre of these vessels due to the unopposed sympathetic tone which further aggravates distal ischaemia. Spasm occurring in isolation as a cause of distal ischaemia is exceptionally rare and in our own series, which numbers well in excess of 1000 cases of arterial trauma, it has been found to be the sole cause of the problem in less than 1%. Spasm as a cause of distal ischaemia is therefore a retrospective diagnosis made at the time of surgical exploration.

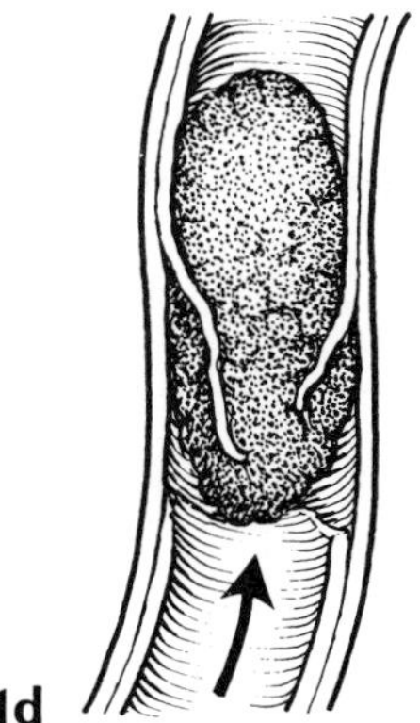

1d

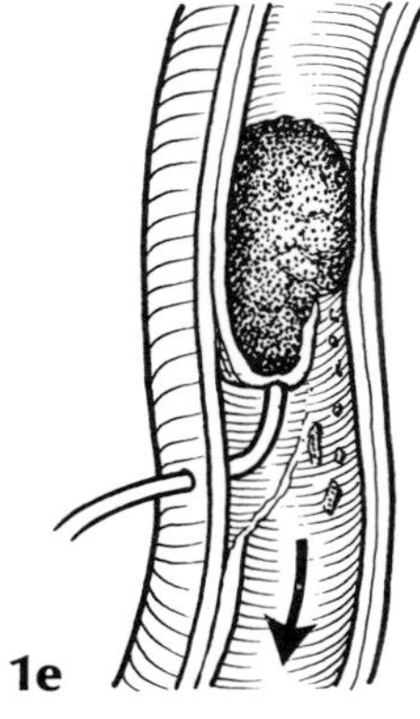

1e

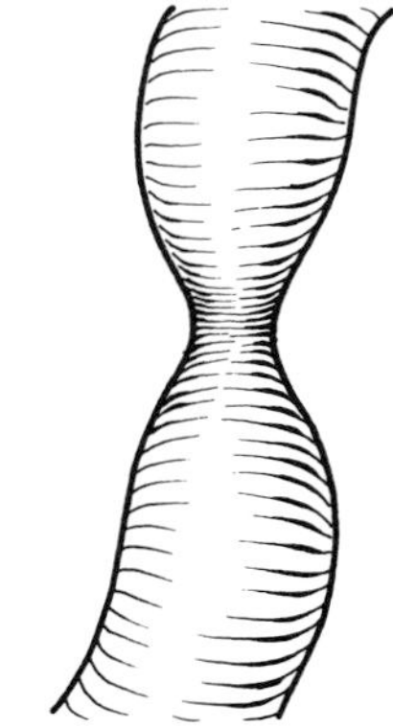

1f

Preoperative evaluation and diagnosis

Diagnosis rests upon a high index of clinical suspicion, and vascular injury should be entertained in every patient who has a penetrating wound of the neck and extremities and in every long-bone fracture or joint dislocation. In patients with multiple injuries, once ventilatory and haemodynamic deficits have been stabilized, every injury must be considered on its particular merit and remote injuries should not be allowed to distract from the possibility of an arterial injury, particularly in the extremities. An accurate assessment of peripheral perfusion cannot be made in a hypovolaemic peripherally vasoconstricted patient and it is important to reserve final clinical assessment of peripheral perfusion until the patient has been adequately volume resuscitated.

Arterial injuries *per se* present in principle with either occlusion, haemorrhage or arteriovenous fistulation. Occlusion invariably results in a pulse deficit with or without significant signs of ischaemia. It must be re-emphasized that in isolation, arterial spasm will never cause significant peripheral ischaemia. Another important pitfall which must be avoided in patients who have sustained blunt trauma is the entity of delayed thrombosis, as it may take several hours of occlusive thrombus to develop on an area of intimal disruption and patients with high-risk injuries such as knee dislocation or lower third femoral fractures must be continually reassessed during the first 24 h following injury.

Haemorrhage may be overt with obvious arterial or venous bleeding occurring through a wound; contained haemorrhage may manifest as a false aneurysm. Bleeding may also be concealed and occur into the pleural or peritoneal cavity or the retroperitoneum. A fairly frequent occurrence, particularly in patients with penetrating wounds, is the finding of unexplained shock or a low haematocrit with no obvious site of haemorrhage, which is encountered in patients who have sustained transection of a major vessel which has ultimately thrombosed. Arteriovenous fistulae are always associated with a machinery-type murmur. However, this may be subtle, and unless specifically sought will be missed. This is the most common pathology found in patients with arterial trauma who present late.

Place of preoperative angiography

While Doppler ultrasound is an extremely useful screening test when there is doubt, angiography provides the definitive diagnosis. In addition, angiography is essential for the localization of, and hence operative planning in, inaccessible areas such as the superior mediastinum, the base of the skull and the abdominal vasculature. In general, in the presence of focal trauma to the mid-cervical region or the extremities, the performance of angiography is time-wasting, as the injury is easily located on clinical grounds. However, in an ischaemic limb which has multiple fractures, it is essential to image the vascular tree at every fracture site as it is not uncommon to find arterial disruption in more than one area. It is best under these circumstances to perform the investigation on the operating table before embarking upon exploration. It must be emphasized that the patient must be volume resuscitated and haemodynamically stable before angiography is performed. In our own experience, the retrograde femoral route is usually preferable utilizing the digital subtraction technique. In young healthy adults, the complication rate is negligible. In children, as far as possible, digital subtraction angiography via the intravenous injection technique has been found adequate. An overview of the indications for preoperative angiography in our practice is summarized in Table 2.

Table 2 Indications for arteriography in trauma

Suspected cervicomediastinal injury
Pulse deficit
False aneurysm
Haemorrhage
Overt
Unexplained shock
Low haematocrit/haemoglobin value
Bruit
Injury to anatomically related nerves
First rib fracture
Widened mediastinum on chest radiograph
Suspected renal artery injury
Upper quadrant/loin pain
Proteinuria
Non-function on intravenous pyelography
Suspected intraperitoneal haemorrhage
Pelvic fracture
Ongoing haemorrhage
Pulsating or expanding retroperitoneal haematoma
Ischaemic extremity
Severe soft tissue injury
Multiple fractures

Indications for operation and prioritization

The urgency for the operative procedure ranges from the 'crash' exploration in the 'clinically dead' patient, to the stabilized patient in whom a planned urgent procedure can be conducted, to the individual who presents months or years later with the long-term complications of a misdiagnosed or conservatively treated lesion. The question often arises in the stable patient without distal ischaemia or any other significant manifestations of arterial disruption other than an abnormal arteriogram, whether repair should be undertaken. While the precise incidence of complications in injuries that have been misdiagnosed or treated non-operatively is not known, when they do occur they may be life-threatening and indeed cause considerable morbidity. With penetrating wounds, secondary haemorrhage may occur between 5 days and 3 weeks after injury. This is probably due to low-grade sepsis with clot lysis resulting in active haemorrhage, or the acute onset of a false aneurysm which compresses surrounding structures. This most frequently applies to nerves and, in particular, to the brachial plexus. The prognosis for nerve recovery under these circumstances is guarded and when it does occur it may take anything up to 1 year for full function to be restored. Similarly, neglected false aneurysms or haematomas are susceptible to infection. Arteriovenous fistulae with a significant shunt may return with cardiac problems, due to the hyperdynamic circulation and when situated in the extremities with associated distal ischaemia and venous hypertension. Claudication or growth disparity in children are important long-term considerations with occluded arteries in the extremities.

Contraindications to reconstruction

Limb salvagability in the presence of extensive trauma may be an extremely difficult decision to make and should certainly not be left to the junior staff. In general terms, it is probably better to give the patient the benefit of the doubt and to proceed with revascularization under most circumstances. However, in the presence of extensive crush trauma associated with bone comminution and neurological dysfunction, the outlook is generally poor.

Similarly, the decision whether an extremity is irreversibly ischaemic or not may considerably exercise clinical judgement. Fixed skin staining and muscle rigidity in all compartments obviously preclude vascular reconstruction. However, in the presence of localized muscle compartment rigidity, such as the extensor compartment in the lower extremity, for example, a good functional result can still be obtained.

The general approach to the patient with a vascular injury should comprise concerted combined effort on the part of the involved disciplines with rapid resuscitation and definitive therapy as soon as possible. In virtually all instances we believe that the vascular injury should take priority over orthopaedic or plastic surgical intervention. The proviso however is that the vascular surgeons remain in attendance until the procedures are concluded. In our experience, it is exceptionally uncommon for orthopaedic manipulations to disrupt the vascular repair. We believe that this approach is preferable to the use of temporary shunts which serves to prolong the operative procedure considerably.

Operative procedure

Access and positioning

2

Besides meticulous surgical technique the basis for successful surgery is to be on the alert for the unexpected and to provide wide access to the area of injury. It is certainly preferable to overexpose than the converse and there is no place for 'keyhole' or cosmetic surgery. In principle, the aim should be to plan operative exposure to the major vessels in a definitive way in order to obtain control of the vessels proximal and distal to the site of injury. It is ill-advised to attempt to approach the injury by enlarging pre-existing stab wounds, particularly in the root of the neck, because the bony confines of the superior mediastinum make rapid access difficult if torrential haemorrhage from a superior mediastinal vessel is initiated by manipulation through an inadequate incision. The most difficult anatomical areas to deal with from the access point of view are injuries near the base of the skull, the root of the neck and superior mediastinum and the major abdominal vessels, particularly the aorta and its branches above the level of the renal artery. The optimum utility incisions for injuries in these various areas are shown in *Illustration 2*.

In principle, for cervico-mediastinal injuries, the entire neck, sternum and left thoracic cage down to the posterior axillary line should be prepared and draped with the neck in extension and a bolster placed between the scapulae in order to brace the shoulders and thrust the aortic arch and mediastinal vessels forward. An oblique incision placed along the anterior border of the sternomastoid muscle, and extending from the mastoid process to the suprasternal notch is the best utility approach to neck wounds. To expose the distal internal carotid, the sternomastoid muscle can be divided close to its origin from the mastoid process. The incision can be readily extended into a median sternotomy which provides the best access to the superior mediastinum and heart. Left thoracotomy via the fourth or fifth intercostal space provides good exposure of the descending thoracic aorta and structures in the pulmonary hilum. Under certain circumstances the proximal subclavian artery is best approached in this manner.

Similarly, when intra-abdominal vascular injuries are suspected, the entire abdomen and thoracic cage should be prepared and draped and both lower limbs should be free-draped and prepared down to the level of the knee. The initial utility incision is a mid-line from xiphisternum to pubis. There should be no hesitation to extend this incision either by subcostal incisions into the flanks or into the lower

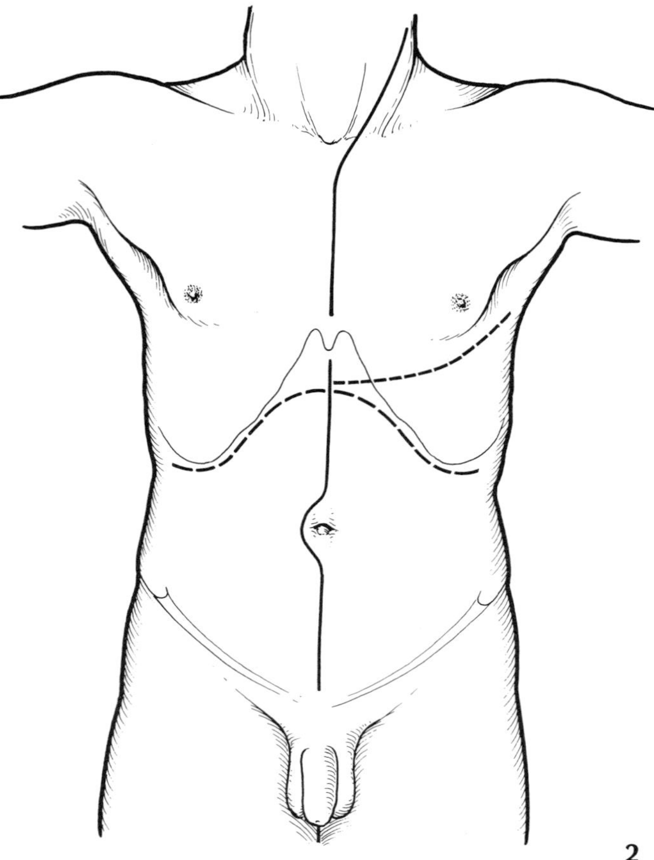

2

thoracic cavity via one of the lower intercostal spaces should this become necessary. The proximal abdominal aorta and its branches are exposed by mobilization of the left colon, spleen and pancreas towards the right side of the patient. The suprarenal inferior vena cava is exposed by mobilization of the right colon to the left, together with Kocher's manoeuvre to the duodenum. For access to the retrohepatic IVC, the right lobe of liver must be mobilized in addition by division of the right triangular ligament.

3a & b

When the injuries are confined to the extremities the entire limb should be prepared and free-draped and there should always be access to the groins in order to obtain a long saphenous vein graft should this be necessary. In every case, arrangements should be made for the ready availability of on-table angiographic facilities. The upper limb should be abducted to 90° and we find it most convenient to place it on a narrow arm board rather than to use a conventional arm table (*a*). It is also helpful to place a bolster behind the shoulder which serves to thrust the axillary vessels forward. The major access problem is provided by vessels in the vicinity of the shoulder girdle and it is usually necessary to divide the insertions of both pectoralis minor and major muscles in order to obtain adequate exposure and control of the proximal axillary vessels. This applies particularly if the anatomy is distorted by the presence of a large aneurysm which fills the axilla, a frequent accompaniment of penetrating injury. Adequate exposure of the distal subclavian vessels usually requires division of the clavicle mid-shaft. We have never found resection of the clavicle, in part or whole, necessary. The brachial is easily approached directly as illustrated.

The lower limb should be positioned with the knee slightly flexed on a bolster (*b*). The femoral vessels can be directly exposed via an overlying incision. The optimum approach to the popliteal vasculature is via a medially placed incision. When the injury is situated in the artery behind the knee the hamstrings should be detached as a unit from their insertion on the tibia, together with a cuff of periosteum which can be stapled back into position.

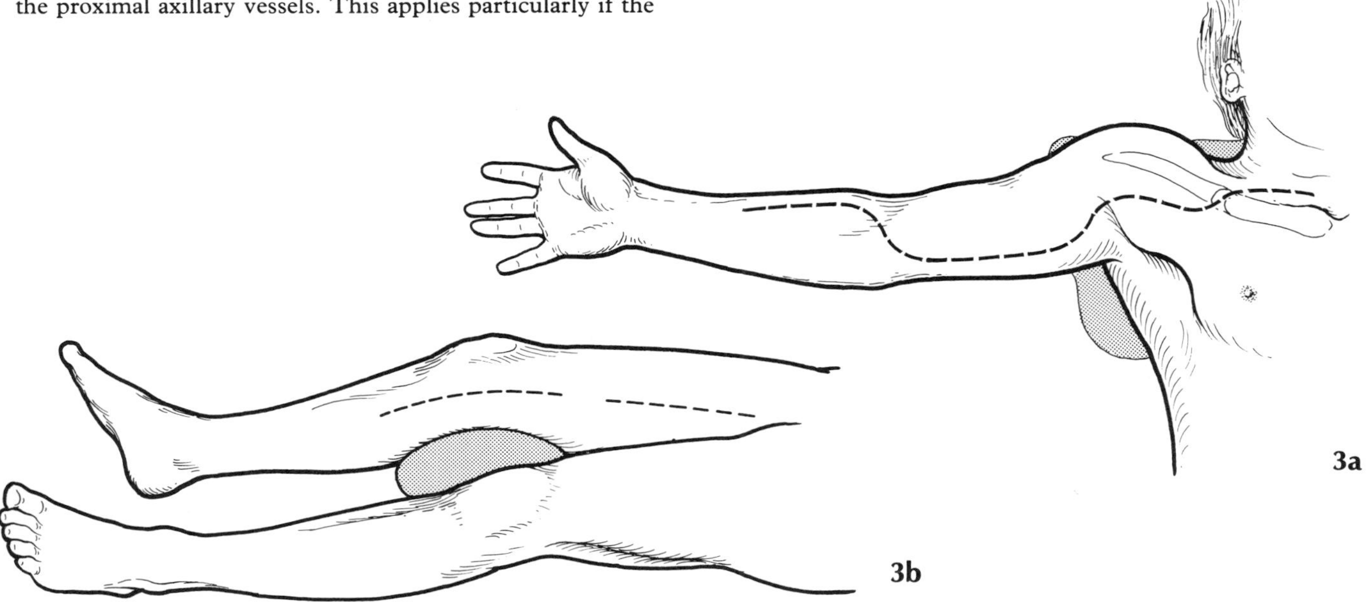

3a

3b

Control of active haemorrhage

Should active bleeding be initiated during dissection it is essential to avoid the blind application of clamps as this will frequently cause unnecessary associated injuries to surrounding nerves or veins. It is usually possible to control bleeding by judicious application of pressure using a finger or sponge stick while resuscitation proceeds, and definitive proximal and distal control can be obtained by dissecting out the relevant vessels and applying atraumatic vascular clamps. Under certain circumstances it may be possible or even desirable to pass intraluminal balloon catheters and to control haemorrhage in this way until more definitive control is obtained.

Principles of repair

Once the pathology has been identified and the vessel controlled the options for repair include lateral suture, patch angioplasty, end-to-end reconstruction and interposition grafting. Under certain circumstances, arterial ligation may be necessary. In order to fully appreciate the significance of the various manoeuvres involved in the techniques or repair, it is important to understand the common reasons for early failure of arterial reconstruction. These may be summarized as follows:

1. Narrowing at the suture lines.
2. Inadequate calibre graft.
3. Anastomotic tension.
4. Failure of intimal apposition with the formation of a distal flap.
5. Adventitial incorporation into the lumen.
6. Inadequate distal run-off due either to undetected thrombosis or additional distal injury.
7. Infection causing thrombosis or disruption of the suture lines.

4

Assessment of inflow and the distal arterial tree

Backbleeding is not a reliable sign of distal patency, as a short collateral network may result in considerable backbleeding even in the presence of propogated thrombus distal to the collateral network. A small (size 3) balloon embolectomy catheter should be routinely passed into the distal vessel, gently inflated with air and withdrawn. This serves to extract any distal thrombus and to break gently co-existing arterial spasm. We do not believe that there is any place for the use of topical vasodilators such as papaverine or local anaesthetic agents. Should the catheter fail to pass the full length of the extremity, an intraoperative angiogram should be obtained. It is also advisable to pass the embolectomy catheter into the proximal artery and ensure that any proximal propagated thrombus is removed and that good pulsatile inflow is obtained. Both proximal and distal segments should be copiously irrigated with dilute heparin solution (10 000 u/litre normal saline); systemic heparin is not recommended in the trauma context.

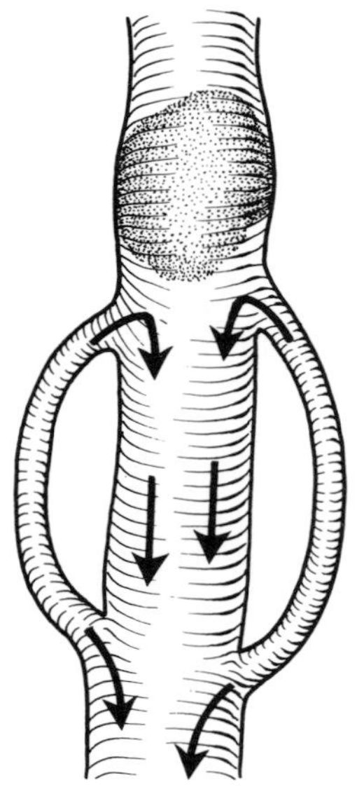

4

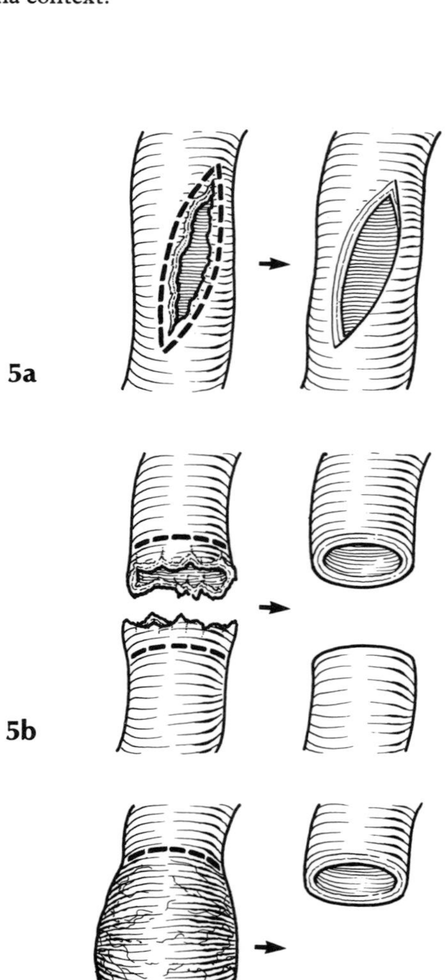

5a

5b

5c

5a, b & c

Preparation of artery for repair

The edges of the artery at the site of injury should be debrided back to healthy intima. The adventitia should be trimmed sufficiently by sharp dissection to prevent incorporation into the suture line; however, care must be taken to avoid excessive adventitial stripping which may result in the sutures cutting out. Thrombosed segments should be excised back to healthy non-oedematous arterial wall; this usually comprises 2–3 cm of vessel wall.

6 & 7

Lateral suture

This can only be performed when closure will not result in narrowing at the site of the suture line. It is important to pick up all layers of the vessel wall and the sutures should be spaced approximately 2 mm apart and about the same distance from the edges. In this way, blocks of tissue are opposed and intimal apposition is secured. The principle applies to any vascular suture line.

Puncture wounds in the aorta compatible with survival are usually relatively small. *Illustration 7* illustrates a useful technique. Bleeding is controlled by digital pressure and the laceration is closed by means of interrupted mattress sutures placed deep to the finger. This technique is, however, not applicable to smaller calibre vessels as it would result in significant narrowing.

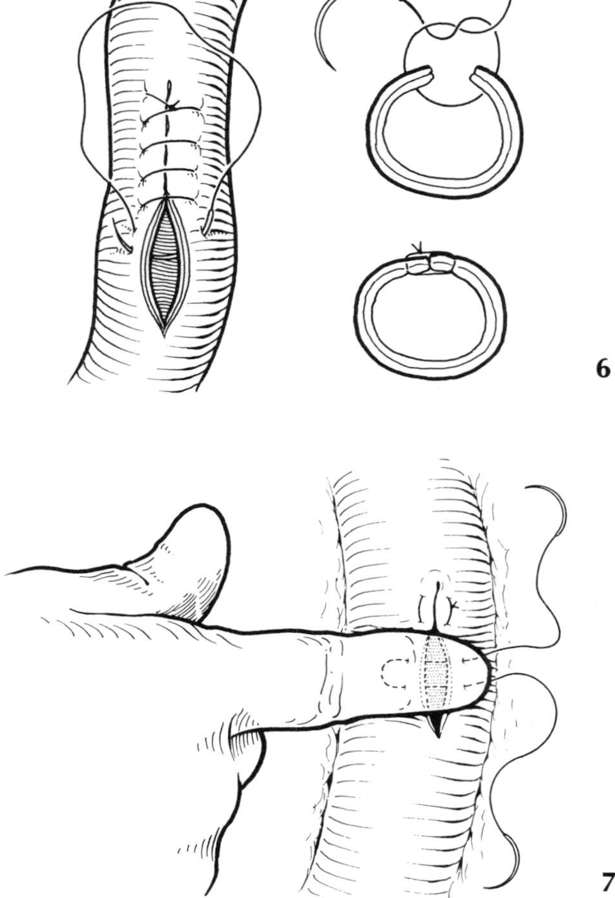

6

7

8a, b &c

Patch angioplasty

This should be used whenever simple lateral suture will result in narrowing. Any regional subcutaneous vein may be used and cut to size. Prosthetic material should be avoided in view of the danger of infection. The initial corner suture is of the mattress type in order to evert the suture line and ensure intimal apposition (*a*). The suture line is then completed by an over-and-over technique at approximately 2-mm intervals using the principles described for lateral suture (*b*, *c*).

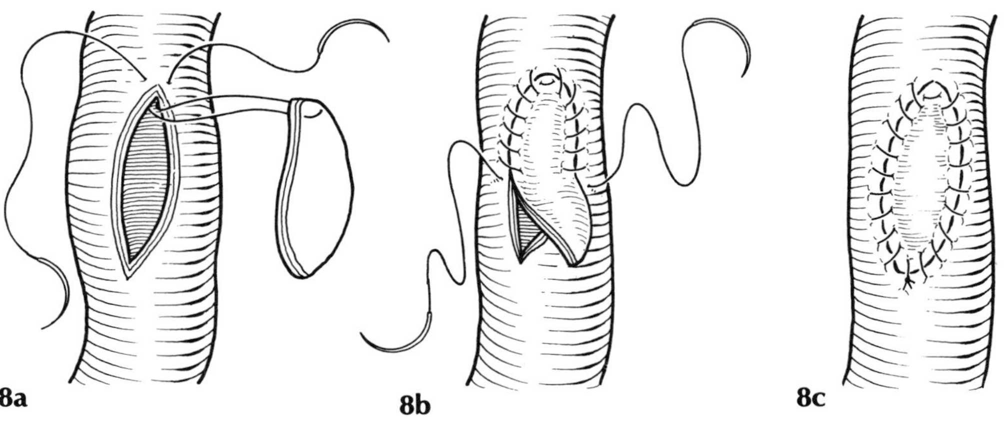

8a 8b 8c

9a–d

End-to-end anastomosis

This can only be performed when apposition between the vessel ends can be maintained without tension. The best parameter to use in this regard is whether the single corner tethering stitch can maintain apposition of the ends with the limb in full extension. If tearing out results under these circumstances it is preferable to insert an interposition graft. After adequate debridement the ends of the vessel are fish-mouthed at opposite ends to prevent narrowing (*a*). It is best to commence the suture line at the posterior corner with a mattress tethering suture (*b*), and it is preferable not to simultaneously tether the opposite corner so that the intimal surface of the suture line can be inspected at all times while the artery is being sutured. In general, interrupted sutures are preferable, placed approximately 2 mm apart as described for lateral suture (*c*). In larger vessels a continuous over-and-over suturing technique may be used. In deeply situated vessels in which ready access to the posterior wall is difficult, e.g. the great vessels in the superior mediastinum, it is possible to suture the posterior third of the anastomosis intraluminally (*d*). The initial suture is placed posterolaterally at approximately the four o'clock point on the circumference and knotted outside the lumen. The lumen is re-entered and a full thickness over-and-over suture placed from within the lumen. Once the posterior part of the suture line is complete (approximately one-third of the circumference) this can be knotted on the adventitial surface at about the seven o'clock point on the circumference and the anastomosis completed in the conventional manner, preferably with interrupted sutures. Whatever technique is used, it is important that the ends be accurately approximated without obliquity of the suture line, the sutures should be evenly spaced, and should always lie at right-angles to the cut ends of the artery.

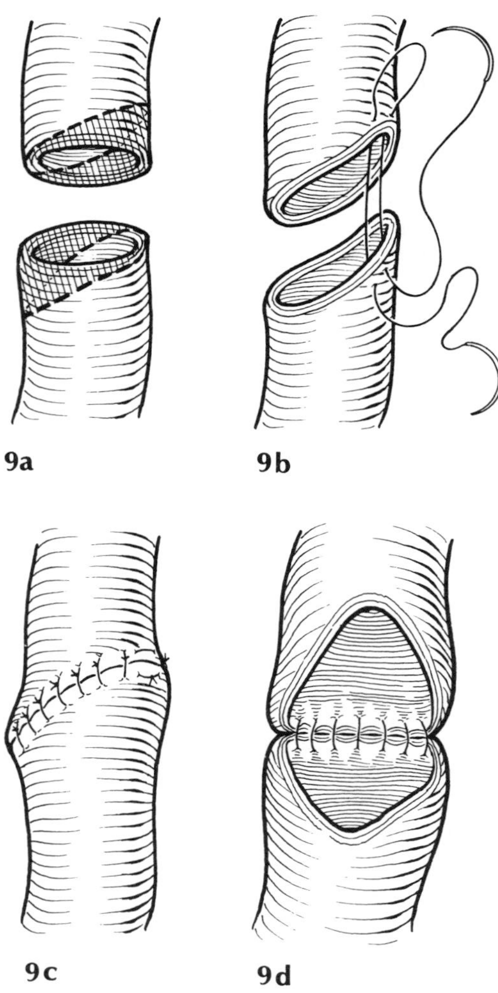

9a 9b

9c 9d

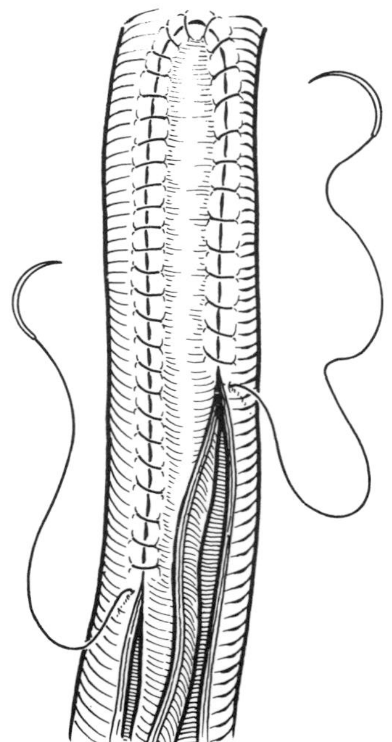

10

Interposition graft

10

The long saphenous vein taken from the groin area provides the most suitable graft in terms of calibre and ease of handling. We have used the cephalic and internal jugular veins on occasion, but found these to be too thin-walled and, in the case of the cephalic vein, too small under most circumstances. Regarded as being of adequate calibre for reconstruction in the extremities is a vein which measures 4–6 cm in diameter in its native state. It is possible on occasion to fashion a larger calibre vein graft by suturing a panel taken from another vein into the circumference. In most instances, the graft is short and can be seen in its entirety at completion of the procedure, so that in preparation it is not necessary to distend it with saline but preferable to allow arterial blood pressure to distend the graft once the clamps have been released, thus avoiding excessive trauma to the graft. It is also unnecessary to totally denude the graft of adventitia and just sufficient should be dissected free from the anastomotic areas to allow suture without adventitial incorporation into the lumen. The principles of anastomosis are identical to those described for end-to-end reconstruction.

11a & b

As a general rule, prosthetic grafts should be avoided in view of the hazards of infection, particularly following penetrating wounds. An exception to this rule is to be found with injuries to the great vessels close to the aortic arch, particularly when a through-and-through perforation of both anterior and posterior walls has occurred (*a*). Attempts to restore in-line continuity invariably results in difficulty in closing the posterior wall as the aorta tends to slip out of the clamp as the medial layer retracts. It is therefore preferable to obtain initial control by means of a side-biting clamp and to oversew the origin of the vessel. Continuity is then restored by means of a Dacron graft which takes origin from the intrapericardial ascending aorta (*b*). Should a prosthetic graft be required elsewhere as a last resort, we have found PTFE to be the most satisfactory substitute.

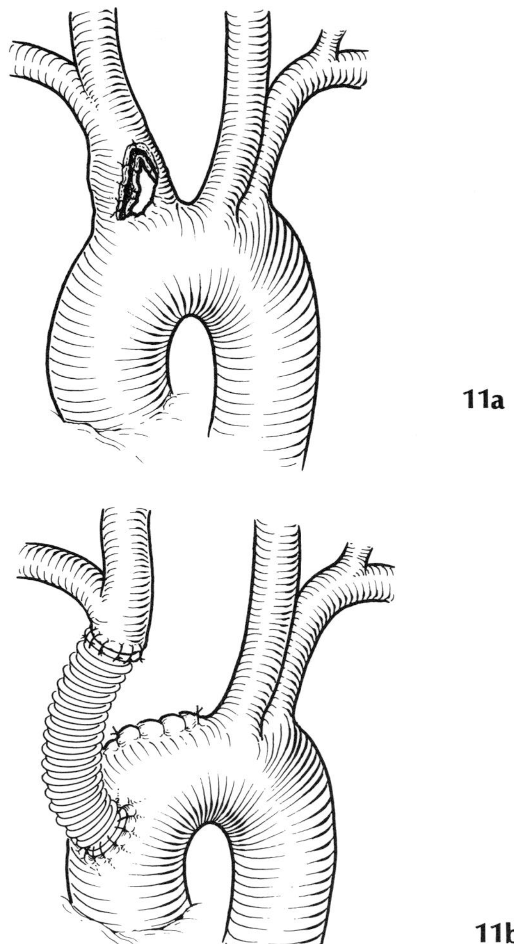

11a

11b

Ligation

Arterial ligation should be limited to 'non-essential' vessels, e.g. branches of the external carotid, or an intercostal vessel. An additional consideration is the situation in which prolonged reconstructive operation is inappropriate to the general clinical condition of the patient ('life or limb').

In a grossly contaminated operative field, attempts at in-line reconstruction are ill-advised. A fairly common example would be the combination of colonic and iliac vessel disruption with gross faecal soiling. When this situation pertains, the injured artery should be ligated and flow to the lower limb restored by means of an extra-anatomical bypass, such as an axillofemoral graft. Once the infection has settled the latter may be taken down and anatomical continuity restored, which may be many months later. The same principles apply in any grossly contaminated operative field and ingenuity may be sorely taxed in finding an extra-anatomical route.

Venous reconstruction

In general, repair in the venous system does not yield equivalent results to arterial construction. This is due mainly to the slower blood flow velocity which makes any technical errors such as stenosis, adventitial invagination or intimal irregularity assume far greater significance in terms of subsequent thrombosis. In addition, the thin-walled delicate structure of the venous system makes it far more susceptible to trauma from clamps or rough handling. There is also a tendency for these vessels to collapse because of their low intraluminal pressure which makes localization and hence control of the bleeding area more difficult. Bleeding from large veins should in most cases be controlled by the use of proximal and distal pressure using sponge sticks or intraluminal balloons in order to avoid tearing collaterals and small branches which aggravate the bleeding and make localization still more hazardous by attempts to encircle and mobilize the vein proximal and distal to the injury. An additional important consideration in dealing with injuries to the neck, mediastinum and abdomen is the danger of significant air embolism. Definitive repair of venous lacerations follows the principles outlined for arterial trauma and entails debridement of the edges and closure by means of lateral suture, patch angioplasty or reanastomosis. Suture technique must be fine and meticulous with close attention to detail. Complex injuries present a great problem and if an interposition graft is required the long saphenous or jugular system make the best grafts. We have found prosthetic grafts in the venous system to be uniformly unsatisfactory and thrombosis is the inevitable result. However, the use of temporary arteriovenous fistulae to improve flow has been shown to be effective in improving patency rates. An example of this technique is the anastomosis of the long saphenous vein to the superficial femoral artery to maintain patency in the iliac system or inferior vena cava. Haemodynamic problems may, however, result if these fistulae exceed 5 mm in diameter and they should be closed within 4–8 weeks. Prolonged reconstructive manoeuvres for complex venous injuries are seldom indicated, as these patients frequently have associated arterial and other injuries that mandate reconstruction and, under most circumstances, ligation of the major veins may be performed without immediate adverse effects. For example, in the superior mediastinum, an extensive analysis of our own experience has shown that any major veins cephalad to the azygous confluence may be ligated with safety, with minimal, if any, postoperative sequelae with regard to oedema. An additional problem in treating inferior vena caval and iliac venous injuries is that a thrombosed repair might theoretically result in pulmonary embolism. The morbidity from chronic venous insufficiency in the lower extremity following failure to repair femoral and distal venous injuries is well established, and every attempt should be made to repair these. On the other hand, more recent reports on long-term follow-up of these patients in civilian practice has indicated a more benign course in those in whom veins have been ligated at this level. Following venous repair to the great veins, in view of the theoretical possibility of pulmonary embolism, it is probably advisable to heparinize these patients until they are fully mobile.

Arteriovenous fistula

In our own experience, these have always occurred as a complication of penetrating trauma and the usual pathology is a lateral perforation of adjacent artery and vein with or without an interposed false aneurysm. Perforations are usually relatively small and the most frequent area involved is the neck and mediastinum. In most instances, the diagnosis is made soon after injury, but in a significant proportion in whom arterial haemorrhage is not a major presenting feature due to immediate decompression into the vein, the fistula only becomes evident some time later with the emergence of haemodynamic complications or the detection of a bruit. Patients frequently notice the latter themselves. The sooner repair is effected after injury, the easier it is technically. Once fibrosis has become established, it adds greatly to the difficulty of control and repair of the component vessels and the concept of waiting for a fistula to mature is historical. Ideally, control of both afferent and efferent arterial and venous components should be obtained and can usually be performed without difficulty in the recently acquired lesion. However, when extensive fibrosis has occured, this may prove hazardous or, indeed, impossible. Under these circumstances, the venous components can usually be readily identified and isolated by palpation of the thrill as they lie on a more superficial plane to the artery. In addition, in the extremities and cervico-mediastinal areas, no vital structures cross the major veins. The thrill pinpoints the situation of the fistula which can then in most cases be occluded by direct transvenous pressure using a finger. Arterial control may then be obtained by sharp dissection proximal and distal to this site. Distal control may on occasion prove difficult, especially when the vessels involved are close to the base of the skull. Under these circumstances, once arterial inflow has been isolated and controlled, and proximal and distal venous control obtained, the fistula should be exposed transvenously and arterial backbleeding controlled digitally. More definitive distal control may then be obtained by means of an intraluminally placed inflated balloon embolectomy catheter. Arterial and venous injuries should be repaired on their respective merits as described in some detail earlier.

While recurrent fistulae undoubtedly occur, in our own experience we have found this to be usually due to a second fistula which remained undetected at the original operation. These have more frequently been a consequence of gunshot or, in particular, shotgun wounds. It is therefore important to study and trace the trajectory of the penetrating agent and ensure that the machinery bruit has disappeared at the conclusion of the operation. While the classically held concept is that soft tissue should be interposed between the arterial and venous repairs, we have not made this standard practice as this proves difficult on occasion unless considerable tissue mobilization is performed.

Interventional radiology

Occlusion of fistulae by embolization using thrombin pellets, detachable balloons or various coil devices via transarterial catheters are well adapted to the treatment of surgically inaccessible post-traumatic arteriovenous fistulae involving smaller vessels. Particular application is found in the kidney, smaller intra-abdominal vessels such as the pancreatico-duodenal, and the vertebral and carotid near the skull base. In the latter instance, virtually all afferent flow enters the fistula with very little distal flow into the brain, which makes occlusion safe from the point of view of cerebral blood supply.

These embolization techniques have also proved invaluable in arresting haemorrhage arising from branches of the internal iliac artery as a complication of pelvic fracture or penetrating wounds in the buttock or perineal area.

Wound management

Primary closure of a contaminated wound invites septic complications. The most serious of these is disruption of suture lines with massive exsanguinating secondary haemorrhage. In the presence of a compound wound with false aneurysm formation, significant associated blunt tissue injury, multiple foreign bodies (e.g. shotgun wound), and patients with penetrating trauma presenting more than 8–12 h after injury, primarily suture of the wound is inadvisable. Under these circumstances, the deep fascia and skin should be left unsutured and the wound covered with an absorbent, non-adherent dressing. Copious irrigation with antiseptic or antibiotic solution should be performed. Vascular repairs must not be left exposed in the wound but should be covered with muscle or, under certain circumstances, a split skin graft.

The wound should be inspected under sterile conditions 48 h later and further debridement performed if necessary. This should be repeated at regular intervals until the wound is healthy, at which stage formal closure is effected. This regimen significantly reduces the infection rate and hence secondary haemorrhage from the repair site in our own experience.

Postoperative management and complications

Careful monitoring of peripheral pulse status and for evidence of excessive haemorrhage is essential during the postoperative period as a routine. Early complications occur within 5–10 days of operation and may be local or systemic. Local complications are thrombosis, haemorrhage, compartment syndrome, infection and recurrent arteriovenous fistula. Graft thrombosis usually has a mechanical cause and occurs within 24–48 h of operation. Haemorrhage may result from inadequate haemostasis due often to reperfusion of traumatized tissues, but may also occur 5–7 days later due to infection with disruption of the anastomosis. Compartment syndrome may become manifest within the following 6–24 h and must be anticipated, particularly if there has been prolonged preoperative ischaemia or extensive soft tissue injury; its development demands urgent fasciotomy. Compound injuries are contaminated by their very nature and significant infection usually supervenes in the presence of non-viable tissue. Open wound management and frequent inspections with a view to debridement are important. Recurrent arteriovenous fistula as such is rare and persistence of the physical signs usually indicates failure to detect additional fistulae which are not uncommon after missile wounds.

Systemic complications such as adult respiratory distress syndrome and disseminated intravascular coagulation are complications of severe multiple trauma and massive blood transfusion must be anticipated in these patients. The myonephropathic syndrome (crush syndrome) accompanies severe crush trauma or revascularization of necrotic tissue. The major issue is acute renal failure due to the deposition of myoglobin crystals in the renal tubules. In addition, at the time of allowing reperfusion to occur, the patient undergoes a severe metabolic insult in that a bolus of 'metabolic debris' including potassium and lactic acid which in turn may cause diffuse vasodilatation and myocardial depression with hypotension. It is therefore vital to anticipate this complication in the severely traumatized patient in the appropriate clinical setting. Prior to release of the clamp with reperfusion of the limb, the patient should be well volume resuscitated, should be rendered alkalotic by means of bicarbonate infusion and an osmotic diuresis initiated by means of mannitol infusion. The clamp should then be gradually released and reapplied should the blood pressure fall. At this stage the metabolic acidosis should also be carefully monitored. During the postoperative period, diuresis must be maintained at a level of at least 150–200 ml/h by means of adequate crystalloid volume replacement and, if necessary, mannitol administration. The urine should also be carefully monitored for the presence of myoglobin which has a characteristic brown discolouration. Renal failure can be largely eliminated by this regimen.

References

Costa, M. and Robbs, J.V. (1988). Nonpenetrating subclavian artery trauma. *Journal of Vascular Surgery* **8**(1), 71.

Hirshberg, A., Thomson, S.R. and Robbs, J.V. (1988). Vascular complications of diagnostic angiography via limb arteries. *Journal of Royal College of Surgeons of Edinburgh* **33**, 196.

Meek, A.C. and Robbs, J.V. (1984). Vascular injury with associated bone and joint trauma. *British Journal of Surgery* **71**, 341.

Robbs, J.V. and Baker, L.W. (1979). Late revascularisation of the lower limb following acute arterial occlusion. *British Journal of Surgery* **66**, 129.

Robbs, J.V. and Baker, L.W. (1984). Cardiovascular trauma. *Current Problems in Surgery* **XXI**(4).

Robbs, J.V. and Costa, M. (1984). Injuries to the great veins of the abdomen. *South African Journal of Surgery* **22**(4), 223.

Robbs, J.V. and Naidoo, K.S. (1984). Nerve compression injuries due to traumatic false aneurysm. *Annals of Surgery* **200**(1), 80.

Robbs, J.V. and Reddy, E. (1987). Management options for penetrating injuries to the great veins of the neck and superior mediastinum. *Surgery, Gynecology, and Obstetrics* **165**, 323.

Robbs, J.V. *et al.* (1981). Cervicomediastinal arterial injuries: A surgical challenge. *Archives of Surgery* **116**, 663.

Cervical trauma

MALCOLM O. PERRY MD
M. KATHLEEN REILLY PhD, MD
Department of Surgery, Division of Vascular Surgery, Texas Tech University, Health Sciences Center, School of Medicine, Lubbock, Texas

Introduction

Most cervical injuries are caused by penetrating trauma, usually from knives or low-velocity bullets and the damage therefore is usually confined to the wound tract. High-velocity weapons are capable of causing considerable damage because of the blast effect. Vascular injuries caused by blunt trauma are more difficult to manage and can be easily overlooked because often there is no superficial evidence of injury to the neck. Moreover, patients sustaining blunt trauma sometimes have associated closed head injuries and other wounds that require an array of diagnostic tests.

Most patients sustaining penetrating cervical trama are males. In the authors' series, 14% of the vascular wounds were in the cervical region, but there is a trend seen in recent publications suggesting that the incidence of penetrating cervical trauma may be as high as 38% (Fry and Fry, 1987; McCormack and Burch, 1979).

1

In evaluating patients with penetrating cervical trauma it is useful to divide the neck into three zones as described by Monson *et al.* (1969). Zone 1 extends from 1 cm above the clavicle down to include the base of the neck and the thoracic outlet. Zone 2 is from 1 cm above the clavicle to the angle of the mandible and Zone 3 extends from the angle of the mandible to the base of the skull.

It is the authors' practice to explore all penetrating wounds of the anterior triangle of the neck that pierce the platysma muscle (Perry, 1981). This is controversial, and if the patient does not have an obvious injury, some surgeons prefer to observe the patient and perform various diagnostic manoeuvres. Patients with injuries of the oesophagus or trachea may have subcutaneous air or drainage; surgical exploration is mandatory. In patients who do not have clear evidence of injury to the aerodigestive tract, endoscopy and contrast studies have been used to exclude injury. These tests have an incidence of false-negative results and cannot be relied upon to exclude damage, particularly to the hypopharnyx.

A thorough neurological examination is mandatory in all patients because of the anatomic relationships of the major nerves and vessels. It is important to identify injuries to the cranial nerves or brachial plexis preoperatively, not only to assess the extent of injury, but to document pre-existing damage prior to an operative procedure.

Arteriography may be used to exclude the need for an operation in patients with no obvious injuries. In others, an arteriogram may be helpful in planning the operation, or perhaps will identify a clinically unsuspected injury (Perry *et al.*, 1980). It is the authors' practice to obtain four vessel arteriography in all patients in stable condition who have penetrating trauma to the neck in Zones 1 and 3, as well as in patients with neurological deficits from injuries in Zone 2. Patients with penetrating injuries in Zone 2, but who have no neurological deficit, can safely undergo operative exploration without arteriography.

Because the main concern in these patients is the possibility of a carotid artery injury, it is useful in planning treatment to divide them into three neurological groups (Thal *et al.*, 1974) (Table 1). The majority of patients fall into the first group – those who have no neurological deficit. Their prognosis is good and one can anticipate a successful surgical repair. The second group contains those patients with a moderate neurological deficit, generally manifested by hemiparesis or monoparesis, or transient episodes of cerebral ischaemia. Repair of carotid injuries in these patients is also expected to be successful. Group 3 consists of patients who have severe neurological deficits, and often have carotid artery occlusion. In this group the eventual outcome is directly related to the severity of the neurological deficit before surgical treatment. It is the authors' practice to repair all carotid injuries in patients in Groups 1 and 2. We recommend repair of carotid injuries in Group 3 if prograde arterial flow is preserved and if the patient does not have an acute severe stroke with coma.

Most injuries of the vertebral artery are treated by ligation, but if the injured artery is a large dominant vessel it should be repaired. Those methods described for the carotid artery are used in this situation as well (Fry and Fry, 1987).

Jugular vein wounds are also usually treated by simple ligation. If both veins are damaged, it is prudent to repair the larger of the two. The vessel is often of a size that will permit lateral venography, but vein patch venoplasty may be needed.

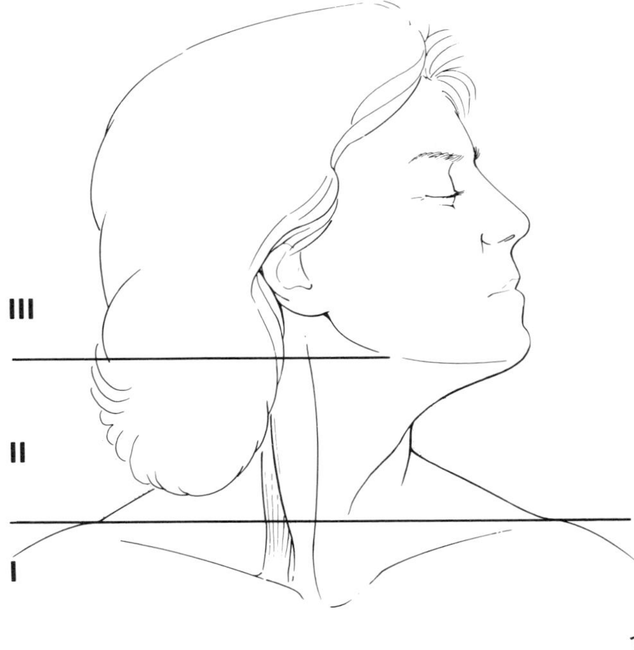

1

2

A standard oblique neck incision is made along the anterior border of the sternocleidomastoid muscle. The dissection continues through the plastysma muscle, reflecting the sternocleidomastoid muscle posteriorly, thus exposing the carotid sheath. The exposure of the carotid artery is begun at the base of the neck. If haematoma is identified in the sheath or in the periadventitial tissue surrounding the carotid artery at this level, the incision may be extended as a median sternotomy as demonstrated by the dotted lines. This will enable the surgeon to obtain proximal control of the great vessels in the thoracic outlet.

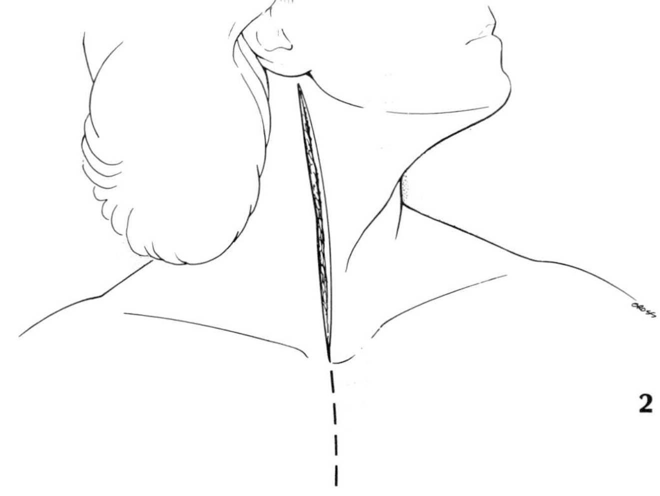

2

3

As the bifurcation of the carotid artery is approached, the jugular vein and sternomastoid muscles are retracted laterally. Beginning the dissection of the common carotid artery first enables the surgeon to establish proximal control. This step also centres the dissection at the proper depth (deep to the visceral fascia) to identify and protect the vagus and hypoglossal nerves, and their branches. The superior laryngeal nerve is hidden by the carotid bifurcation, and if the artery must be freed from its bed, that nerve is protected – it passes forward and medially adjacent and behind the bulb.

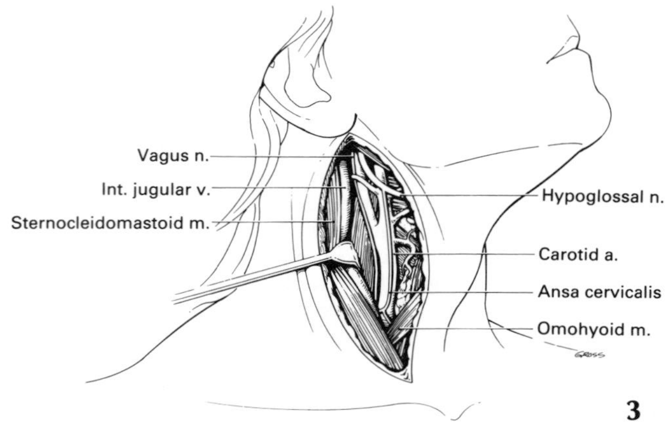

3

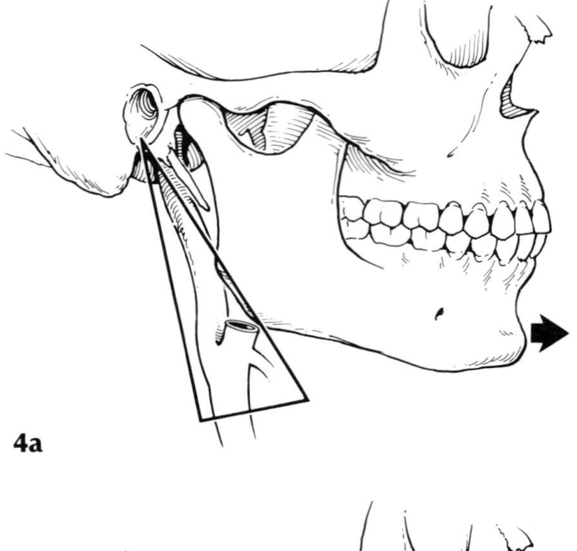

4a

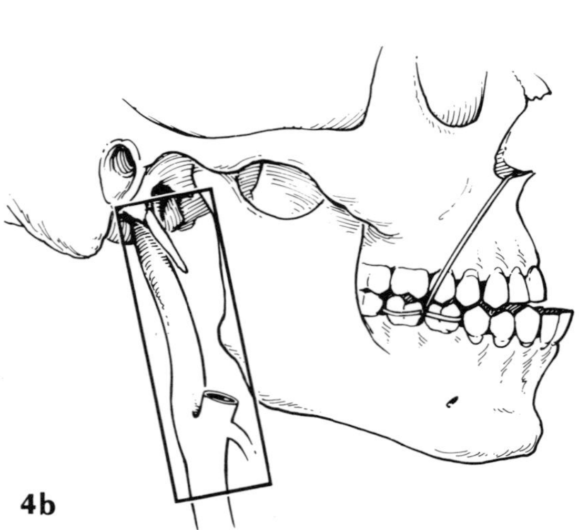

4b

4

This demonstrates the exposure obtained by anterior subluxation of the mandible. This manoeuvre is useful when arteriograms show injuries to the internal carotid above the level of the angle of the mandible. With the mandible in the normal anatomic position (*a*), the dissection enters a progressively smaller area at the apex of the triangle near the base of the skull. If the mandible is moved anteriorly (*b*), this narrow apex of the triangle can be expanded by 1.5–2 cm, thus facilitating exposure up to the base of the skull. This eliminates the need for mandibular osteotomies. It is usually helpful to divide the digastric muscle and perhaps excise the styloid process.

There are several methods of obtaining and holding mandibular subluxation. The maxillary wires shown eliminate the need for continuous traction that is required when only mandibular wires are placed at the mentum.

The mandible should be brought directly and evenly forward, and not permitted to assume an angled position because this may compress the opposite carotid artery. Little disability has been seen in these patients after subluxation, although the procedure is rarely needed.

5

Simple oblique lacerations – the kind often seen from a knife injury – are best repaired by simple suture repair after debridement of devitalized wound edges. Intimal coaptation is particularly important in the carotid artery because of the damage to the brain from microemboli.

Most surgeons prefer small monofilament sutures. Often these lacerations are best managed by interrupted suture techniques.

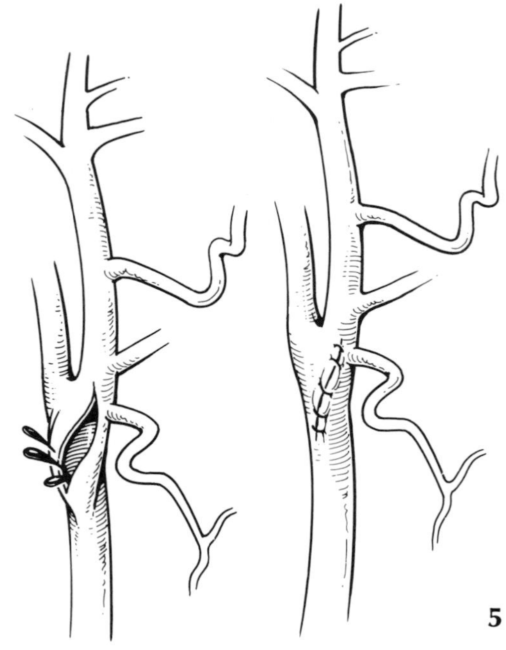

5

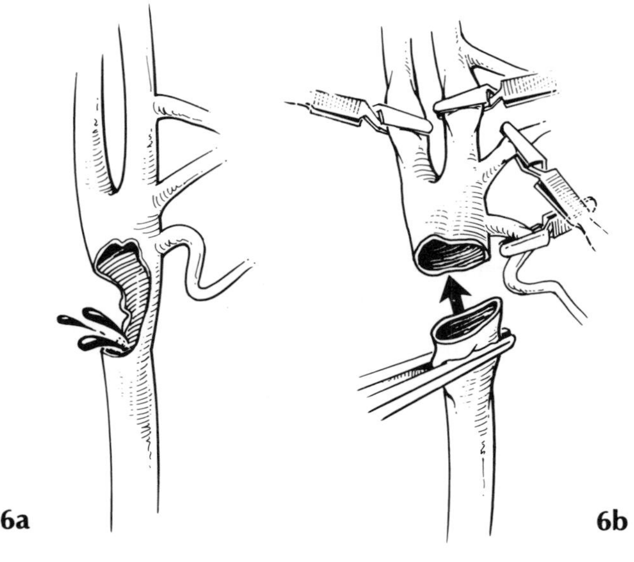

6a 6b

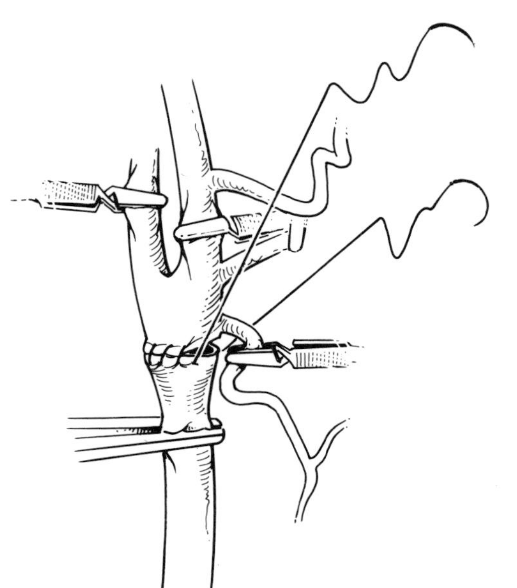

6c

6

An extensive injury involving the carotid bifurcation, with loss of most of the circumference of the vessel, generally results from a bullet wound. It is most easily treated by resection of the involved segment as shown in (*b*), and then a simple end-to-end anastomosis is performed (*c*). Injuries to the internal carotid artery involving extensive loss of vessel may be treated by similar technique.

If the artery has a small diameter (4 mm), interrupted sutures are preferred but, alternatively, a spatulated, running suture anastomosis may be chosen.

7

When the internal carotid artery cannot be repaired directly, continuity may be obtained by substituting the external carotid artery. A standard end-to-end anastomosis is constructed between the proximal external carotid and the undamaged distal part of the internal carotid artery. In patients who have multifocal arterial occlusvie disease, the external carotid may be an important collateral pathway, and should be preserved. In this situation, an interposition saphenous vein graft is preferred.

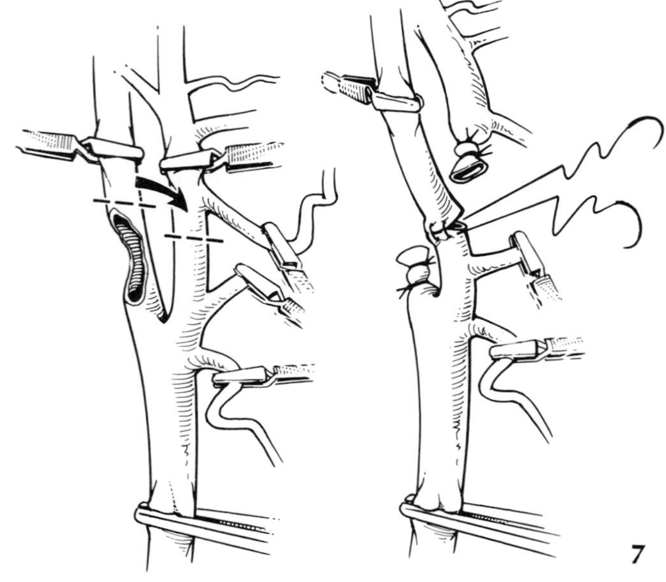

7

8

When the internal carotid artery is severely damaged, direct repair or vein patch graft angioplasty may not be possible. An interposition saphenous vein graft is obtained from the groin (these areas should be prepared in all of these cases, since vein grafts may be needed in several situations).

If there is scanty backflow from the internal carotid artery, rather than bright red, brisk, pulsatile flow, a temporary inlying shunt is threaded through the prepared vein graft and put in place to support cerebral blood flow. Alternatively, the surgeon can measure the back pressure in the internal carotid artery. If it is greater than 70 torr, it is thought to be safe to proceed without a shunt. Some surgeons do not employ a shunt in any of these situations.

During these operations a dilute heparin-saline solution (1:10) is used to prevent local thrombosis. Since many of these patients have multiple injuries, full systemic doses of heparin my be contraindicated. If there is only the isolated carotid artery wound, 5000 u of heparin are administered intravenously as soon as control of the bleeding is obtained.

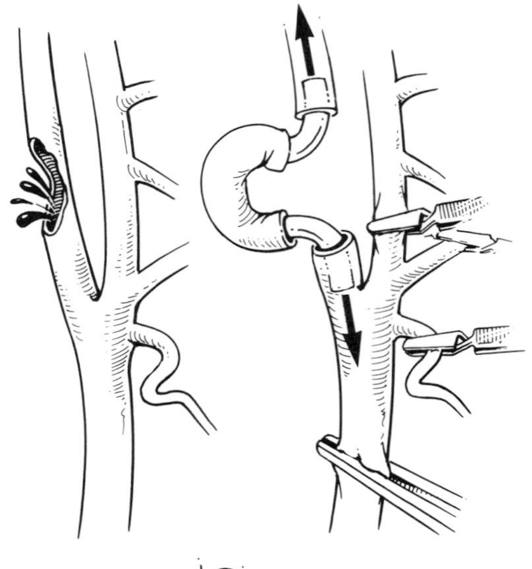

8

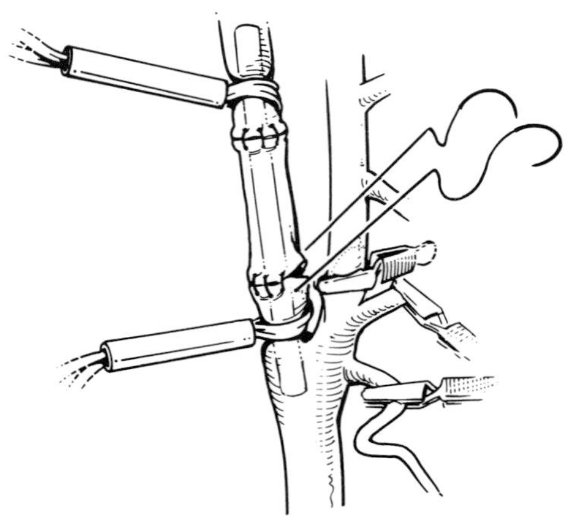

Summary

Although thromboembolic events following the repair of carotid artery injuries are unusual they may cause serious neurological problems on rare occasions if frequent evaluation of the haemodynamic and neurological status of these patients is mandatory. Any alteration in the neurological findings is a clear indication for further studies, usually arteriograms. If a build-up of thrombus in the arteries is suspected, some of the non-invasive tests may be helpful, but often an arteriogram would be required to be certain. If a patient has a frank stroke it is best not to delay for confirmatory studies, but return the patient to the operating room for exploration and restoration of cerebral blood flow as rapidly as possible. The problem is most likely a clot at the site of the repair, and if this is treated before cerebral infarction supervenes, the outcome is usually satisfactory.

Long-term results of repairing carotid artery injuries are quite good (Table 2). In the absence of infection and if the patient does not have a neurological deficit prior to operation, a majority of the patients recover without incident. As seen in Table 2 carotid injuries caused by penetrating trauma have a more favourable outlook than those caused by blunt trauma (Table 3). As indicated in the preliminary remarks of this section, if the patients can be successfully operated upon prior to the develpoment of a neurological deficit, the prognosis is usually favourable. Once the patient has a cerebral infarction then the amount of recovery will depend on the extent of brain damage.

Table 1
Carotid injuries

Group	Degree of neurological deficit	n
1	None	49
2	Mild	8
3	Severe	15

Table 2
Carotid injuries: penetrating trauma

Group	Mortality	
	n	%
1	0	0.0
2	1	1.3
3	5	6.9

Table 3
Carotid injuries: blunt trauma

	Mortality	
	n	%
All cases	4/17	23
Carotid operations	2/14	14
Successful repair	0/7	0

References

Fry, W. J. and Fry, R. E. (1987). Management of carotid artery injury. In *Vascular Surgical Emergencies*. Bergan, J. J. and Yao, J. S. T., eds. New York: Grune and Stratton.

McCormack, T. M. and Burch, B. H. (1979). Routine angiographic evaluation of neck and extremity injuries. *Journal of Trauma* **19**, 384.

Monson, D. O., Saletta, J. D. and Freeark, R. J. (1969). Carotid-vertebral trauma. *Journal of Trauma* **9**, 987.

Perry, M. O. (1981). *The Management of Acute Vascular Injuries*. Baltimore: Williams and Wilkins.

Perry, M. O., Snyder, W. H. and Thal, E. R. (1980). Carotid artery injuries caused by blunt trauma. *Annals of Surgery* **192**, 74.

Thal, E. R., Snyder, W. H., Hays, R. J. and Perry, M. O. (1974). Management of carotid artery injuries. *Surgery* **76**, 955.

Upper and lower limb vascular trauma

AIRES A. B. BARROS D'SA MD, FRCS, FRCSEd
Consultant Vascular Surgeon, Vascular Surgical Unit, Royal Victoria Hospital, Belfast, UK

Introduction

Vascular injuries of the limbs which once occurred almost exclusively in wartime, are now observed not only on the field of battle and following criminal violence so typical of large conurbations, but also as a consequence of road traffic and industrial accidents. Blood vessel injuries of the extremities represent approximately two-thirds of all vascular trauma. Confronted with these undoubtedly challenging injuries, the vascular surgeon must swiftly control life-endangering haemorrhage and initiate resuscitation which proceeds in concert with definitive operative treatment. The objective of surgery is to preserve the viability of a limb by precise repair of damaged arteries and veins using accepted principles in the knowledge that failure may lead to crippling disability, amputation and sometimes to death.

The scenario within which penetrating vascular injury of the extremities takes place, i.e. the nature of the wounding agent, the mode of injury and the lapse of time before admission, will strongly influence operative management. Knives, splinters of glass, shards of metal, bullets, shrapnel and fragments from a variety of explosive devices, account for injuries ranging from mere contusion or puncture to complete transection of a vessel. Stab wounds, usually sustained by the upper limb, may sever major vessels quite cleanly with minimal soft tissue injury. In contrast, a missile has a considerable wounding capacity which is proportional to its mass, muzzle velocity and distance before impact. Whereas a low-velocity missile usually only disrupts a vessel segment lying in its path, the temporary cavitational effect of a high-velocity missile will cause traumatic displacement and destruction of tissues sufficient to stretch and tear neighbouring arteries. If bone is struck, dissipating most of the energy of such a missile, the resulting fragments of bone, now behaving as secondary missiles, will wreak havoc on the soft tissues. A shotgun fired at close range can inflict massive damage to a limb, particularly to soft tissues, including blood vessels. Survivors of bomb explosions sustain a multiplicity of injuries with widespread destruction of all body tissues caused not only by the blast wave, initially faster than the speed of sound, but also by flying fragments, secondary missiles, and falling masonry. A few of the thousands of transfemoral and transaxillary diagnostic procedures undertaken by cardiologists and radiologists in modern hospital practice, represent a further iatrogenic source of penetrating limb vascular trauma.

In road traffic accidents, a sharp bony fragment may directly lacerate a vessel, but more frequently indirect damage may ensue as a result of the intense shearing forces generated by the sudden fracture of long bones. Particularly vulnerable arterial segments are those which lie adjacent to a long bone or at points of relative fixity, especially in close proximity to joints. Sudden violent angulation of the shaft of a long bone or the traction associated with fracture dislocations at the knee, progressively disrupts the layers of the vessel wall beginning with the intima. Crush injuries caused by falling masonry after air raids and bomb explosions are observed in peacetime following industrial, mining and train accidents, and earthquakes. The ischaemia consequent upon injury, whether in the form of extrinsic compression and contusion or division of a vessel, will accelerate the progression of a 'crush syndrome' and renal failure.

Limb vascular trauma may result in blood loss, and hypovolaemic hypotension which compounds the ischaemia of arterial injury. These effects and the impaired drainage due to concomitant vein injury are rapidly overtaken by complex and interdependent pathophysiological events (Barros D'Sa, 1980, 1988). If resuscitatory measures and vascular repair are not forthcoming, the protracted hypoxia will increase capillary permeability, causing a rise in intracompartmental pressure, which may herald a disastrous outcome either in the form of Volkmann's ischaemic contracture or amputation.

Preoperative measures

A firm pad and pressure bandage is preferable to a clamp which, when blindly applied, may add to the injury. The principal resuscitative measure must be the re-expansion of the circulating volume. Prophylactic tetanus toxoid and broad-spectrum antibiotics are prescribed. If the patient is not hypotensive a narcotic analgesic will decrease vasospasm and assist peripheral perfusion.

The surgeon runs through a mental checklist of clinical signs of limb vascular injury: a tense and expanding haematoma in blunt closed injuries, persistent arterial or venous bleeding in penetrating injuries, the presence of a thrill or bruit suggestive of incomplete occlusion or an acute arteriovenous fistula. It should be remembered that pulses may still be palpable beyond an injured artery which on exploration almost invariably reveals intimal damage and mural thrombosis. Doppler ultrasound assessment of pulse waveform and ankle systolic pressure is helpful. Evidence of concomitant bone and nerve injury should be documented.

In the shocked patient, delay in the radiology department may endanger life but in most instances plane films which define the bony injury and identify foreign bodies are of value in planning the best incisional approach. Preoperative angiography wastes valuable time in situations of impending loss of life or limb, whereas a policy of selective angiography based on clinical judgement will rule out arterial injury and prevent unnecessary surgery. In these times the medico-legal implications of not having obtained an arteriogram when the ultimate outcome turns out to be less than ideal, should be emphasized. In institutions unaccustomed to a round-the-clock emergency angiography service, the simple alternative of one-shot percutaneous angiography represents a fast, efficient and effective way of using resources. In certain circumstances such as delayed admission, persistent ischaemia after fracture reduction or doubt as to the trajectory of the wounding agent, a negative angiogram supports the surgeon's decision not to explore the wound and, by the same token, a positive angiogram makes operation mandatory. Biplane arteriograms of good quality will define the site and type of injury, and a lateral projection is of particular value in demonstrating a potentially sinister popliteal injury such as an intimal tear, often missed in an anteroposterior view.

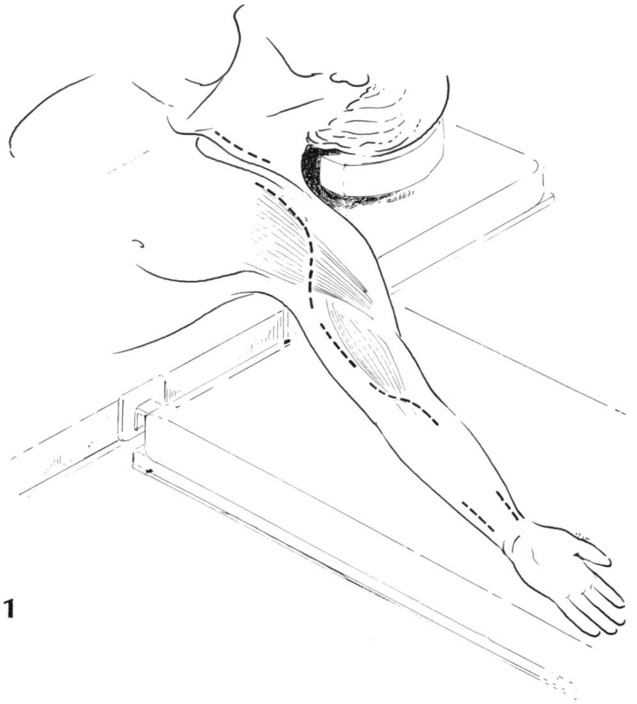

1

The operation

The operation must be undertaken with the least possible delay, the objectives being control of bleeding, wound toilet, restoration of circulation and prevention of complications. Delay in diagnosis or improper management may result in amputation or lasting functional disability. All wounds in anatomical proximity to a major vessel should be explored.

Emergency amputation

If tissue death and gangrene have supervened due to delayed admission, amputation at the appropriate level must be carried out expeditiously. Following massive destruction and irreparable mutilation of a limb, for example following a bomb explosion, it may be prudent, after careful deliberation, to proceed to immediate amputation so avoiding gas gangrene, sepsis, haemorrhage and renal failure. In such cases, amputation should include vigorous wound toilet and excision of all devitalized tissue, doubly ligating the vessels within viable boundaries and leaving the stump to drain. After inspection, delayed closure, no earlier than 5 days later, is undertaken, using whatever tissue has been preserved to fashion definitive flaps in order to create a functioning rather than cosmetic stump.

Incisions and exposure

1

In upper limb injuries, peripheral and central venous lines should not be inserted on the injured side. The patient lies supine, the upper limb is abducted and extended palm-upwards at right-angles to the body and the draping should provide an operative field with access to the chest, neck and arm if needed. One lower limb should also be prepared and draped in case donor vein is required. The incisional approaches are illustrated.

2

In injuries such as stab wounds of the first part of the axillary artery it is wise to secure proximal supraclavicular control of the subclavian artery. Partial division of the clavicular head of the sternocleidomastoid, and identification and delicate retraction of the phrenic nerve medially before careful division of the scalenus anterior will reveal the subclavian artery which can be encircled.

3

The incision to approach the axillary artery commences below the clavicle and is extended laterally down the deltopectoral groove and continued distally if required along the course of the brachial artery. This means that the axillary artery can be approached either above or below the margins of the pectoralis major or by separating the fibres of this muscle, as shown. The pectoralis minor tendon has been divided. For rapid access in occasional exsanguinating situations the pectoralis major tendon may be divided at its insertion. Dissection in this area should be meticulous in view of the intimate proximity of nerves and collateral vessels.

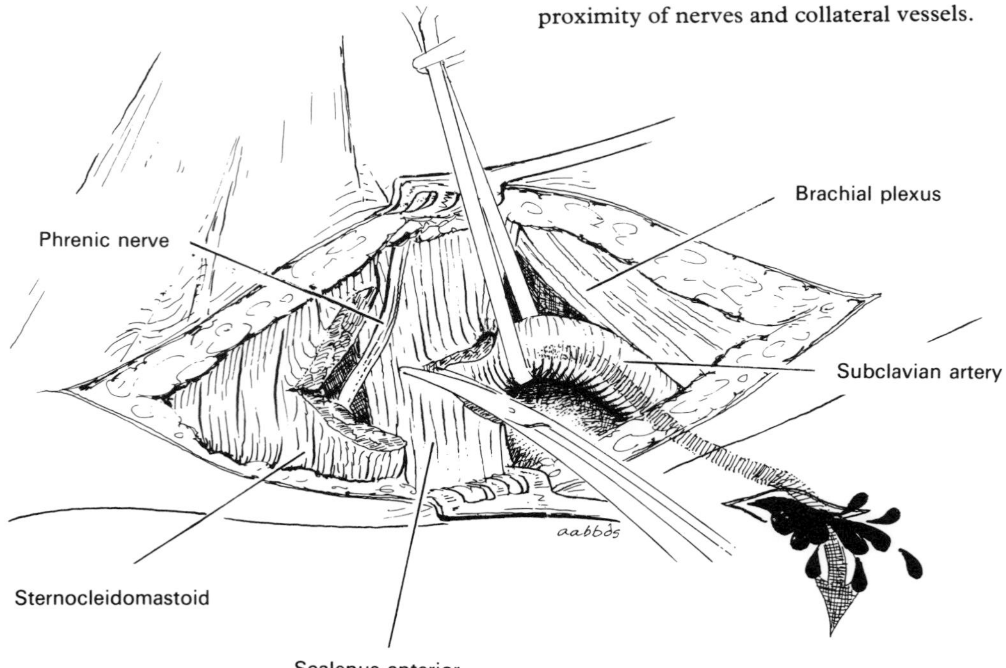

2

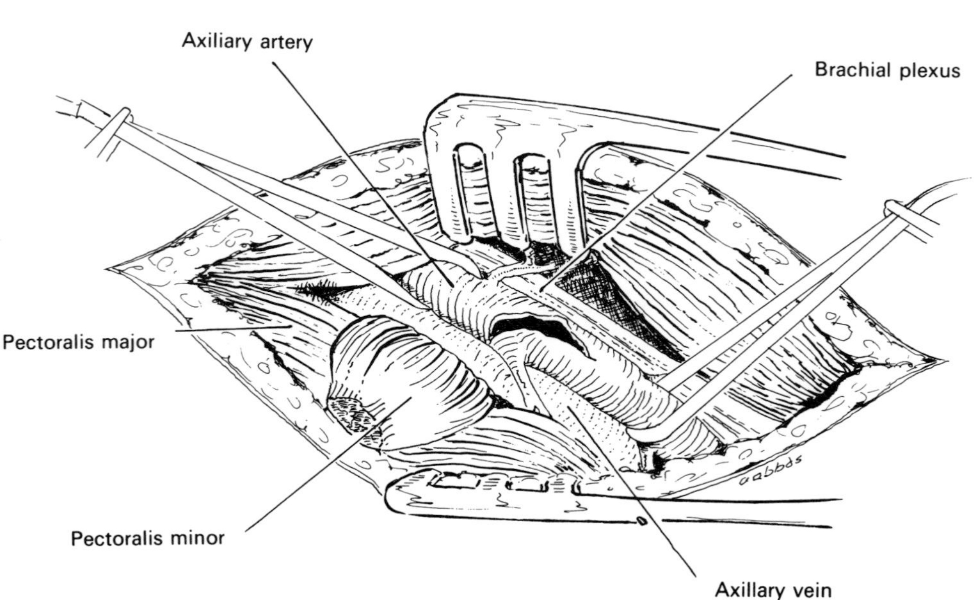

3

4

The brachial artery in the upper arm or at the elbow is exposed via a standard longitudinal incision of sufficient length to expose the injured segment and to establish control. Diagnostic cannulation of this vessel may cause intimal fracture, dissection and thrombosis. Short longitudinal incisions over radial and ulnar arteries are usually quite adequate.

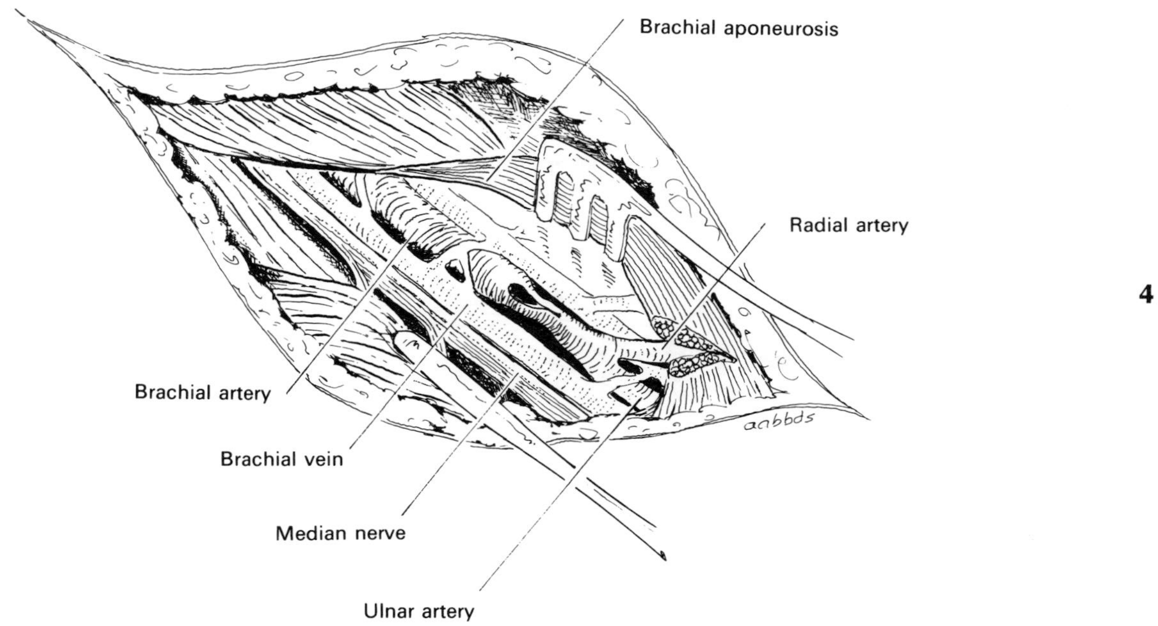

4

5

In most instances of lower limb vascular injury the patient lies supine and both lower limbs are prepared and draped to permit proximal and distal extension of longitudinal incisions in the injured leg and to enable the procurement of a donor vein from the contralateral leg.

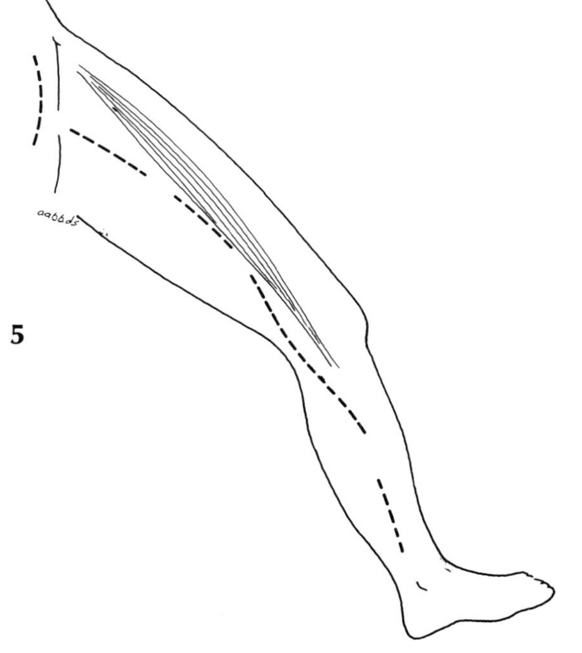

5

6

Of particular importance are vascular injuries of the groin associated with torrential bleeding, where control of the external iliac artery may have to be established through an oblique muscle-splitting incision affording retroperitoneal access above the inguinal ligament. While this is in progress, digital pressure over the bleeding artery is maintained and only after the external iliac artery has been clamped can the groin incision be made.

7

Classical longitudinal incisions are employed in the approach to vessels of the lower limb. The common femoral artery and adjacent vein are exposed. Injuries at the common femoral artery bifurcation will also require encirclement and control of the superficial and deep femoral arteries.

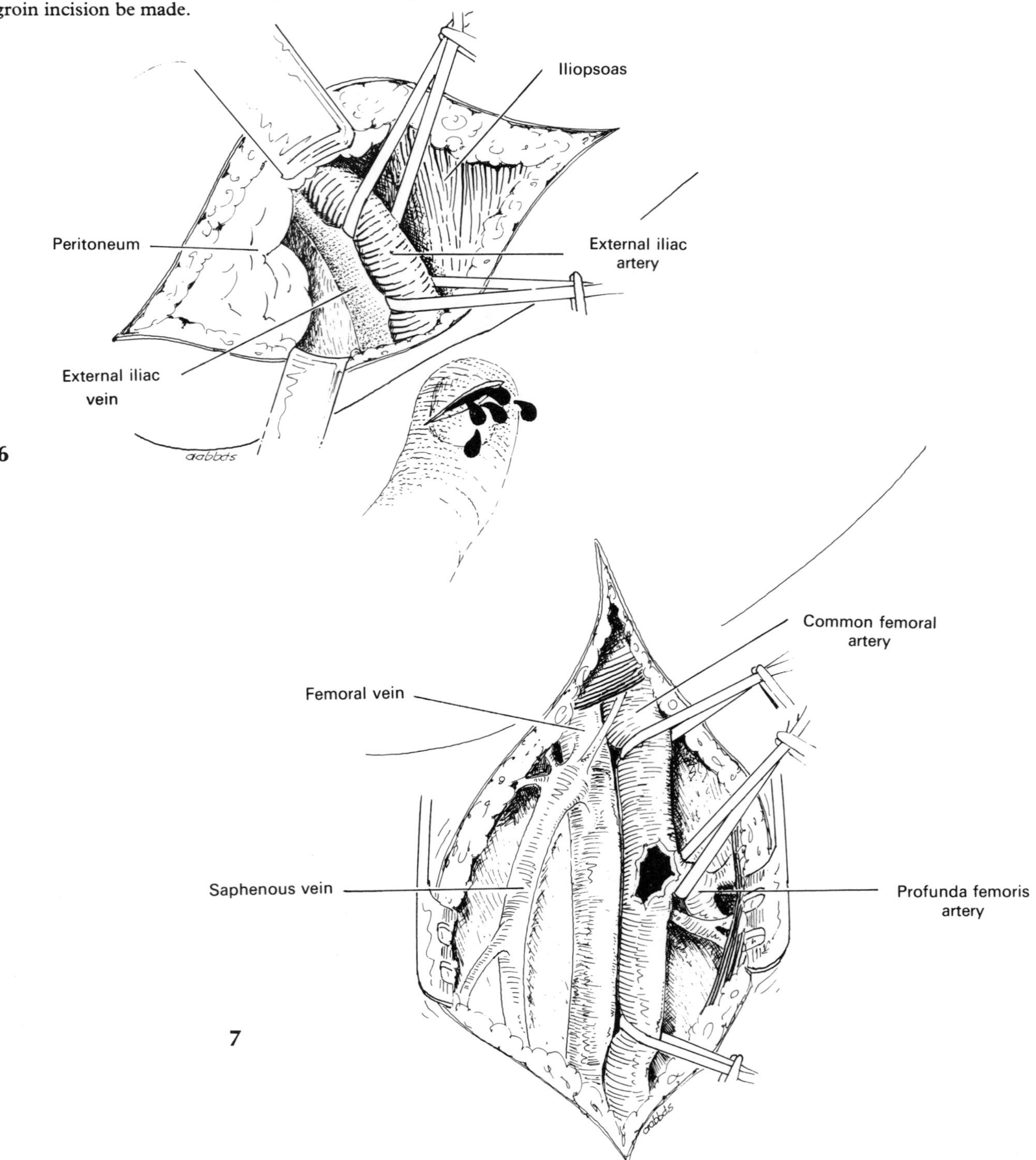

8

The medial approach parallel to and preserving the long saphenous vein will expose the entire length of the popliteal vessels. External rotation of the thigh and 50° knee flexion using a pack of two sterile gowns for lateral support at the hip, is the ideal position. This exposure usually necessitates division of the medial head of the gastrocnemius.

9

A posterior approach with the patient lying prone is convenient for localized mid-popliteal artery injuries. A gentle 'S'-shaped incision in an oblique axis, commencing medially above and proceeding laterally downwards provides adequate exposure. In these instances, both legs are routinely prepared enabling a segment of distal long saphenous vein to be removed with moderate ease from the opposite leg when it is flexed at the knee. Alternatively, with the patient supine, the upper long saphenous vein is harvested and the incision closed before turning the patient over for a posterior approach to the popliteal artery. The deep fascia is incised, watching for the short saphenous vein which may be ligated as it enters the popliteal vein. The tibial nerve should be handled gently as it crosses the vessels in the distal fossa. The popliteal vessels lie on the floor of the fossa, the vein superficial to the artery and united to it by dense areolar tissue, which may be carefully snipped to facilitate encirclement.

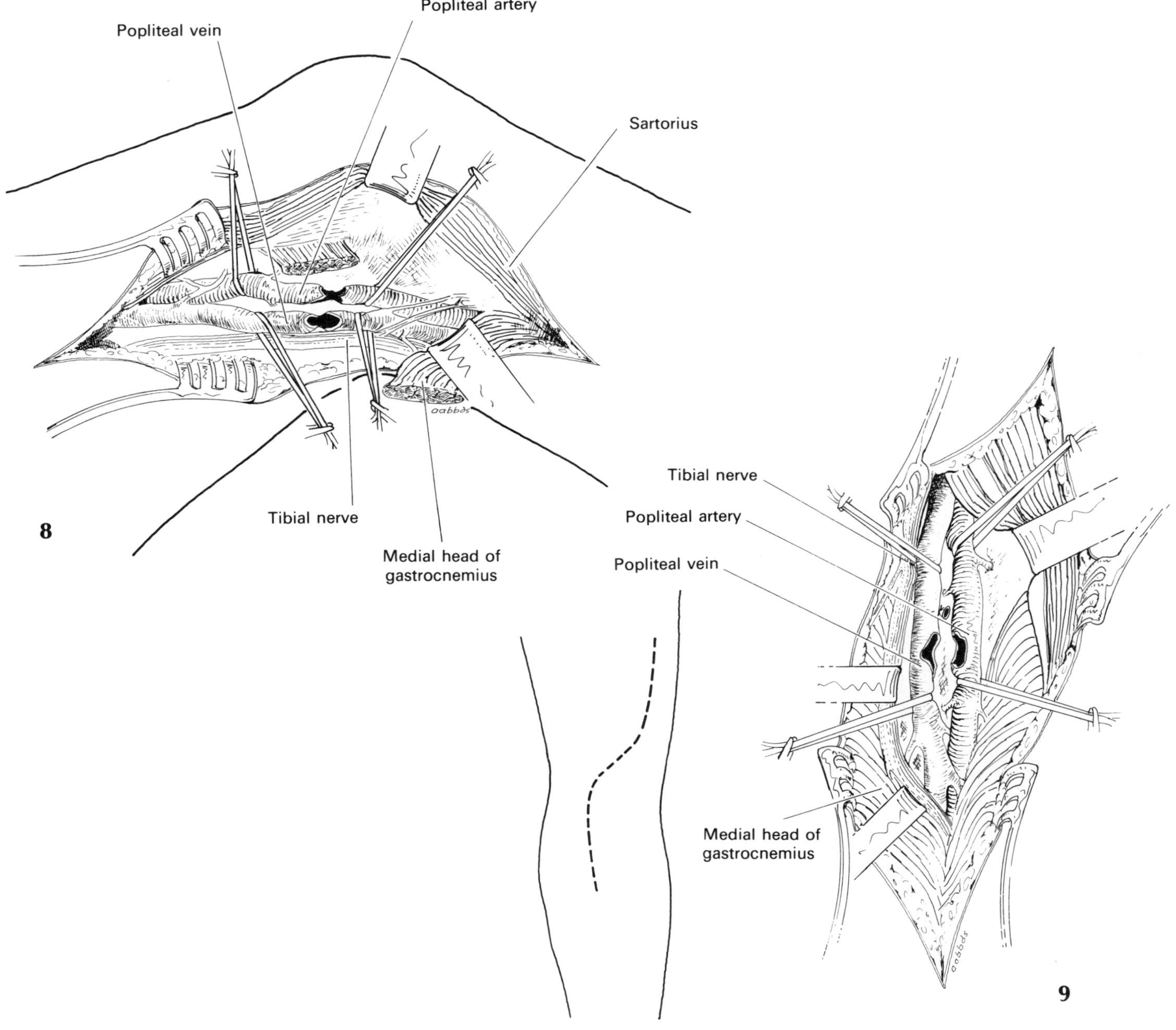

8

9

Control and preparation of vessels

10

The damaged vessels in a wound are quickly exposed and bleeding controlled initially by digital pressure. Using sharp dissecting scissors the segments of an artery above and below are dissected free before encircling them with silastic loops of suitable thickness before clamping. Care is taken to preserve significant branches, which in turn are doubly encircled for control. A sufficient length of artery on either side of the injury is exposed so that it can be trimmed back if necessary to a point where the wall is intact. Minor venous tributaries can be ligated.

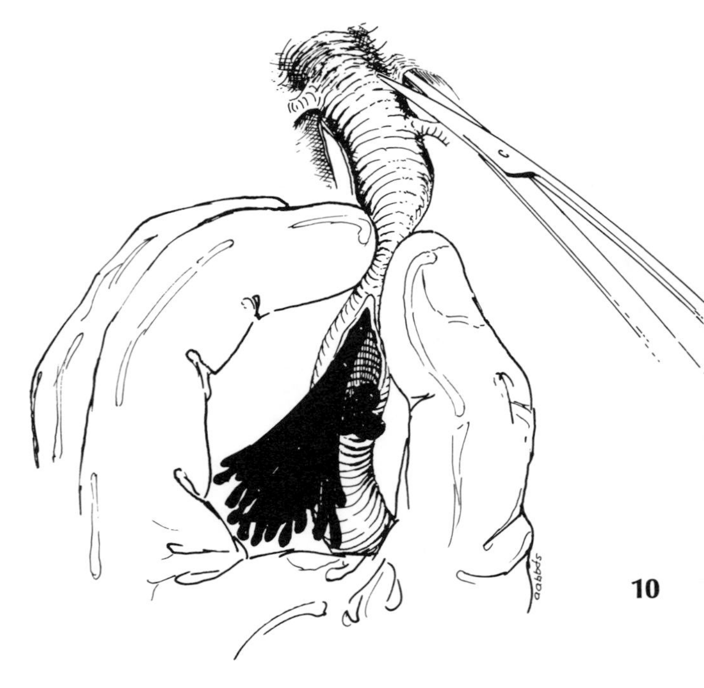

10

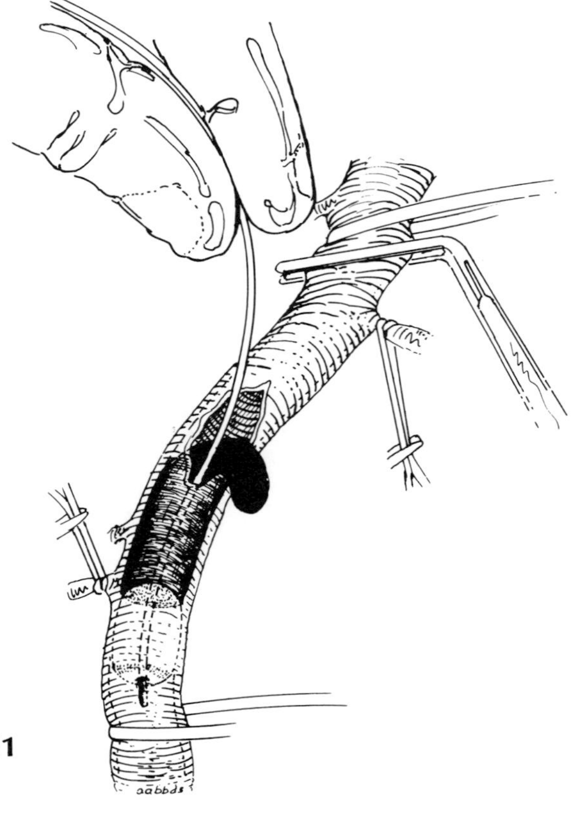

11

11

If ischaemia has been prolonged, release of the upper clamp may wash out a plug of clot but a balloon catheter may also be required. Distal balloon exploration, delicately employed, will often recover clot, especially when backbleeding is poor or absent. Lack of backbleeding is ominous, and in these circumstances vigorous upward milking of the limb musculature distal to the injury may express recent propagated clot. In the young patient lacking an established collateral network, backbleeding will be limited making arterial repair even more essential if the limb is to be salvaged. The distal arteries are then perfused with heparinized saline in a ratio of 5000 u of heparin to 250 ml saline. In the absence of other injury, systemic heparinization is both reliable and easily reversible.

Shunting

When flow through an artery or vein has been interrupted, a policy of routine intraluminal shunting has contributed to improved operative technique, a reduction in complications and enhanced viability (Barros D'Sa, 1982; 1988). Intraluminal shunts of the Brener, Sundt and Javid type of appropriate size, employed in carotid artery surgery, are reasonably effective and a new purpose-built shunt system for vascular trauma has been designed (Barros D'Sa, 1989). When shunts are used, demarcation between viable and dead muscle is more clearly apparent, facilitating accurate debridement and ensuring better haemostasis. In the event of a patient being admitted with multiple injuries, limb-threatening vascular trauma can be safely ignored after shunt insertion, so buying valuable time to complete life-endangering surgery first.

12

A Brener shunt inserted in a torn popliteal artery revitalizes the distal limb and a Javid shunt placed in a severed vein prevents the inevitable rise in intracompartmental pressure, thereby limiting tissue damage and in consequence significantly reducing the need for fasciotomy. The side arm of a Brener shunt forms a convenient port for the delivery of heparinized saline and antibiotics and also for blood sampling, pressure monitoring and on-table angiography if distal injury is suspected.

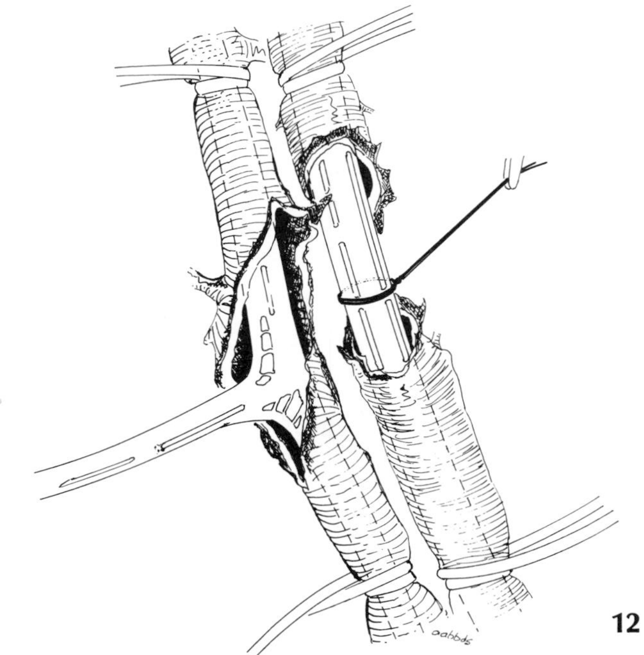

12

13

When a long arterial segment in either upper or lower limb is associated with extensive soft tissue trauma, much time may elapse before restoration of flow. In such cases, a long outlying Pudenz shunt, picking up flow proximal to the injured segment and inserted beyond the injury, will revitalize the limb, and if bleeding through damaged veins is excessive the shunt may be clamped intermittently.

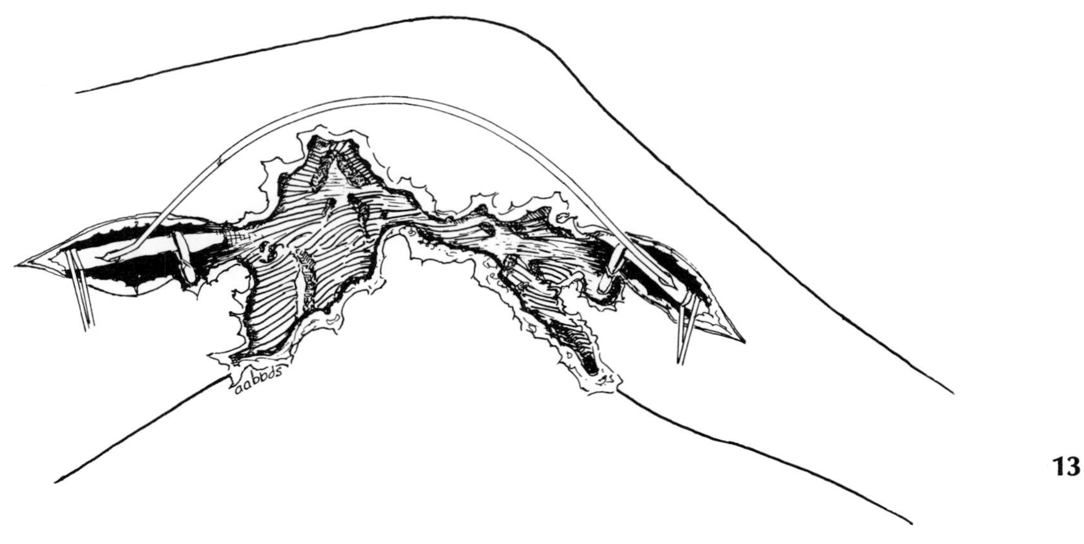

13

14

When skeletal and vascular injuries co-exist a logical policy formulated around the use of inlying shunts streamlines and co-ordinates operative management. After an agreed incisional approach, if necessary by extending an open wound as when confronted with a case of virtual dismemberment just below mid-thigh level, the vascular surgeon re-establishes flow through artery and vein by means of shunts. He is then relieved by the orthopaedic surgeon who can proceed methodically without undue haste approximating the bone ends and using the most suitable method of fracture stabilization, which in penetrating trauma is usually by external fixation.

15

The vascular surgeon then returns to execute the vascular repair using long vein grafts to bridge the gaps in the confident knowledge that they will not be disturbed. A great deal of debate still takes place about the order of repair when artery and vein are injured concomitantly, but such controversy is dispelled if both vessels are shunted. In the past an understandable desire to restore limb flow speedily led to exhortations to repair the artery before bony fixation, but this policy was attended by the real fears of suture line disruption of a delicate vessel repair during the robust manipulations necessary to achieve alignment of bone fragments. Shunts render this approach almost obsolete.

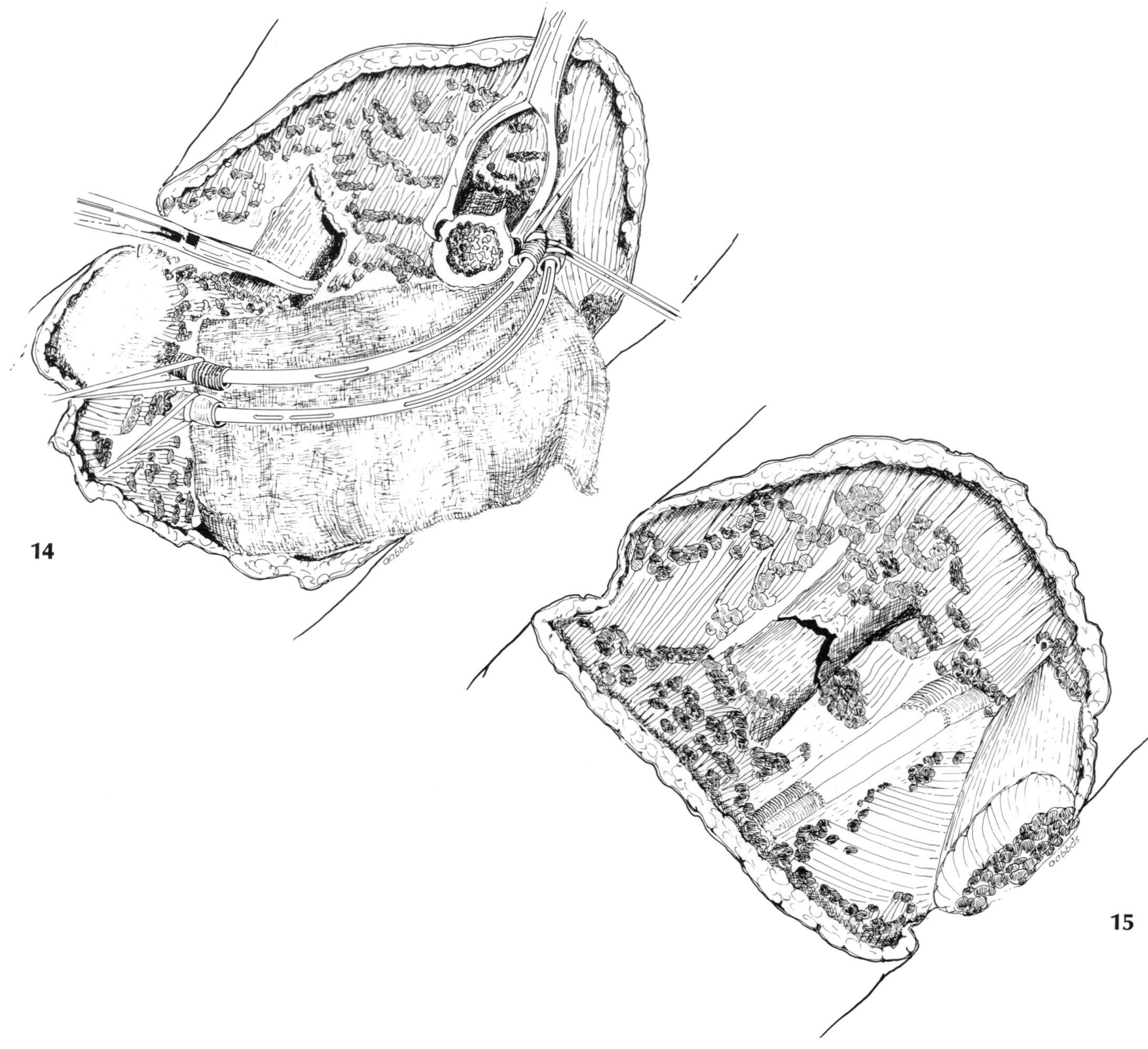

14

15

Care of the wound

Excision of knife wounds is usually unnecessary and only a small margin of devitalized tissue around the edge of a low-velocity bullet wound is removed. Debridement of high-velocity wounds must be adequate if infection is to be averted, and therefore a liberal longitudinal incision dividing the investing fascia is required. All devitalized muscle, recognized by its deep purplish colour and failure to bleed and contract, is trimmed back to a point where it does. Bone fragments are detached from periosteum and foreign bodies, missiles and contaminants are meticulously removed, aided by copious and if possible pulsatile irrigation. A contused nerve is simply left alone, but if transected in a clean wound accurate primary repair is advisable. If damage is extensive following severe blunt injuries and gunshot wounds, the sheath of each nerve end is simply tagged so that delayed secondary repair can be undertaken as an elective procedure.

Arterial repair

While it may be reasonable to ligate minor arteries and veins, in principle all damaged vessels should be repaired, a precept which is particularly applicable to the small calibre brachial or femoral artery of a child whose limbs require sufficient blood flow for proper growth and development. Tibial arteries should be reconstructed, especially if two of them are known to be damaged. The presumption that axillary or brachial artery ligation will not lead to upper limb amputation due to the protective presence of adequate collateral blood flow should be diminished. Brachial artery injuries should not be regarded as innocuous and left to be repaired by a novice, as opportunities to obtain a good result diminish with each repeated attempt. The Allen test should be used in determining the importance of repairing injured radial and ulnar arteries. The choice of vascular repair indicated will obviously depend on the nature of the injury. The morphological types of injury (Barros D'Sa, 1988) include varying degrees of intimal fracture and dissection with thrombic occlusion, laceration or a lateral defect sometimes complicated by false aneurysm and arteriovenous fistula formation, transection and complete disruption by avulsive forces. In practice, various permutations of these morphologically simple subdivisions may be present in a single vascular injury. The diagnosis of 'spasm' is both presumptive and dangerous if it leads to inactivity in the presence of limb-threatening arterial injury.

16

Lateral suture

Lateral suture is acceptable in a small puncture wound, especially if it can be performed transversely using interrupted sutures. Transverse and short oblique lacerations with sharp edges may be repaired similarly. When the laceration is longitudinal and particularly if it is contused, adequate excision followed by lateral suture will narrow the lumen and could endanger the extremity, notably in critical vessels such as the brachial and popliteal.

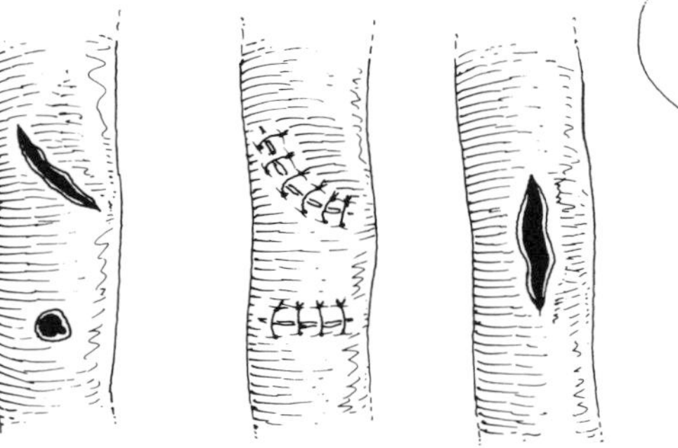

16

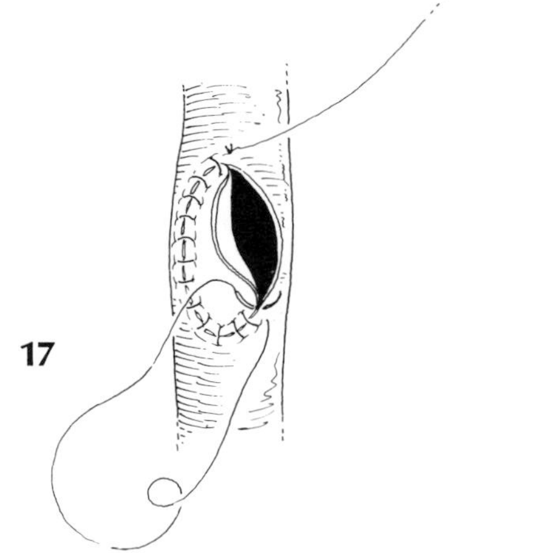

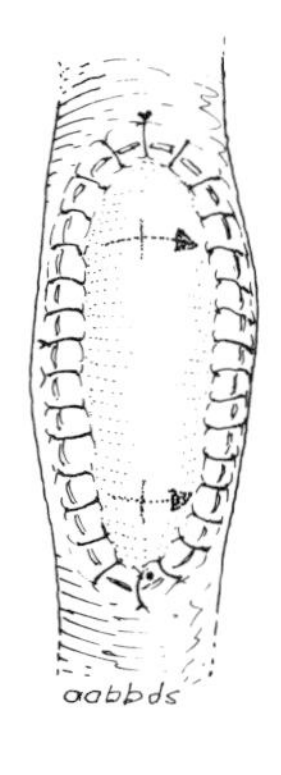

17

17

Patch angioplasty

In order to preserve the calibre of the artery an angioplasty using a vein patch is preferable to lateral suture. In a closed or uncontaminated injury to a large vessel such as the iliac or common femoral artery, it would be quite acceptable to employ a suitable prosthetic patch graft in the knowledge that it will heal with an endothelialized flow surface in a matter of a few weeks (Barros D'Sa *et al.*, 1980).

18

Direct anastomosis

Direct end-to-end anastomosis is possible after stab wounds or after excising the edges with limited loss of length. The presence of excessive anastomotic tension may well lead to disruption or thrombotic failure. If a joint has to be flexed and if major collateral channels, particularly in an atherosclerotic artery, have to be sacrificed to permit approximation, then excision and vein grafting is indicated. These limitations are once again particularly applicable to the popliteal artery.

Vein grafts

Autogenous tissue is durable, resistant to infection and can develop nutrient flow from surrounding viable tissue. Long-term promise of patency makes vein the most desirable graft, especially as vascular trauma largely afflicts the young. The indiscriminate use of prosthetic arterial grafts in combat wounds predisposes to infection, secondary haemorrhage and a high amputation rate, and has been avoided with beneficial results (Barros D'Sa, 1980, 1982; Barros D'Sa *et al.*, 1980). An institutional policy of using substitute arterial conduits in the form of polytetrafluorethylene (PTFE) prostheses in gunshot wounds has shown early promise (Feliciano *et al*, 1984), but should not lead to complacency.

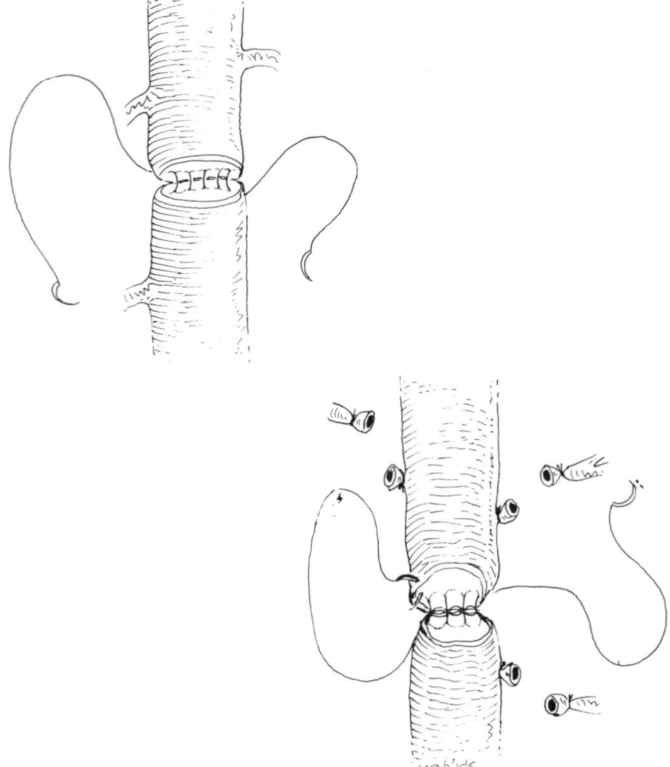

18

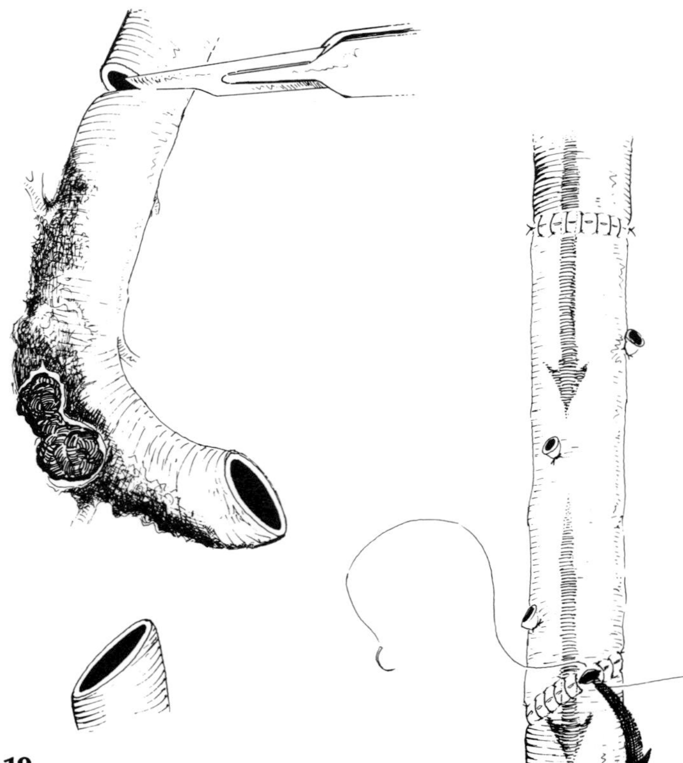

19

19

The excision of only a centimetre of apparently normal vessel with a No. 15 scalpel blade on either side of an obvious vascular injury may be inadequate, particularly in high-velocity bullet trauma or the complex traction injury of the popliteal vessels in a motor-cycle accident. The external appearances of an injured artery often belie the extent of damage to the intima, and therefore the arterial wall may have to be trimmed back further with sharp scissors to a point where it is visibly intact. The practice of interposing a reversed vein graft which is easily available encourages adequate excision of a damaged artery. The long saphenous vein of the opposite leg is the usual source for donor graft, the ipsilateral vein representing a precious drainage channel in circumstances where the deep vein may be injured. The vein graft is reversed and is usually used at once but may be stored temporarily in cold Hank's solution or heparinized saline.

20

In larger vessels such as the axillary and femoral, a polypropylene everting suture commenced at diametrically opposite points is continued along the suture line, access to which is gained by a measure of rotation on the axis of the vessel. If a shunt is in place, the vein graft can be drawn over it. The shunt then acts conveniently as a stent, permits a more disciplined suture technique and prevents purse-stringing of the anastomosis.

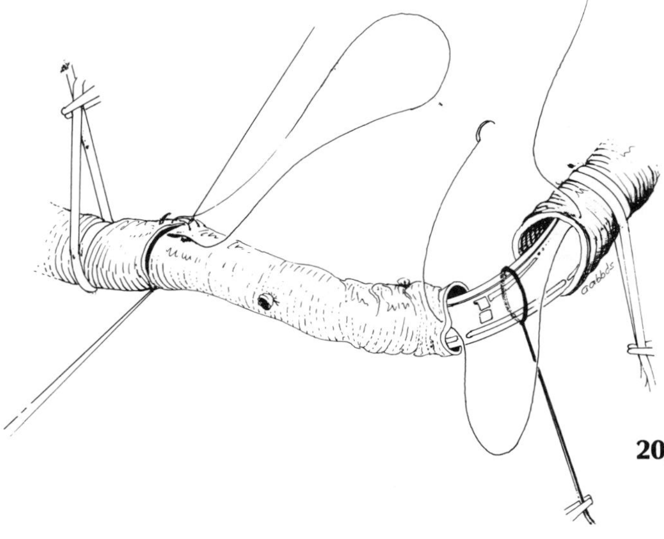

20

21

If the arterial diameter is less than 4 mm, careful thrombectomy using a size 2 balloon catheter is essential. Meticulous attention is paid to technique in executing the anastomosis using loupes and fine instruments. Small arteries of children are prone to vasospasm which may be abolished by judicious inflation with a fine rounded catheter. The ends of the vein graft and host vessel are cut obliquely and spatulated, a necessary step which will accommodate increasing vessel diameter without stenosis as the child grows. Repair is then undertaken by interrupted 6/0 to 8/0 polypropylene sutures carefully placed without tension so as to prevent constriction at the suture line. Accurate coaptation of intimal surfaces while everting the edges will prevent inward protrusion of adventitial strands.

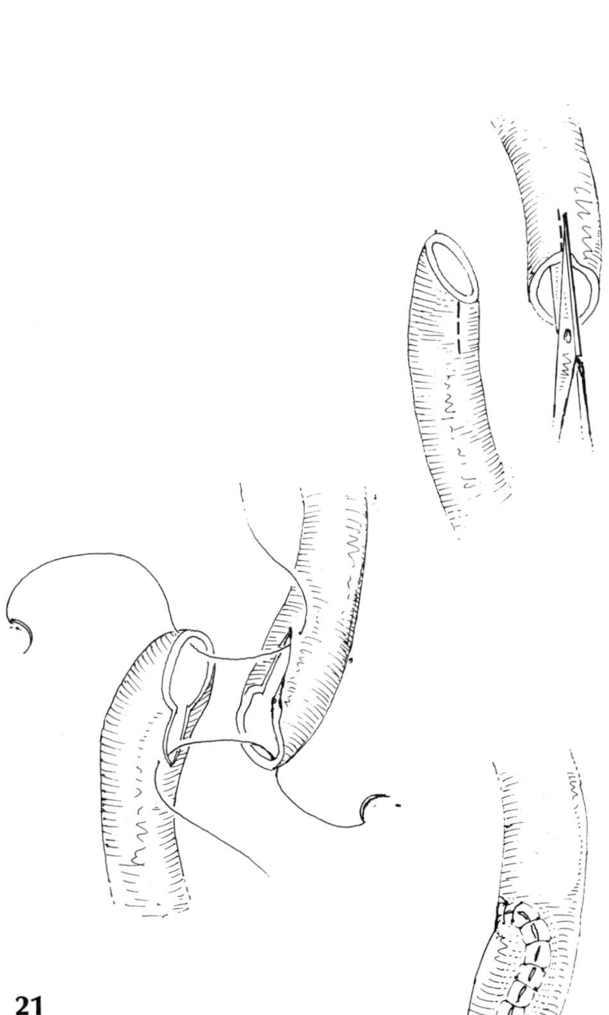

21

22

If a lengthy segment of atherosclerotic artery is damaged, emergency bypass surgery may be necessary. If soft tissue loss is extensive and if contamination is extreme, then an extra-anatomic vein bypass through clean tissues should be considered. If, for example, a lengthy femoropopliteal segment has been destroyed in a large contaminated wound, the trimmed ends are ligated and an extra-anatomic vein graft, unreversed but with its valves disrupted, is inserted subcutaneously from the common femoral to, for example, the anterior tibial artery.

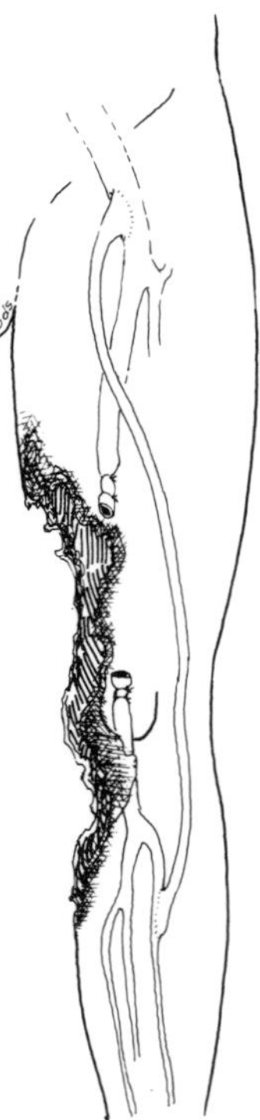

22

23

When the calibre of the donor vein is much smaller than that of the host vessel – often a vein – the graft will fail unless a panel compound graft of larger diameter can be constructed to ensure laminar flow. It is fashioned 'on the bench' by taking two segments of vein opened longitudinally to form panels and these are sewn together side by side with 6/0 polypropylene to achieve proportions comparable to the host vessel (Livingston and Wilson, 1975). These grafts have to be made slightly longer than the gap to be bridged.

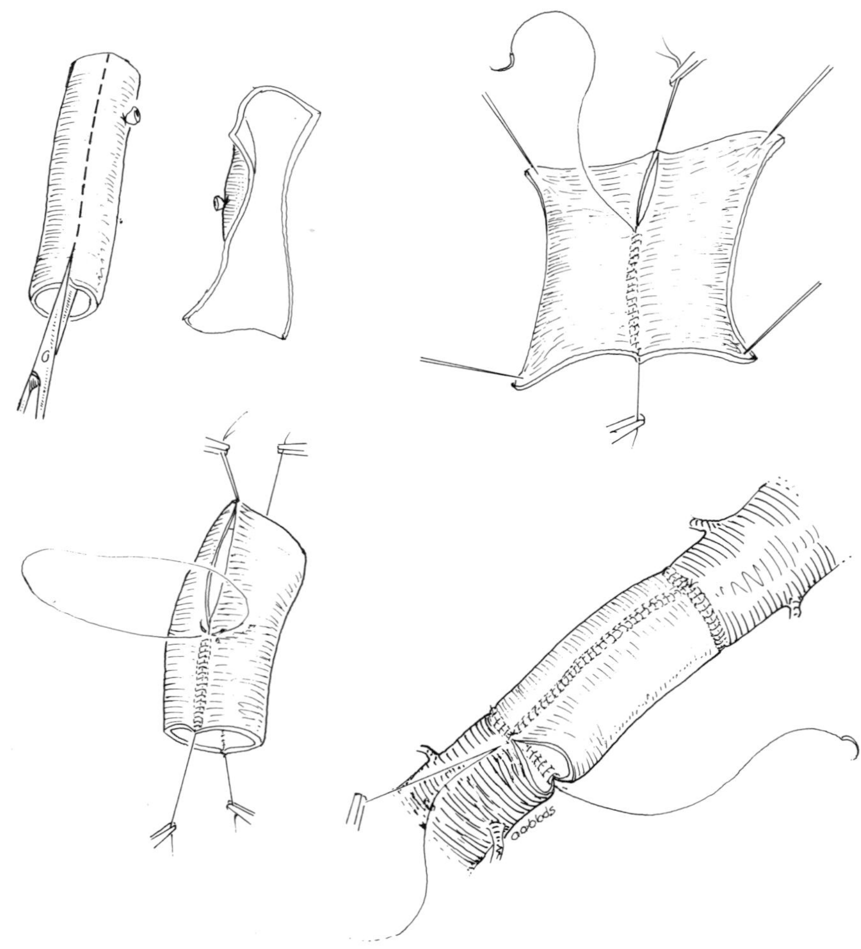

23

24

For larger vessels such as the femoral vein, three rather than two panels may be required. Alternatively, a technique used to replace a segment of the vena cava can be employed and it may have particular value in contaminated wounds. A length of vein is slit open longitudinally and wrapped spirally over a shunt of sufficiently wide bore to act as a stent and then the adjoining margins of vein are sewn together using a continuous 6/0 polypropylene suture.

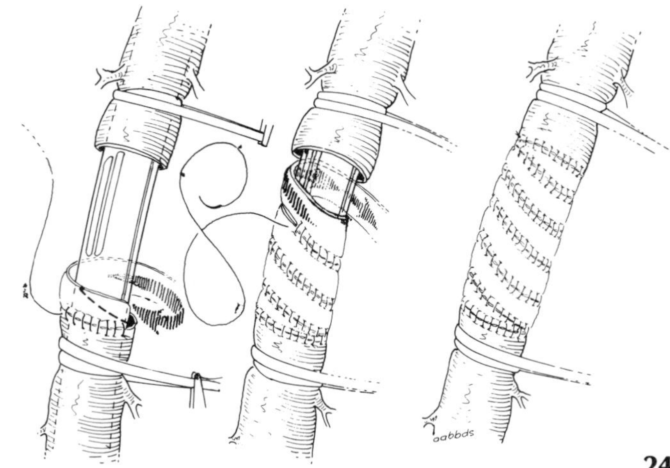

24

25

False aneurysms

A false aneurysm may develop in a partially penetrating injury which has been missed usually because distal flow did not appear to be compromised. Most frequently, false aneurysms follow diagnostic transfemoral cardiac catheterization. For obvious reasons, these patients may not be fit for general anaesthesia and regional or local anaesthesia may have to be used. After establishing proximal and distal control, the aneurysm is opened and the profunda femoris which could not be exposed initially is now clamped. The thrombus is removed and the aneurysm excised. The vessel lumen is inspected for intimal damage, if necessary by transverse extension of the opening. If a loose atheromatous flap is present on the posterior wall, it is tacked down with a 5/0 or 6/0 polypropylene suture. The laceration is repaired transversely with interrupted 5/0 double-ended sutures, picking upper and lower edges from within outwards. In the case of a chronic larger fusiform aneurysm, patch angioplasty or segmental excision and replacement with an interposed vein graft or prosthetic conduit is preferred.

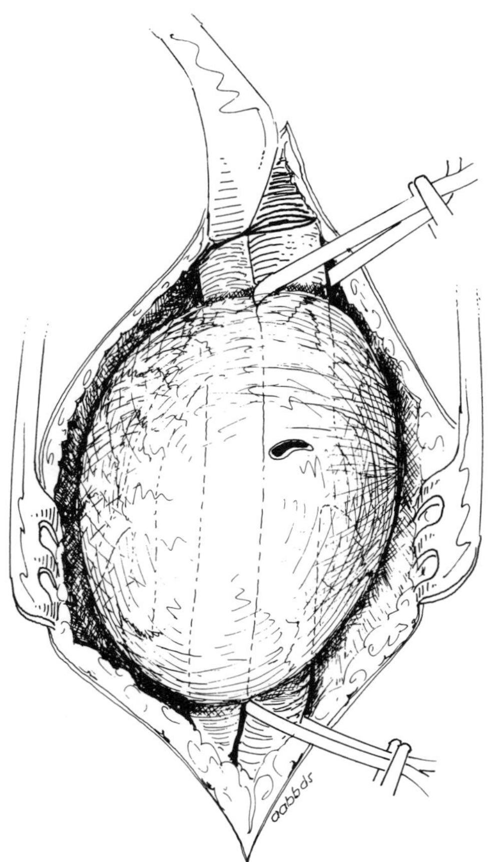

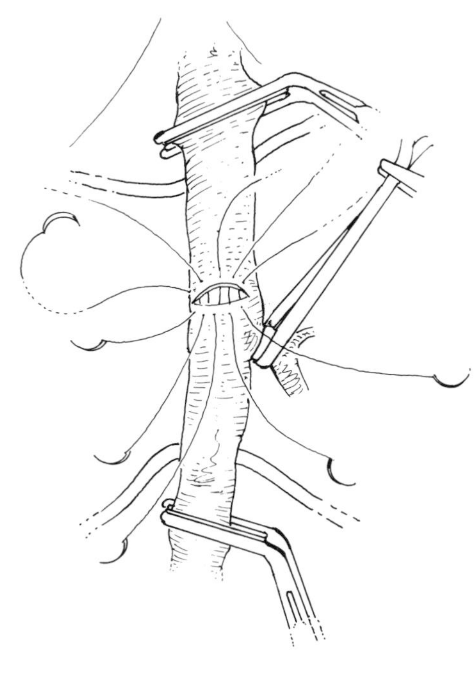

25

26

Arteriovenous fistulae

Arteriovenous fistulae may be missed both clinically and at operation due to inadequate exploration and will present much later, usually accompanied by one or two false aneurysms. The intraoperative use of a sterile stethoscope may have some value, especially in cases of shotgun wounds, to ensure closure of all fistulae. The artery and vein are exposed, brought under control, the fistulous communication separated by means of a fine scalpel and the false aneurysms excised. The edges of the defects are trimmed back to intact vessel wall. The openings in the artery are best repaired by vein patches and, if required, by excision of a segment and vein graft replacement. The vein is usually repaired successfully either by lateral suture or by insertion of a vein patch. Finally, a flap of fascia may be interposed between adjacent suture lines to prevent recurrence.

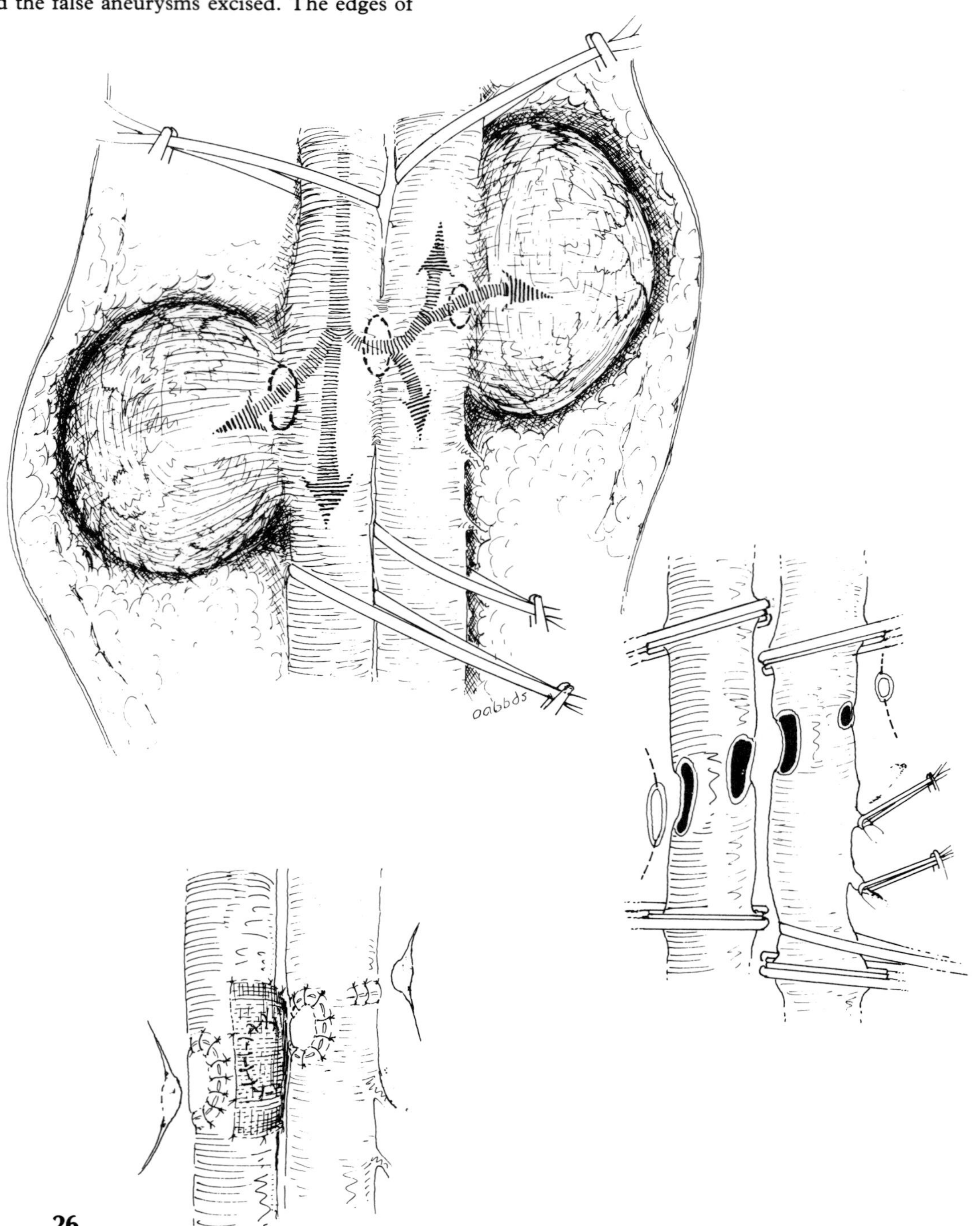

26

On-table angiography

Clinical evaluation of the quality of arterial repair in a severely injured and hypotensive patient whose core temperature has fallen may be difficult simply because distal pulses are weak or absent, and even Doppler ultrasound cannot be relied upon. The only way of excluding technical error or distal thrombotic obstruction is by on-table angiography which takes a few minutes and provides visual evidence of the adequacy of surgery.

Venous repair

The mistaken attitude that ligation of a damaged vein, while not helpful, would do no harm, or that venous repair is possibly less important than arterial repair, should not be perpetuated. When both vessels are injured, vein ligation may result in amputation even after successful arterial reconstruction. Conversely, venous repair will enhance arterial patency. Ligation of a main vein causes venous hypertension and can result in acute massive oedema, in some cases leading to gangrene and amputation and in others to deep vein thrombosis and pulmonary embolism or to disabling chronic odema and postphlebitic changes. Every effort must be made to secure at least one good venous channel at axillary, femoral or popliteal level. A vein tolerates lateral suturing much better than an artery, but loss of diameter must still be guarded against. Repair of a major vein is quite valuable when tissue loss is massive and lymph damage is compromised.

27

If both artery and vein are injured and each is shunted, the order of repair of these two vessels is immaterial, but if neither vessel has been shunted then preliminary vein repair will prevent a serious rise in venous pressure when arterial flow is eventually re-established. With shunts in place in this wound, a simple vein graft has been reversed and interposed perfectly adequately to replace a damaged arterial segment of similar calibre, but it would have been too narrow for the adjacent vein of much larger diameter. As time is not of crucial importance, a panel compound vein graft is constructred to match the host vein, drawn over the shunt and sutured in position.

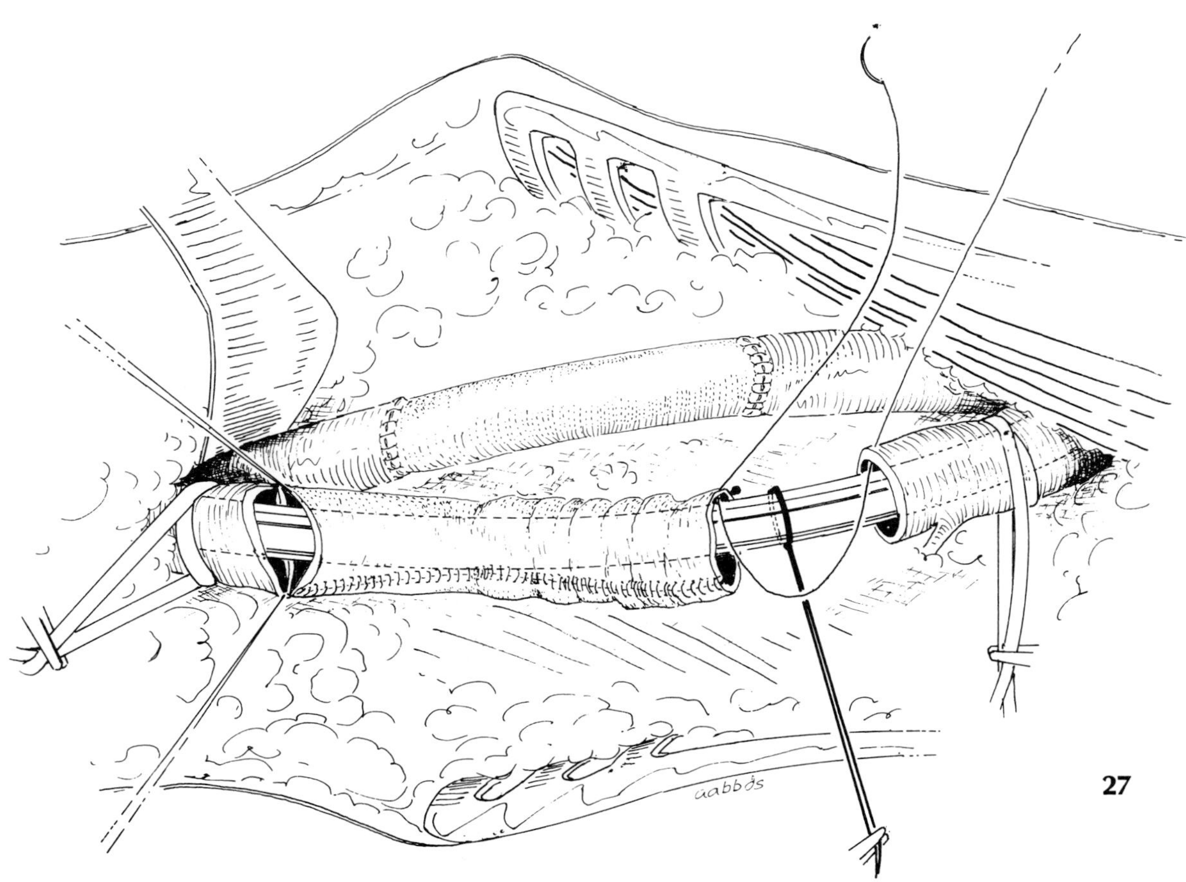

27

Fasciotomy

Restoration of arterial flow, especially if delayed, increases intracompartmental pressure, which in turn aggravates peripheral ischaemia. These considerations are of particular importance in brachial and popliteal artery injury, and in the latter case the anterior compartment which lies within rigid confines is most vulnerable. Adequate pedal pulses, good skin flow and satisfactory Doppler signals may be observed, although the muscle within the compartments is dying. Fasciotomy, if carried out early and effectively, is an invaluable adjunctive measure aimed at forestalling the serious complications of muscle ischaemia. The early use of intraluminal shunts in both artery and vein diminishes the need for fasciotomy. If shunts have not been employed, fasciotomy should be considered if any one of the following several factors is present: sustained hypotension, an interval of more than 4 h between injury and surgical intervention, evident oedema or patchy muscle necrosis, concurrent injury to a main vein, marked injury of distal soft tissue, subfascial haematoma and bleeding, muscle paralysis and fixed flexion deformity after initial vascular repair or a compartment pressure in excess of 40 mmHg.

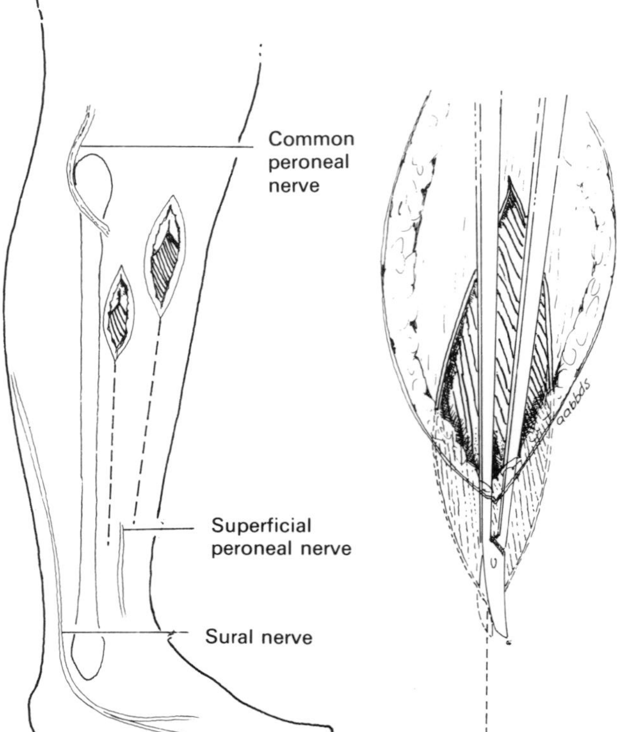

28

28

The classical percutaneous or closed fasciotomy is employed as a rule by using 5-cm vertical incisions into the deep fascia through which muscle tends to bulge. These incisions are made in the centre of the upper anterior compartment, further laterally in the middle of the upper lateral compartment and, finally, medial to the short saphenous vein over the upper posterior compartment. A pair of long curved blunt-tipped scissors is held slightly open to grasp the lower corner of the divided fascia and advanced, slitting it down the length of each compartment. Care is taken to avoid damaging the common peroneal nerve at the neck of the fibula as well as the distal superficial peroneal and sural nerves.

29

If the muscle is pale, grey and firm, or if obvious compartmental tension is still present, the skin and subcutaneous tissues are incised converting it to an open fasciotomy. As tension decreases, these transcutaneous fasciotomy incisions will gradually approximate, but during this period utmost care must be taken to prevent infection within relatively ischaemic tissues.

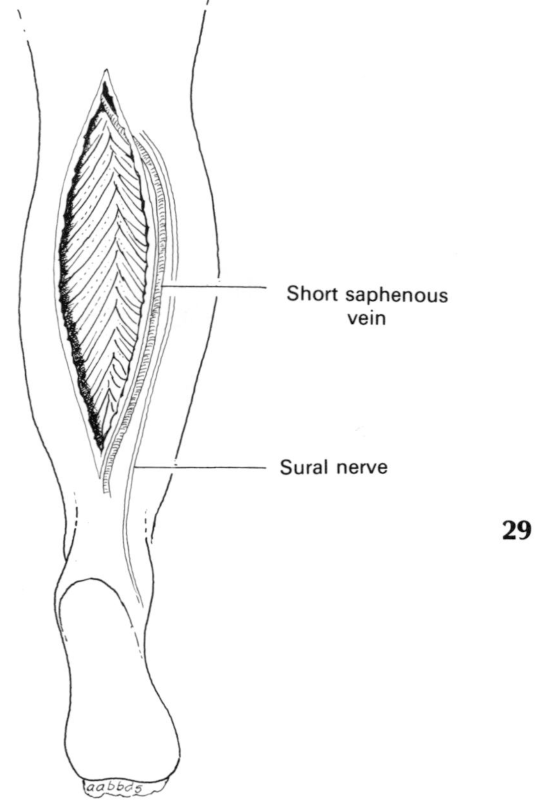

29

30

Open fasciotomy is the technique of choice in severe compression of the muscles of the forearm. The extensor compartment is released by a longitudinal centrally placed incision, while the flexor compartment is decompressed by a long curvilinear incision commencing in the antecubital fossa and crossing the wrist onto the palm along the thenar crease.

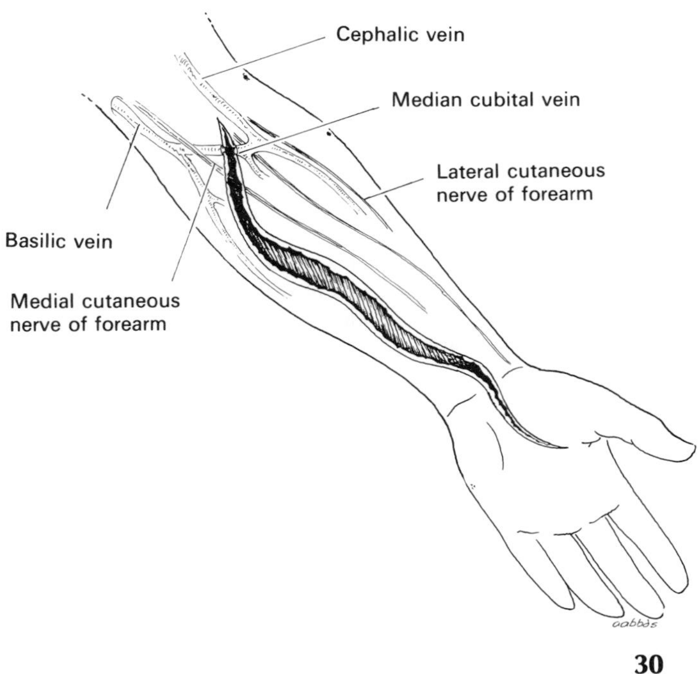

30

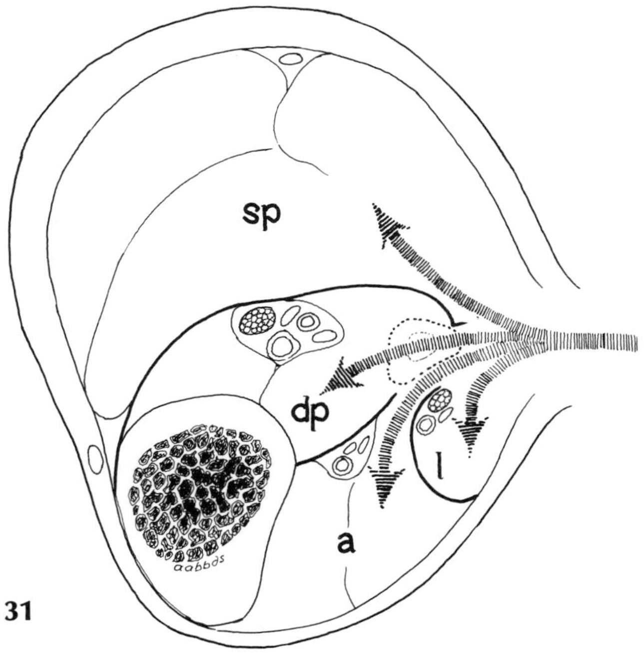

31

31

It should be remembered that a fourth deep posterior compartment is present in the lower leg in addition to the other three, and all four can be decompressed simultaneously after first resecting the mid-third of the shaft of the fibula subperiosteally (Patman and Thompson, 1970). The relationship of the superficial posterior (sp), deep posterior (dp), anterior (a) and lateral (l) compartments to the fibula when imagined in transverse section show how this route of entry can achieve the desired result.

Wound closure and vessel cover

It is important to ensure adequate cover of repaired vessels by adjacent tissues. In closed injuries primary suture of the wound is acceptable, leaving a vacuum suction drain *in situ* for a short period. In contaminated wounds the wisdom of a policy of delayed primary suture 5–7 days later has been borne out by experience (Barros D'Sa, 1980), but that should not be an excuse for slipshod wound excision and toilet.

In situations of extensive loss of skin and soft tissue over a site of arterial repair, the wall of a vein graft or adjacent artery may conceivably undergo ischaemia, desiccation and degeneration followed by catastrophic haemorrhage. While prosthetic grafts are immune to these influences they still represent alien material and if the field is contaminated then infection, thrombosis and suture line dehiscence could follow. This observation has a special bearing on the management of large dirty wounds which have to be left open to drain, making graft cover difficult. Biological dressings, such as porcine heterografts and amniotic membrane, have been tried but the alternative of a vascularized muscle flap requiring the skills of a plastic surgeon is preferable. Many of these difficulties will, of course, have been countered by the employment of the extra-anatomic vein bypass described.

Postoperative management

Ordinarily, following arterial repair, a limb is nursed in a horizontal position, but when the adjacent vein has been repaired, some degree of elevation is justified. As the patient rewarms, a deficiency in fluid replacement, evident from general observation and vital signs, must be corrected to ensure adequate flow through the reconstructed vessels. Anticoagulation with low-dose heparin (5000 u every 6 h subcutaneously) will aid graft patency and prevent deep vein thrombosis.

Failure of repair

Utmost vigilance must be exercised in monitoring flow by checking pulses, skin circulation and Doppler signals. Their absence may be a prelude to amputation unless urgent angiography and further reconstruction are undertaken. In such cases, classical weaknesses of technique are observed, namely, constriction caused by lateral suture, tension at the suture line of a direct anastomosis, insufficient excision of damaged artery, too narrow or too long vein grafts, 'purse-string' effect of a continuous anastomotic suture and poor intimal coaptation. In dealing with graft failure the most reliable sequence of measures is as follows: excise the segment concerned liberally, confirm the quality of the freshly trimmed vessel, perform an adequate balloon thrombectomy, reperfuse the distal artery with heparinized saline and very precisely revise the repair with a fresh vein graft of suitable calibre and length. Systemic heparinization and close observation will avert an unfavourable outcome.

In summary, a number of factors play a role in minimizing the complication rate and incidence of limb loss: routine use of intraluminal shunts in both injured artery and vein, vascular repair after skeletal fixation, early and definitive repair of both artery and vein injury, avoidance of lateral suture and direct anastomosis, use of vein grafts and of panel compound grafts of appropriate diameter when required, immediate fasciotomy when indicated, postoperative vigilance and, in cases of graft failure, expeditious re-exploration and fresh repair.

References

Barros D'Sa, A. A. B. (1980). Missile-induced vascular trauma. *Injury* **12**, 13.

Barros D'Sa, A. A. B. (1982). A decade of missile-induced vascular trauma. *Annals of the Royal College of Surgeons of England* **64**, 37.

Barros D'Sa, A. A. B. (1988). How should we manage acute ischaemia associated with trauma? In *Limb Salvage and Amputation for Vascular Disease*. Greenhalgh, R. M., Jamieson, C. W., Nicolaides, A. N., eds. London and Philadelphia: W. B. Saunders.

Barros D'Sa, A. A. B. (1989). The rationale for arterial and venous shunting in the management of limb vascular injuries. *European Journal of Vascular Surgery* **3**, 471.

Barros D'Sa, A. A. B., Berger, K., DiBenedetto, G., *et al.* (1980). A healable filamentous Dacron surgical fabric. *Annals of Surgery* **192**, 645.

Feliciano, D. V., Carmel, G., Bitondo, P. A. C., *et al.* (1984). Civilian trauma in the 1980's. A 1-year experience with 456 vascular and cardiac injuries. *Annals of Surgery* **199**, 717.

Livingston, R. H. and Wilson, R. I. (1975). Gunshot wounds to the limbs. *British Medical Journal* **1**, 667.

Patman, R. D. and Thompson, J. E. (1970). Fasciotomy in peripheral arterial injury. *Archives of Surgery* **101**, 633.

Portacaval and splenorenal shunts for portal hypertension

MARTIN BIRNSTINGL MS, FRCS
Consultant Surgeon, St Bartholomew's Hospital, London, UK

Introduction

The rationale for using portal-systemic shunting procedures for variceal haemorrhage is their effect in reducing pressure and flow in the gastro-oesophageal collateral veins. Unfortunately, total shunts, which are the most effective in producing permanent lowering of portal venous pressure, also tend to cause the highest incidence of portal-systemic encephalopathy (PSE). They also lead to progressive deterioration in liver function in patients with cirrhosis. However, the more selective shunts are not only difficult to construct, but also more likely to thrombose, and are therefore less reliable in securing permanent protection against recurrent variceal bleeding. These disadvantages have to be set against a probable lower incidence of PSE.

Direct portacaval shunts are appropriate for emergency procedures, where the shorter operating time and reliable decompression are advantages (Orloff *et al.*, 1974). The end-to-side procedure is usual, side-to-side portacaval anastomosis is used in the Budd-Chiari syndrome and occasionally in the presence of refractory ascites. Splenorenal shunts are used when the portal vein is unsuitable, for instance following congenital or neonatal thrombosis (extrahepatic portal obstruction).

The selective splenorenal (Warren) shunt is appropriate as an elective procedure in certain instances (Warren, Zeppa and Fomon, 1967). It is tedious to perform and its claimed low incidence of PSE and improved maintenance of liver function are still unconfirmed by good follow-up studies. The author's preference is for end-to-side portacaval anastomosis as the most effective shunting procedure for variceal haemorrhage. A hospital mortality of 18% has been achieved in a series of 56 consecutive emergency operations (Birnstingl, 1980).

The mortality of elective shunt operations is of course much lower than this (2% in Orloff's series of 612 patients), although much influenced by the type and severity of the underlying liver disease. End-to-side portacaval anastomosis is the most likely to remain patent, most likely to stop the bleeding and to prevent later rebleeding and the easiest to perform quickly. It remains the best standard with which to compare other shunt operations.

In selecting patients for shunt operations the most important considerations are the pathology of the underlying liver disease, which varies greatly in different countries, and the degree of impairment of liver cell function, assessed by a classification such as Child's (Child, 1954). In emergency shunts, the duration and severity of the current bleeding episode also influence survival.

Portacaval shunt

1

The patient is positioned lying on the left side with a 30° lateral tilt towards the right side. The knee is bent up and the right arm carried on a rest across the front of the neck. The long thoracoabdominal incision is preferred. This extends through the bed of the right 10th rib nearly to the midline. A long right subcostal incision is also fairly satisfactory, provided the liver is not too large.

A self-retaining retractor is inserted, the diaphragm partially divided and then sutured to the edge of the wound to improve access. An open or trucut needle biopsy of the liver is taken and the presence of portal hypertension confirmed, if necessary, with a saline manometer after tying a plastic cannula into a jejunal vein in the mesentery.

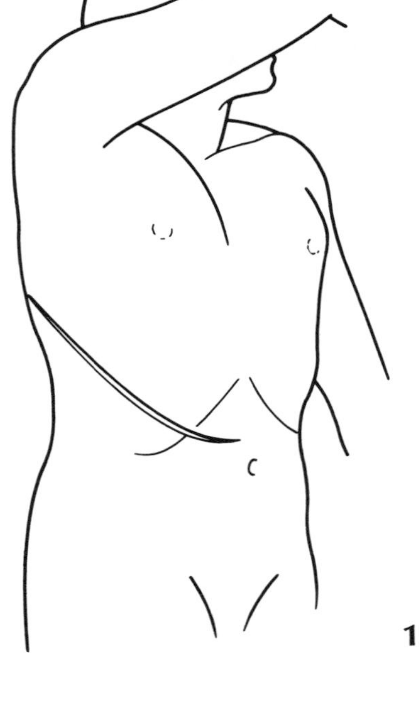

1

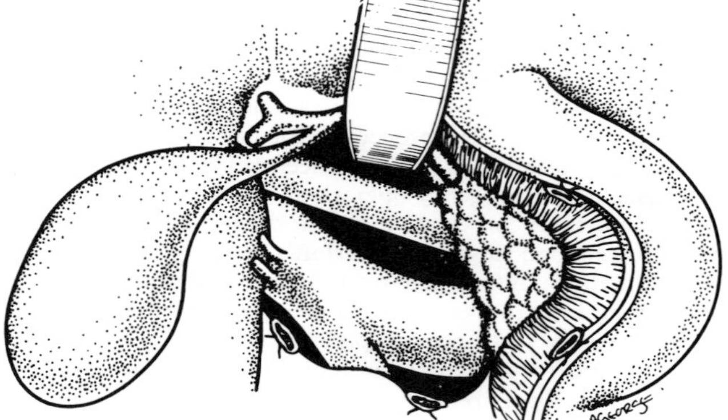

2

2

The lateral reflection of the peritoneum is divided along the margin of the second part of the duodenum to expose the inferior vena cava as far up as the caudate lobe of the liver. The peritoneum must be clamped and tied, and it is usually very vascular and thickened in portal hypertension. Oedema of the retroperitoneal tissues is also often striking. The front and both lateral aspects of the inferior vena cava must be displayed, taking care to avoid the right adrenal vein and inferior hepatic veins, when present.

The shunt will usually be positioned just above the entry of the right renal vein, which is clearly evident.

It is essential to identify the common bile duct and retract this forward and medially before searching for the portal vein, which lies behind the duct on a deeper plane and may be difficult to find. The portal vein is carefully exposed by very gentle dissection in the hepatoduodenal ligament.

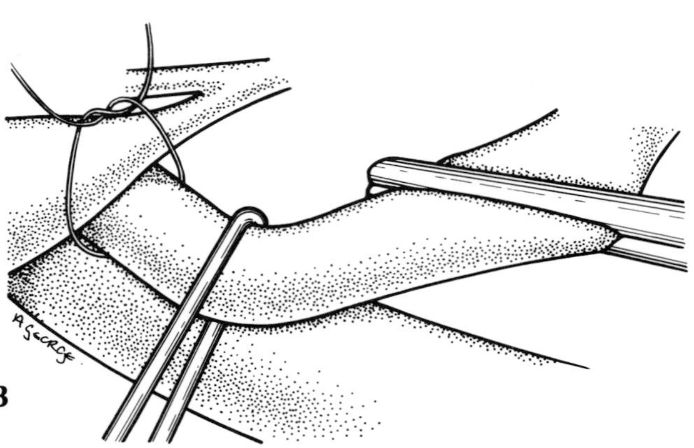

3

3

A plastic sling is carried round the portal vein, which is gently freed nearly to the lower border of the liver, although its bifurcation is not always seen. Care must be taken not to tear the left gastric (coronary) vein which joins the left side of the portal vein. The portal vein is now securely tied just proximal to its bifurcation, using 2/0 linen thread or silk.

4

A straight vascular clamp is applied to the portal vein where it emerges from the pancreatic bed. Some areolar tissue may need to be divided at this point to prevent kinking of the vein. The portal vein is then cleanly divided at an appropriate level near to the bifurcation ligature.

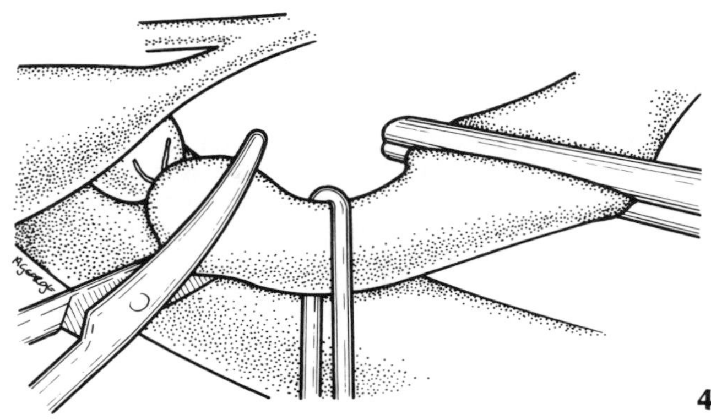
4

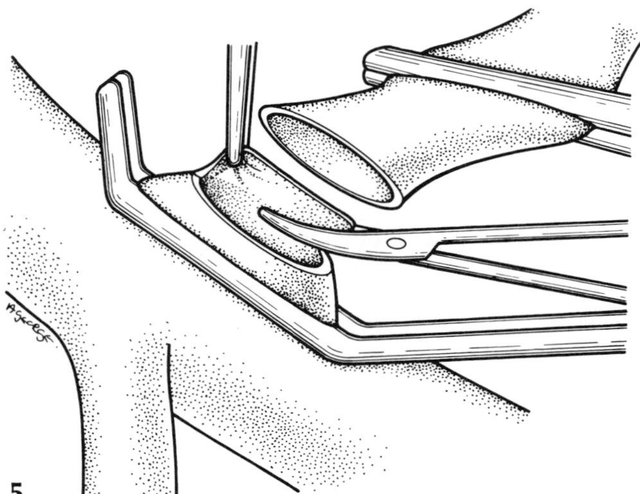
5

5

A Satinsky partial exclusion vascular clamp is next applied to the front of the vena cava. The precise siting of the stoma needs great care, to prevent angulation or flattening of the portal vein. The best level is usually at or just above the right renal vein and it should be well towards the left side of the vena cava, at the junction of the anterior and left lateral aspects. With the vascular clamp in place, an opening is made in the vena cava and an ellipse of vein wall carefully removed with scissors.

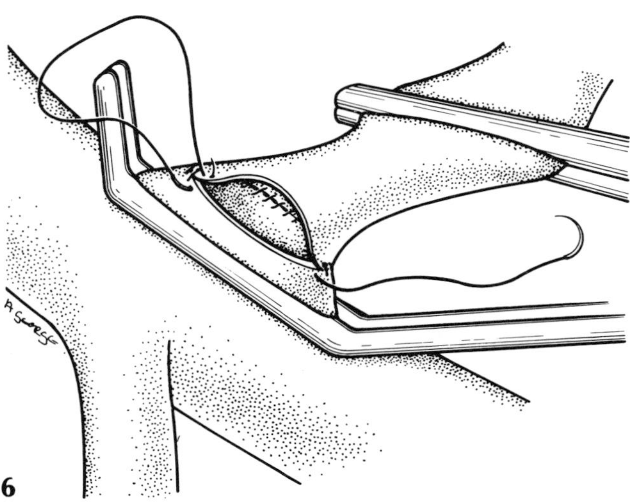
6

6

A double-ended 4/0 polypropylene suture is used for the anastomosis. The suture is passed through the lower margin of the opening in the portal vein and the lower end of the caval incision and then tied. A single running, everting suture is then inserted from within the lumen of the two channels, since the back of the anastomosis is otherwise inaccessible. The illustration shows the posterior run completed and the beginning of the front run, which of course is constructed from the outside. Care must be taken not to pick up the earlier row of stitches since the stoma is rather flattened at this stage. The suture can either be continued as far as the initial knot and tied there as shown, or the unused needle can complete the anastomosis.

When the anastomosis is finished the Satinsky clamp on the vena cava is opened and, provided there is no leakage, it is withdrawn. Should any leak occur, the clamp is reapplied and additional interrupted sutures placed. Finally, the portal vein clamp is removed and the shunt should be seen to be open.

7

The shunt should be wide and there must be no suspicion of kinking, twisting or angulation of the portal vein. This is largely a matter of choosing the right site on the vena cava. Occasionally, a small wedge of pancreatic tissue or part of the caudate process of the liver must be excised to allow proper positioning, and this may require division of inferior hepatic veins (*see Illustration 2*).

The incision is closed in the usual way. An underwater seal pleural drain should be used for the thoracotomy, but the abdomen should not be drained as this may lead to serious protein loss if ascites develops during the postoperative period. Ascites can also be avoided by reduction of sodium intake in the intravenous fluid to a minimum.

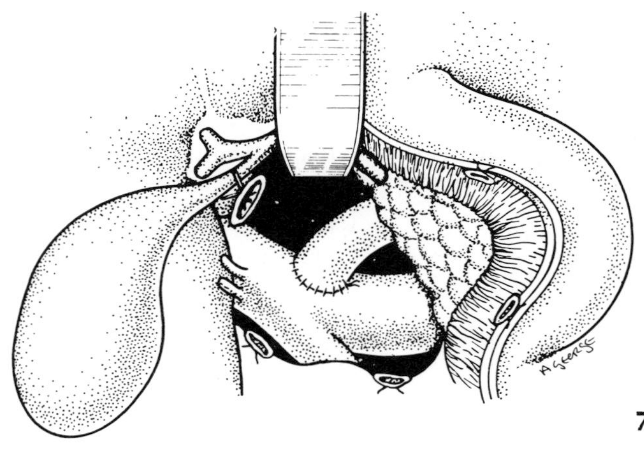

7

8

Side-to-side portacaval shunt

This shunt is seldom appropriate. The essential steps are similar to those in end-to-side anastomosis. It is often necessary to resect some of the caudate lobe of the liver and it is not always possible to approximate the two veins to allow a tension-free shunt. In such cases, the procedure is abandoned or an interposition graft of jugular vein or Dacron is used.

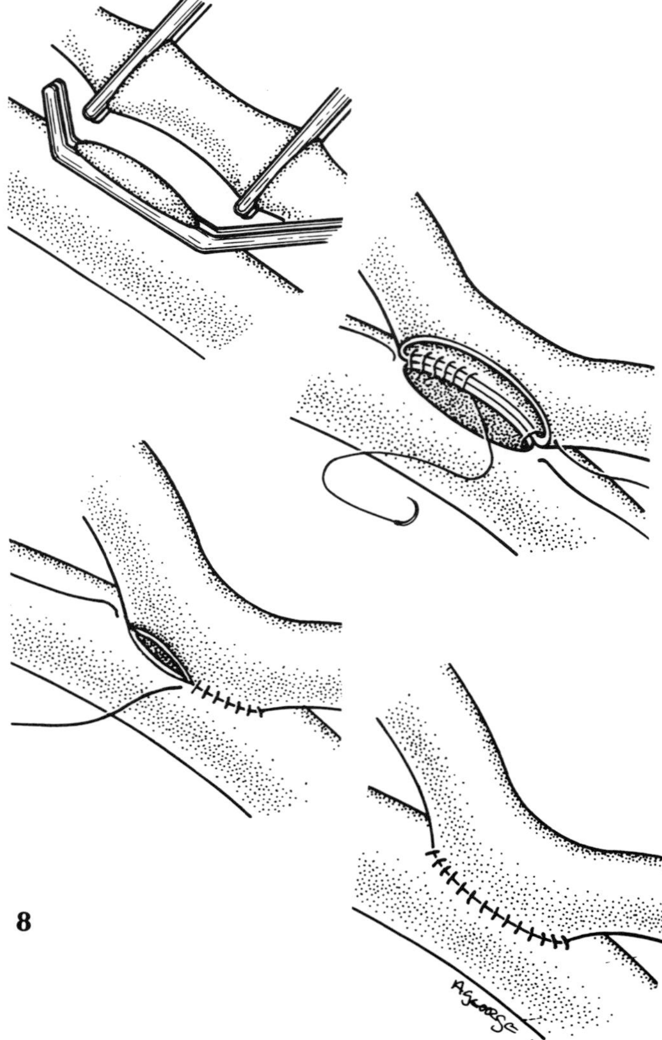

8

Splenorenal shunts

Selective distal splenorenal (Warren) shunt

9

The right gastric (coronary), left gastric, right gastroepiploic and splenic veins are ligated. The intention is to allow hepatic perfusion from the superior and inferior mesenteric veins, while diverting the flow from the gastro-oesophageal varices through the shunt. However, the fall in portal pressure produced by the shunt, combined with the increase in hepatic resistance due to the liver disease, produces a pressure gradient between the portal vein and the rest of the portal bed. The result is a gradual resumption of collateral flow towards the shunt, as shown by portal venography at various times after selective shunting (Rikkers *et al.*, 1978). In spite of obvious theoretical advantages and a low incidence of early PSE, selective portal shunting requires long-term evaluation before it can be recommended.

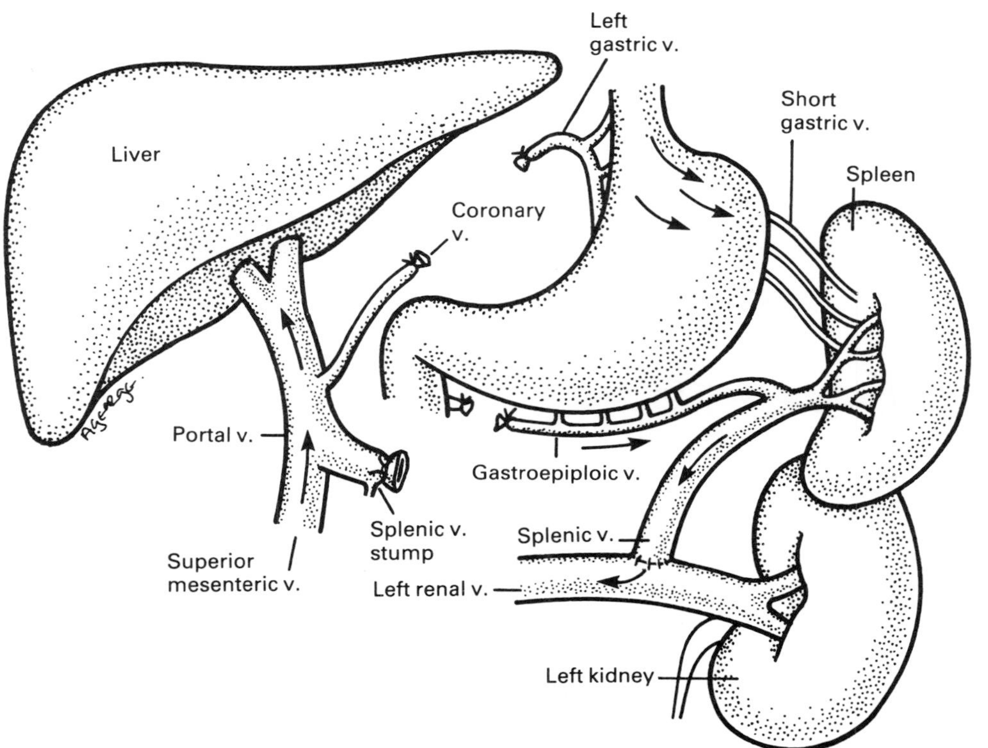

9

10

Before the operation it is important to have angiographic evidence of patency of the splenic vein. For the procedure, the patient lies prone and a midline upper abdominal incision is used.

The splenic vein can be exposed above or below the transverse mesocolon. The author prefers to retract the transverse colon upwards. The posterior parietal peritoneum is then opened along the lower border of the pancreas. Three or four 3/0 silk sutures are placed at intervals along the lower border of the pancreas and tied to provide slings to hold it forward.

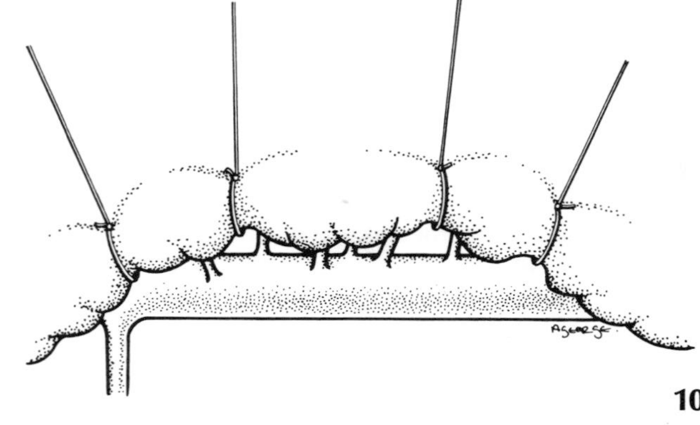

10

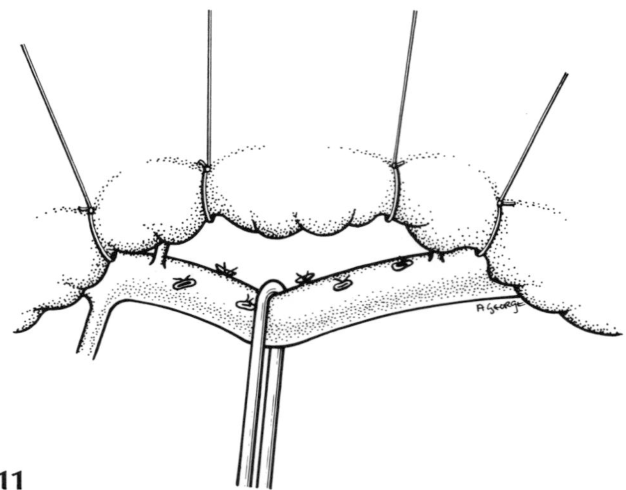

11

11

The splenic vein is identified and gradually mobilized, which necessitates the division of many small veins joining it from the pancreas. This is tedious and difficult, as they must be tied with 3/0 silk before division and they are easily torn.

12

When several centimetres of splenic vein have been freed, the vein is ligated and after applying a covered bulldog clamp, divided well to the right, close to the junction of the inferior mesenteric vein. The latter vein is a useful guide to the splenic vein if it proves difficult to find.

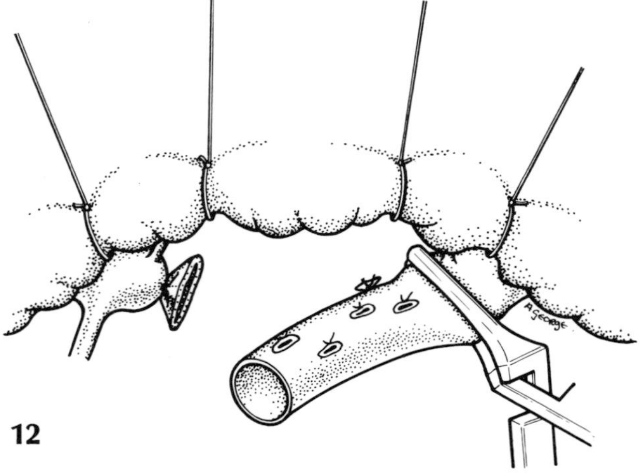

12

13

The left renal vein is identified in the retroperitoneal tissues and it may be necessary to divide a large adrenal vein. If the renal vein is difficult to find, the kidney can be felt and the hilum identified. The renal vein usually needs two straight vascular clamps. This has never caused detectable effects upon the kidney, presumably because of adequacy of collateral veins in the renal hilum.

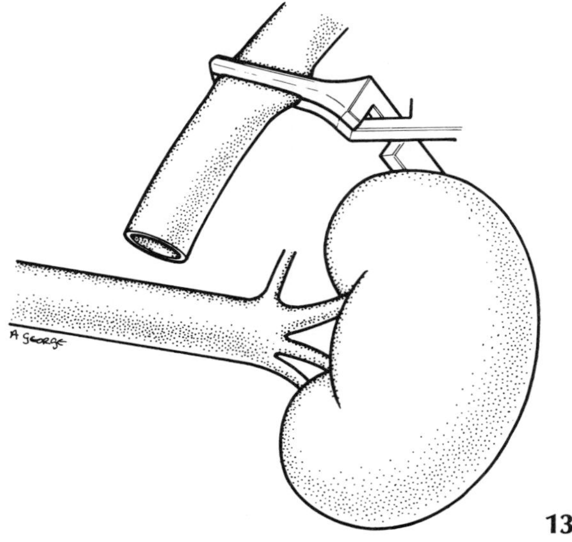

13

14

14

An ellipse of renal vein is removed at an appropriate site on its upper border and an end-to-side anastomosis constructed using a double-needle 5/0 polypropylene suture. Occasionally, positioning demands that the renal vein must be tied and the left end turned up and anastomosed to the side of the splenic vein. Ligation of the renal vein seems to cause no harm in such cases.

15

Central splenorenal shunt

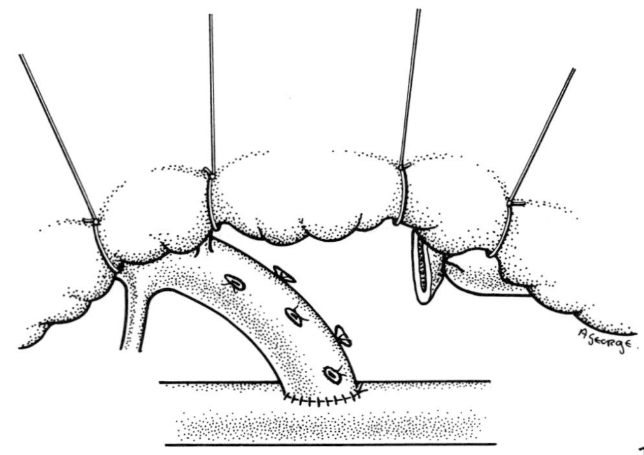

15

This is a non-selective shunt, suitable when the portal vein is not available. The infrapancreatic site is more accessible than that used in the older approach which entailed splenectomy, followed by mobilization of the much smaller and branching distal part of the splenic vein.

Isolation of the splenic vein is performed as in the selective operation, but the vein is ligated towards the left and the central (right) end of the vein is used for the anastomosis, as shown. The right and left gastric and gastroepiploic veins are not ligated.

This shunt probably has a lower incidence of PSE than portacaval anastomosis, but the advantage is offset by less complete portal decompression and a tendency to shunt thrombosis leading to variceal bleeding. These disadvantages also apply to the mesocaval shunt, which for this reason is not described here.

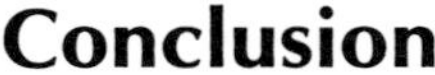

Conclusion

The complications of these procedures can be severe. Portal-systemic encephalopathy is a great concern and the problem of bleeding during surgery has been stressed. The mortality rate of these procedures has to be weighed against the natural history of the condition without surgery. Shunting is not justified as a prophylactic procedure and should only be undertaken for recent or continuing significant variceal haemorrhage.

References

Birnstingl, M. (1980). Surgical treatment of emergencies. In: *Medical and Surgical Problems of Portal Hypertension.* Orloff, M. J., Stipa, S. and Ziparo, V., eds. London and San Diego: Academic Press.

Child, C. G. (1954). *The Hepatic Circulation and Portal Hypertension.* London and San Diego: W.B. Saunders.

Orloff, M. J., Charters, A. C., Condon, J. K. *et al.* (1974). Emergency portocaval shunt for bleeding oesophageal varices. *Archives of Surgery* **108**, 293.

Rikkers, L.F., Rudman, D., Warren, W. D. *et al.* (1978). A randomized controlled trial of the distal splenorenal shunt. *Annals of Surgery* **188**, 271.

Warren, W. D., Zeppa, R. and Fomon, J. J. (1967). Selective trans-splenic decompression of gastro-oesophageal varices by distal splenorenal shunt. *Annals of Surgery* **166**, 437.

The endoscopic management of gastro-oesophageal varices

S. G. J. WILLIAMS MA, MRCP, *Research Registrar*
D. WESTABY MA, FRCP, *Consultant Physician*
N. A. THEODOROU MS, FRCS, *Consultant Surgeon*
Gastrointestinal Unit, Charing Cross Hospital, London, UK

Introduction

Variceal bleeding, the most serious complication of portal hypertension, occurs in approximately 30% of patients with chronic liver disease (Cales and Pascal, 1988). The mortality is as high as 50% for the index bleed (Christensen *et al.*, 1981), and 30% for subsequent recurrent bleeds. Survival is inversely proportional to the number of blood transfusions required and directly proportional to the patients' functional hepatic reserve as expressed by the Child's classification. The rate of recurrent haemorrhage for those surviving the initial bleeding episode is as high as 100% over a 2-year period.

Emergency surgical intervention is associated with a high operative mortality (up to 56%) (Langer, Greig and Taylor, 1990) and despite a documented reduction in rebleeding has no long-term survival benefits when compared with endoscopic techniques (Cello *et al.*, 1987).

Diagnostic endoscopy and injection sclerotherapy is the establishment treatment of choice in the initial management of these very ill patients (Terblanche, Burroughs and Hobbs, 1989). Recently developed techniques and new injectates have increased the endoscopist's options for instituting therapy at the time of the initial endoscopy.

Prophylactic treatment of varices confers no benefit with respect to bleeding or survival and is not recommended (Kleber, Ansari and Sauerbruch, 1992).

Aims of treatment

1. To resuscitate the patient with adequate appropriate fluid replacement and support of vital organ function whilst protecting the airway, particularly in the encephalopathic patient.
2. To perform an emergency endoscopy to confirm the source of bleeding and initiate appropriate treatment to arrest haemorrhage.
3. To enter patients into a long-term programme of elective endoscopic therapy to prevent recurrent haemorrhage and achieve variceal obliteration.

Pre-endoscopic management

1. The mainstay of management is early therapeutic endoscopy within 4 hours of suspected variceal haemorrhage. This allows early control of bleeding.
2. Adequate venous access should be established with large-bore peripheral cannulae, and a central venous line. In patients with ascites, the elderly, and those with associated medical conditions a Swan-Ganz catheter should be inserted for accurate monitoring of fluid replacement. Avoiding hypovolaemia will help protect renal and hepatic function. A urinary catheter should be passed.
3. Fluid replacement should be with colloid or cross-matched whole blood. Crystalloid in the form of saline should be avoided due to impaired renal sodium handling and the development of ascites in patients with chronic liver disease. Vitamin K 10–20 mg should be given intravenously. Fresh frozen plasma should be used if the prothrombin or partial thromboplastin times are more than 50% prolonged, and platelets should be transfused if the platelet count falls below $50 \times 10^9/1$.

When adequately resuscitated the patient should be taken to the endoscopy unit/theatre to undergo diagnostic/therapeutic endoscopy.

5. Endotracheal intubation of the patient, particularly if encephalopathic, should be considered in order to protect the airway from aspiration.

Anaesthesia

1. In the co-operative patient the endoscopy is preferably performed under light intravenous sedation with a benzodiazepine. Very occasionally a general anaesthetic may need to be considered.

2. Supplemental nasal oxygen is used throughout the procedure. The patient is monitored with a pulse oximeter and continuous ECG and blood pressure recording are used.

The procedure

A full diagnostic oesophagogastroduodenoscopy (OGD) should be performed in all patients suspected of variceal haemorrhage to establish the precise source of bleeding.

1

The endoscopy is performed with a forward-oblique or end-viewing endoscope. The oblique viewing endoscope has the advantage that the injection needle can be elevated towards the varix by a bridge which facilitates more accurate and rapid needle placement. However, the oblique viewing endoscope cannot be used for the technique of banding ligation (see below).

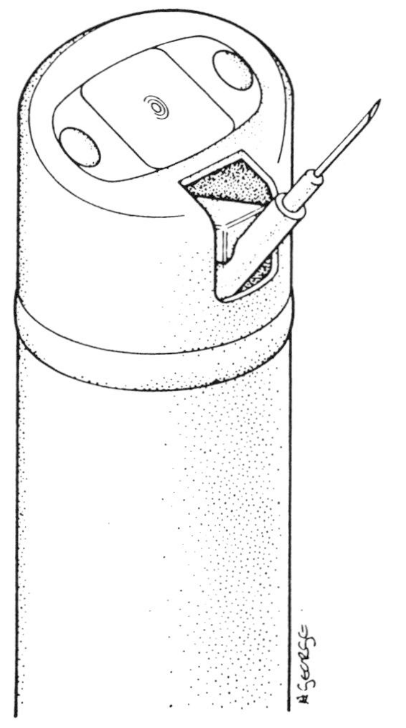

1

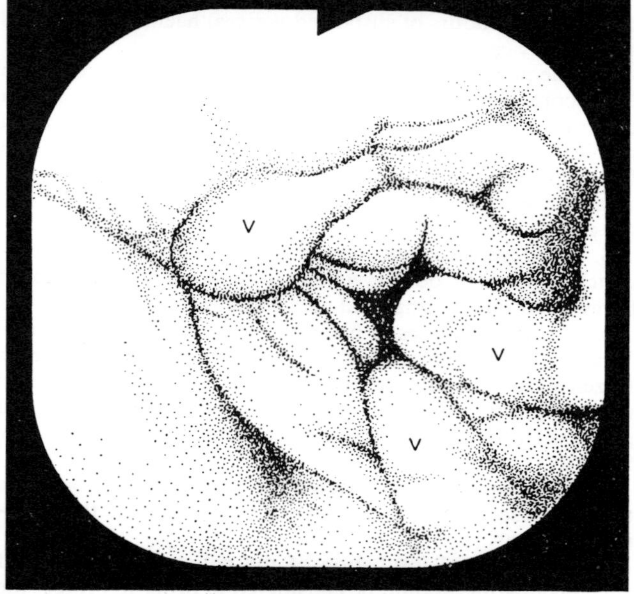

2

2

In the emergency situation it is important that varices are confirmed to be the source of haemorrhage. The prominent tortuous variceal columns (V) are seen to extend proximally from the cardio-oesophageal junction. The extent of the variceal columns should be accurately documented for later assessment of the efficacy of treatment.

3

The varices (V) are followed to the squamo-columnar junction or 'Z' line. Actively bleeding oesophageal varices should be treated with injection sclerotherapy. Injection should begin close to the cardio-oesophageal junction to obliterate the intrinsic vessels at this point, proceeding proximally for at least 3–5 cm to ensure the obliteration of the perforating vessels.

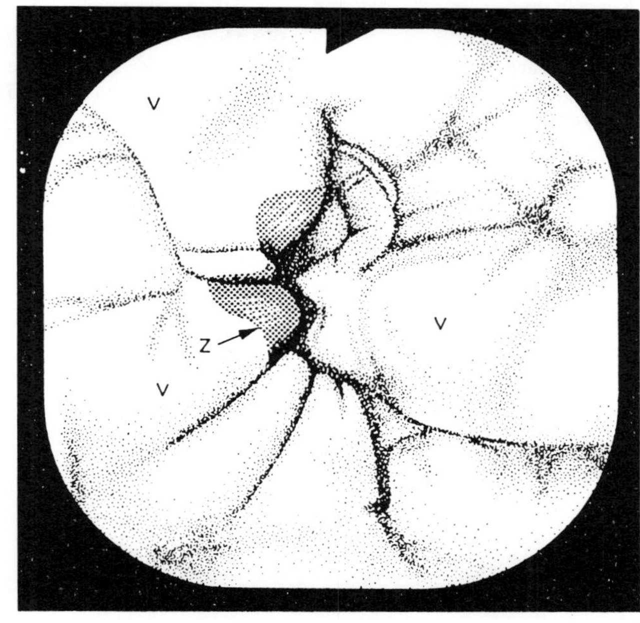

3

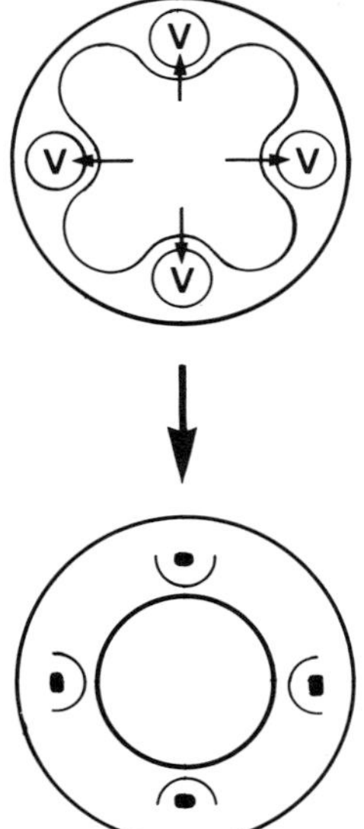

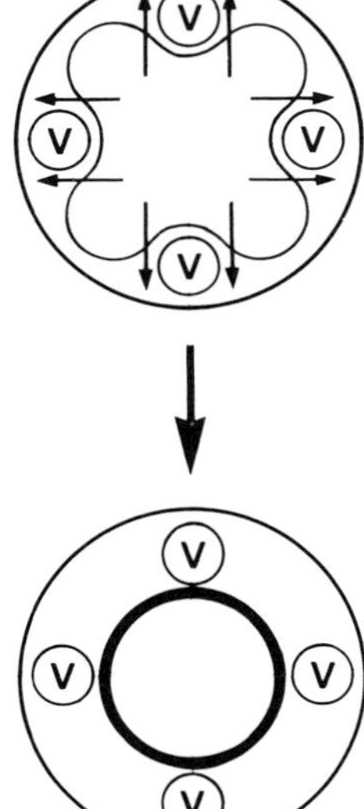

4

4

In the UK and USA intravariceal injection, with the aim of luminal obliteration is favoured. In Austria and Germany the paravariceal approach, with the intention of initiating local fibrogenesis and creating a protective covering over the intact varix (V), is favoured. Both techniques, in experienced hands, achieve similar results.

5

In intravariceal injection 5% ethanolamine should be injected, using a disposable Teflon sheathed needle (N), into each variceal column (V) in 0.5–1 ml aliquots.

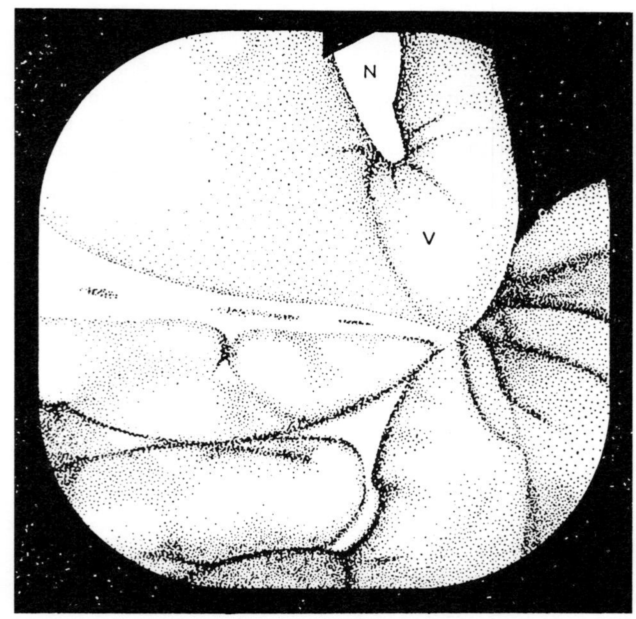

5

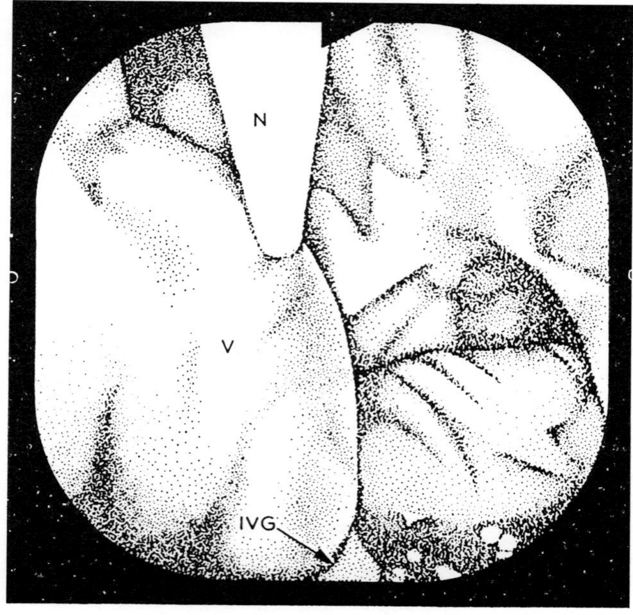

6

6

Successful intravariceal injection is recognized by a gentle distension of the varix (V), without the formation of a submucosal blister or obliteration of the intervariceal groove (IVG). Up to 5 ml of sclerosant per varix can be used but there is a trend towards using smaller volumes resulting in fewer complications.

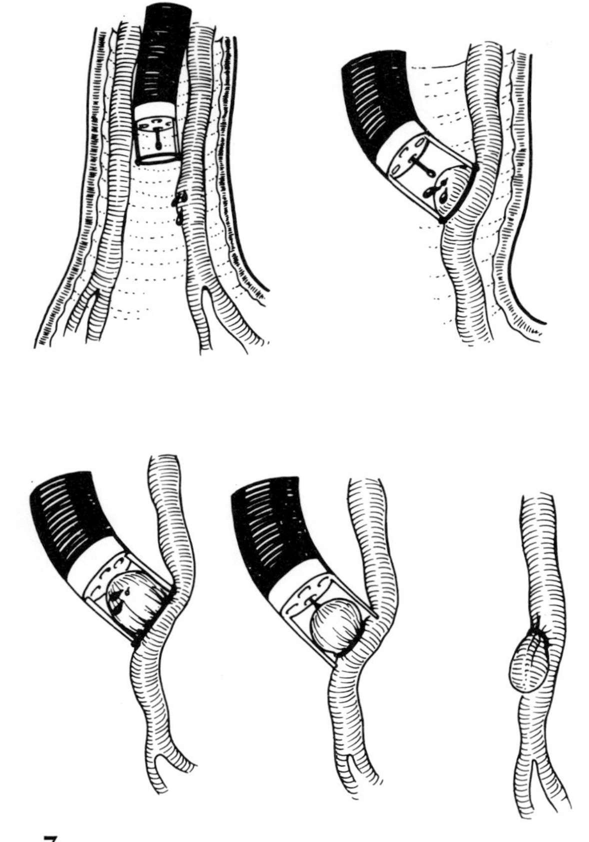

7

7

Oesophageal varices, which are clearly the source of haemorrhage, but which have stopped bleeding spontaneously are best treated using endoscopic banding ligation (EBL).

This technique is a modification of that used for band ligation of internal haemorrhoids. A cylindrical device is attached to the end of a forward viewing endoscope. A second cylinder with a pre-stressed rubber band attached is inserted into the first cylinder and held in place by a trip wire running through the biopsy channel of the endoscope. The endoscope, with banding device attached, is passed through an oesophageal overtube positioned at the time of the initial endoscopy. The banding device is apposed to a variceal column, suction applied through the suction channel of the endoscope and the band rolled onto the entrapped varix by retraction of the trip wire. The entrapped varix will slough off within 5–7 days leaving a small discrete ulcer.

Bands are applied from the distal oesophagus proximally for approximately 5 cm until all the variceal columns have received at least one application. A median of 6–8 bands are applied at the first session.

EBL is a highly effective technique which needs fewer sessions to achieve variceal obliteration and has been associated with fewer complications. Its use in the acute setting is limited by the reduced views that the banding device allows which, in the presence of blood within the oesophageal lumen, increases the technical difficulties of the therapeutic endoscopy.

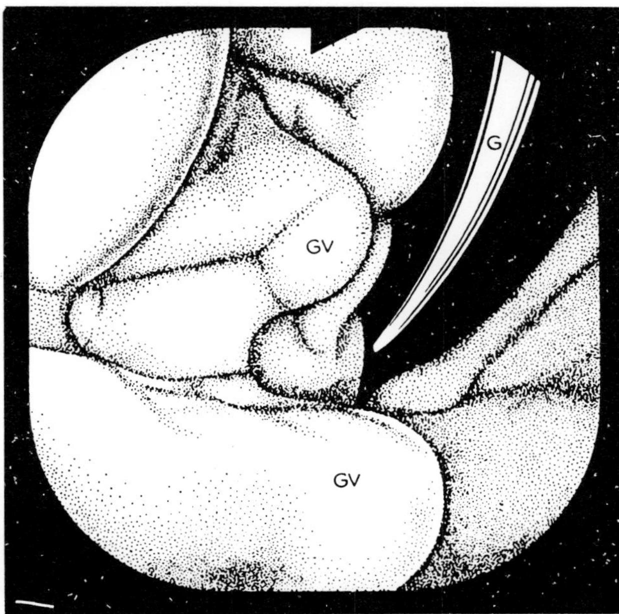

8

8

As part of the diagnostic endoscopy the gastroscope (G) is retroflexed within the stomach (the 'J' manoeuvre) to determine the presence of gastric varices (GV). Gastric varices account for 10–25% of all episodes of variceal bleeding. If views of the gastric fundus are obscured by the pooling of blood repositioning the patient usually allows adequate visualization.

The three endoscopic options for the management of gastric varices are:

(i) Conventional sclerosants. Injection of small volumes of 5% ethanolamine for the treatment of bleeding lesser curve varices or those within a hiatus hernia. However, the use of conventional sclerosants in fundal/cardiac varices has a high complication rate and poor efficacy.

(ii) The tissue adhesives histoacryl and bucrylate may be injected through a standard sclerotherapy needle following preliminary injection with 1 ml of distilled water to ensure that the needle is placed intravariceally. 0.5–1.0 ml of the tissue glue is rapidly instilled. The needle is withdrawn from the varix, rinsed with distilled water and retracted into the Teflon sheath. The injector must not be drawn back into the endoscope for 20 seconds to ensure that the injector is not cemented into the working channel of the endoscope. Two to three injections may be required for a large polypoid fundal varix.

(iii) Bovine thrombin, reconstituted to 1000 u/ml and injected in 1 ml aliquots into the varix, has been used for the eradication of gastric varices.

Postendoscopic management

1. The patient must be managed in a high dependency or intensive care unit.

2. The patient's haemodynamic status is carefully monitored for continued bleeding and to ensure adequate volume replacement.

3. In the alcoholic patient alcohol withdrawal should be anticipated and managed appropriately with chlormethiazole or benzodiazepines. Vitamin B complex, thiamine and folate should be administered.

4. Patients who are encephalopathic should receive titrated doses of lactulose orally. Sucralfate (preferably as a gel or suspension) should be administered prophylactically to reduce the risk of mucosal damage at the site of endoscopic therapy. Omeprazole should be given to those in whom extensive mucosal damage is observed.

5. Treatment of ascites should be deferred until the patient is haemodynamically stable. Massive ascites causing respiratory embarrassment may occasionally require small volume paracentesis.

6. The patient is entered into a programme of endoscopic therapy to achieve variceal obliteration. Early obliteration of varices with banding ligation (three to four sessions) supports this as the long-term treatment of choice.

It is more difficult to recognize the obliteration of gastric varices as they remain visible even after thrombosis. Patency of the varix can be assessed using the injector needle. The use of tissue adhesives is usually considered a single therapy treatment, while bovine thrombin injection can safely be repeated.

References

Cales, P. and Pascal, J. P. (1988). Histoire naturelle des varices oesophagiennes au cours de la cirrhose (de la naissance a la rupture). *Gastroenterologie Clinique et Biologique* **12**, 245.

Cello, J. P., Grendell, J. H., Crass, R. A. *et al.* (1987). Endoscopic sclerotherapy versus portacaval shunt in patients with severe cirrhosis and acute variceal haemorrhage. Long-term follow up. *New England Journal of Medicine* **316**, 11.

Christensen, E., Fauerholdt, L., Schlichting, P. *et al.* (1981). Aspects of the natural history of gastrointestinal bleeding in cirrhosis and the effect of prednisolone. *Gastroenterology* **81**, 944.

Kleber, G., Ansari, H. and Sauerbruch, T. (1992). Prophylaxis of first variceal bleeding. *Baillères Clinical Gastroenterology* **6**, 563.

Langer, B., Greig, P. D. and Taylor, B. R. (1990). Emergency surgical treatment of variceal haemorrhage in management of variceal haemorrhage. *Surgical Clinics of North America* **70**, 307.

Terblanche, J., Burroughs, A. K. and Hobbs, K. E. F. (1989). Controversies in the management of bleeding oesophageal varices. *New England Journal of Medicine* **320**, 1393.

Surgical techniques in the treatment of varicose veins

SIDNEY S. ROSE MB, ChB, FRCS

Consulting Surgeon, University Hospital of South Manchester, Withington Hospital, Manchester, UK

Introduction

The surgical treatment of varicose veins has in the past even in experienced hands, produced notoriously bad results. This is due to a number of factors among the commonest of which is the inexperience of the surgeon and the natural prevalence of recurrence. It is felt that it is also attributable in part to the unquestioning acceptance of the hitherto established aetiological concept of primary valvular incompetence and the influence this has on surgical technique. In particular this has led to concentration of operative techniques on proximal ligation of main stem superficial veins and/or ligation of incompetent deep perforators. It is obvious that proximal ligation is necessary in the case of irreversible incompetence at the confluence of the main deep and superficial veins but the necessity for ligation of the deep perforator has been called into question. Full-length stripping has had its advocates and been found wanting because of failure to remove varicose bunches. Routine stripping often removes a saphenous vein which is largely normal and deprives the patient of a possible future bypass conduit.

Our concept of the aetiology based on a series of examinations of the vein wall by transmission electron microscopy is somewhat different and has led us to adopt our present techniques. We believe that the primary lesion is in the muscle cell of the vein wall where a degenerative fibrosis develops, producing first of all loss of tone and then dilatation not only of the vein wall in between the valves but of the valve ring itself. Dilatation at this point leads to secondary valvular incompetence because the valve cusps can no longer meet and eventually undergo disuse atrophy. This applies to both the superficial veins and the deep perforators. The surgical treatment is therefore based on removal of the varicose veins themselves combined if necessary with proximal ligation at the main saphenofemoral or saphenopopliteal junction if incompetence exists at these points. We maintain that meticulous removal of the superficial varices renders it unnecessary to ligate deep perforators as most of the connections to the superficial veins will be interrupted by this procedure, and the veins into which they feed will be eliminated surgically.

The modern technique has been variously described in the centres where it has been developed *viz* 'winkling', multiple excision, ligation-excision, but has now become known for convenience as stab-avulsion although micro-incision would be more descriptive in many circumstances.

Preoperative

Indications for surgery

Relief of symptoms

Varicose veins are often asymptomatic but the sensation of heaviness of the legs and chronic aching in the calves may be so severe as to require treatment. The other symptoms which cause patients to seek advice are night cramps, 'restless' legs, localized pain and tenderness over localized blow-outs, even in the absence of phlebitis. Itching and irritation of the overlying skin may occur. Any of these symptoms may be severe enough to require treatment by surgery.

To treat complications

The common complications of varicose veins are haematoma, possible even after slight trauma, haemorrhage which may be spontaneous or traumatic, eczema which may be local or generalized, recurrent superficial phlebitis, the development of subcutaneous and intradermal induration and varicose ulceration. Deep venous thrombosis may occur although the relationship to varicose veins is not as clear-cut as might be expected. Pulmonary embolism has also been recorded although this may be considered to be related to a subclinical deep venous thrombosis. A history of any of the above complications is an indication for surgery, although an interval of 3 months should be allowed after an attack of superficial thrombophlebitis before surgery is undertaken.

Cosmetic considerations

There is no doubt that varicose veins can be extremely ugly, both from a subjective and objective point of view. The development of a cosmetic procedure which also provides efficient and long-lasting relief justifies operating for cosmetic reasons. It must be noted here that a purely cosmetic complaint has difficulty in finding a place on a hospital waiting list and some health insurance companies specifically exclude such complaints from benefit.

Contraindications

1. Age and general condition. General condition is more important than age in this respect but it is obviously unwise and unnecessary to carry out operative procedures requiring long anaesthetics in the aged. Removal of symptomatic bunches under local anaesthetic may be carried out in the elderly if otherwise quite fit.
2. Obesity. This increases the hazards of any surgical procedure, and may produce special difficulties in removing varicose veins. This should be corrected if feasible before proceeding.
3. Active superficial thrombophlebitis. This must always be controlled before embarking upon surgery for varicose veins.
4. Subcutaneous induration (lipodermatosclerosis). It is often impossible to remove veins from these areas. The local condition may be improved by support (firm bandaging or pressure-graded elastic stockings), elevation of the legs at night, calf muscle and ankle exercises, and stanozolol in acute cases. The feeding veins may then be dealt with by ligation, sclerotherapy, or a combination of the two.
5. Infected ulceration. The presence of an ulcer alone is not a contraindication to surgery provided it is clean, but infection must be treated first.
6. Pregnancy. It is inadvisable to operate during pregnancy and in any event many of the veins regress within 3 months of parturition.
7. Arterial insufficiency. Peripheral pulses must always be recorded and the state of the peripheral circulation must be identified in patients at risk.
8. The presence of a large intra-abdominal tumour which may be the cause of venous back pressure and will require primary treatment.

Both the latter conditions will have been excluded by the preliminary examination.

Preoperative preparation

A pubic shave is only necessary where the groin is to be explored. The leg must be shaved, especially in men, and the patients are instructed to do this themselves before admission.

The veins are marked with the patient standing using a black or blue fine-point felt pen, the sites of maximum discomfort being marked with a circle, so that special attention may be given to the underlying vein. If the veins are extensive in one leg, both legs are not operated on unless the contralateral limb is only slightly involved. This is because an extensive procedure on both sides will hinder the postoperative walking ability, necessary to minimize phlebitis, and will involve an unjustifiably long anaesthetic.

Anatomy

1

Normal distribution of main superficial veins of the lower limb with common sites of deep perforators (after *Gray's Anatomy*). A similar chart is used to record the distribution of the varicosities at the first examination.

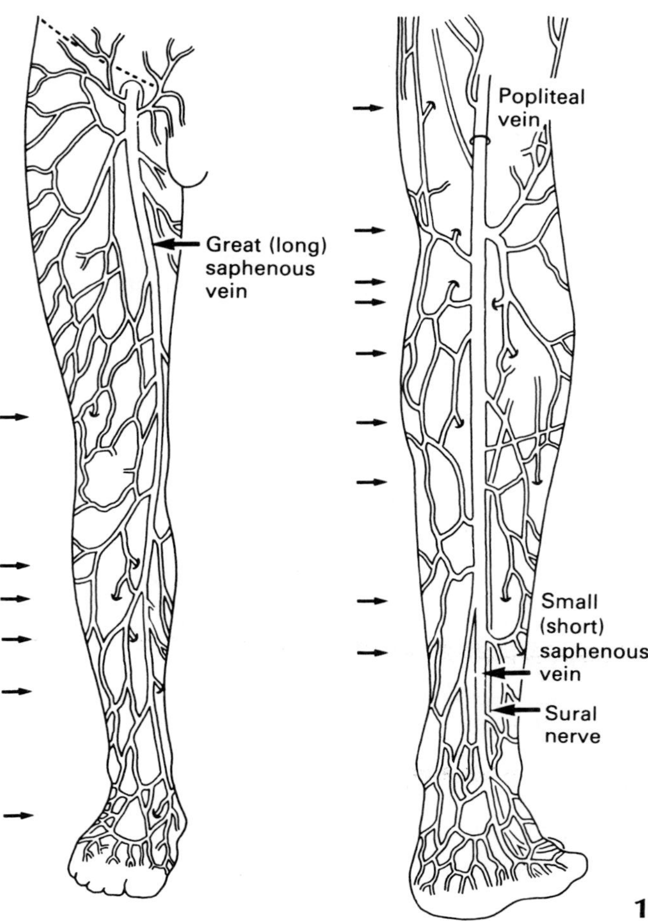

2

Normal anatomy of the saphenofemoral junction (after *Gray's Anatomy*). The position of the inguinal ligament is shown dotted, but this is not synonymous with the groin crease. This is usually lower than the inguinal ligament, the distance increasing with obesity.

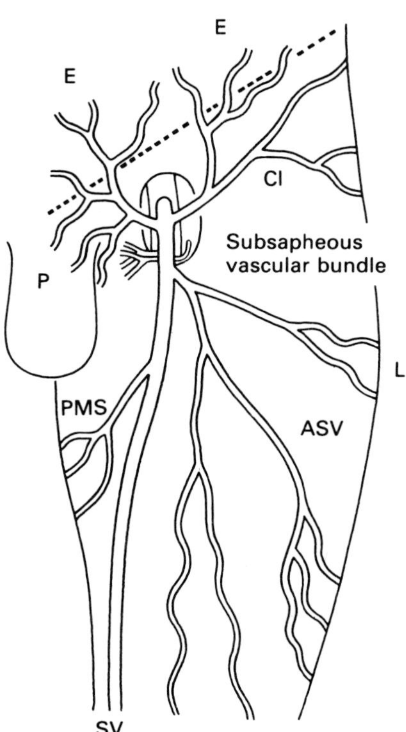

2

SV = long saphenous vein; ASV = anterior saphenous veins; PMS = posterior medial saphenous veins; P = superficial internal pudendal veins; E = superficial epigastric veins; CI = superficial circumflex iliac veins; L = lateral saphenous veins

The operation

Position of patient

The patient is positioned on the table with a sandbag under the contralateral buttock to rotate the affected limb outwards to improve access to the groin, and this is further improved by having the knee moderately flexed.

Most aspects of the limb can be reached by judicious rotation but exploration of the saphenopopliteal junction and veins at the back of the thigh must be carried out with the patient in the prone position. If this is necessary, this part of the procedure is carried out first. It must be remembered that pressure on the abdomen in the prone position causes some obstruction to the vena cava and will increase venous bleeding unless the chest and pelvis are raised off the operating table.

The groin incision

Exploration of the groin is indicated where there is a pronounced cough impulse at the groin on palpation. Reflux may be confirmed by Doppler examination. This may be confined to the immediate vicinity of the saphenofemoral junction or propagated down the leg in more advanced cases. The incision must be placed so that an adequate exposure of the saphenofemoral junction is obtained. Its position and length will be governed by the degree of obesity of the patient since the groin fold only approximates to the inguinal ligament when there is a minimum of subcutaneous fat. It will be appreciably lower in obese patients, in whom the incision needs to be above the groin crease. In any event, the incision is parallel to the inguinal ligament, using the femoral pulse as the lateral landmark, and will be on average 3.5–7 cm long.

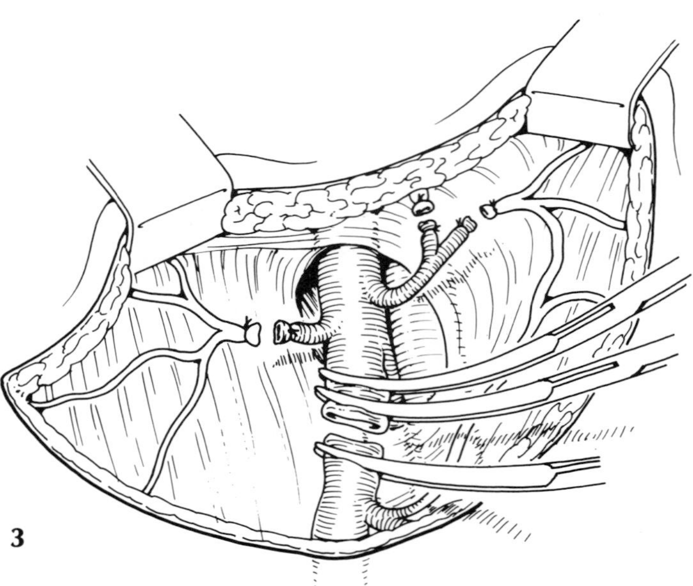

3

3

The saphenous vein and its tributaries are identified by blunt dissection, remembering that it lies much more superficially in the male. The saphenofemoral junction must be clearly visualized before the clamps are applied, since considerable anatomical variation may occur. Two clamps are applied proximally and one distally and the vein is divided between them. It is safer to leave a small proximal stump than to carry out a flush ligation, because if a clamp slips it can be picked up without difficulty. The term flush ligation should be abandoned as it can be misleading for the uninitiated. A short stump cannot be the site of significant thrombus formation. The tributaries are divided and ligated as gentle traction brings them into view.

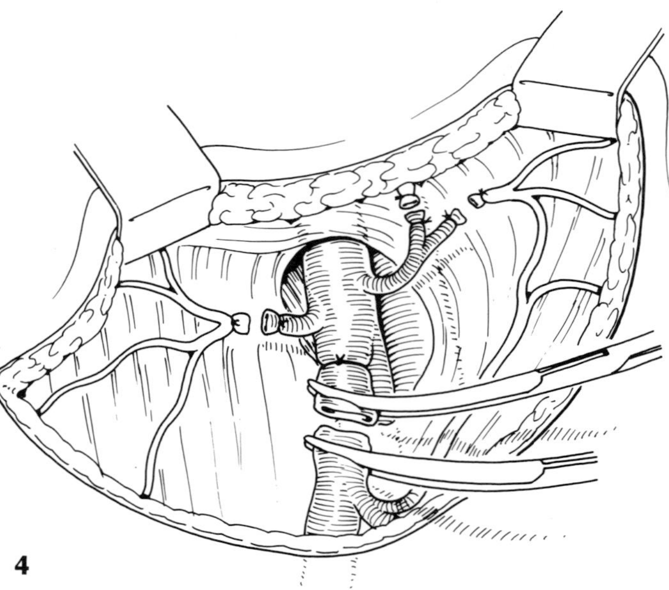

4

4

The saphenous vein is ligated with No. 1 linen thread and the most proximal clamp is removed.

A second ligature of 2/0 linen thread is placed above the second proximal clamp which is then removed.

In cases where there is no downward propagation of the cough impulse, ligation of the distal end with 2/0 linen thread completes the groin operation. The rest of the operation is then completed by multiple removal of the varicosities by the technique described below (*see Illustrations 11–16*).

Where the impulse is propagated down the leg, limited stripping of the long saphenous vein is indicated and is carried out as follows.

Limited stripping of long saphenous vein

5

The stripper is inserted into the upper cut end of the saphenous vein. Mosquito forceps are applied as shown to make this easier.

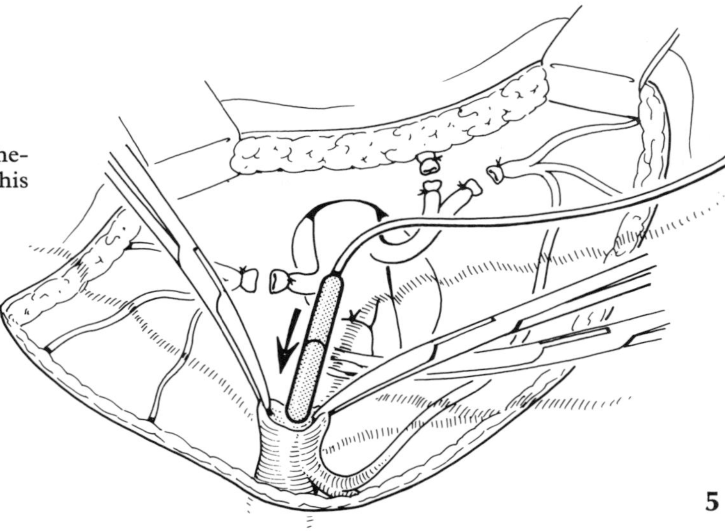

5

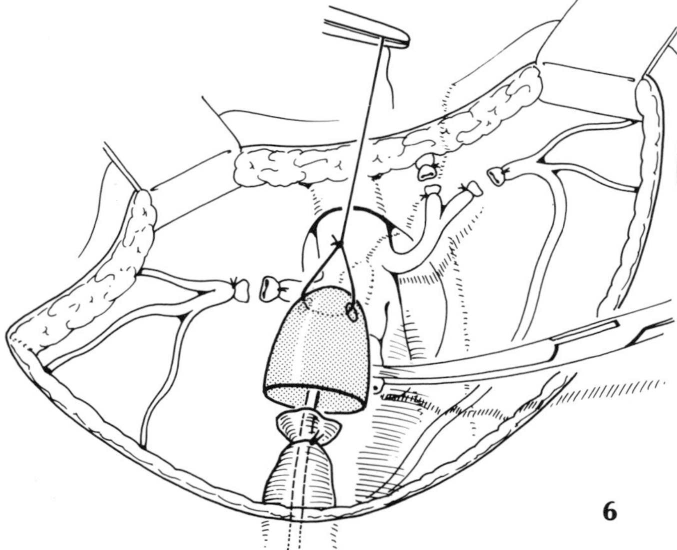

6

6

The vein is tied round the stripper head with 1/0 linen thread, leaving one end of the thread long enough to follow the stripper all the way down to the lowest point of the strip. Preferably, the acorn of the stripper is drilled as shown and the long end of the thread is tied through the hole. This prevents the stripper angling at the junction with the acorn when it is drawn upwards. The end of the thread is secured with an arterial clamp.

7

The lower end of the stripper is identified by palpation and the vein is dissected out through a small transverse incision using curved mosquito forceps. The vein is doubly clamped and the tip of the stripper is drawn out through a small incision in the vein just above the proximal clamp.

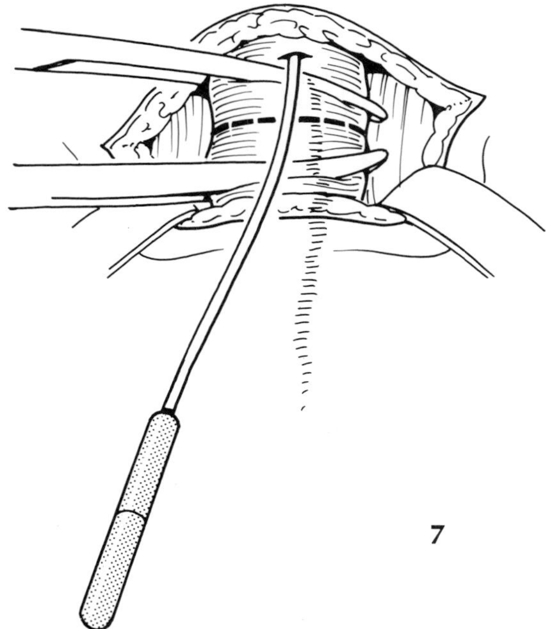

7

8 & 9

The vein is divided between the clamps and the stripper is now pulled gently downwards keeping the proximal retaining thread taut until the head of the stripper is just above the lower incision. The end of the vein is freed by traction on the retaining forceps which is now removed.

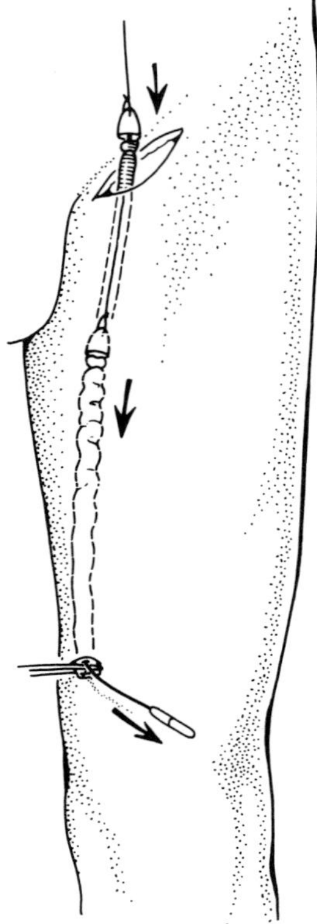

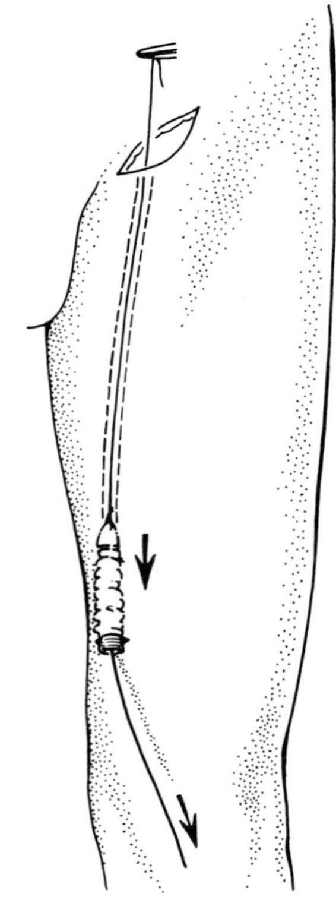

9

10

The vein is then removed by upward traction on the retaining thread so that the head of the stripper is removed through the groin incision, thus avoiding enlarging the incision at the lower end to pull the head through.

Firm pressure is applied over the whole length of the stripped channel for a few minutes to prevent haematoma formation. This part of the operation is now completed by removing the lower end of the saphenous vein by firm traction until it breaks in the manner shown in *Illustration 14*. Haemostasis is again secured by firm pressure.

This method of stripping ensures that only the incompetent saphenous vein is removed and incidentally avoids damage to the saphenous nerve at the ankle – a frequent cause of lingering postoperative discomfort.

Routine orthograde stripping has been abandoned in favour of this technique, since not only does that method endanger the saphenous nerve but it often removes long lengths of normal saphenous vein which should be preserved whenever possible.

10

Multiple excision of varicose veins

11

Multiple tiny (2–3 mm) transverse incisions are made over the previously marked veins, at such intervals that the maximum length of vein can be removed through the minimum number of incisions. The number will be dictated by the size and the fragility of the veins and by familiarity with the technique. A No. 65 Beaver blade and handle have made extremely small incisions possible. It is often possible to make a tiny stab incision which should go right through the dermis, but if there is any underlying fibrosis or previous scars or a blow out lying very close to the surface it is necessary to make a careful microincision which can be almost as small. Once all the incisions are made, the marking ink is rubbed off with spirit to avoid tatooing of the scars. The incision is opened up using sharp mosquito forceps which are then laid aside in favour of a blunter instrument which is less liable to perforate the vein.

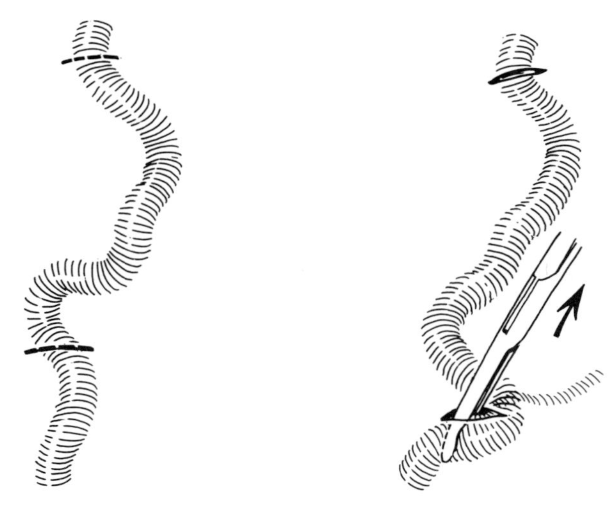

11

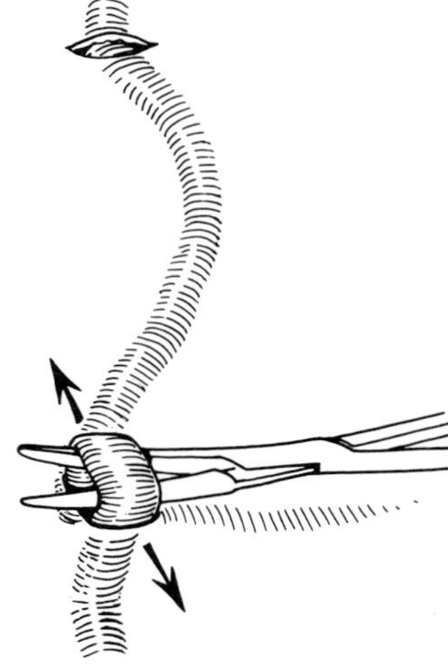

12

12

Using the blunt curved mosquito forceps, a loop of vein is drawn out through the incision.

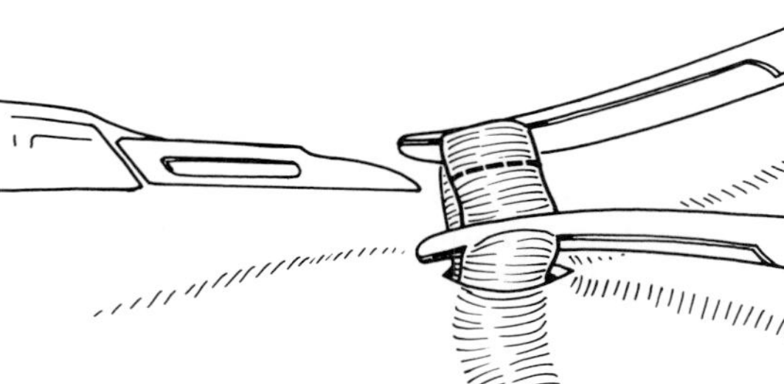

13

The vein is now divided between the forceps and each end is 'winkled out' in turn by firm but gentle traction.

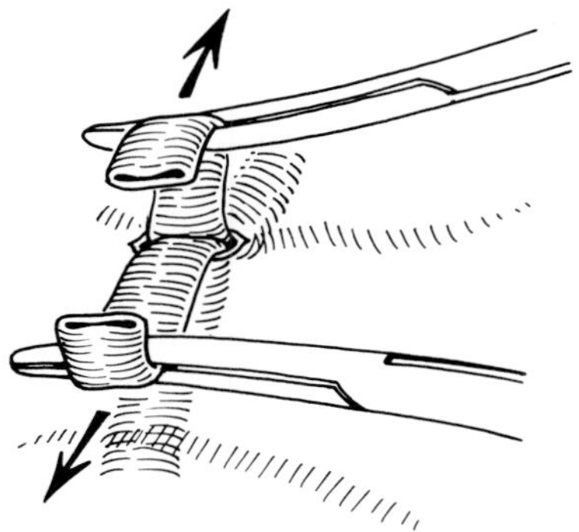

13

14

The vein is always pulled in the direction shown and never across the incision, which would otherwise become enlarged. Heavier curved forceps (Cairns) should be used to apply traction as the broader grip will prevent the vein from breaking prematurely. Sometimes a deep perforator will come into view if traction continues, and it may be grasped and broken by traction in the usual way. No ligatures are required.

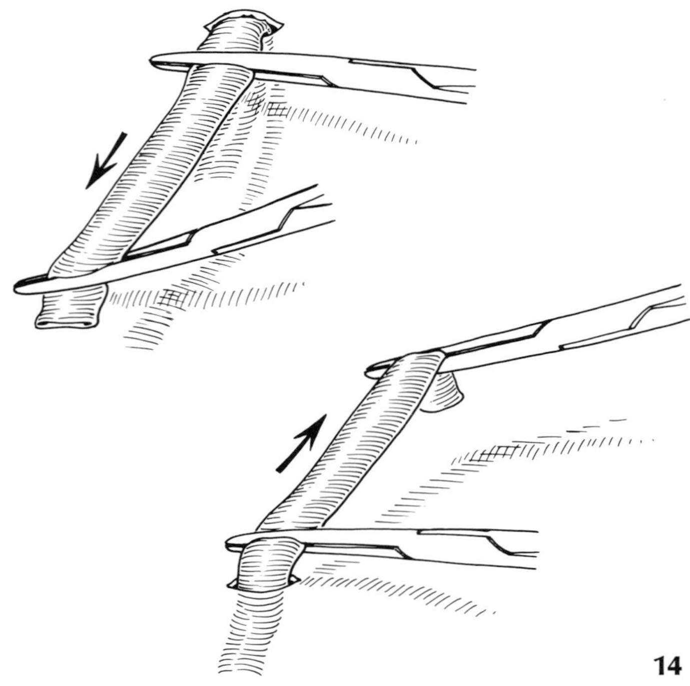

14

15

Haemostatis is secured by firm pressure over each incision as before while the next incision is being explored.

Skin sutures are not necessary and the incisions, when dry, are sealed with Steristrips, applied in the line of the incision without tension and reinforced by a plastic spray. This minimizes blister formation. A gauze roll is applied with the limb elevated.

Firm pressure is maintained by the application of Gamgee pads to include all the operated areas. The limb is firmly bandaged from foot to groin using 15-cm crêpe bandages.

In patients over 50 years of age, 1 unit of Rheomacrodex 40 is given intravenously at the end of the operation to minimize the possibility of postoperative venous thrombosis. The incidence of this complication has been cut to less than 1% since the introduction of this technique.

15

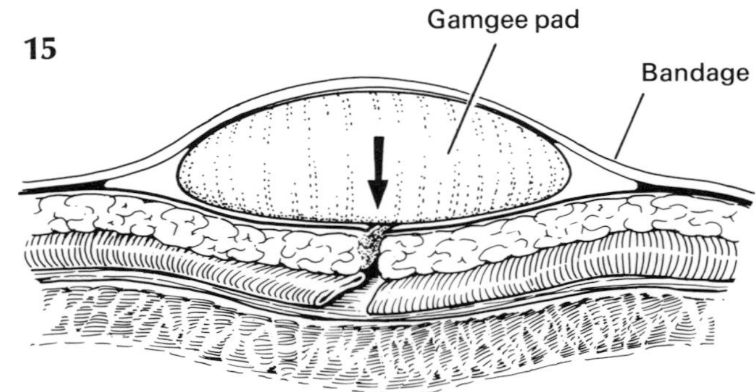

Postoperative care

The limb is elevated for 8 h postoperatively and this is followed by immediate brisk ambulation. The patient may be treated as a day case or as an outpatient but if the procedure has been extensive an overnight stay is advisable. The limb is rebandaged firmly before discharge after the Gamgee pads are removed. This encourages freer movement of the leg and allows the patient to undertake brisk walking exercise. Patients are advised to do this for 10 min at a time, at least six times a day, for the first 2 postoperative weeks. This is preferable to time-consuming walks of 5–8 km (3–5 miles) and is more likely to be adhered to.

The patient takes a bath on the 7th postoperative day and the strips are allowed to come off with each succeeding bath. A firm tubular bandage support should be worn for a further 4 weeks. Continued pressure helps to accelerate healing. A postoperative instruction sheet is given to the patient as an *aide-mémoire*. The multiple avulsion technique may be carried out under a local anaesthetic as an out-patient procedure. The average patient is able to tolerate as many as 15–20 incisions without difficulty and follows the same postoperative regime. The patient should be kept under observation for about half an hour postoperatively with the leg elevated. In the event of bleeding a firm pressure bandage is applied over the dressings. If bleeding occurs later the patient should be instructed to lie down with the limb elevated while a firm bandage is applied.

Operative treatment of varicose veins with tourniquet

JOHN P. ROYLE MB BS, BS, FRCS(Ed), FRCS, FRACS, FACS

Director of Vascular Surgery Unit, Austin Hospital, Heidelberg, Victoria, Australia;
Senior Associate, University of Melbourne, Victoria, Australia;
Consultant Vascular Surgeon, Fairfield Hospital, Melbourne, Victoria, Australia

Introduction

1a & b

The preoperative assessment of a patient with varicose veins should include Doppler evaluation of the saphenofemoral and saphenopopliteal junctions. These should not be ligated as a routine, but their ligation is required when reflux is present. Clinical examination, particularly in obese patients, often fails to reveal any abnormality at these sites, but such abnormality is revealed with ease by a Doppler (Chan, Chisholm and Royle, 1983).

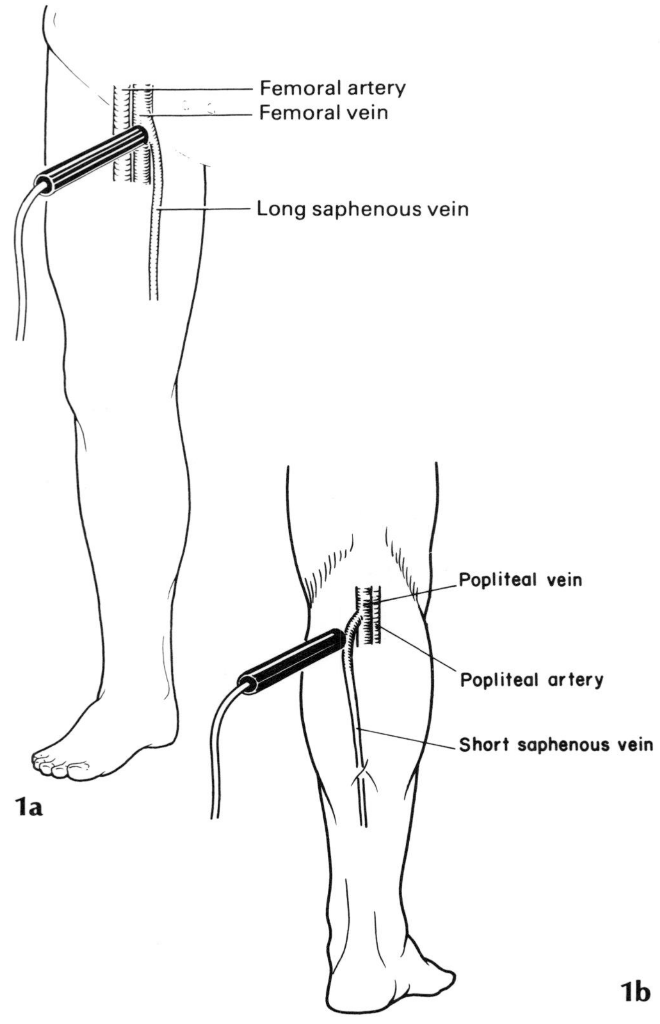

1a

1b

2a & b

Marking the veins

Very careful preoperative marking of the varices is performed with the patient in a standing position in a good light. All visible varices are marked and in particular the most superficial portions of the varices are marked clearly (these will be the sites for subsequent stab avulsion). The obvious normal veins on the dorsum of the foot are not marked for removal, but genuine varices on the dorsum of the foot are so marked.

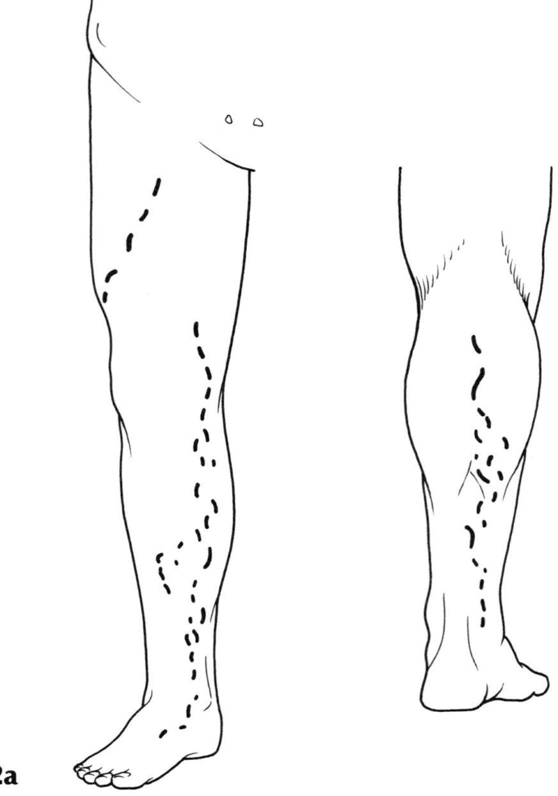

Long saphenous vein

3

Skin incision

The groin incision should be made directly over the saphenofemoral junction, i.e. *above* the groin skin crease. The incision is made in a line parallel to the skin crease centred over a point 1 cm medial to the femoral pulse and 1 cm distal to the line of the pubic tubercle. Except in obese patients, the incision does not need to exceed 4 cm. A small self-retaining retractor is inserted to spread the skin edges apart. The fat separates easily, revealing Scarpa's fascia.

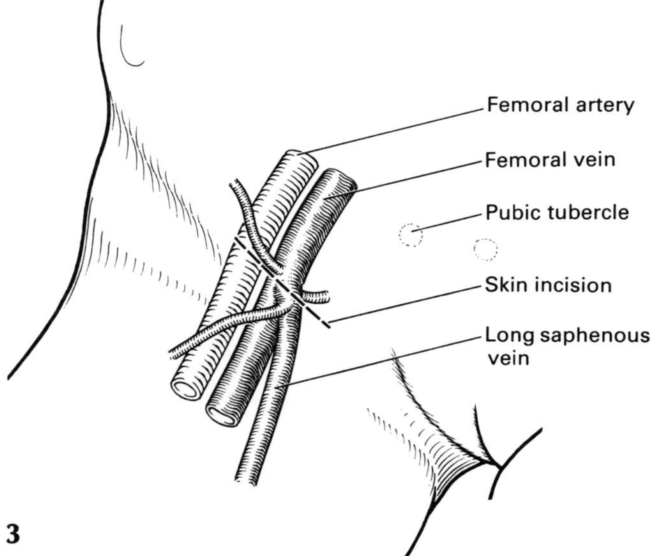

4

Scarpa's fascia

The incision is deepened through Scarpa's fascia and the self-retaining retractor is placed in a deeper plane to spread this layer. At this stage the long saphenous vein is usually visible. The vein is grasped with forceps and gently pulled outwards.

4

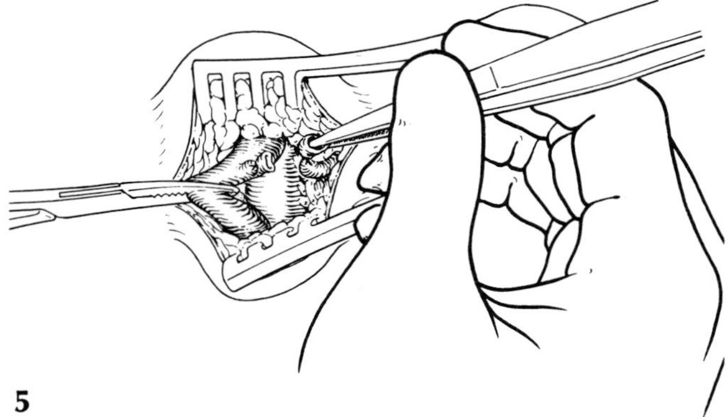

5

5

Division of tributaries

Thereafter dissection takes place in the immediate perivenous plane. The plane immediately alongside the vein is avascular and consists only of loose areolar tissue. The tributaries of the terminal portion of the long saphenous vein are all identified at the site where they drain into the long saphenous vein and pass across this loose areolar tissue. They are ligated and divided.

6

Saphenofemoral junction

The junction of the long saphenous vein with the femoral vein must be clearly identified before the saphenous vein is divided. The junction on the medial side must be carefully inspected, along with the medial aspect of the femoral vein at this point to check for the point of entry of the deep external pudendal vein. This may enter the long saphenous vein itself, the junction of the long saphenous vein and the femoral vein, or the femoral vein itself (as illustrated). It should be ligated and divided (Royle, Eisner and Fell, 1981).

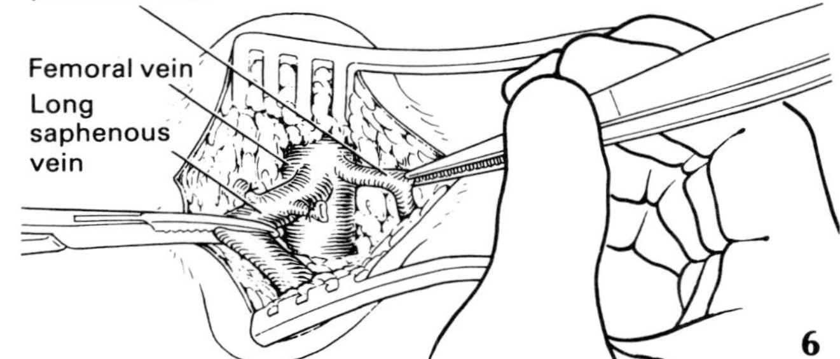

6

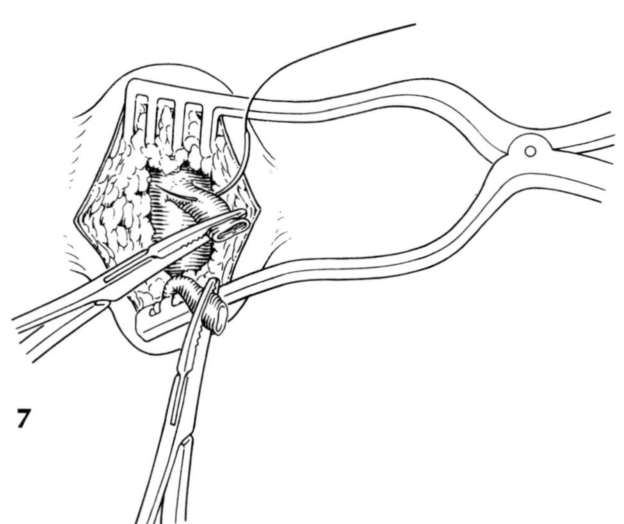

7

7

Flush ligation

The long saphenous vein is divided some 2 cm from the junction, and is then transfixed and tied. To provide a flush ligation, the needle of the transfixion suture enters the long saphenous vein one-half of the diameter of the long saphenous vein away from the saphenofemoral junction. The ligature is then tied, looped around the vein and tied again. The transfixion suture will then lie flush with the femoral vein, and constriction of the femoral vein by the suture is avoided.

8

Long saphenous vein removal

When it is intended to remove the long saphenous vein, traction is applied to its cut end, so that the vein can be identified farther down the leg. A small incision is made with a No. 11 blade over the long saphenous vein, the vein is grasped with toothed mosquito forceps and extracted through the wound. The vein is removed down the leg by similar traction, identification, stab incision and extraction (as described below).

As the long saphenous vein is pulled towards the groin, and also when a portion of the long saphenous vein is being removed through stab incisions, tributaries emerge, still attached to the long saphenous vein. These are clipped with a haemaclip before severing the tributary adjacent to the long saphenous vein. Clipping of tributaries in this manner helps to lessen thigh bruising.

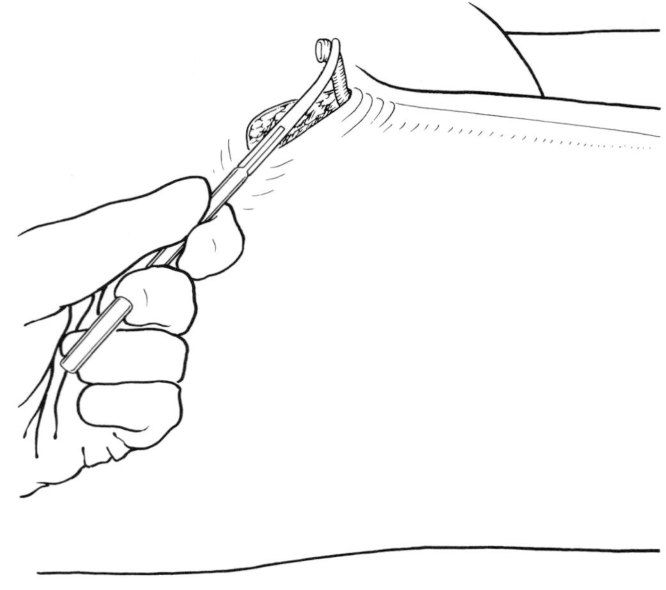

8

Groin wound closure

The orifice left by the removal of the long saphenous vein is closed over. This prevents any haematoma from passing up to the groin wound. The subcutaneous tissue in the groin is approximated with an absorbable deep suture. The skin is closed with a subcuticular absorbable suture. The wound edges are infiltrated with 0.5% Bupivacaine HCl local anaesthetic solution. There is then little discomfort in the leg for some hours (even when multiple varicose tributaries are also removed through stab incisions as in *Illustrations 9–16*).

9

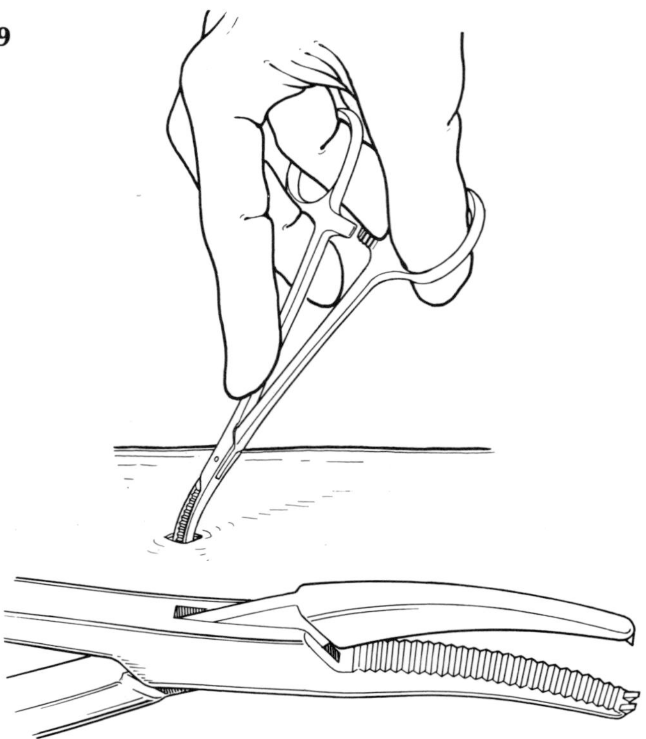

Varicose tributaries

Thigh veins are approached in the following manner.

9

A small stab incision 3 mm long is made directly over the vein in the long axis of the limb and passing through the dermis only. A pair of toothed mosquito forceps (shown magnified) is passed through the incision and the underlying vein grasped.

10

The grasped vein is pulled to the surface and the toothed forceps are replaced by stronger artery forceps.

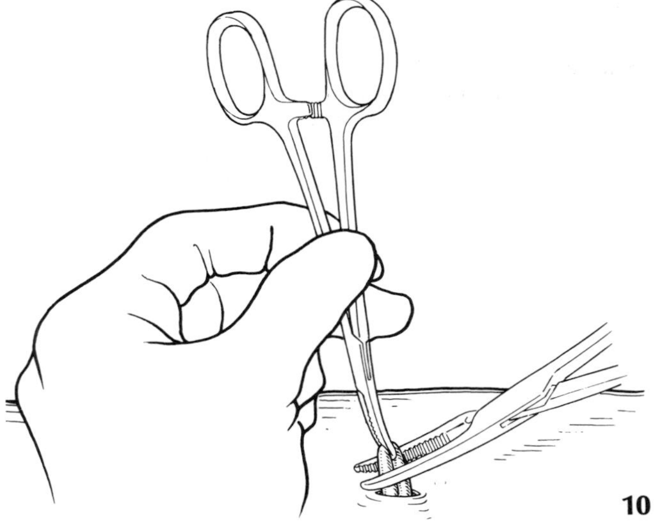
10

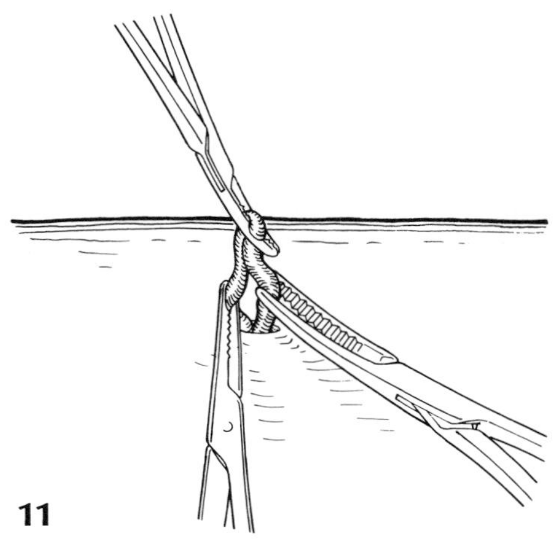
11

11

The vein is pulled further until it emerges as a loop. A pair of forceps is placed on each limb of the loop.

12

Taking one limb of the loop at a time, the vein is pulled gently.

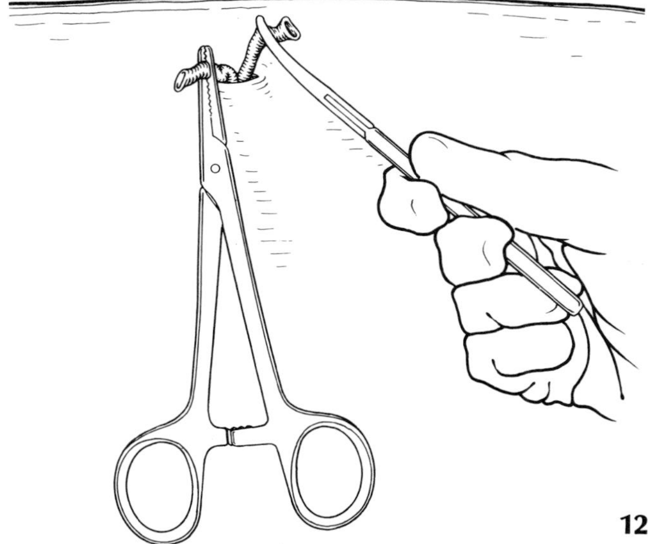
12

13

As it emerges through the skin, the vein is grasped with another pair of forceps near the skin and pulled farther, a new pair of forceps being placed on nearer the skin as every 2 cm or so is extracted.

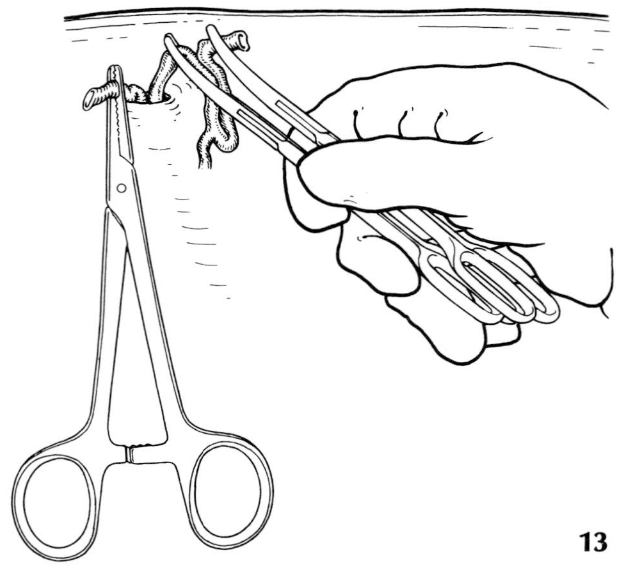

13

14

This process is continued until the vein breaks off. A new incision is then made farther down the marked vein to pick up the vein again. In this manner the whole of the superficial varicosity is removed.

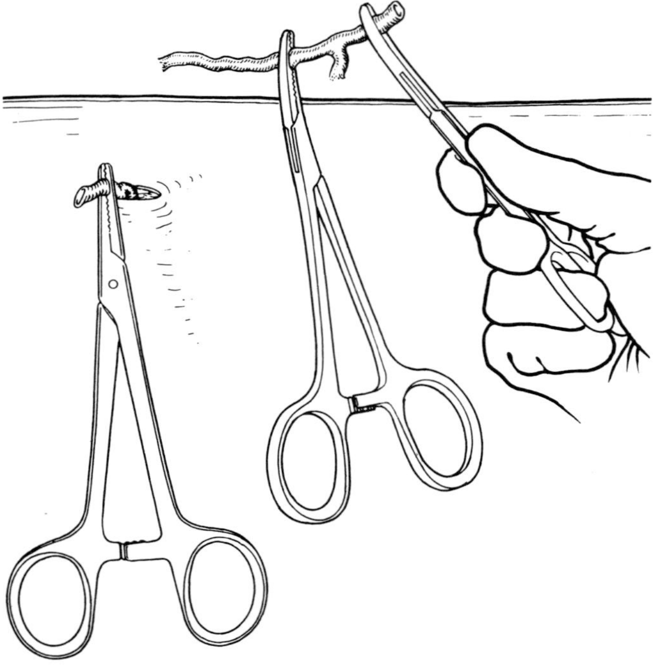

14

15 & 16

Tourniquet

When sufficient thigh veins have been dealt with so that a tourniquet can be positioned higher than all the remaining veins, an Esmarch's bandage is applied from medial malleolus to thigh. The upper turns are used on the thigh as a tourniquet and the lower turns are then removed. After application of the tourniquet, the remainder of the varices in the leg are removed from the now avascular field through multiple small stab incisions as described above (*see Illustrations 9–14*).

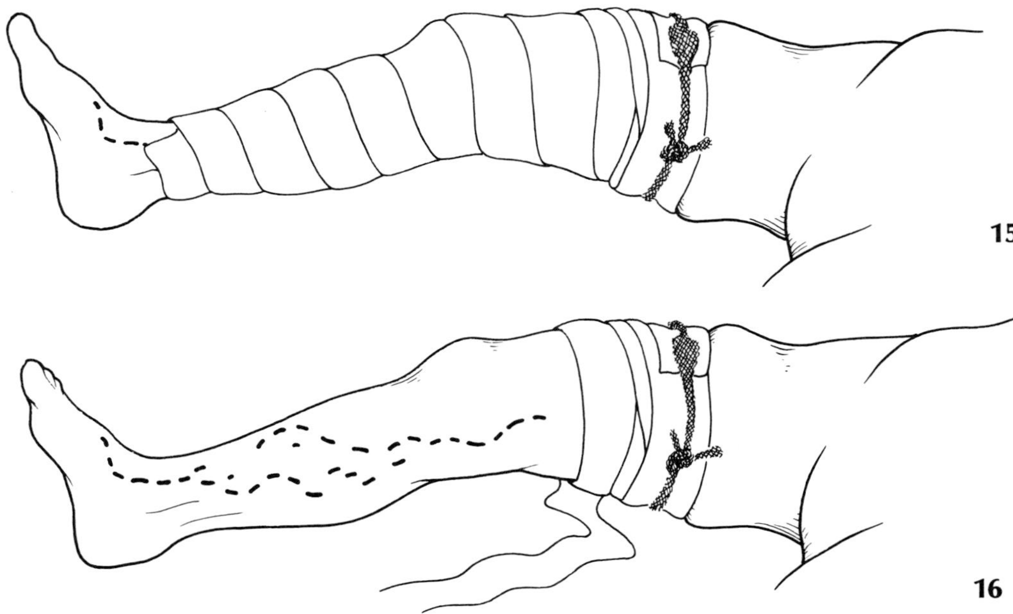

15

16

17

Wound dressings

The incisions are *not sutured*; they are dressed with tulle gras, gauze, cotton wool and a crêpe bandage. The bandage must be firm enough to occlude the surface veins, as no venous connections have been ligated except in the groin incision. The wounds distal to the tourniquet are dressed and bandaged while the tourniquet is still in place. The tourniquet is removed and any thigh wounds are then dressed and bandaged. If any bloody ooze comes through the bandages after removal of the tourniquet, an extra, firmer crêpe bandage is applied over the top of the original bandage.

Finally, a TED elastic stocking is placed over the top of the bandages. This keeps the bandages in good position and prevents them from slipping. There is less thigh bruising when such a stocking is used.

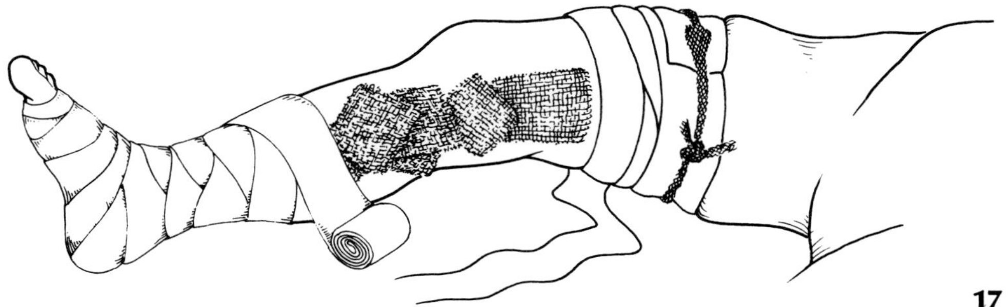

17

Short saphenous vein

18

Duplex scan

When short saphenous vein incompetence is found with a continuous wave Doppler, it is useful to obtain a duplex scan of the popliteal fossa. This will ascertain whether there are multiple sources of reflux (e.g. gastrocnemius veins) and to enable preoperative marking of the level of the saphenopopliteal junction.

Venography

In the absence of a duplex scan, a venogram can be performed. The venogram will confirm whether the reflux heard with the Doppler has been from the saphenofemoral junction or from a communication with the long saphenous vein (Hoare and Royle, 1984), but it will not demonstrate multiple sites of reflux as can be shown by duplex scan and is therefore inferior to examination with a duplex scan. The skin crease is marked with a radiopaque marker (a needle will do for this). The venogram is performed by introduction of the needle into a prominent varix adjacent to the popliteal fossa.

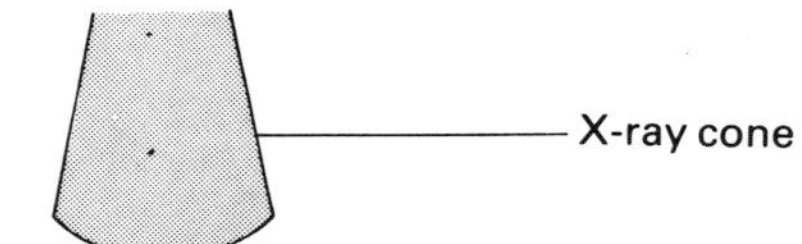

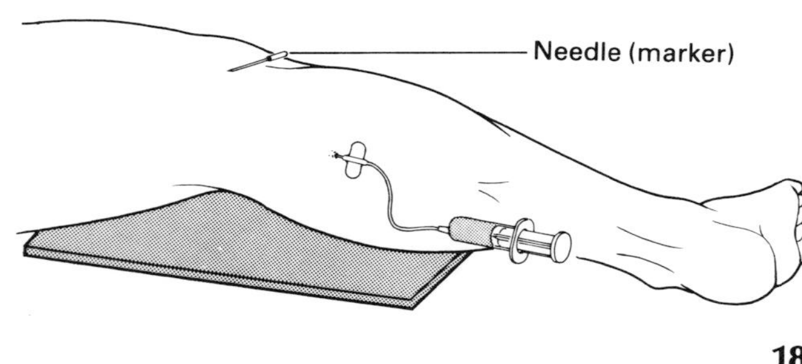

18

Saphenopopliteal ligation

When only the short saphenous vein is abnormal, the patient may be placed in the prone position and an Esmarch's tourniquet applied. When the saphenopopliteal junction is being ligated as part of a more generalized operation on other veins, the flush ligation of the saphenopopliteal junction is usually delayed until after the tourniquet has been applied and all the superficial varices have been removed by stab avulsions as described above (*see Illustrations 9–14*). In these circumstances the patient is turned on his side.

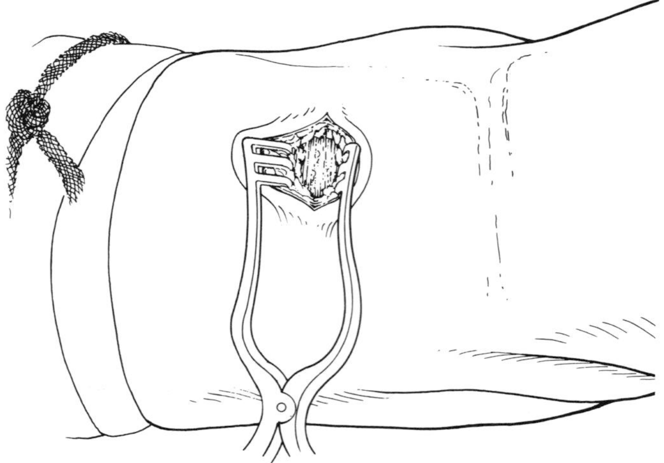

19

19

The skin incision is made transversely at the level indicated by venography and a small self-retaining retractor is inserted to separate the skin. The fat usually parts to reveal the deep fascia.

20

The deep fascia is opened transversely in the line of its fibres. The short saphenous vein can then usually be seen easily.

The short saphenous vein is grasped with forceps and dissection is conducted in the immediate perivenous avascular plane. Care is taken to avoid damage to the sural nerve. All patients undergoing short saphenous vein surgery should be warned of the possibility of postoperative numbness over the sural nerve distribution as this is quite common.

The vein that passes upwards from the short saphenous vein to form the posteromedial vein of the thigh is ligated and divided. Gastrocnemius veins joining the incompetent short saphenous vein are ligated and divided. The dissection of the short saphenous vein is continued down to the saphenopopliteal junction.

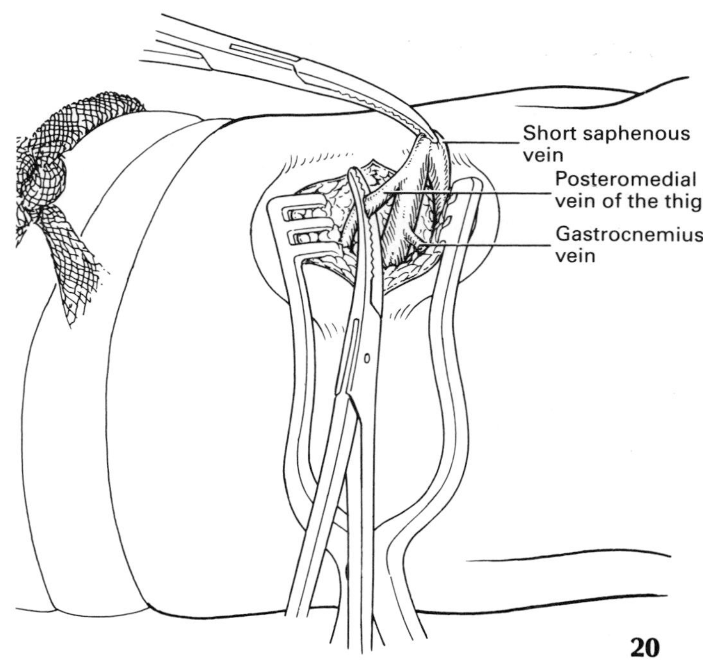

20

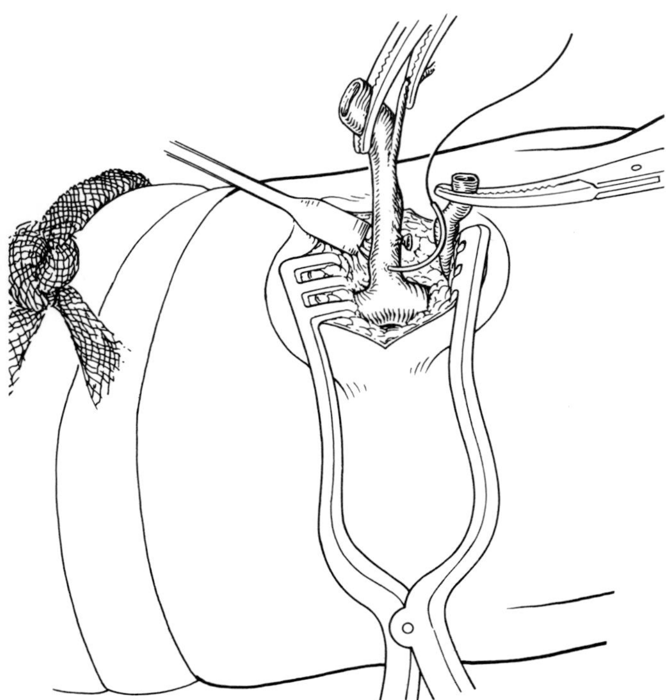

21

21

Flush ligation

A transfixion flush ligation is performed as described for the saphenofemoral junction, with the needle passing through the saphenous vein one-half of the diameter away from the popliteal vein in order to produce a flush ligation without constriction. Any incompetent gastrocnemius vein or popliteal area vein separately draining into the popliteal vein, is divided and ligated adjacent to the popliteal vein.

Short saphenous vein removal

The short saphenous vein can be removed by putting tension on the vein and locating it at a lower level through small stab incisions as described for long saphenous vein removal (*see Illustration 8*). More often just the ligation and excision of the length of short saphenous vein in the wound itself is performed. This lessens the incidence of sural nerve hyperaesthesia and anaesthesia postoperatively. The fascia is closed with an absorbable deep suture. The skin is closed with a subcuticular absorbable suture. The wound edges are infiltrated with 0.5% Bupivacaine HCl local anaesthetic solution as for a groin wound.

Postoperative management

The patient is returned to the ward with the foot of the bed elevated. Narcotic analgesia is seldom necessary. The patient is ambulated later the same day. If there is any bloody ooze through the bandages and stocking, an extra reinforcing bandage is applied. The patient leaves hospital later the same day or on the following day.

The bandages and dressing are left in place for 5–7 days and then removed. After removal of the dressings, occasionally one or two of the stab wounds may not be quite healed and a small dressing may be used over such wounds for several days.

Because the wounds have not been sutured the scars tend to be more prominent than usual for the first few weeks after surgery. However, the cosmetic result after 6 months is generally better when the wounds have not been sutured than when they have been.

References

Chan, A., Chisholm, I and Royle, J. P. (1983). The use of directional Doppler ultrasound in the assessment of saphenofemoral incompetence. *Australian and New Zealand Journal of Surgery* **53**, 399.

Hoare, M. C. and Royle, J. P. (1984). Doppler ultrasound detection of saphenofemoral and saphenopopliteal incompetence and operative venography to ensure precise saphenopopliteal ligation. *Australian and New Zealand Journal of Surgery* **54**.

Royle, J. P., Eisner, R. and Fell, G. (1981). The saphenofemoral junction. *Surgery, Gynecology and Obstetrics* **152**, 282.

Ligation of perforating veins

F. B. COCKETT MS, FRCS
Consulting Surgeon, St Thomas's Hospital, London, UK

Introduction

The perforating veins referred to here are the so-called 'direct' perforators – defined as those veins which perforate the *deep fascia* of the limb to enter directly into a main deep vein (such as the femoral or posterior tibial). These veins are few in number and in definite regular anatomical sites. The termination of the long saphenous vein at the groin and of the short saphenous vein in the popliteal vein behind the knee are the two most well-known perforator sites. There is also the 'Hunterian' or mid-thigh perforator.

This chapter deals with the important direct perforators in the lower half of the leg, which normally drain the venous blood from the subcutaneous tissue and skin of the ankle directly into the posterior tibial and peroneal veins.

1

On the inner side of the limb there are two main direct perforating veins (*2*) emerging from holes in the deep fascia. They are situated behind the long saphenous vein (*1*). The upper one is approximately halfway up the leg. The lower one is four fingers' breadth above the medial malleolus. Note that the perforating veins communicate by fine venous arches, and with the long saphenous vein by a large constant posterior arch vein (*3*) arising at knee level.

On the outer side of the limb there is only one constant large perforator (*5*) which communicates directly with the short saphenous vein (*4*). Much less constant is the so-called midcalf perforating vein (*6*) emerging close to the insertion of the gastrocnemius into the soleus tendon. When present, however, it is often large and important.

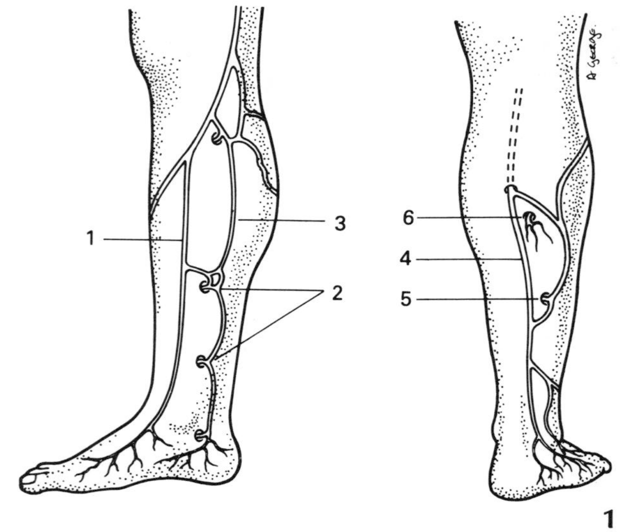

1

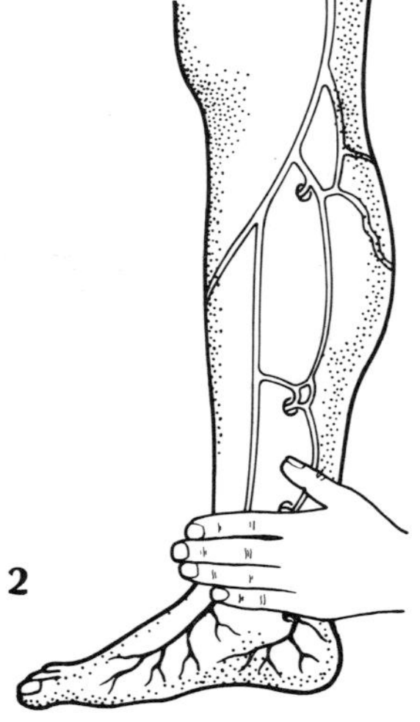

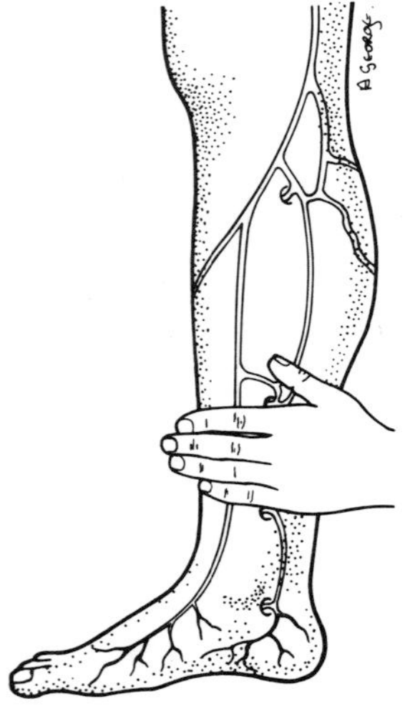

2

2

Clinically, these perforators are easily located by the 'hand's breadth' rule. In other words, the perforating veins on the medial aspect are separated by approximately the breadth of a hand as shown.

3

In the normal erect exercising limb, very high pressure (about 100 mmHg) develops in the deep calf veins during the contraction phase of the calf muscles. Blood is normally prevented from leaking out into the skin and subcutaneous tissue by the valve in the perforating vein, but when this valve is destroyed or becomes incompetent for any reason, the high pressure is exerted directly on to the fine mesh veins on the inner side of the ankle. These veins dilate rapidly, giving rise to the typical and important sign called 'ankle flare'. This process eventually leads to sclerosis and skin destruction – the lesion we know as a venous ulcer.

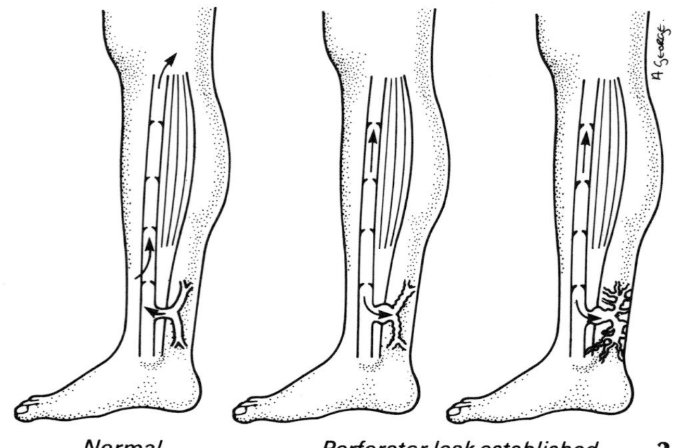

Normal *Perforator leak established* 3

Essential diagnostic points

There are three distinct groups of cases in which incompetent ankle perforators occur. In the first two groups, they are the main cause of the steady deterioration of the ankle skin and subcutaneous tissues which leads eventually to venous ulceration.

4

Group 1: Incompetent ankle perforators occurring as a late complication of primary varicose veins

In many longstanding cases of primary hereditary long saphenous incompetence, as the varicose veins of the posterior arch branch become bigger and more prominent, they connect with and drain into a competent medial ankle perforator. This competent perforator 'drains off into the deep veins', the high pressure coming down the long saphenous system, and thus protects the ankle skin. However, in many cases, as time goes on, the ankle perforator enlarges and its valve is either destroyed or becomes inefficient. When this occurs a massive venous hypertension from the perforator is added to that coming down the saphenous system, and rapid deterioration of the ankle occurs, leading to ulcer (hence the old name, 'varicose ulcer').

These cases are fairly common, and give the best results after long saphenous ligation and stripping, combined with ankle perforator exposure and ligation. In this group, associated varicose veins will be seen and should be marked as they must be dealt with when the perforating veins are tied.

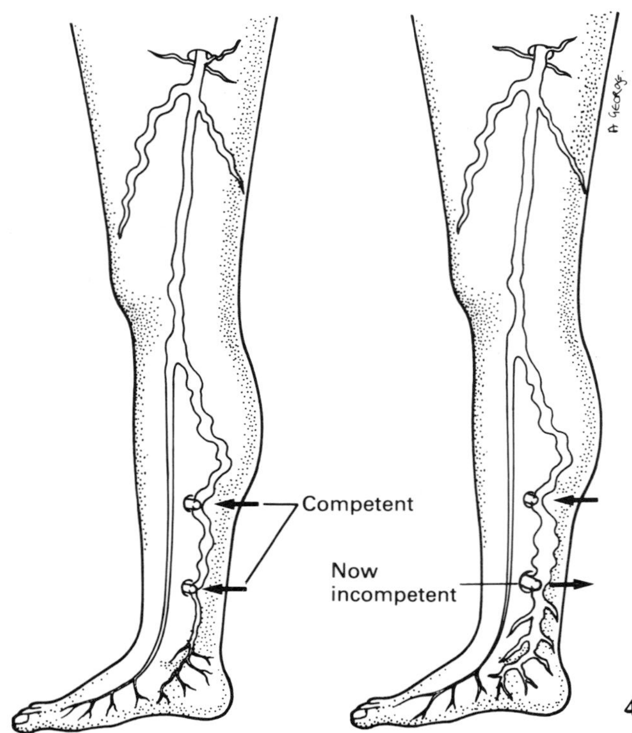

4

5

Group 2: Incompetent ankle perforators occurring late (2–5 years) after an acute venous thrombosis of the peripheral type

In this type, the thrombosis starts deep in the calf, either in the calf sinusoids or in the posterior tibial or peroneal veins. It spreads upwards into popliteal or femoral veins, but rarely higher. Usually, the clot spreads into the perforator up to its valve. During the recanalization phase the valve is destroyed and a 'perforator leak' is established. This causes swelling, venular dilatation, sclerosis and pigmentation of the ankle (the classic post-thrombotic syndrome), eventually leading to ulcer.

Often, in these cases, there is a remarkable degree of recanalization of the main deep veins in the post-thrombic phase. Also in the profunda vein and its branches there is usually an efficient collateral channel from the lower leg, so that there is often very minimal deep vein obstruction after a peripheral type of thrombosis, leaving the incompetent perforator as the main lesion responsible for the ankle ulcer. It is essential to discover any past history of possible deep vein thrombosis in order to recognize this state of affairs, because it implies that the only surgery required is ligation of these perforating veins.

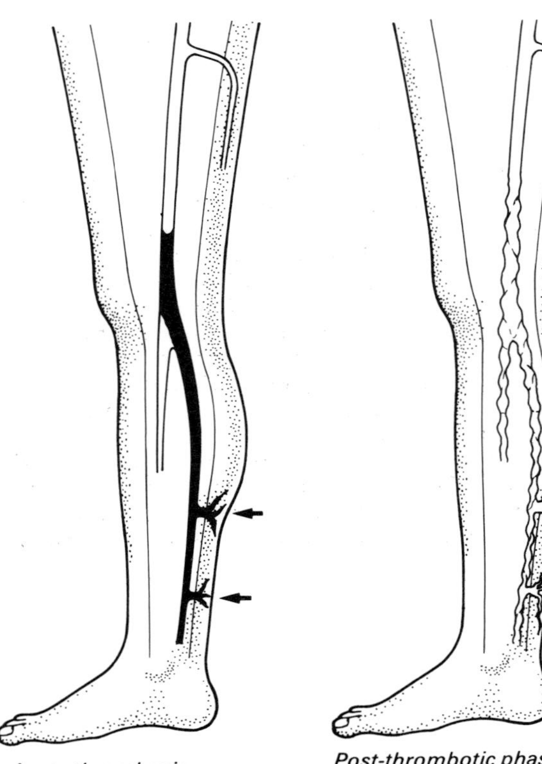

5

6

Group 3: Incompetent ankle perforators occurring after a patient has had a proximal or iliofemoral type of thrombosis

In these cases the thrombosis starts in the iliac vein segment; usually, patients are young and have the developmental anomaly known as the 'iliac compression syndrome'. The left iliac vein is partly (or sometimes wholly) obstructed by the right common artery passing over it and compressing it against the promontory of the sacrum. When this partly obstructed left iliac vein thromboses, the thrombosis usually spreads down to the groin. After this resolves and attempts recanalization, the patient is left with an obstructed iliac vein, but a *normal* calf pump and perforators.

Occasionally, the thrombus extends peripherally right back into the calf, producing a very severe clinical picture (phlegmasia caerulae dolens). When this resolves and recanalizes, there may be extensive deep vein obstruction *plus* incompetent ankle perforators. These patients develop the worst and most intractable ulcers and even though incompetent perforating veins are detected, ligation in this situation gives poor results, because the venous hypertension due to obstructed deep veins is unrelieved. More frequently, venous reconstructive surgery is required.

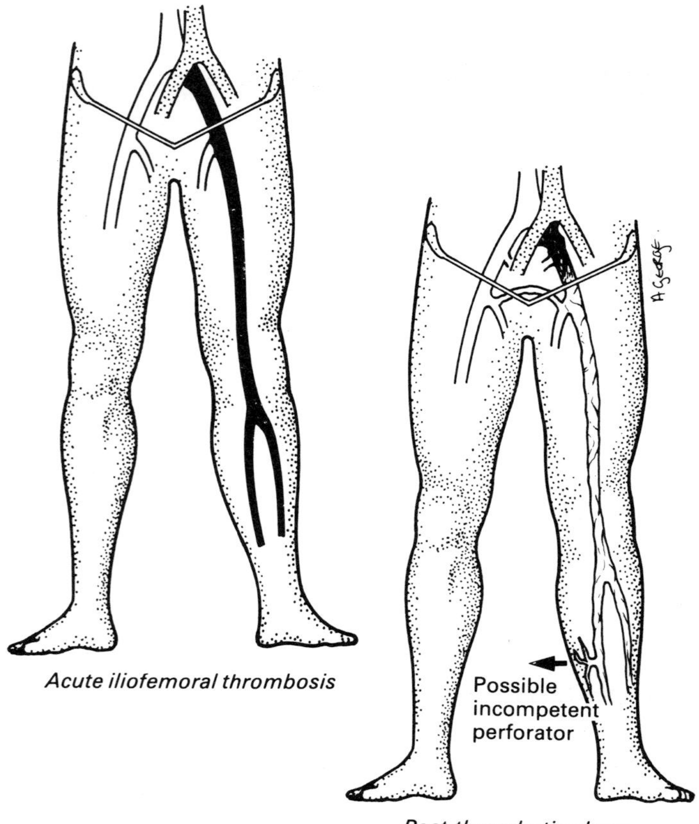

Acute iliofemoral thrombosis

Post-thrombotic phase

6

Editorial comment

Preoperative management and the operative procedure

At present venous ulceration healing is usually achieved by firm compression and ambulation. The four-layer bandage technique requires change of bandages weekly or sometimes twice weekly. Colour duplex scanning pinpoints the underlying abnormality and surgery relates to this. Perforating veins are usually located by colour duplex scan and the incision is placed just over the perforation. The long incision for extrafascial ligation or subfascial ligation (Linton) or stocking incision (Dodd) is seldom required. The great contribution of these pioneers, however, was to recognize the relative constant situation of the perforating veins. The ligation of perforating veins is now usually performed in conjunction with surgery for primary varicose veins as described by Royle (pp. 479-488) or Rose in other chapters. The patient is usually admitted on the day of operation and stays in hospital at most for one night postoperatively. Compression bandaging continues in the postoperative period for patients with unhealed ulcers.

References

Cockett, F. B. (1955). Surgery of venous ulcers. *British Journal of Surgery* **43**, 179.

Cockett, F. B. and Jones, D. E. (1953). Ankle blow-out syndrome. *Lancet* **1**, 17.

Cockett, F. B., Lea Thomas, M. and Negus, D. (1967). Iliac vein compression – its relation to iliofemoral thrombosis and the post-thrombotic syndrome. *British Medical Journal* **2**, 14.

Dodd, H., and Cockett, F. B. (1976). *Pathology and Surgery of the Veins of the Lower Limb*, 2nd ed. Edinburgh: Churchill-Livingstone

Edwards, J. M. (1976). Sherry operation for incompetent perforating veins. *British Journal of Surgery* **63**, 885.

Linton, R. R. (1953). *Annals of Surgery* **138**, 415

Moffatt, C. J., Franks, P. J., Oldroyd, M., Bosanquet, M., Brown, P., Greenhalgh, R. M. and McCollum, C. N. (1992). Community clinics for leg ulcers and impact of healing. *British Medical Journal* **305**, 1389.

Negus, D. and Friedgood, A. (1983). Effective management of venous ulceration. *British Journal of Surgery* **70**, 623.

Venous reconstructive surgery

JOHN J. BERGAN MD

Clinical Professor of Surgery, North Coast Surgeons Medical Group Inc., La Jolla, California, USA

JAMES S. T. YAO MD, PhD

Professor of Surgery and Director, Blood Flow Laboratory, Northwestern University Medical School, Chicago, Illinois, USA

Introduction

Direct surgery of veins has lagged behind direct arterialization of the extremities and viscera partly because surgeons have been more fascinated with the drama of cardiac and arterial surgery and partly because of the genuine difficulties which attend venous reconstruction and anastomosis. The standard operations with expected good results are bypasses of venous obstruction. Kistner has been successful with valveplasty (Ferris and Kistner, 1982), but others have found it to be a technically difficult procedure (Sottiurai, 1988). Kistner's technique of segment transfer is less demanding and enables venous flow to be directed through competent valves; unfortunately, it is applicable to a very small number of patients. The procedure championed by Taheri, Lazar and Alias (1982) of transplantation of valve-containing venous segments must await long-term evaluation before it is considered acceptable. Free-segment venous transfer must also be regarded as experimental. This chapter presents our current techniques of direct venous reconstruction.

Femorofemoral cross-over grafts

1 & 2

In this procedure, the saphenous vein is used as a conduit to bypass contralateral common and external iliac venous occlusion. Exposure is gained through vertical incisions over the femoral veins; one-third of the incision extends above the inguinal ligament. The saphenous vein is removed from the thigh under direct vision, through multiple, discontinuous incisions. Preparation of the graft must be meticulous to avoid venous trauma. As much adventitia as possible is carefully removed to allow maximum venous dilation. All tributary veins are ligated and divided at least 2 mm from the main trunk, in order to avoid constriction of the trunk during dilation. The graft is gently distended with heparinized saline solution to check for inadvertent tears or leaks. Localized varicosities, if present, must be dealt with either by resection or external support using normal vein tissue as recommended by Palma (1976).

The junction of the saphenous vein with the femoral vein is left intact. The superficial epigastric and external pudendal tributaries must be maintained so that angulation of the saphenofemoral junction is prevented.

The tunnel is made deeply, but subcutaneously, in the suprapubic region by digital dissection. The saphenous vein is passed through the tunnel using a long vascular clamp. Twisting of the vessel must be avoided. If possible, the graft should gradually curve into Scarpa's triangle on the affected side, and if necessary the vein can be stitched to the deep fascia using adventitial stitches.

The anastomosis should be 2–3 cm in length. It can be made to the saphenous vein on the affected side, but is best made to the common femoral vein, if possible. The venous intima should not be traumatized.

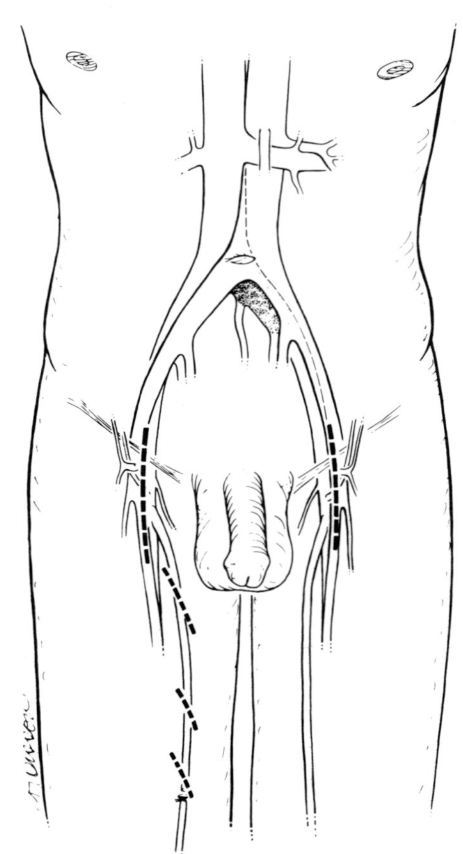

1

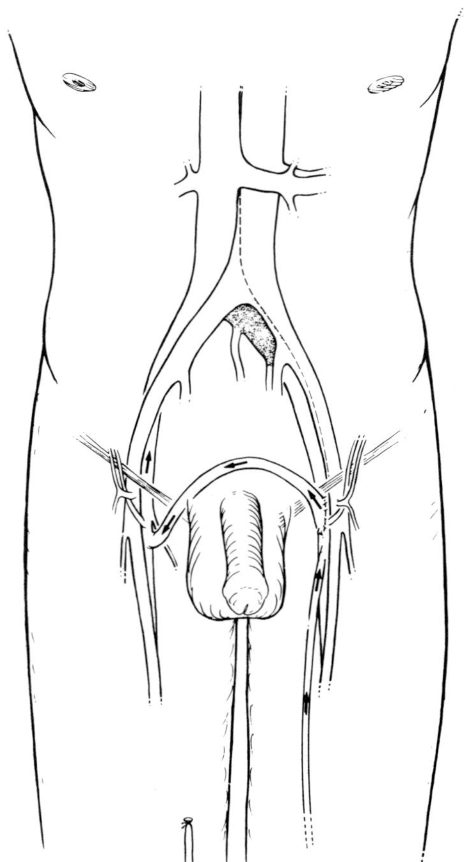

2

3a & b

Illustration 3(a) shows the orientation of the structures after mobilization. Atraumatic clamps, as shown here, or siliconized rubber slings can be used for venous occlusion. *Illustration 3(b)* indicates the anastomotic technique, with careful atraumatic eversion of the venous edges and approximation with 6/0 or 7/0 monofilament suture.

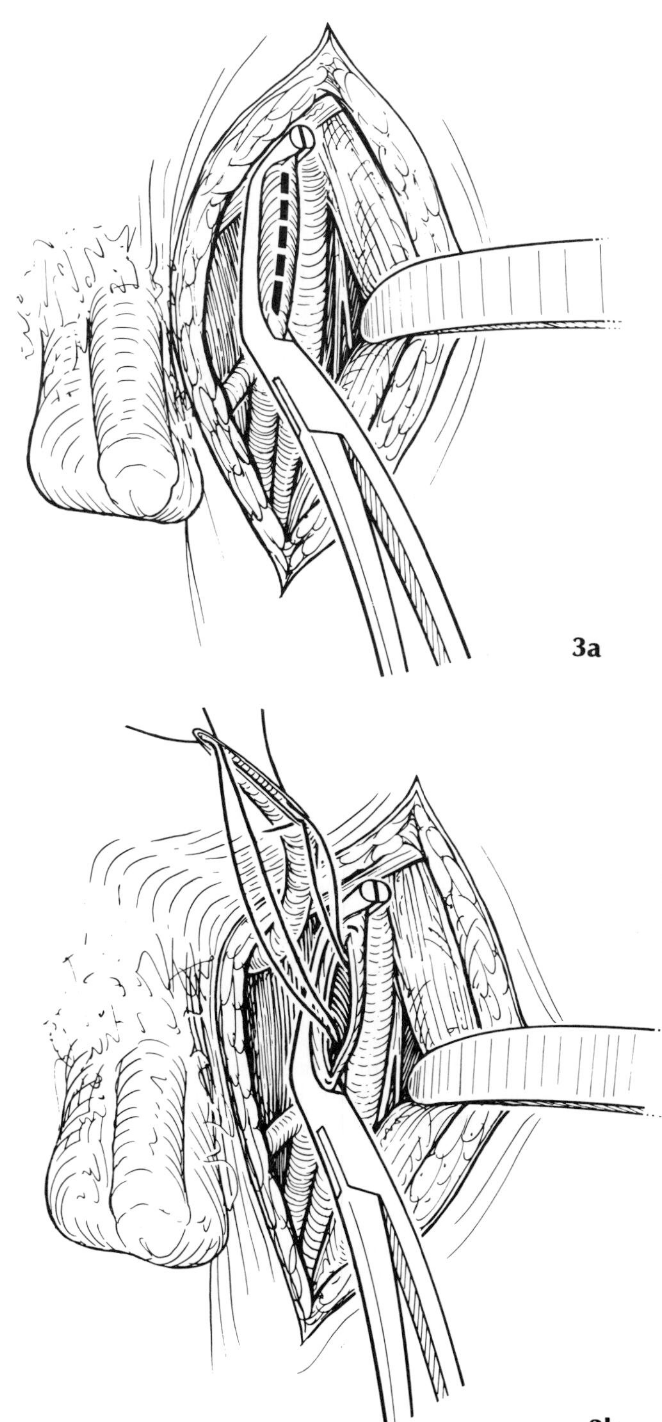

The wounds are closed in several layers to obliterate dead space. On our service, the arteriovenous fistula has been abandoned; instead, intermittent calf compression boots are applied using a 15-second on-cycle and 45-second off-cycle. Anticoagulants are not used.

Late results of the procedure are comparatively good. Harris *et al.* (1988), reporting from Sydney, Australia, described a 17-year experience, ending in 1982, involving 40 cross-saphenous bypasses. The cross-over bypass graft managed symptoms in all patients, except two who required some distal reconstructive or ablative surgery. There were five late deaths, all unrelated to venous disease; three patients were lost to follow-up. The 5-year cumulative patency rate was 83%, but this was based on clinical judgement only. It is known that 8 of the 41 grafts have occluded. In this study, 11 patients had surgical interruption of perforating veins or removal of distal varicosities, either concomitantly (8) or following the bypass (3). The remaining 28 patients constituted a follow-up group: 11 have normal legs, 9 confirmed by photoplethysmography (PPG), and 9 have residual calf symptoms controlled with stocking support. Only one patient has had recurrent ulcerations. The eight patients with occluded grafts continue to have swelling, pigmentation and ulceration of the affected limb.

Saphenopopliteal bypass

When deep venous thrombosis of the superficial femoral vein is poorly recanalized, severe distal venous stasis may appear. When wearing of supportive bandages or well-fitted elastic stockings does not relieve stasis symptoms, direct surgical bypass of the obstruction is required. The calf muscle pump is relatively ineffective when working below an obstruction, and the long saphenous vein is inefficient because it is not connected to the muscle pump mechanism. Therefore, the objective of the operation is to provide a conduit to connect the deep venous system of the calf with a patent proximal venous pool.

In the United States, first Warren (Warren and Thayer, 1954), and then Husni (1970) performed saphenopopliteal bypass. May (1979), in Innsbruck, also advocated this procedure. In 50% of Warren's patients, the saphenous vein was transplanted deep to the sartorius muscle.

As time has passed, we have become increasingly disappointed with this procedure.

For this procedure the poorly recanalized venous segment must be confined to the superficial femoral vein, the iliac system being spared, and the saphenous vein must be of good calibre preferably with functioning valves and no varicosities.

Careful ascending venography should show at least the distal half of the popliteal vein to be completely patent. There should be no evidence of smouldering, sub-acute venous thrombosis, as this will cause the procedure to fail.

Operative procedure

4

The patient lies supine on the operating table, with the leg slightly externally rotated and the knee moderately flexed. An incision is made parallel to the tibia, distal to its crest. The vein is marked prior to the operation, so that the skin incision can be made directly over it. The saphenous vein is mobilized and transected 2–3 cm distal to the distal end of the operative incision. The deep fasica is divided. The medial head of the gastrocnemius muscle is retracted medially. The soleus is exposed. The popliteal vein may be doubled, but the larger portion will lie posterior to the artery, with the anterior tibial veins crossing that structure.

Additional exposure can be gained by cutting the semitendinosus and semimembranosus muscles. These do not have to be repaired.

Once an adequate segment of vein for anastomosis has been mobilized, attention is turned to the anteromedial aspect of the thigh. A 6-cm incision is made at the junction of the middle and distal thirds of the thigh and is carried through the deep fascia, displacing the sartorius posteriorly and incising the fascia over the popliteal space. A tunnel is made between the thigh and calf wounds, so that the mobilized saphenous vein can be inserted parallel to the popliteal vessels from above downward and thus lie in a gentle curve in the thigh, without tension behind the knee joint.

The leg is extended to make sure that the saphenous vein is of adequate length, and a site is chosen for the distal anastomosis. Thin, siliconized vessel loops are used to encircle the popliteal vein. A venotomy is created, and the venotomy and the distal end of the saphenous vein are irrigated with heparinized saline solution. The distal end of the saphenous vein is fishmouthed to conform exactly to the venotomy in the popliteal vein. A long anastomosis, 1.5 cm in length, is then made using 6/0 or 7/0 monofilament polypropylene suture.

Following the attainment of haemostasis, the wounds are closed, leaving the fascia open, both in the calf and in the thigh. The skin is approximated with synthetic, absorbable intradermal suture. Suction drainage may be used, but an arteriovenous fistula is not created.

Postoperatively, the patient is not anticoagulated but may receive 500 ml of 10% Rheomacrodex each day for the first 5 days. An intermittent compression pump is applied to the calf, with a cycle of 15 seconds on, 45 seconds off.

The patency of the anastomosis is monitored by the transcutaneous Doppler technique.

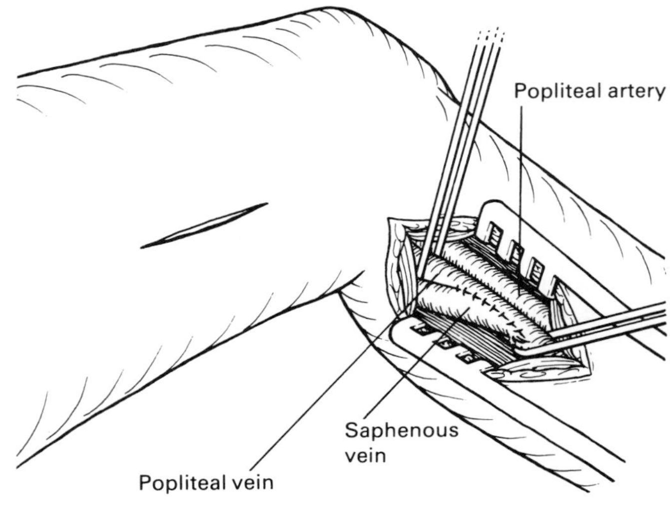

4

Prostheses in venous reconstruction

Anecdotal reports have been received about the use of polytetrafluoroethylene (PTFE) grafts in the cross-over femorofemoral position. None of these has been successful below the femoral vein.

Investigators using prosthetic grafts have been encouraged by experimental models which have used short-segment venous interposition grafts in the portal and vena caval systems, yet the clinical application of PTFE has been limited. There are reports of successful cross-over grafts (Clowes, 1980), but these are few, and the operation should be applied with great caution.

As externally reinforced grafts have become available, they have been used clinically although, admittedly, in situations of great difficulty. A 1983 report from Japan (Takaba *et al.*, 1983) included a follow-up of 3–15 months in five patients requiring such femorofemoral cross-over grafts. The grafts used were 16, 12, 8 and 6 mm, the last two being externally reinforced.

Direct venous valve surgery

Operations to correct valvular incompetence include direct valvuloplasty, transposition of the venous stream through a competent valve system, and valve transplantation.

Valvuloplasty, as invented by Kistner (Ferris and Kistner, 1982), can be a technically difficult operation. It is performed under magnification, using a 7/0 to 9/0 sutures. It is used in patients who have demonstrated a grossly incompetent superficial femoral valve, through which retrograde flow is visualized on descending venography.

5a, b & c

The femoral vein is exposed through a linear incision extending from the inguinal ligament. After complete mobilization of the superficial femoral vein, the anterior aspect is studied carefully, so that the incision in the vein can be made from below upward exactly through the valve commissure. It is very easy to carry the incision through a valve cusp and destroy the valvuloplasty operation.

6a, b & c

It is essential not to tear the valve cusp while sutures are being placed, and the reefing sutures must be placed precisely, in order to shorten the valve cusp but not excessively.

The venotomy may be closed from above downward to test the competence of the valve under direct vision. A dental mirror may be inserted into the venotomy to check the status of the reconstruction further or, alternatively, as the venotomy is being created from below upward, to assist in placing the venotomy precisely through the valve commissure (Samuels, P., 1983, personal communication).

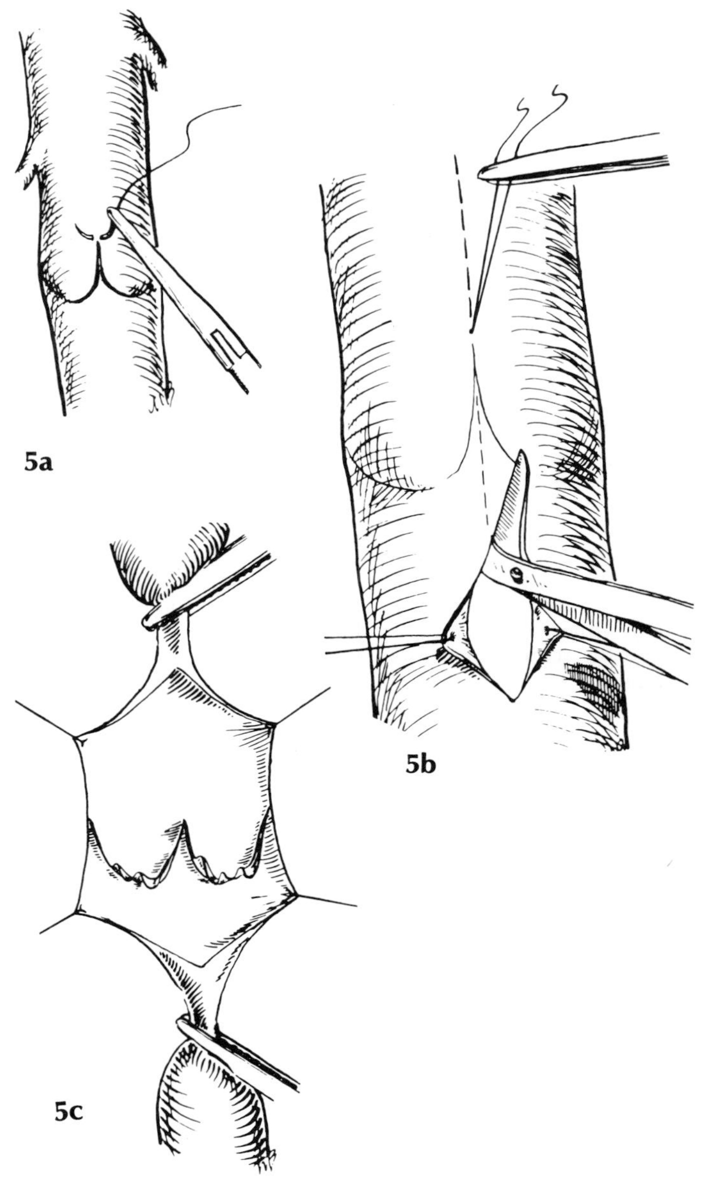

5a

5b

5c

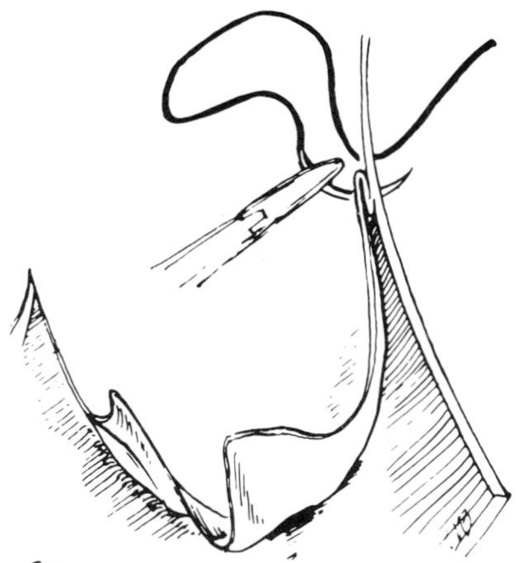

6a

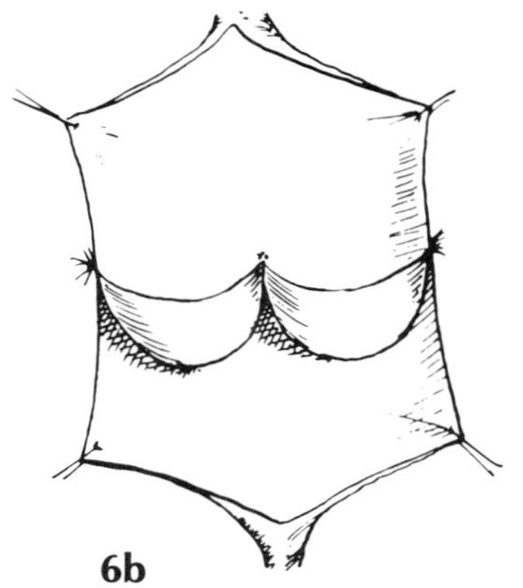

6b

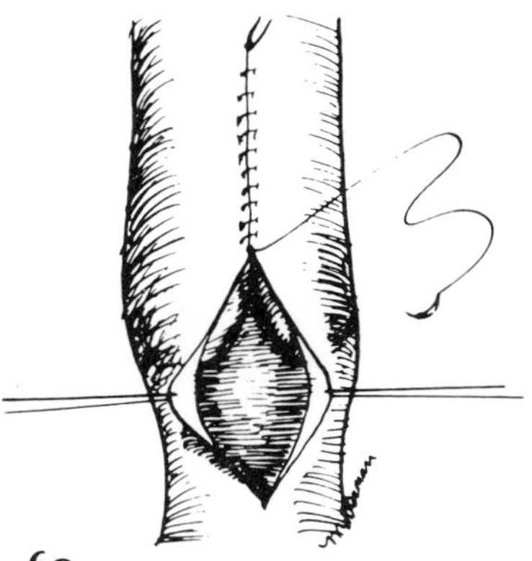

6c

Transposition of the venous stream

7a, b & c

Kistner made a second major contribution to direct venous surgery by inventing the procedure of transposition of the venous stream through a demonstrably competent valve. He has called this redirection of venous flow through competent proximal valves the 'segment transfer operation'.

In this procedure, competent valves are identified in the profunda femoris vein, the saphenous vein or the superficial femoral vein by means of descending phlebography. After a competent valve is identified, an adjacent deep vein is transected and anastomosed to the venous segment containing the competent valve. An example of this is transection of the superficial femoral vein, which contains only incompetent valves, and anastomosis of this to the saphenous vein, which contains a competent saphenofemoral valve (*a*). Another example is anastomosis of the divided superficial femoral vein to a profunda femoris vein which contains a competent valve (*b*). Otherwise, the superficial femoral vein can be ligated and the saphenous vein anastomosed end-to-side below the ligature (*c*).

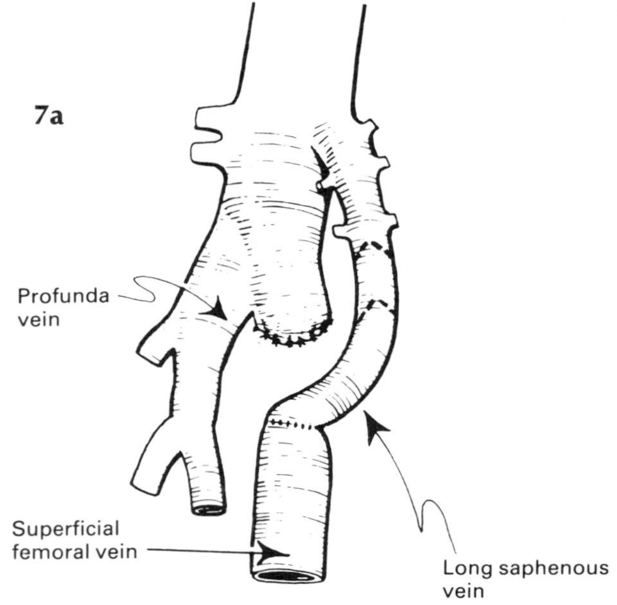

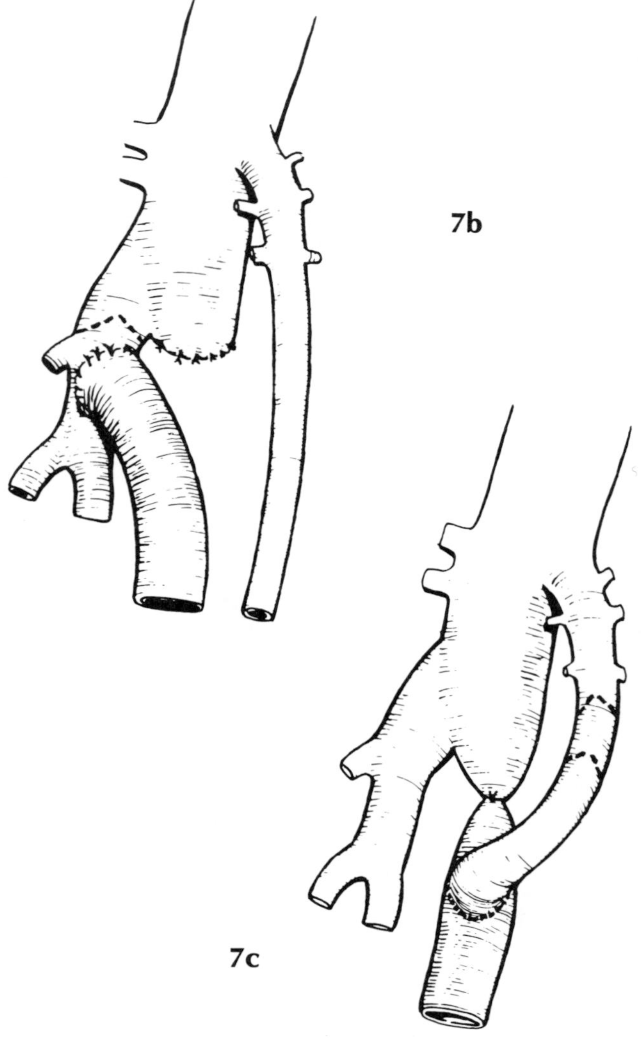

The femoral venous confluence is approached through a linear incision made directly over the veins. One-third of the incision should be above the inguinal ligament, and two-thirds below. The saphenous vein and its tributaries are isolated, the common vein is skeletonized, and the profunda and superficial femoral veins are mobilized for a distance of 3–6 cm. The patient is systematically heparinized prior to the application of atraumatic clamps or occlusion of the major veins with siliconized rubber slings. Anastomosis is done with 7/0 polypropylene suture, ensuring that there is no tension between the structures to be anastomosed. Continuous stitching is utilized.

Competence of the valve is checked by emptying the distal vein through the valve and observing the distal vein for refilling. Wound closure is done in layers to avoid dead space. The skin edges are approximated using intradermal sutures of synthetic absorbable material, such as polyglycolic acid. Suction drainage may be used, but anticoagulants have been abandoned on our service.

Intermittent calf compression can be applied to maintain venous velocity through the reconstructed segment.

Kistner's late 1982 report (Ferris and Kistner, 1982) included 53 venous reconstructions in 46 patients, performed over a 14-year period. Seven of these reconstructions were excluded from evaluation. In two of these, superficial femoral vein ligation was required because of haemorrhage. In two others, superficial femoral vein ligation was required because of valve injury during repair or irreparable valve due to postphlebitic state. In another case, external plication rather than valve repair was done. Two patients had lymphoedema but underwent repair of a leaking superficial femoral vein valve; their symptoms of lymphoedema persisted.

In the remaining 46 extremities, there were 32 valve repairs and 14 venous segment transpositions. The results were good-to-excellent in 80% of both groups. Patients with stasis and ulceration had better results than those with pain and oedema. Interestingly, descending postoperative venography was performed in 41 of 46 cases, and thrombosis of the reconstructed segment has not occurred in any patient. Improvement of venous competence was demonstrated in 39 of the 41 cases.

It should be noted that incompetent perforators have been treated in conjunction with femoral vein reconstruction in this series. In another series (Queral *et al.*, 1980), in which incompetent perforators were not treated, good results were only achieved in 11 of 16 patients, and excellent results in only 1 patient. This experience is similar to ours.

Valve transplantation

Taheri has had the greatest experience with valve transplantation. In the original procedure described by him the superficial femoral vein was exposed through a longitudinal incision below the inguinal ligament. Later, he implanted the new segment in the above-knee popliteal vein. The brachial vein is approached through a longitudinal incision 5 cm below the axilla. A 2-cm segment of brachial vein, including valve, is tested for competence and removed. A segment of popliteal vein is excised, and the brachial vein, including the valve, is sutured to the popliteal vein with 7/0 or 8/0 polypropylene suture, using a continuous, everting or interrupted technique.

Taheri uses continuous heparin administration and suction drainage of both the arm and the thigh wound. Oral anticoagulation is used for 3 months.

Taheri, Lazar and Alias (1982) described 38 patients having valve transplantation. Postoperative venography (16 ascending, 12 descending) showed 13 patients with normal venous systems and 3 patients with thrombosis of the superficial femoral system.

The only other large experience with valve transplantation is that of Raju (1983), who reported 20 valvuloplasties, 22 vein valve transplantations and 3 Kistner segment transfer operations. Thrombosis of a valve repair was only found in 1 of 17 patients who had venographic examination of the repair after operation. The valve transplant operation seemed quite satisfactory, with resolution of the primary symptom in 13 limbs (9 ulcers, 2 oedema, 2 chronic pain). Of this group, 10 limbs showed improvement in the venous haemodynamics, as measured in the laboratory, and in 3 limbs, despite subjective improvement, the laboratory parameters remained unchanged. Eight patients were surgical failures: there was a technical problem in one small axillary vein; in the other seven patients there was recurrence of reflux through the transplanted axillary vein segment, proved by venography/venous testing.

Superior vena cava bypass

8

Superior vena cava obstruction may have a variety of causes, including granulomatous mediastinitis, tuberculosis and malignant tumour. When cerebral insufficiency syndromes occur, consideration may be given to the performance of a bypass of the superior vena cava (Chiu, Terzis and MacRae, 1974; Wright and Doty, 1980). A suitable graft for such bypass may be obtained by removing the long saphenous vein, ligating all of its branches, distending the vein with heparinized saline solution under gentle hydrostatic pressure, and splitting the vein longitudinally throughout its length. The open vein is then wrapped around a previously chosen stent of appropriate size (No. 40 chest tube). The continuous anastomosis can be made utilizing 6/0 or 7/0 polypropylene suture.

A median sternotomy incision is made, and the innominate vein exposed and mobilized throughout its length. The pericardium is then opened through a vertical incision, retracted laterally and held in place with stay sutures. Biopsy of the upper mediastinum can be obtained at this time. The distance between the innominate vein and atrial appendage is measured. The distal anastomosis can be made end-to-end, as preferred by Doty and Wright, or end-of-graft to side-of-innominate vein. Meticulous performance of the anastomosis is eased by use of loop magnification. The suture material is 6/0 polypropylene.

The anastomosis to the right atrial appendage can be done using a partial occlusion clamp. The trabeculated portion of the atrial appendage is excised and the anastomosis constructed with 6/0 polypropylene. The clamps are removed, and the blood flow through the graft is checked. As in all venous surgery, meticulous technique must be utilized for construction of the spiral graft and both of the anastomoses. Fibrous adventitial strings must not be allowed to cross the suture lines; neither should purse-stringing of either anastomosis be allowed to occur.

The pericardium is not closed, but the median sternotomy is closed by peristernal wire, in order to immobilize the sternum entirely. Drainage tubes are left in the mediastinum, but anticoagulation is unnecessary.

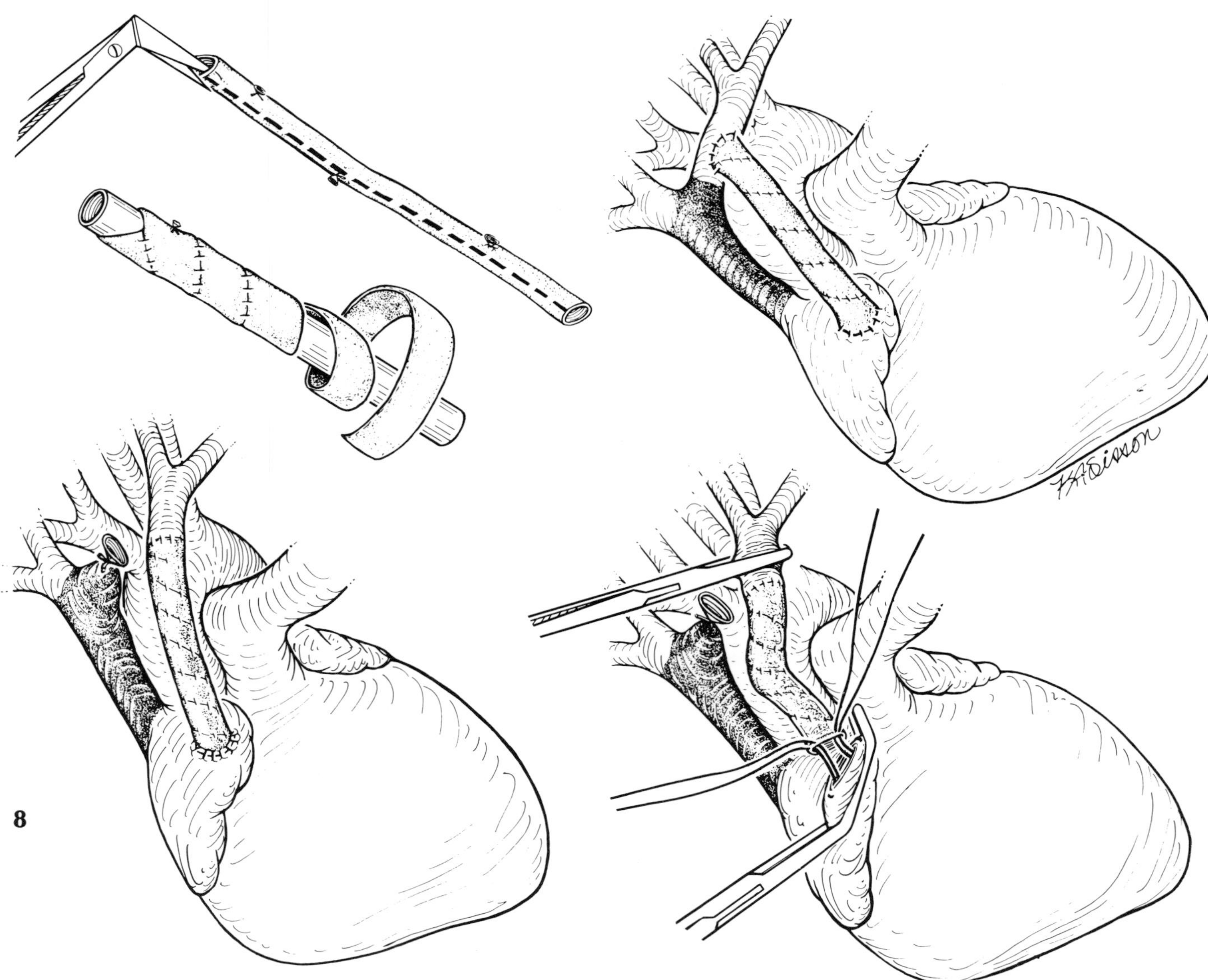

8

Acknowledgements

Supported in part by the Conrad Jobst Foundation, the Seabury Foundation and the Northwestern Vascular Research Foundation.

Illustrations 5 and *6* are from Kistner and Ferris (1980, pp. 293 and 295). *Illustration 7* is from Queral (1980, p. 304).

References

Chiu, C. J., Terzis, J. and MacRae, M. L. (1974). Replacement of superior vena cava with the spiral composite vein graft. *Annals of Thoracic Surgery* **17**, 555.

Clowes, A. W. (1980). Extra-anatomical bypass of iliac vein obstruction. *Archives of Surgery* **115**, 767.

Ferris, E. B. and Kistner, R. L. (1982). Femoral vein reconstruction in management of chronic venous insufficiency. *Archives of Surgery* **117**, 1571.

Harris, J. P., Kidd, J., Burnett, A. and Halliday, P. (1988). Patency of femorofemoral venous crossover grafts assessed by duplex scanning and phlebography. *Journal of Vascular Surgery* **8**, 679.

Husni, E. A. (1970). *In situ* sapheno-popliteal bypass grafts for incompetence of femoral and popliteal veins. *Surgery, Gynecology and Obstetrics* **130**, 279.

Kistner, R. L. and Ferris, E. B. (1980). Technique of surgical reconstruction of femoral vein valves. In *Operative Techniques in Vascular Surgery*. Bergan, J. J., Yao, J. S. T., eds. London and San Diego: Grune and Stratton.

May, R. (1979). *Surgery of the Veins of the Leg and Pelvis*. London and Philadelphia: W. B. Saunders, p. 150.

Palma, E. C. (1976). Vein grafts for treatment of post-phlebitic syndrome. In: *Vascular Surgery: Principles and Techniques*. Haimovici, H., ed. New York: McGraw Hill, p. 857.

Queral, L. A. (1980). Correction of deep venous insufficiency by valvular transposition. In *Operative Techniques in Vascular Surgery*. Bergan, J. J., Yao, J. S. T., eds. London and San Diego: Grune and Stratton.

Queral, L. A., Whitehouse, W. M. Jr, Flinn, W. R. *et al.* (1980). Surgical correction of chronic deep venous insufficiency by valvular transposition. *Surgery* **87**, 688.

Raju, S. (1983). Venous insufficiency of the lower limb and stasis ulceration. *Annals of Surgery* **197**, 688.

Sottiurai, V. S. (1988). Techniques in venous valvuloplasty. *Journal of Vascular Surgery* **8**, 646.

Taheri, S. A., Lazar, L. and Alias, S. (1982). Status of vein valve transplant after 12 months. *Archives of Surgery* **117**, 1313.

Takaba, T., Yamamoto, N., Fumami, M., *et al.* (1983). Reconstruction with expanded polytetrafluoroethylene (EPTFE) for iliac venous obstruction (abstract). *Journal of Cardiovascular Surgery* **24**, 422.

Warren, C.B. and Thayer, T. P. (1954). Transplantation of the saphenous vein for post-phlebitic stasis. *Surgery* **35**, 867.

Wright, C. B. and Doty, D. B. (1980). Spiral vein grafting: the technique. In: *Operative Techniques in Vascular Surgery*. Bergan, J. J., Yao, J. S. T., eds. London and San Diego: Grune and Stratton, pp. 307–310.

Repair of venous valves using silicone cuffs

RODNEY J. LANE MS, FRCS, FRCSE, DDU, FRACS

Visiting Vascular Surgeon, The Royal North Shore Hospital, St Leonards, New South Wales, Australia; Visiting Vascular Surgeon, North Harbour Private Hospital, Harbord, New South Wales, Australia

Introduction

The present indications for the use of silicone valve cuffs are to correct chronic deep venous insufficiency usually associated with ulceration unresponsive to other forms of therapy. Similar silicone cuffs may be used for varicose veins. The underlying aetiology of lower limb venous insufficiency is first determined using non-invasive testing. If deep venous incompetence is thought to be the problem it is confirmed by venography. Grades of III or IV (Kistner) of reflux must be demonstrated and the best results are obtained when the whole venous system is uniformly dilated with multiple valves. These must be clearly demonstrated by venography, particularly by descending venography. Both cusps must be seen to be present and the attachment of the cusps on to the wall must be symmetrical. Radio-opaque markers are essential during all forms of venography in order to allow accurate location of the valves at the time of operation.

There are reservations about this technique in patients with extensive deep venous thrombosis and associated inflammatory changes with destruction of valve cusps. However, patients who have venographically intact valve cusps either above or below a previous thrombosis do not necessarily have to be excluded. At present, at least three valves in more than one area (i.e. popliteal or femoral level) should be corrected. The distal repairs are always performed initially, because one of the operative tests for valve function requires maximal hydrostatic pressure with anaesthetic-induced valsalva. Additional back pressure is created by elevating the head as much as possible and clearly this is best achieved without having interposing competent valves. Main axial valves are selected in order to minimize distal alternate retrograde flow. In patients where the function of a particular valve cannot be totally corrected (but a good pressure gradient can be maintained), additional valves should be repaired. It is essential that all valves are tested at operation usually via the 'milking' and the 'proximal occlusion' techniques to check competence visually. Typically, complete competence is obtained with reduction of the lumen by apparently one-third.

Preoperative precautions

Microbiological examination of swabs from the ulcer is used to determine the presence of pathogens and patients are covered with the appropriate antibiotics during the anaesthetic induction. Heparin is also given. Our practice is to give 5000 u subcutaneously and 2000 u intravenously. The level of the valve is marked on the skin with an indelible pencil based on preoperative venogram with magnification taken into account.

The operation

1

The popliteal fossa or thigh is prepared and draped in the usual manner and the skin covered with a suitable plastic drape. The incision is curved to minimize contracture at the skin fold.

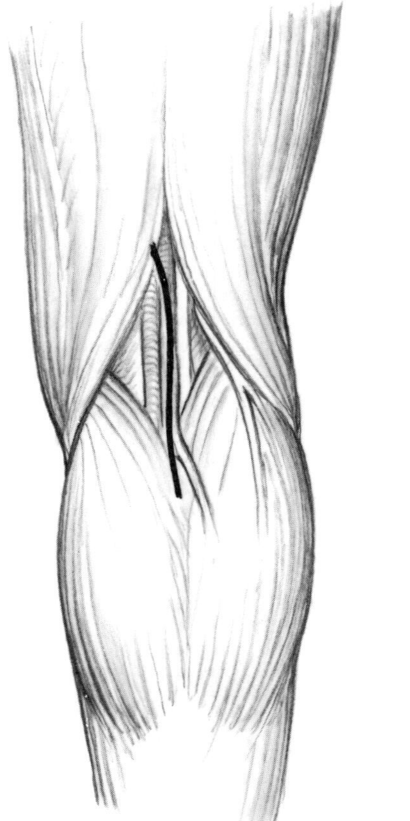

1

2

The incision is carried through the deep fascia and the vein is located adjacent to the artery. Minimal dissection is required in order to obviate or minimize lymphatic interruption. The segment of vein above and below the valve is isolated and minor tributaries are ligated and divided. If there are major tributaries then these are slung.

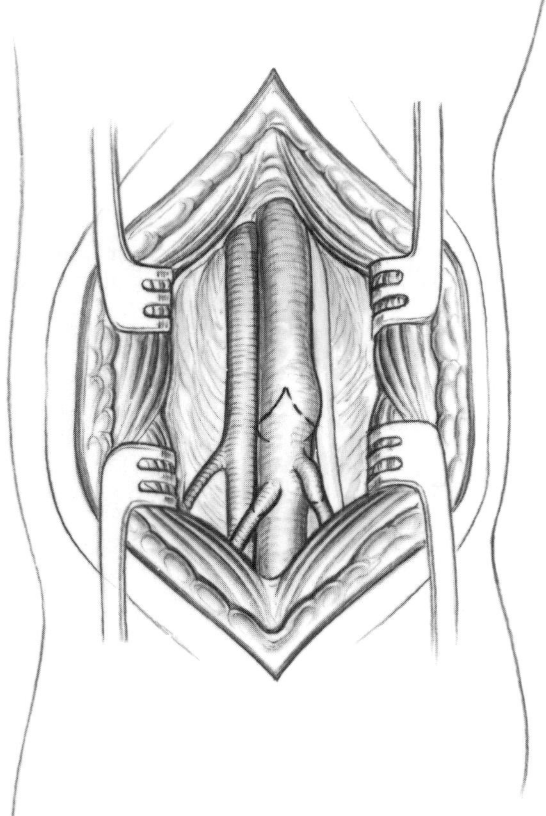

2

3

During the dissection the valve is located and appears as an oblique curvilinear line of attachment joining in a proximal apex. There is commonly a bulge just proximal to the valve cusp and it may be necessary to refer to the venogram and remeasure the actual site of the valve from a bony prominence.

If the valve cannot be identified by these means, intraoperative B-mode imaging may be used. Occasionally, to decide finally on the presence or absence of a valve, the vein is narrowed to see if competence is achieved. Very gentle dissection is essential as spasm of the valve may occur and cause temporary competence interfering with testing. This can always be overcome, however, by proximal occlusion and digital pressure between the occlusive loop and the valve.

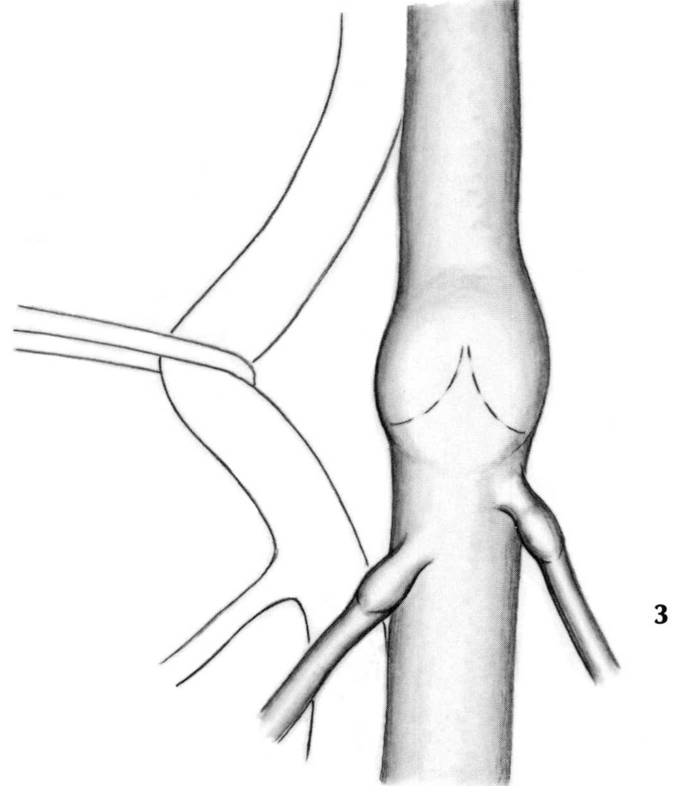
3

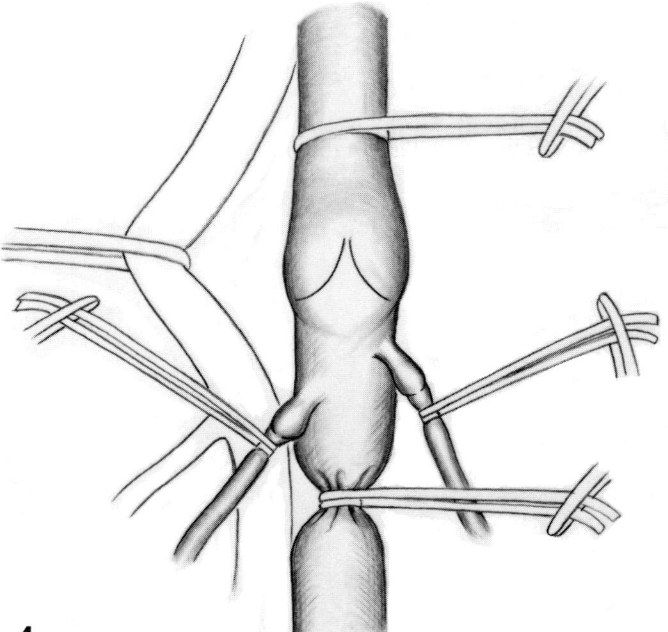
4

4

Having identified the valve and dissected at least 3 cm distally and 1 cm proximally, silastic vessel loops are placed around the vein in order to control inflow and outflow.

5

The silicone cuff used is called the 'Venocuff'. A right-angle forceps is used to pass one end of the 'Venocuff' around the vein. The other end of the 'Venocuff' is already attached to its applicator. Sometimes the end of the 'Venocuff' may impinge upon the vein wall and great care should be taken.

6

The free end of the 'Venocuff' is engaged into the applicator 'Venocuff' slot. The 'Venocuff' is now wrapped around the vein and is positioned at the valve site.The buckle action is similar to a car seat belt. At this stage, irrigation solution containing antibiotics in saline is used to irrigate the wound to maintain asepsis. The 'Venocuff' should not be allowed to touch the patient's skin.

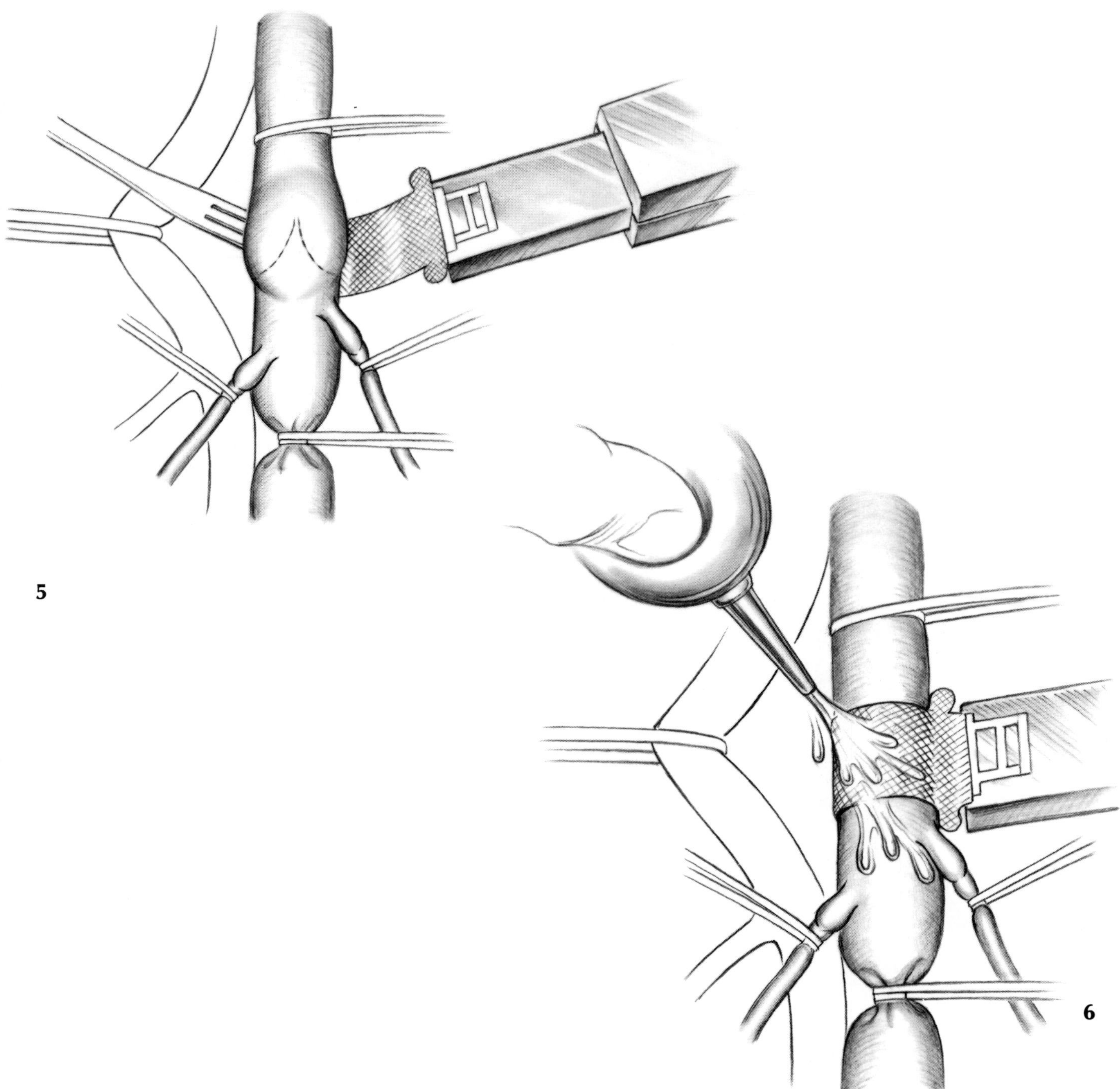

5

6

7

The applicator tensioning bar is then activated to decrease the valve ring circumference and so bring valve cusps closer together to produce competence. This is checked frequently during the tightening using the 'milking technique'. The inflow is first occluded with the distal silastic slings and the segment up to the valve ring is milked free of blood with the finger and thumb. Maximum 'head up' of the patient on the operating table is required during this testing. A 'valsalva manoeuvre' is performed by the anaesthetist to obstruct venous return and further stress the valve being tested. It becomes clear if the valve withstands the downward force of venous pressure if the distal vein segment stays collapsed. The distal silastic loop is now released to fill the distal segment and again the test is repeated.

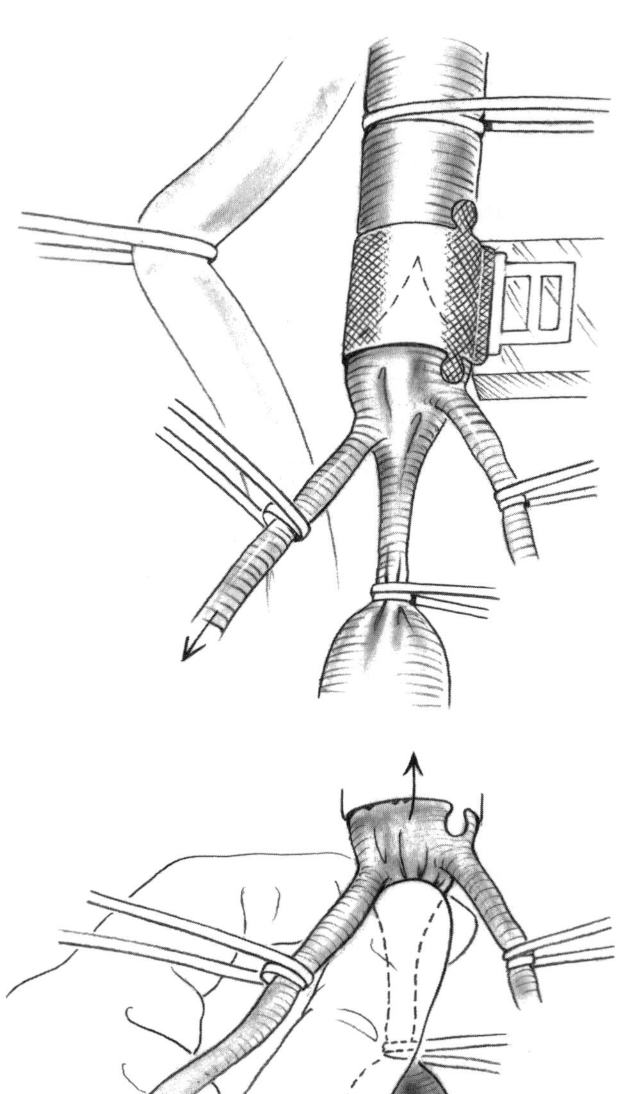

7

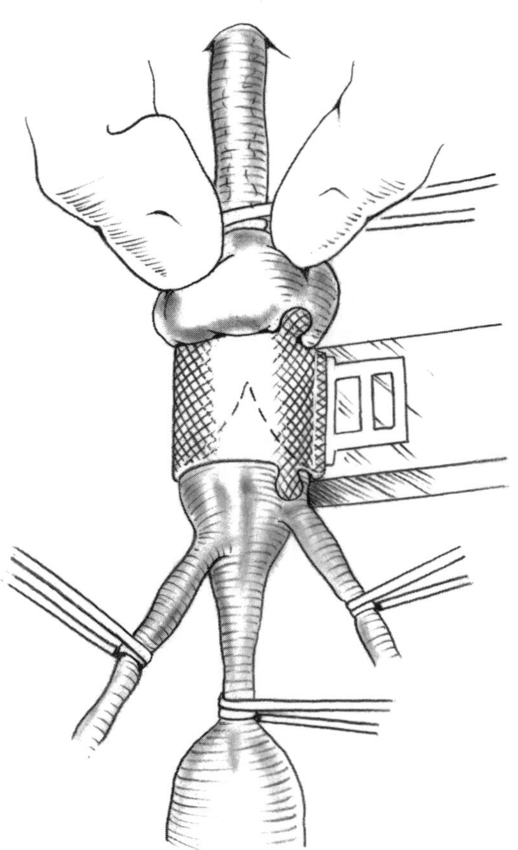

8

8

The proximal compression test or close segment compression test is then performed by obstructing the proximal sling, cranial to the valve being tested and allowing the segment between to fill. Digital pressure then compresses this segment and a competent valve generates a high pressure. This can be compared with the pressure in the distal vein. This test is useful when access to the more distal parts of the vein are not possible because of tributaries or inadequate dissection. If a valve seems to be incompetent following 'Venocuff' application on repeated testing, an unsighted tributary should be sought. In many cases, competence is demonstrated when this hidden tributary is controlled. If the valve is not completely competent under high pressure but clearly maintains a gradient, the 'Venocuff' is left in place.

9

When valve function has been corrected or, at least, improved, the staple trigger on the applicator is fired and the staple automatically fastens the 'Venocuff' at the appropriate diameter and cuts off excess strapping. Occasionally, the operator may place excessive downward pressure on the actual vein, so that when the applicator has been removed, the valve subsequently becomes incompetent again. Therefore, both testing manoeuvres should be repeated after fastening the 'Venocuff'. The diameter of the 'Venocuff' should always be noted using the graduations on the applicator. Hence, if incompetence occurs, a new 'Venocuff' is applied and the diameter is further decreased, which usually imparts competence.

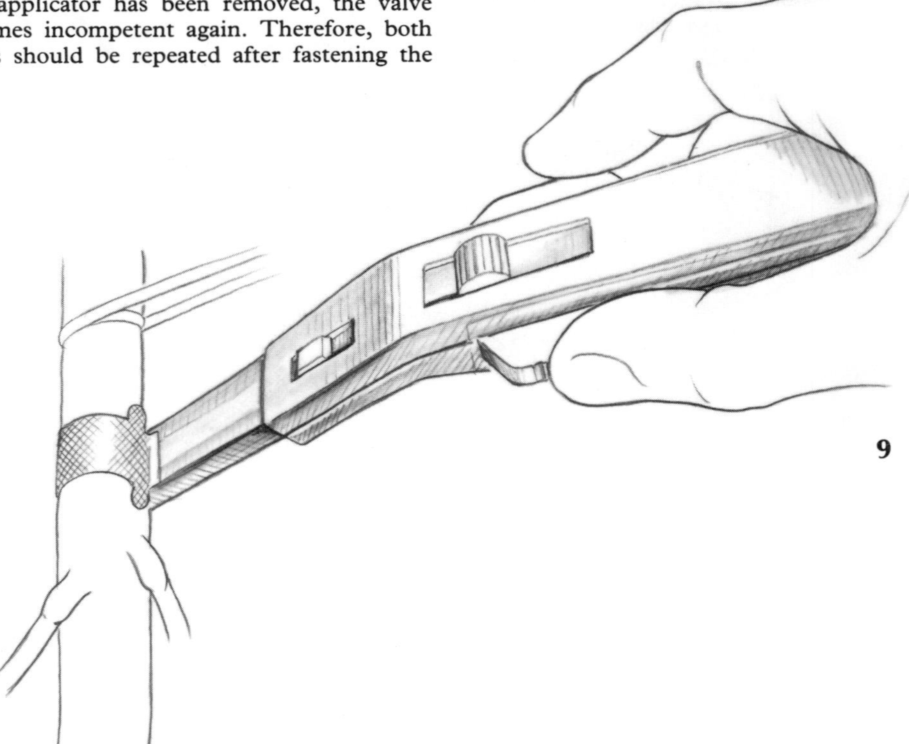

9

10

Occasionally, the ends of the 'Venocuff' require a metal vessel clip at the join of the two straps. These may be inserted at either end above or below.

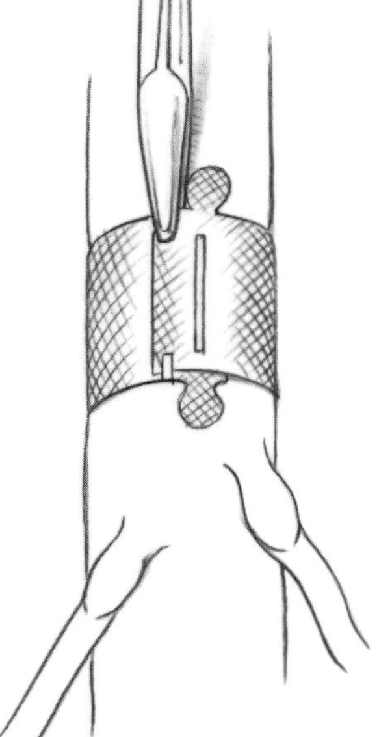

10

11

There are two fixation tags on the 'Venocuff' which are then used to suture the 'Venocuff' to surrounding tissue. A 5/0 polypropylene suture is used to do this. Two further sutures are used to fasten the 'Venocuff' directly to the adventitia of the vein as shown. Sometimes when checking for competence it becomes necessary to cut the distal fixation tag off, and this direct extra suturing to the vein is then mandatory.

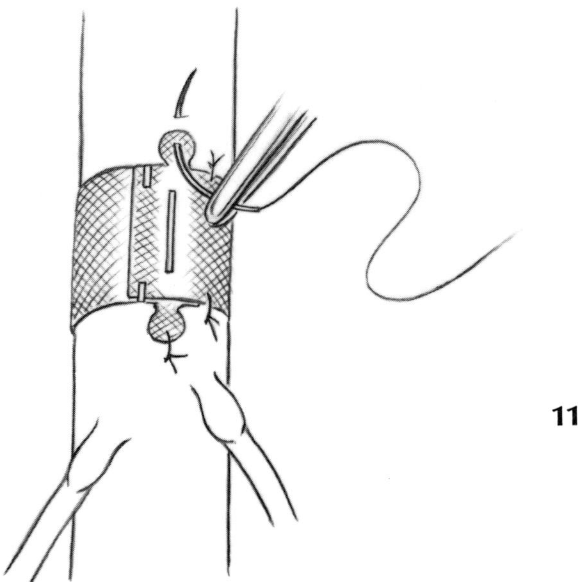

11

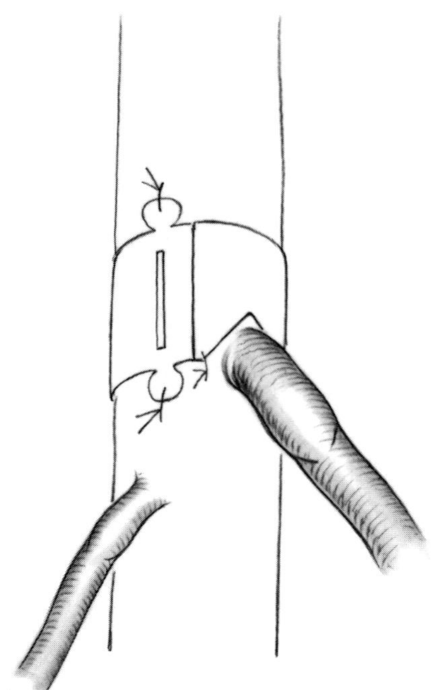

12

In cases of a valve being very close to a tributary, a 'Venocuff' with a V-notch (Venocuff S) can be chosen to allow adequate and suitable reduction of the circumference of the valve. There are two notched 'Venocuffs', the left and right (Venocuff SL and SR), to suit the situation.

It should be emphasized that the corners of the notch must be sutured directly to the adventitia, preferably anteriorly and posteriorly in order to maintain the diameter and tension of the 'Venocuff'.

12

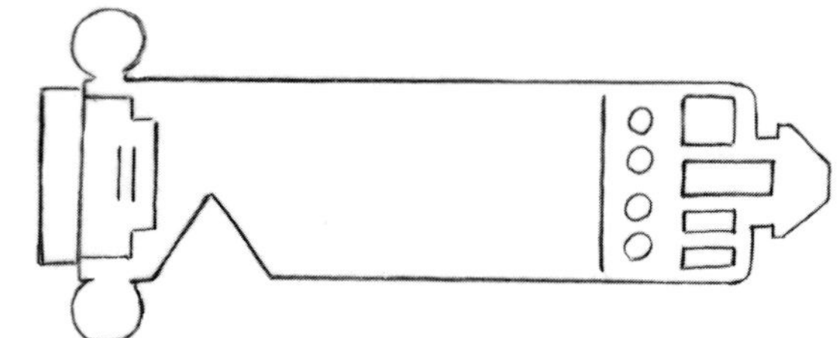

13

Closure is completed in layers and sterility maintained by again irrigating with an antibiotic solution. A suction drain is used routinely and careful haemostasis is essential. Mobilization should begin as soon as possible, preferably the next day, and subcutaneous heparin is administered until ambulation is complete. Intravenous antibiotics are continued for 24 h. The patient is usually discharged at 4 days and ulcer care is continued.

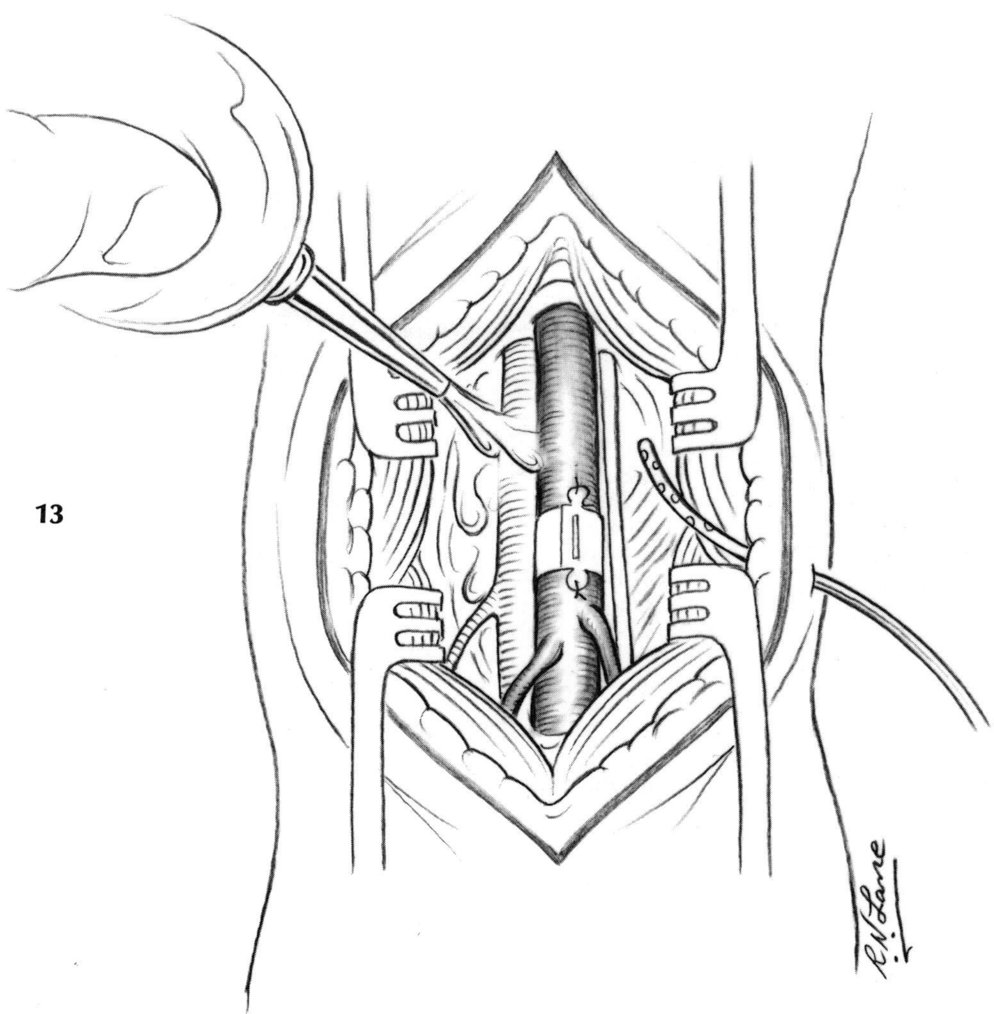

13

Deep venous thrombectomy

O. WAGNER MD

Professor of Surgery, Krankenhaus der Barmherzigen Brüder, Vienna, Austria

Introduction

Intervention for the removal of acute thrombosis of the iliac and femoral veins consists of thrombolysis or venous thrombectomy. The aim of these procedures is the prevention of lethal pulmonary embolism as well as the immediate restoration of venous blood-flow, thereby also preserving the valvular system and preventing a post-thrombotic syndrome. The advantages of these procedures over elevation and heparin therapy are the immediate relief of the compromised venous drainage, lowered and shortened morbidity, venous valve preservation and prevention of the postphlebitic syndrome in a large percentage of these patients. Success of surgical thrombectomy can only be expected in cases of very recent thrombosis, which means that surgery should be performed within the first few days of occurrence. If thrombectomy is performed after a longer interval, adherence of the thrombus to the vessel wall makes removal of the clot increasingly more difficult and enhances the chance of rethrombosis. Surgery performed later than 6 days after the onset of symptoms shows no better results than conservative treatment; thrombolysis, however, may be successful up to 15 days (Minar *et al.*, 1983).

Preoperative

Indications

Surgery is indicated for thrombosis of the deep femoral and iliac veins with a history of onset up to 5 days. However, floating thrombus or segmental femoral or iliac thrombosis can be operated on successfully up to 4 weeks.

Contraindications

Surgery is contraindicated in patients with a short life expectancy (such as those with inoperable tumour) or when postoperative heparin or anticoagulant therapy is inadvisable.

Preoperative assessment

The clinical course with sudden onset of swelling and pain is characteristic. A reliable diagnosis depends on clinical findings only and can be supplemented by ultrasound examinations. Venography is not obligatory but provides helpful information on the extent of the thrombosis. The blood group should be determined and 2 u of blood prepared in case of extensive blood loss.

The operation

This operation was first described in 1937 by Läwen, Professor of Surgery in Königsberg, Germany and followed up by Mahorner, Castleberry and Coleman in 1957.

The operation is performed under general anaesthesia. In slim patients thrombectomy from the common femoral vein is also feasible in local anaesthesia. Systemic heparinization is attained by administration of 5000 i.u. of heparin i.v.

1 & 2

A transverse inguinal incision is made just above the groin crease, and the femoral vein, saphenous vein, deep femoral vein and superficial femoral vein are controlled by Silastic slings.

After heparinization a longitudinal incision of 2–3 cm is made at the entrance of the saphenous vein. First the local thrombus is removed; then each orifice is explored for clots which are removed by forceps and Fogarty catheters. The same procedure is performed on the deep femoral veins. The veins are then controlled by bulldog clamps (Fogarty and Kreppoehne, 1965). Proximal clots are removed by passing Fogarty catheters into the iliac venous system. During this procedure the pressure in the intra-abdominal vena cava is increased by hyperbaric respiration to prevent pulmonary embolism. (A blocking catheter from the collateral side should not be used since this would constitute an added trauma to the normal collateral vein without providing absolute security against embolization.)

Intraoperative phlebography of the iliac veins is helpful when additional information on the completeness of thrombectomy is necessary. In some patients repeated attempts at thrombectomy are necessary before normal venograms can be obtained.

Intraoperative endoscopy is another possibility for checking completeness of clot removal and to demonstrate residual disease in the iliac veins (Loeprecht, Weber and Monnig, 1985).

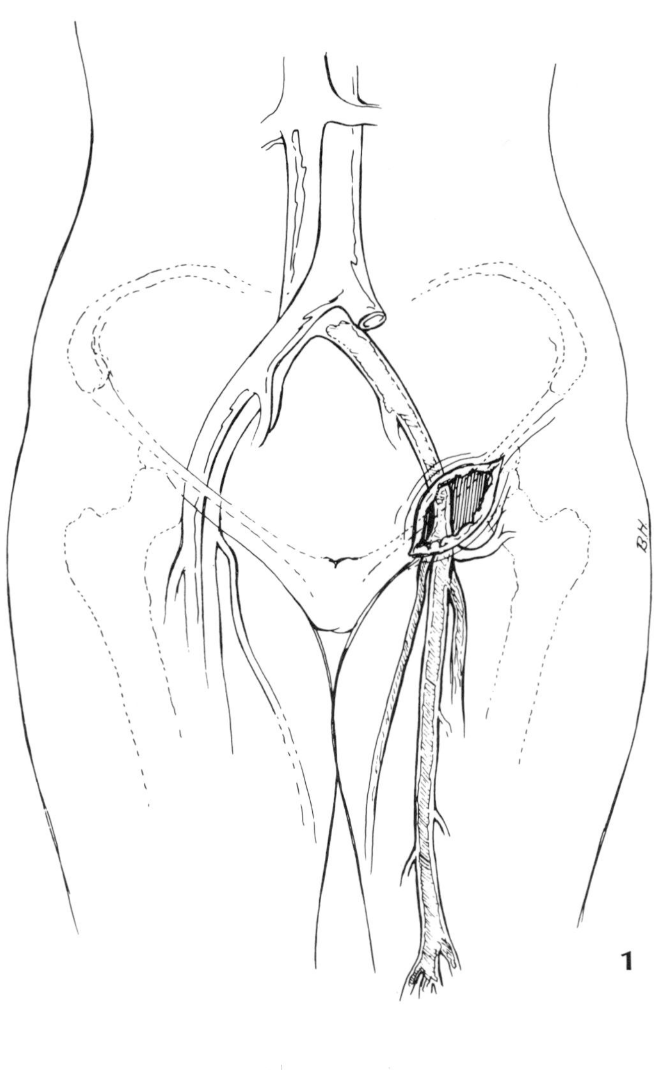

1

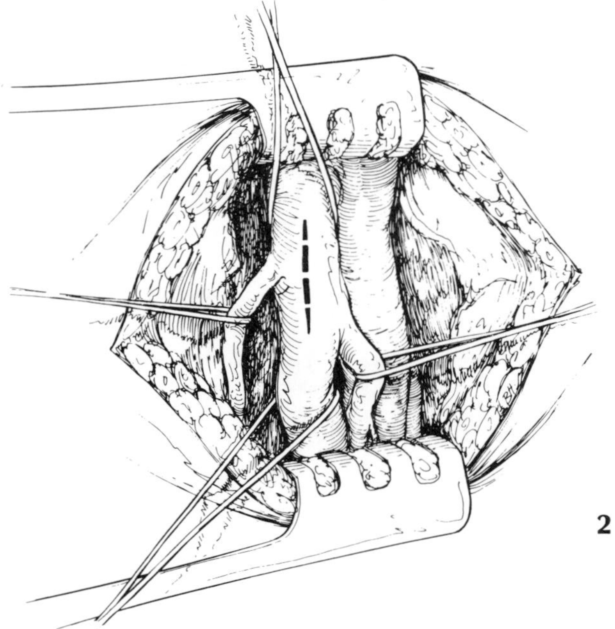

2

3

If a chronic thrombus in the iliac vein cannot be removed with the Fogarty catheter despite successful catheterization, the Fogarty catheter can be guided through the hole of a ringstripper and used to block the entrance of the common iliac vein. Following this procedure, the ringstripper can be used to remove the thrombotic material with gentle force from the vessel wall. When the clots are loosened they can then be removed by retracting the Fogarty catheter.

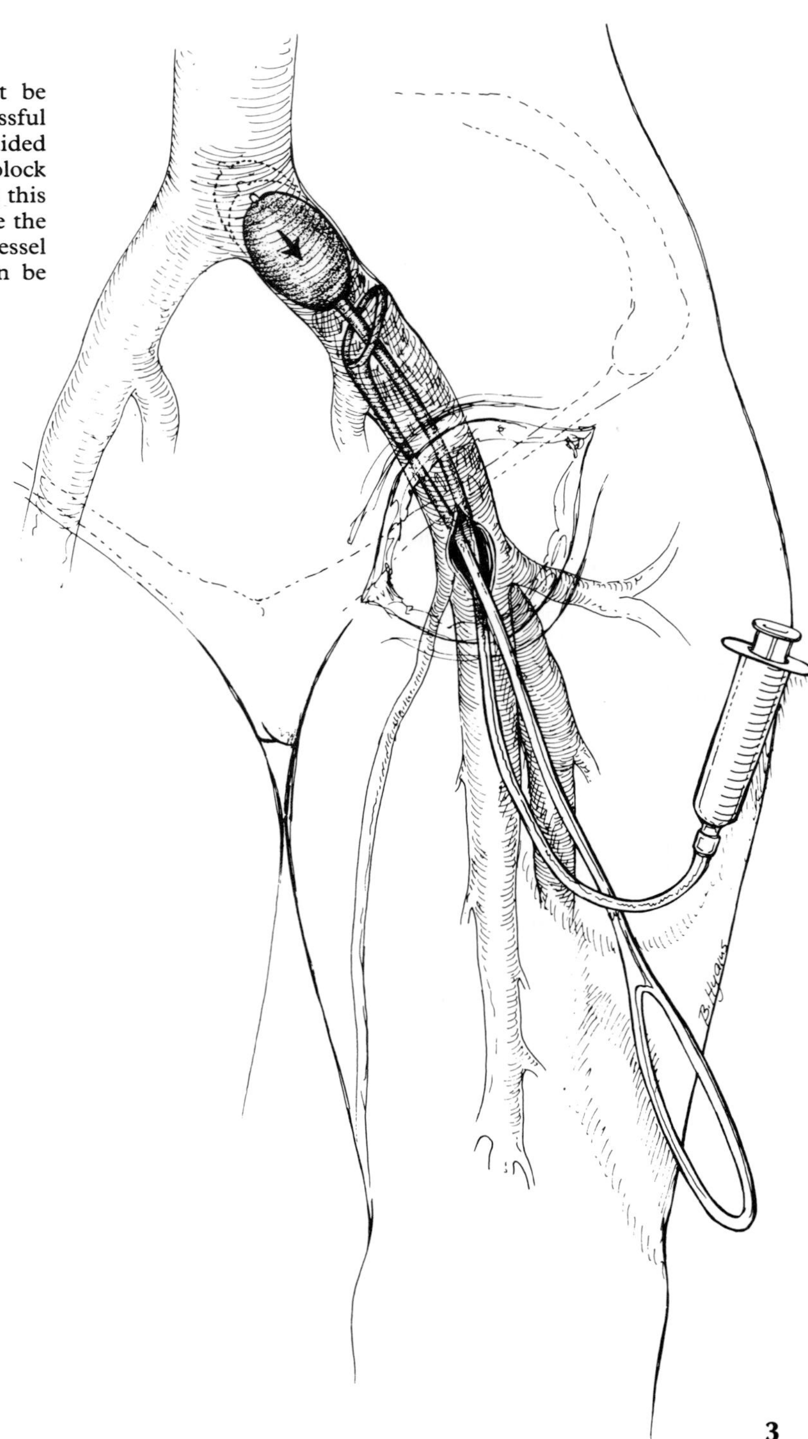

3

4

Finally, the distal clot is removed. When the thrombus is of recent origin and not yet firmly attached to the vessel wall, it can be removed by circumferential manual pressure which is exerted at the calf and gradually advanced upward. In cases of fresh thrombosis, sudden compression of the calf and thigh muscles by hand or with an Esmarch bandage results in complete removal of a thrombus throughout the whole deep venous sytem. The thrombus is then flushed out *in toto* by the bloodstream.

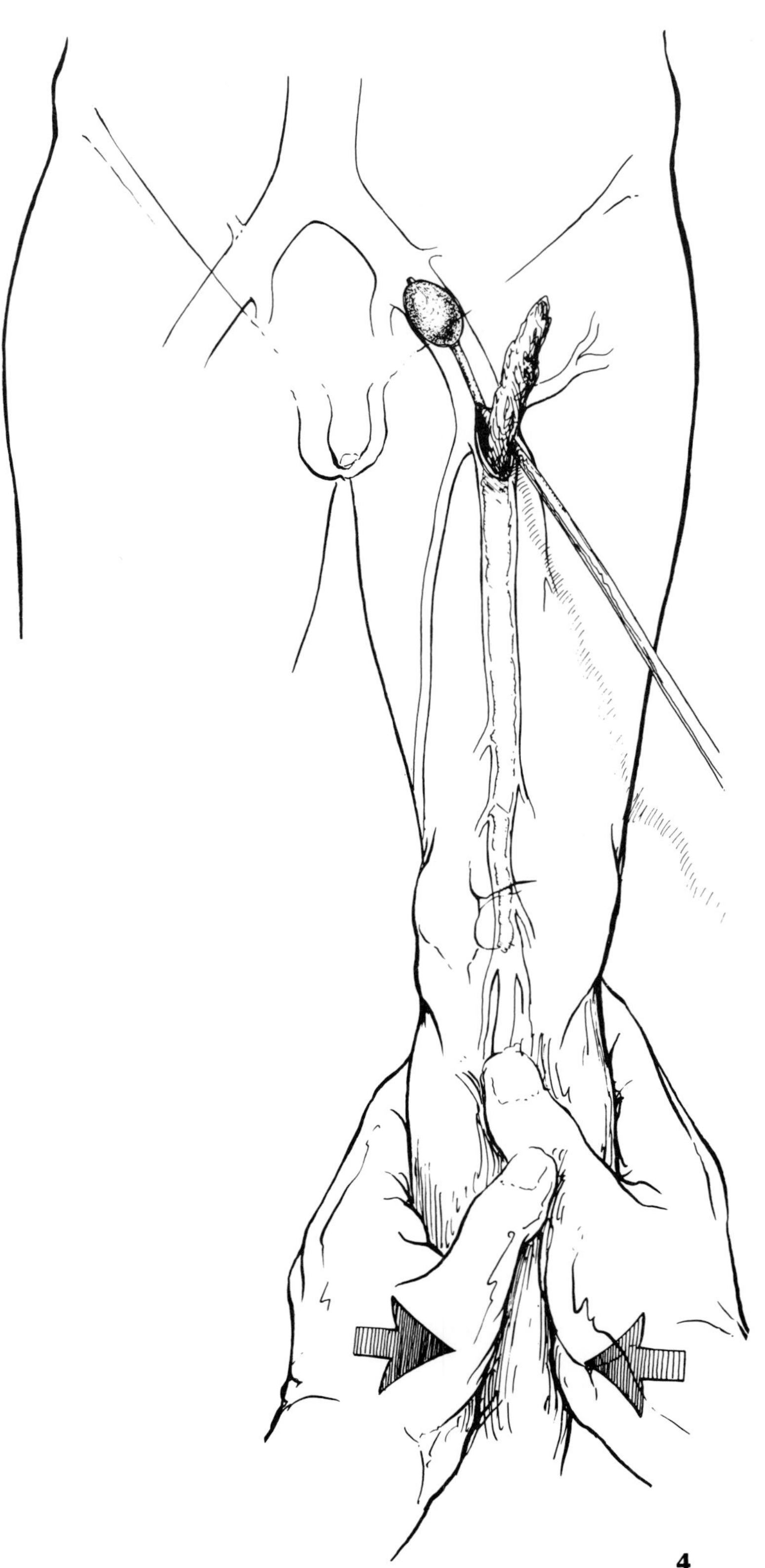

4

5

When the thrombus is adherent and compression does not work, a Fogarty catheter is used. In most cases introduction of this catheter is not possible over a longer distance because of competent valves. In such cases the catheter is attached to a small ringstripper and guided downward through the superficial femoral vein. If this procedure is not successful, because of patent venous valves, an additional incision at the proximal or distal popliteal vein might be helpful. A soft catheter can be brought up from the distal incision, the Fogarty catheter inserted into the lumen of the catheter, moved distally without problems, and the thrombus material can then be removed without interference from the valves.

After satisfactory thrombectomy, the incision(s) is (are) closed with a continuous 6/0 polypropylene suture, a suction drain is inserted and the wound is closed in layers. Postoperative continuous heparin therapy is administered (1000 i.u./h i.v.).

The patient is mobilized on the third postoperative day and anticoagulation with warfarin is started as a longer-term therapy. Anticoagulation treatment should be continued lifelong, because the rate of recurrent thrombosis in the diseased leg is very high (50%) among those patients who stopped anticoagulation even some years after their operation (Polterauer *et al.*, 1988).

Ligation of veins is never performed. If the thrombus cannot be removed during the operation because of its adherence, there is also no danger of pulmonary embolism.

Even if the procedure is not successful because of an unfavourable local situation, the chances of developing a post-phlebitic syndrome are the same as in non-operated cases. The recanalization in coming months or years is probably not adversely influenced by the surgical exploration (Wagner, 1986).

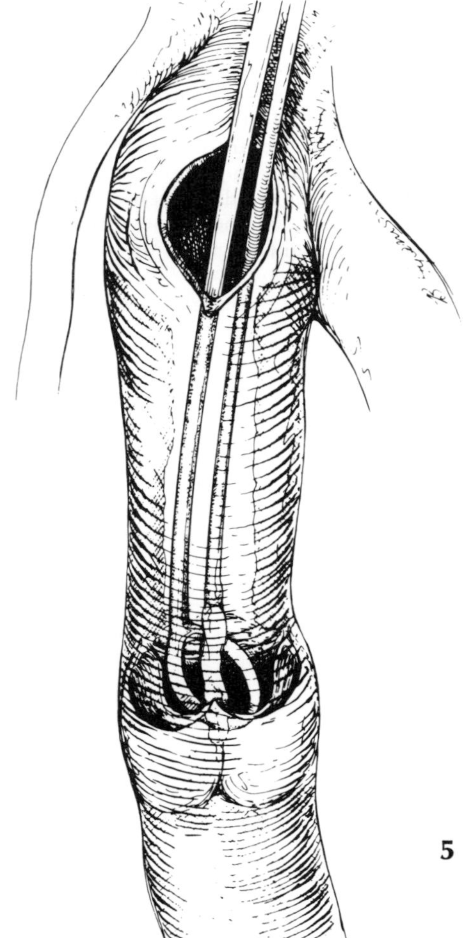

5

Problems

6

Venous spur

In 20–25% of cases a circumscribed stenosis at the entrance of the common iliac vein into the vena cava is found which in many of these cases might be the major cause of thrombosis. This stenosis was described by May and Thurner (1957) and is probably caused by the pulsating irritation of the crossing right iliac artery. It is nearly always possible to pass the stenosis with the balloon catheter and to dilate the spur by balloon dilatation and, if available, a stent might be inserted. Direct exploration of this area and surgical resection of the spur is not advisable as this results in a rather extensive operation. The danger of postoperative haematoma or haemorrhage as a consequence of vigorous interference and heparin therapy is high.

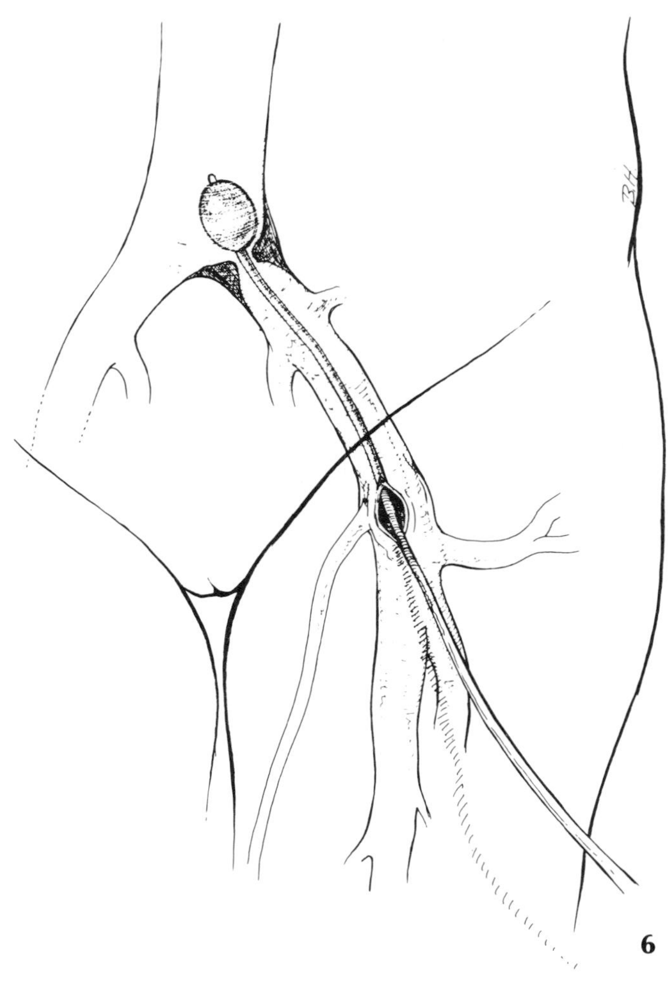

6

7

Impaction in an ascending lumbar vein

Occasionally, the Fogarty catheter, in spite of careful manipulation, repeatedly enters the lumbar ascending vein. In this case the tip of the catheter should be curved (inset). This catheter is introduced for the first few centimetres with the curve backwards and then with the curve towards the medial side of the vein in order to enter the vena cava.

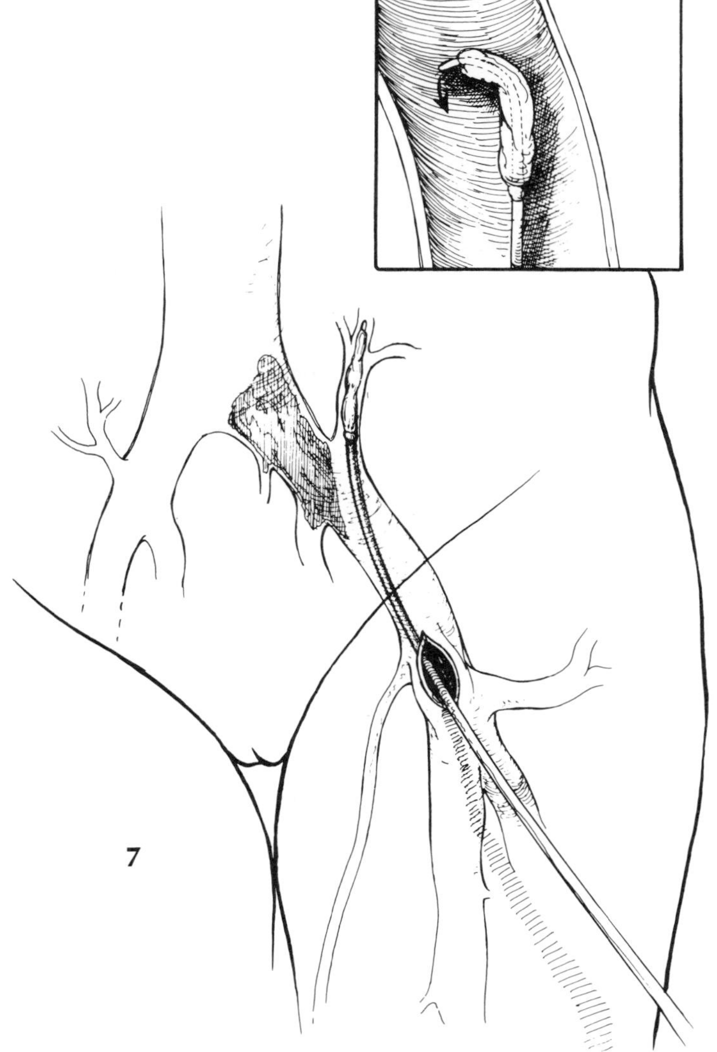

7

Thrombus of longer duration

Even with a history of recent thrombosis, organized clots may be found during the operation, because old thrombi in the major deep veins are sometimes silent. However, acute symptoms follow sudden propagation, and occlusion of small segments (particularly the common femoral vein) as well as of small collateral branches with obstruction of venous drainage may occur. Therefore, even though the indication for venous thrombectomy is restricted to patients with a history of onset up to 5 days, an old thrombosis may be found unexpectedly during operation in the iliac and/or femoral veins in up to 50% of patients. Since the success of clot removal is directly related to intraoperatively determined thrombus age (which may not necessarily correspond to the patient's history), there are definitely two groups of patients with an entirely different prognosis. The most favourable prognosis can be made for patients with a short history of thrombosis and when recent thrombosis is found intraoperatively. The success rate is much lower in patients with a history of over a week or when a chronic thrombosis is found during surgery.

Surgical possibilities

Chronic thrombosis of the superficial femoral vein in combination with fresh iliac vein thrombosis Thrombectomy of the acute thrombus is performed on the iliac vein, thus returning the patient to the preoperative asymptomatic condition. Partial thrombectomy is also beneficial if the venous drainage from the deep femoral veins in iliac veins and vena cava can be preserved.

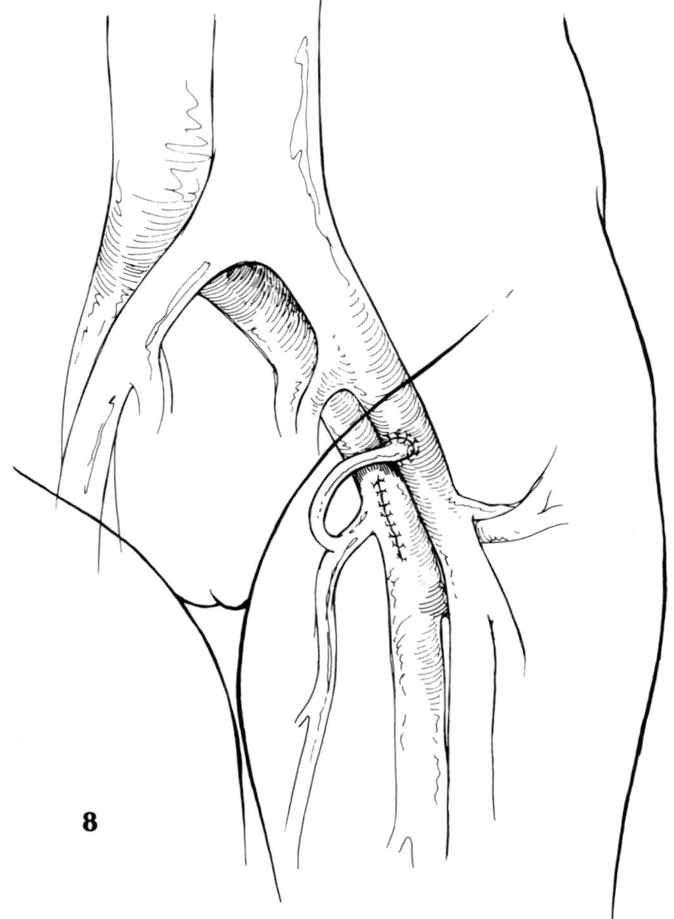

8

Chronic thrombosis of the iliac vein combined with acute thrombosis of the superficial femoral vein In addition to thrombectomy of the acute thrombosis of the superficial femoral vein, thrombectomy of a chronic thrombosis of the iliac vein is often possible. In many of these cases the iliac vein stays patent. If the inflow from the femoral vein is poor, the formation of an arteriovenous fistula at the inguinal level is advisable. This arteriovenous fistula is also indicated when only the deep vein circulation can be obtained. The technique recommended is to mobilize a suitable branch of the long saphenous vein as shown and anastomose its end to the side of the femoral artery.

Additional technical factors

An obstruction in the thigh caused by a doubled superficial femoral vein makes the removal even of a recent thrombus difficult In these cases distal incisions in the proximal or distal popliteal vein are sometimes helpful. The decision can depend on the preoperatively obtained venogram.

9

A still discussed question is, whether thrombectomy should be combined with a temporary arteriovenous fistula (Swedenborg, 1991). If the thrombus is adherent but removable, a distal arteriovenous fistula on a branch of the artery or the vein keeps the thrombectomized vein open in a sufficient number of cases. These fistulae might be located at the level of the proximal or distal popliteal artery, or even at the ankle (between the long saphenous vein and the posterior tibial artery). Arterio-venous fistulae are marked with a silk suture and should be closed after 2–3 months. Arteriovenous fistulae are marked with a silk suture and should be closed after 2–3 months, if they do not close spontaneously. Closure by an operation often presents a difficult technical problem, while occlusion by placing a detachable balloon under radiographic control might be achieved with a very low complication rate (Neglen *et al.*, 1991). During the function of the fistula percutaneous interventions (dilatation, stent implantation) in the arterialized venous system are feasible.

Obstruction of the iliac veins by tumour, pregnancy or chronic fibrosis of the thrombus When a thrombectomy of the femoral vein can be performed but the iliac vein cannot be cleared of thrombosis, distal thrombectomy should be combined with a femoral cross-over saphenous vein bypass (Palma and Esperon, 1960). This procedure was successful in a series of cases of primary undiagnosed pelvic tumour and in cases where pregnancy was the cause of the iliac vein thrombosis (Wagner, Piza and Müller Hartburg, 1973).

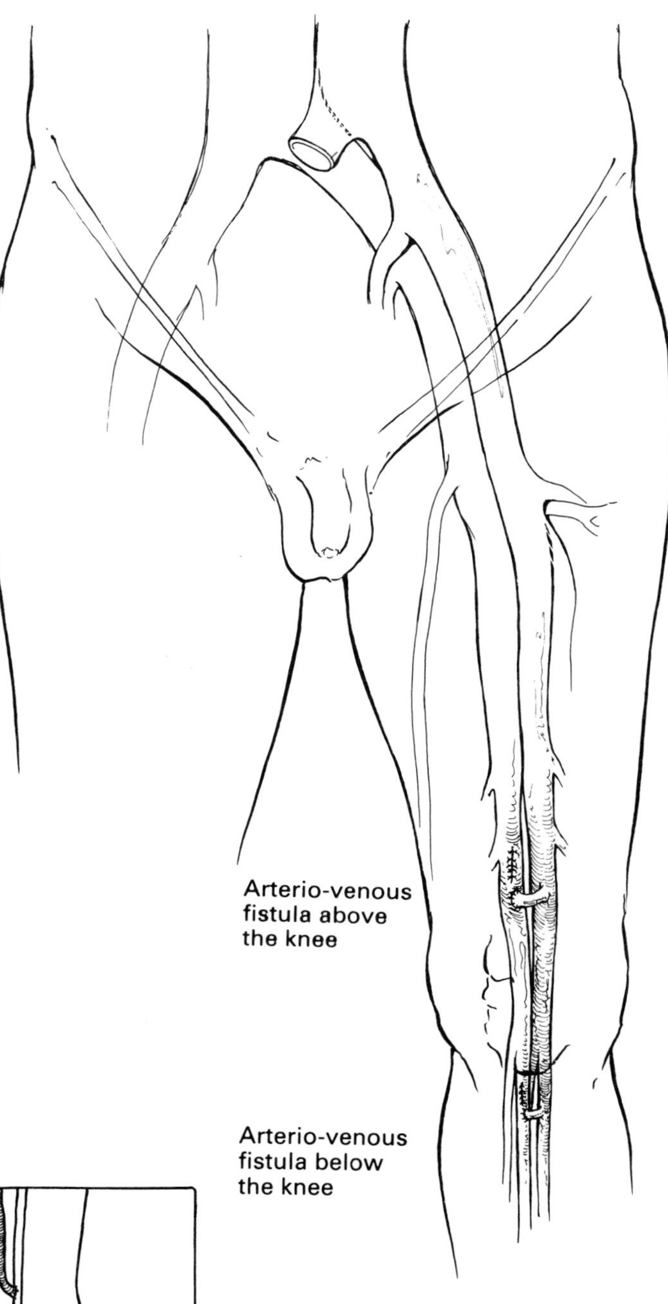

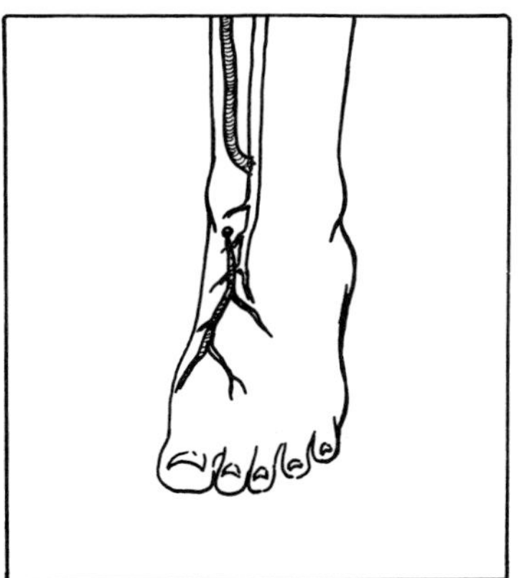

9

Complications

Intraoperative lethal pulmonary embolism is rare (around 0.5%) when appropriate caution is taken. There are some deaths in the postoperative period in patients where peripheral pulmonary embolisms of longer duration are found, but it is difficult to decide whether this embolization occurred before, during or after surgery. It is well established, however, that the pulmonary embolism rate in patients with iliac vein thrombosis is around 75%. The older patient group also shows an additional low mortality in myocardial infarctions. A rare complication is the loss of a transplanted kidney when the unsuspected intubation of the renal vein with the Fogarty catheter and the subsequent inflation results in an arteriovenous fistula and an untreatable haematuria leading to the removal of the otherwise well-functioning kidney transplant.

Rethrombosis is observed in a variable number of cases. In a few of those, restoration of blood flow can be obtained with a second operation and repeated thrombectomy with and without an arteriovenous fistula. In many cases it is advisable to accept the spontaneous course with rethrombosis and not insist on repeated and sophisticated operations.

References

Fogarty, T. J. and Kreppoehne, W. W. (1965). Catheter technique for venous thrombectomy. *Surgery, Gynecology and Obstetrics* **121**, 362.

Läwen, A. (1937). Über Thrombektomie bei Venethrombose und Arteriospasmus. *Zentralblatt für Chirurgie* **64**, 961.

Loeprecht, H., Weber, H. and Monnig, J. (1985). Vascular endoscopy. In *Diagnostic Techniques and Assessment Procedures in Vascular Surgery*. Greenhalgh, R. M., ed. London and San Diego: Grune and Stratton.

Mahorner, H., Castleberry, S. W. and Coleman, W. O. (1957). Attempts to restore functions in major veins which are the site of massive thrombosis. *Annals of Surgery* **146**, 510.

May, R. and Thurner, J. (1957). The cause of the predominantly sinistral occurrence of thrombosis of the pelvic veins. *Angiology* **8**, 419.

Minar, E., Ehringer, H., Marosi, L., Piza, F., Wagner, O. and Czembirek, H. (1983). Klinische, funktionelle und morphologische Spätergebnisse nach venöser Thrombektomie. *VASA* **12**, 346.

Neglen, P., Al-Hassan, H. Kh., Endrys, J., Nazzal, M. M. S., Christenson, J. T. and Eklof, B. (1991). Iliofemoral venous thrombectomy followed by percutaneous closure of the temporary arteriovenous fistula. *Surgery* **110**, 493.

Palma, E. and Esperon, R. (1960). Vein transplants and grafts in the surgical treatment of the postphlebitic syndrome. *Journal of Cardiovascular Surgery* 1, 94.

Polterauer, P., Holzenbein, Th., Huk, I., Kretschmer, G. and Wagner, O. (1988). Die akute tiefe Bëin-Beckenvenenthrombose: Retrospektive Analyse chirurgischen Therapie ergebuisse. *Chirurg*.

Swedenborg, J. (1991). Surgical thrombectomy for ilio-femoral venous thrombosis. *European Journal of Vascular Surgery* **5**, 365.

Wagner, O. (1986). Chirurgischen Thrombektomie. In *Angiologie 86*. Widmer, L. K. and Zemp, E., eds. Bern: Hans Huber.

Wagner, O., Piza, F. and Müller-Hartburg, W. (1973). Zur chirurgischen Therapie der Beckenvenenthrombose in der Schwangerschaft. *Wiener Klinische Wochenschrift* **85**, 17.

Transvenous insertion of the inferior vena caval filter

LAZAR J. GREENFIELD MD
MARY C. PROCTOR MS
Department of Surgery, University of Michigan, Ann Arbor, Michigan, USA

Introduction

Most patients with thromboembolic disease can be effectively managed with anticoagulation; however, there are several situations which require mechanical protection with a vena caval filter. Through the years, the indications for filter placement have remained relatively consistent and address both failures of anticoagulation and individual patient characteristics (Brenner *et al.*, 1992; Greenfield, 1984, 1987). Those who are at risk for bleeding due to injury, physical condition or surgical procedures, those who develop a complication while receiving anticoagulants, or suffer recurrent embolism while therapeutically anticoagulated have a primary indication for filter placement. In addition, those who have undergone pulmonary embolectomy, are noted to have a propagating tail on a thrombus in a major vessel or sustain recurrent embolism after placement of another vena caval device are appropriate candidates for further mechanical protection. A final group of patients to be considered for filter placement include high risk patients with serious, underlying cardiac or pulmonary disease who may not tolerate even small pulmonary embolism. These patients may warrant prophylaxis with both anticoagulant and vena caval filter placement.

Methods

Prior to placement of a vena caval filter, patients should undergo an inferior vena cavagram to determine the level of placement and to identify any anatomical abnormalities of the cava which may affect filter placement such as megacava or extra-anatomic tributaries. Greenfield filters can be safely placed if the diameter of the cava is 28 mm or less in diameter after correction for radiographic magnification.

Multiple factors determine the appropriate level for filter placement. Routinely, the filter is positioned within the inferior vena cava at the level of the L3 vertebral body. If there is thrombus extending to or involving the renal vein or if there is pelvic or ovarian vein thrombosis, the filter should be positioned above the level of the renal veins at T12-L1. This suprarenal location is also appropriate for pregnant patients or young women of child bearing potential. This prevents compression of the filter from the pressure of the gravid uterus. Placement above the renal veins has proved safe and efficacious in long-term studies (Brenner *et al.*, 1992; Stewart *et al.*, 1982; Orsini and Jarrell, 1984; Greenfield *et al.*, 1992). On rare occasions, the filter has been inserted in the superior vena cava in an inverted position when subclavian vein thrombosis has been considered to represent a risk for pulmonary embolism (Owen, Schoettle and Harrington, 1992).

1

The standard Greenfield filter (SGF) is fashioned from stainless steel and designed to be inserted operatively from either the right jugular or femoral vein. Alternative sites include the left jugular or left axillary vein as well as intraoperative insertion via the right atrium. Interventional radiologists have reported their experience with percutaneous insertion of the SGF using the Seldinger technique for progressive dilatation to accommodate a 26 French sheath. This has been associated with a 40% incidence of insertion site thrombosis leading to the introduction of reduced profile vena caval filters designed for percutaneous placement (Kantor *et al.*, 1987; Hye *et al.*, 1990; Rose *et al.*, 1987; Pais, Mirvis and DeOrchis, 1987).

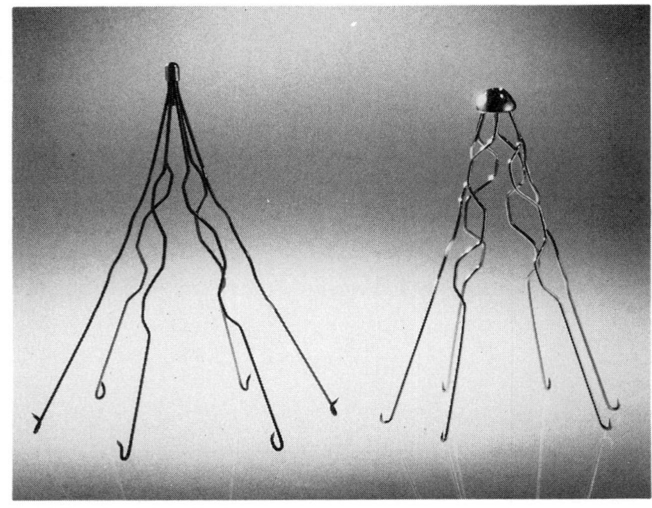

1

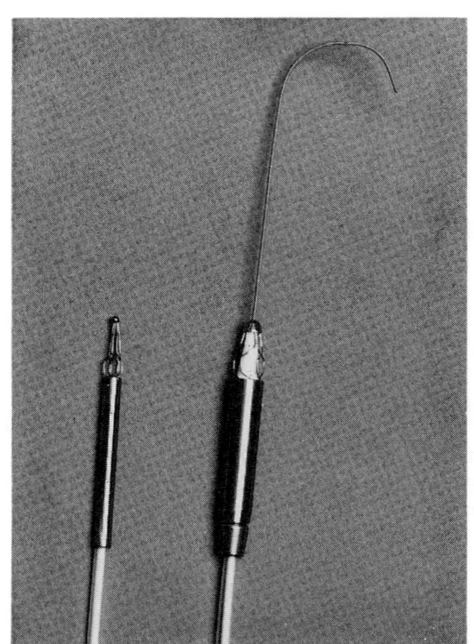

2

2

The smaller titanium Greenfield filter (TGF-MH) is designed to be inserted via a 12 French carrier system, is safer for percutaneous insertion and also allows intraoperative insertion directly into the inferior vena cava.

Operative technique

The technique of operative insertion of the SGF via the jugular vein will be described, then the technique of percutaneous insertion of the TGF-MH via the femoral vein. The open procedure is usually performed in the operating room on a table which allows portable fluoroscopy. Local anaesthesia is preferred, but general anaesthesia may be necessary to prevent air embolism if the patient is not cooperative.

With the head of the table slightly elevated, the patient is placed in the supine position. In order to facilitate exposure of the base of the neck, a small roll is placed under the shoulders and the head is turned to the left. To prevent wound haematoma, heparin should be discontinued 6 h prior to the procedure and may be resumed during the postoperative period.

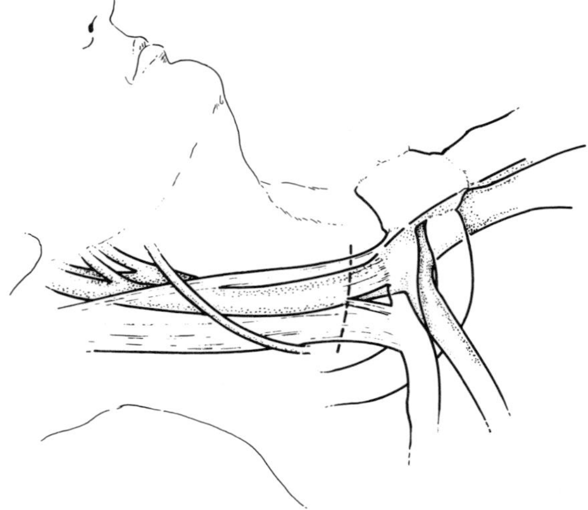

3

3

A transverse incision is made one finger breadth above the clavicle overlying the sternal and clavicular heads of the sternocleidomastoid muscle. Separation of the heads of the muscle allows ready access to the internal jugular vein which is freed for a distance of at least 3 cm. After loops are passed around the vein, a vascular clamp is applied distally, taking care to avoid injury to the vagus nerve. Twill tape is preferred for proximal control to allow repeated clamping by a haemostat.

4

A 0.035-inch flexible tip Teflon-coated guidewire is passed through a No. 14 plastic sheath needle puncture of the jugular vein and threaded under fluoroscopy to the level of the bifurcation of the inferior vena cava. Torque manipulation is usually required in order to pass the eustachian valve at the atriocaval junction. Once the guidewire is in position, the external end is threaded retrograde through the carrier system of the SGF and a clamp applied to it when it emerges from the proximal catheter. The venotomy is enlarged at the point of guidewire entry by incision and clamp dilation after which the carrier is threaded over the guidewire to the desired level of filter discharge. This would be the L3 level for infrarenal discharge and the T12-L1 level for suprarenal discharge.

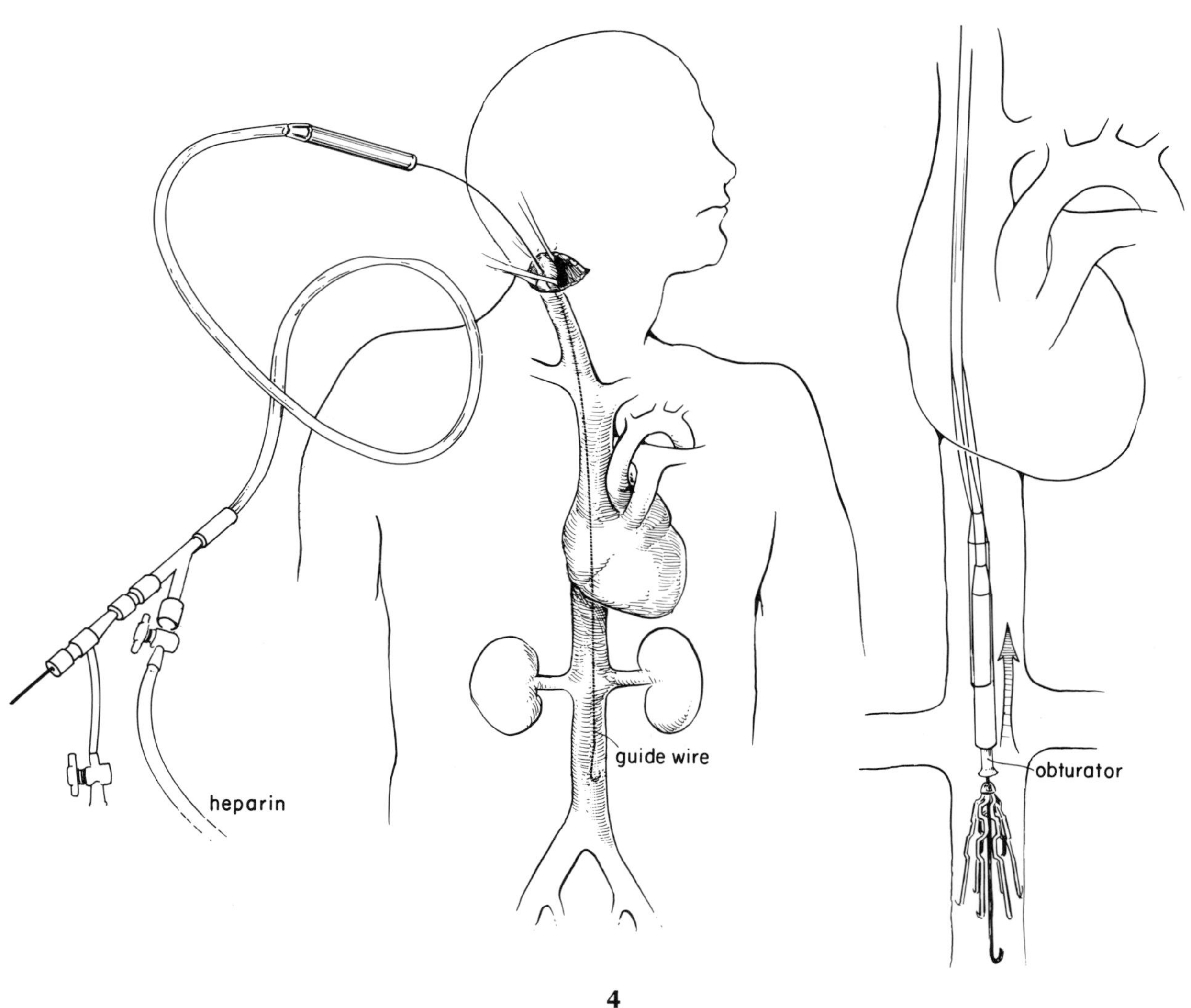

4

5

The locking hub is unscrewed to release the stylet and the main catheter is drawn backward. The filter is uncovered, springs open, and attaches to the wall of the inferior vena cava.

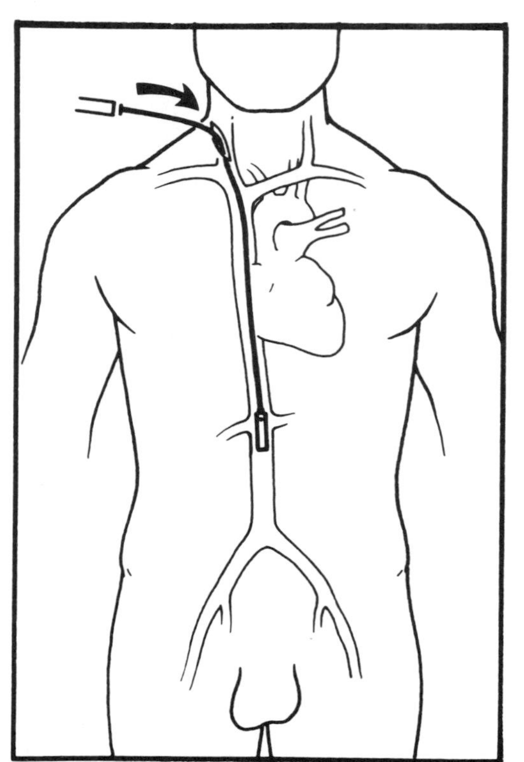

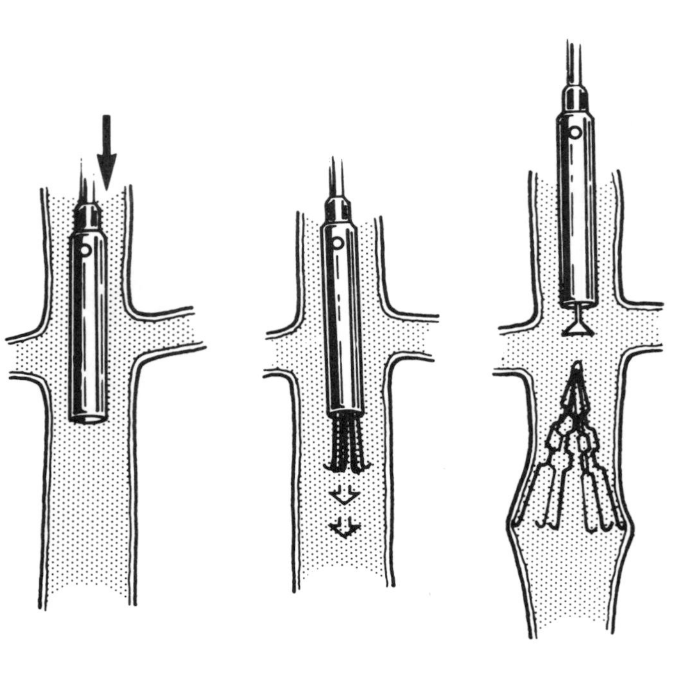

5

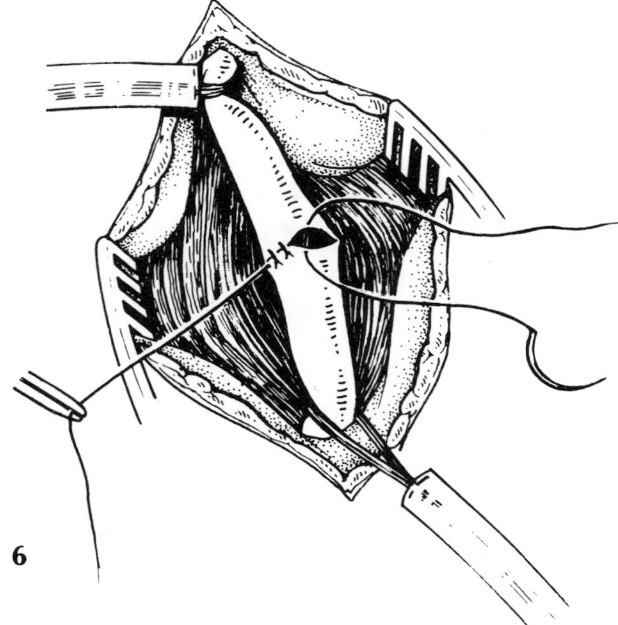

6

6

The carrier system and guidewire are withdrawn and the jugular venotomy is repaired using continuous polypropylene suture. Meticulous haemostasis is obtained and the wound is closed without drainage, usually with subcuticular closure. A compression dressing is applied with elastic adhesive tape.

Percutaneous technique

7

Four percutaneous vena caval filters are currently approved for use by the FDA. These include the Bird's Nest filter (Cook, Bloomington IN), the Simon Nitinol filter (Nitinol Medical Technologies, Worburn, MA), the Vena Tech filter (Vena Tech, Evanston, IL) and the Greenfield Titanium Filter (Medi-Tech, Watertown, MA). Each device offers a low profile delivery system but they differ significantly in design and performance characteristics.

Placement is usually performed in the radiology suite, at the time of pulmonary angiography or venacavography. The presence of iliofemoral venous thrombosis is a contraindication to the use of that side for percutaneous filter insertion. Although the left common iliac vein is usually flattened by the crossover of the right common iliac artery, the smaller size of the TGF-MH carrier system allows it to be inserted from the left if no other route is available.

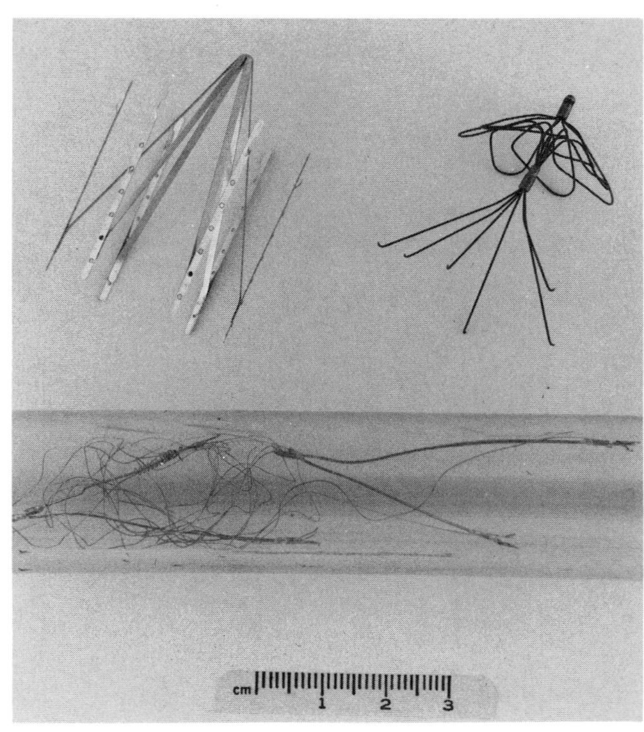

7

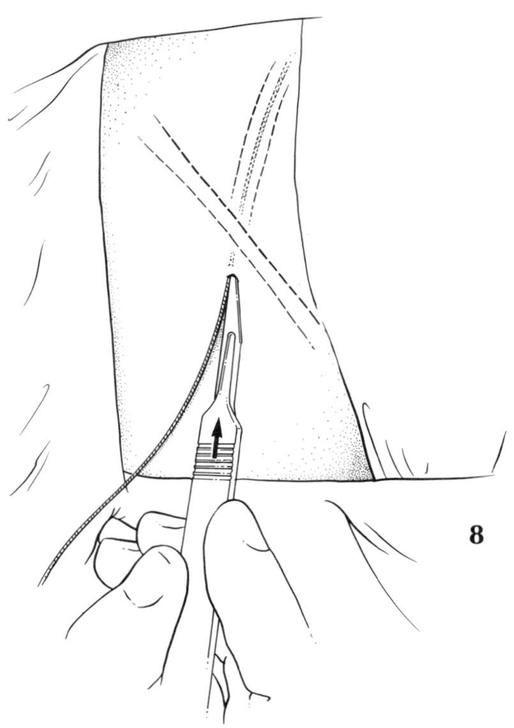

8

8

Under local anaesthesia, percutaneous needle aspiration of the common femoral vein is performed. A guidewire is passed through an attached plastic cannula once the needle is withdrawn. The cannula is removed and a small skin incision is made in order to allow passage of the dilator and sheath over the guidewire.

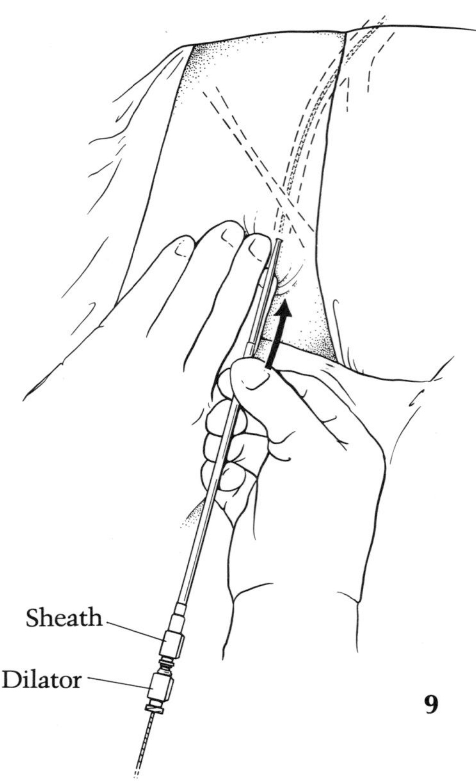

9

The dilator and sheath are passed under fluoroscopy over the guidewire into the inferior vena cava. Once the dilator and sheath are positioned in the vena cava, the dilator and guidewire are withdrawn, leaving the sheath in place.

10

The filter carrier is then introduced into the sheath. Prior to insertion of the carrier system, the sheath should be flushed with heparinized saline to prevent air embolism and thrombus formation within the carrier system. Digital occlusion of the luerlock will avoid excessive blood loss.

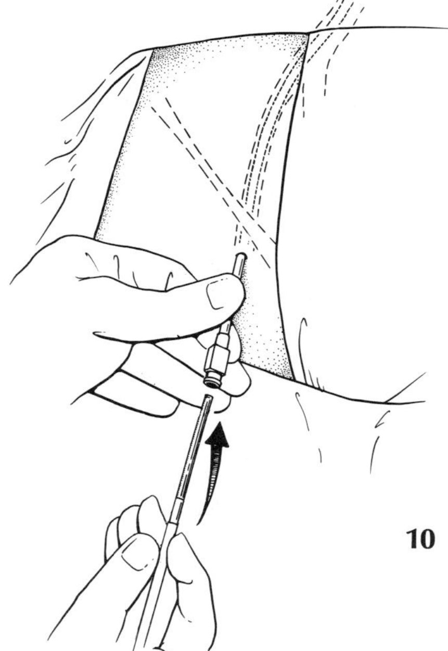

11

In order to prevent accidental release of the filter into the sheath, it is important to advance the carrier through the sheath until the sheath hub contacts the control handle. Using fluoroscopic guidance, the carrier should be positioned at the level of L3. The locking mechanism on the control handle is released by moving the control tab to the unlock position. The control tab is then slid backward which uncovers and discharges the filter. The carrier and sheath are withdrawn and pressure is applied to the puncture site to establish haemostasis. A pressure dressing may be applied.

Regardless of the method of delivery, a follow-up radiograph should be obtained to document filter position.

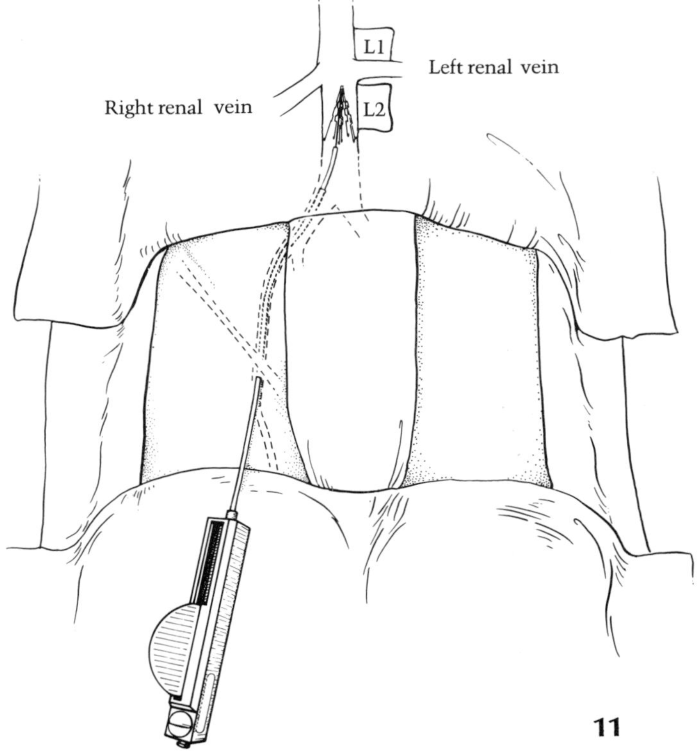

11

12

Long-term patency of the Greenfield filter is in excess of 95% due to its geometry (Greenfield, 1984; Greenfield *et al.*, 1981, 1982; Greenfield and Michna, 1988). The cone shape of the filter allows it to be filled to 70% of its depth by emboli without interfering with flow. Preservation of flow allows for spontaneous resolution of entrapped thrombi, with or without systemic anticoagulation. Anticoagulation should always be used to control the underlying thrombotic disorder, but is not necessary for long-term patency of the filter. The design also enhances entrapment of smaller thrombi, since axial flow is directed into the apex of the filter.

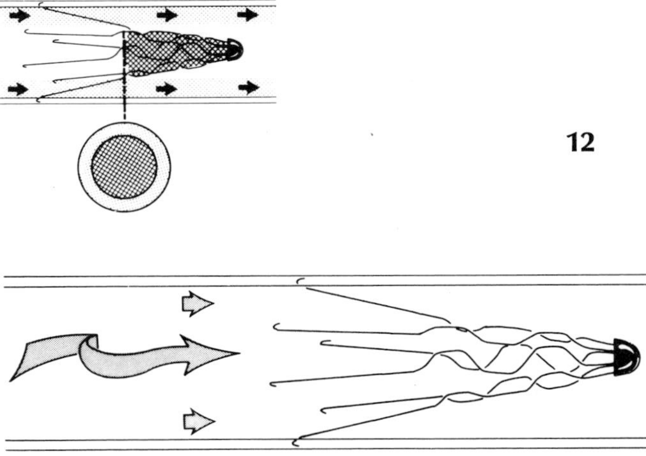

12

Complications

The use of Greenfield vena caval filters is associated with minimal morbidity. Reports of isolated limb penetration have been published but are rarely associated with clinical sequelae. The filter can be deformed and limbs extruded from the cava by external forces at the time of laparotomy or through the flaccid abdominal wall of the quadriplegic during a 'quad cough'. Misplacement of the filter at discharge is rare if the guidewire is used during surgical placement and is eliminated with the use of the sheath during percutaneous delivery. Apparent movement of the filter noted at follow-up is virtually without clinical significance and is often due to radiographic parallax or respiratory variation. Although a few cases of filter tilting have been noted, long-term follow-up studies fail to show a clinical relationship between tilt and the recurrence of PE (Messmer and Greenfield, 1985).

References

Brenner, D., Brenner, C., Scott, J., Wehberg, K., Granger, J. P. and Schellhammer, P. (1992). Suprarenal Greenfield filter placement to prevent pulmonary embolus in patients with vena caval tumor thrombi. *Journal of Urology* **147**, 19.

Greenfield, L. (1984). Current indications for and results of Greenfield filter placement. *Journal of Vascular Surgery* **1**(3), 502.

Greenfield, L. (1987). Vena caval filter placement for prevention of pulmonary embolism: Patient selection and results. *Practical Cardiology* **13**(2), 100.

Greenfield, L. and Michna, B. (1988). Twelve-year clinical experience with the Greenfield vena caval filter. *Surgery* **104**(4), 706.

Greenfield, L., Peyton, R., Crute, S. and Barnes, R. (1981). Greenfield vena caval filter experience: Late results in 156 patients. *Archives of Surgery* **116**, 11451.

Greenfield, L., Cho, K. J., Proctor, M., Sobel, M., Shah, S. and Wingo, J. (1992). Late results of suprarenal Greenfield vena cava filter placement. *Archives of Surgery* **127**, 969.

Hye, R., Mitchell, A., Dory, C., Freischlag, J. and Roberts, A. (1990). Analysis of the transition to percutaneous placement of Greenfield filters. *Archives of Surgery* **125**(12), 1550.

Kantor, A., Glanz, S., Gordon, D. H. and Sclafani, S. J. (1987). Percutaneous insertion of the Kimray-Greenfield filter: Incidence of femoral vein thrombosis. *American Journal Roentgenol* **149**(4), 1065.

Messmer, J. and Greenfield, L. (1985). Greenfield caval filters: long-term radiographic follow-up study. *Radiology* **156**, 613.

Orsini, R. and Jarrell, B. (1984). Suprarenal placement of vena caval filters: Indications, techniques, and results. *Journal of Vascular Surgery* **1**, 125.

Owen, E., Schoettle, P. and Harrington, O. (1992). Placement of a Greenfield filter in the superior vena cava. *Annals of Thoracic Surgery* **53**, 896.

Pais, O., Mirvis, S. and De Orchis, D. (1987). Percutaneous insertion of the Kimray-Greenfield filter: Technical considerations and problems. *Radiology* **165**, 377.

Rose, B., Simon, D., Hess, M. and Van Aman, M. (1987). Percutaneous transfemoral placement of the Kimray-Greenfield vena cava filter. *Radiology* **165**, 373.

Stewart, J., Peyton, W., Crute, S. and Greenfield, L. (1982). Clinical results of suprarenal placement of the Greenfield vena cava filter. *Surgery* **92**(1), 1.

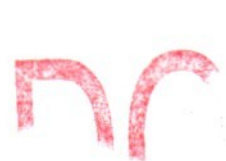